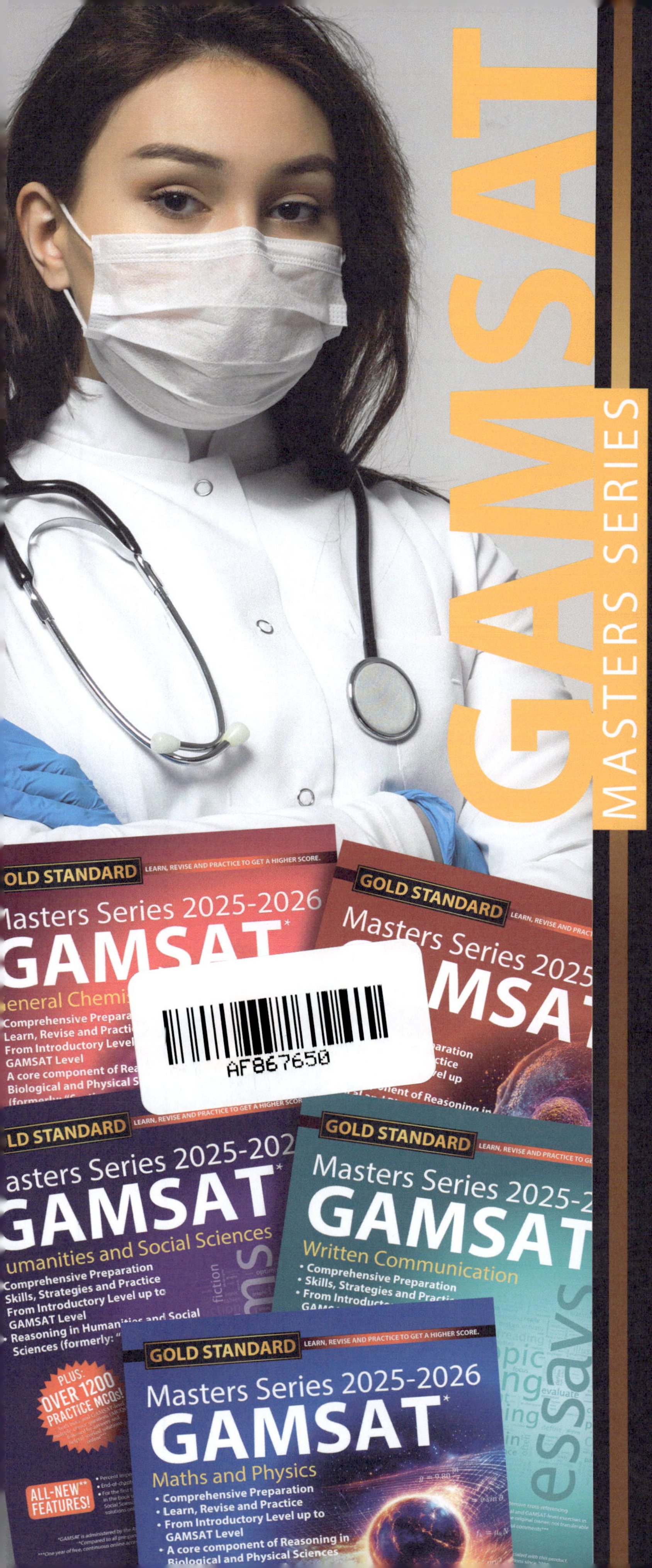

GOLD STANDARD

PERMISSION GRANTED

If you wish to share your study experience in social media (e.g. Instagram, TikTok, YouTube, etc.), Gold Standard GAMSAT gives you the permission to include any of our books (cover and/or interior pages, though never all pages from a chapter), and/or short segments of our videos, in your content. Share your study journey and inspire others!

01 Editor and Author

Brett Ferdinand BSc MD-CM

02 Contributors

Lisa Ferdinand BA MA
Sean Pierre BSc MD
Kristin Finkenzeller BSc MD
Ibrahima Diouf BSc MSc PhD
Charles Haccoun BSc MD-CM
Timothy Ruger BA MA
Jeanne Tan Te

03 Illustrators

Harvie W. Gallatiera BS CompE
Gilbert Rafanan BSc

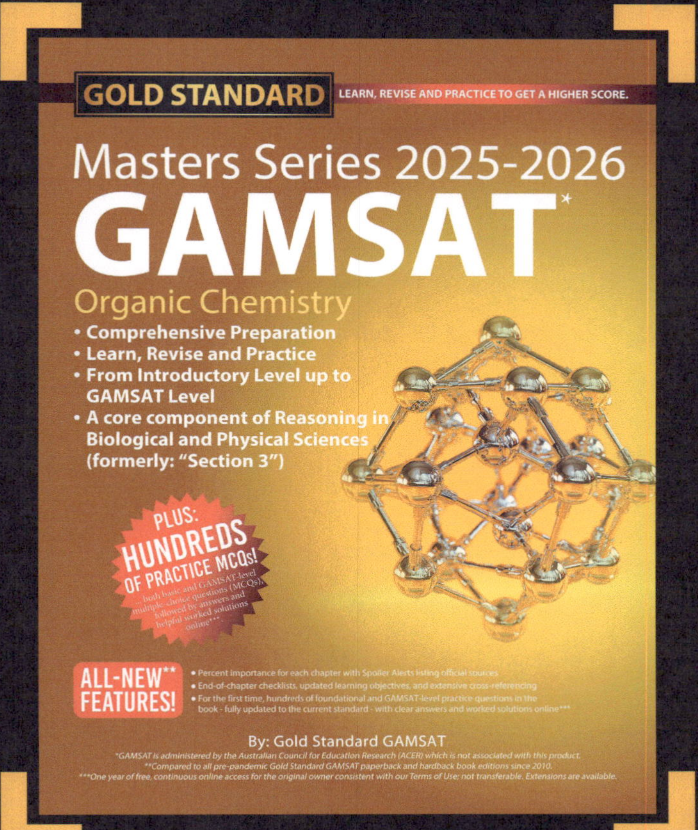

Register your book!

Free Online Access*

Answers and detailed worked solutions for hundreds of end-of-chapter practice questions, as well as the full-length practice test GS-Free which has the new digital GAMSAT format and cross-references to this Masters Series book.

*One year of continuous access for the original owner of this textbook upon online registration at www.gamsat-prep.com/gamsat-organic-chemistry
If you purchased this textbook or the eBook directly from www.gamsat-prep.com, then your online access is automated.

Please note: Benefits last for one year from the date of online registration, for the original book owner only, and are not transferable; unauthorized access and use outside the Terms of Use posted on GAMSAT-prep.com may result in account deletion; if you are not the original owner, or if you are seeking an extension, you can purchase your virtual access card separately at GAMSAT-prep.com.

Online access: reduces digital piracy; allows the addition of relevant multimedia including videos; permits the updating of strategies and content to reflect the evolving GAMSAT; permits more detailed worked solutions; reduces the retail price; and ultimately, saves trees!

ISBN 978-1-927338-86-5

Address all inquiries, comments, or suggestions to the publisher. For Terms of Use go to: www.GAMSAT-prep.com

Gold Standard GAMSAT Product Contact Information

Distribution in Australia, NZ, Asia

Woodslane Pty Ltd 10 Apollo Street
Warriewood NSW 2102 Australia
ABN: 76 003 677 549
learn@gamsat-prep.com

Distribution in Europe

Central Books 99 Wallis
Road LONDON,
E9 5LN, United Kingdom
orders@centralbooks.com

Distribution in North America

RuveneCo Publishing
334 Cornelia Street #559
Plattsburgh, New York 12901, USA
buy@gamsatbooks.com

GAMSAT (Graduate Medical School Admissions Test)

Computer-based exam held at test centres internationally for graduate-entry medicine

Written Communication (Writing Tasks A & B)

- formerly "Section 2"

2 essays responding to 2 different themes using sound reasoning and competent English-writing skills (essays must be typed)

Writing Task A: sociocultural theme (e.g., free speech, justice, social media)
Writing Task B: personal-social themes (e.g., humour, love, happiness)

Reasoning in Humanities and Social Sciences

- formerly "Section 1"

multiple-choice section with stimulus materials requiring comprehension and analysis of non-science content

poetry • proverbs cartoons • novels or play excerpts • travel and/or medical journal entries • social science graphs

Reasoning in Biological and Physical Sciences

- formerly "Section 3"

multiple-choice section with questions mostly based on science passages that require problem-solving and graph analysis

first-year undergraduate level Biology (40%), General Chemistry (20%) & Organic Chemistry (20%) • A-level/Leaving Certificate/ Year 12 level Physics (20%)

Top GAMSAT Score: 100
Average GAMSAT Score: 57

Summary of the new Digital-format GAMSAT Exam Day

	KEY POINTS	EVENT	DURATION
Written Communication	Produce ideas in writing with clarity and soundness; essays are typed with no copy/paste function	2 essays typed on a computer (for all sections including the essays: no longer is there a formal, dedicated reading time)	65 minutes
Arrival and Sitting of Exam	Bring only the acceptable ID documents and permitted items to the test centre as specified in ACER's GAMSAT Information Booklet	Security, identification, health protocols	15-45 minutes
Reasoning in Humanities and Social Sciences	Key skills are reading speed and comprehension of information within socio-cultural contexts	62 MCQs* (the test centre will provide you with 2 sheets of A4 scratch paper; *option*: whiteboard)	100 minutes
Break	Consider packing your own lunch to avoid queues with nervous chatter	–	20 minutes
Reasoning in Biological and Physical Sciences	Analyse and solve problems: 40% Biology, 40% Chemistry (equally split between General and Organic); 20% Physics	75 MCQs* (the test centre will provide you with 2 new sheets of A4 scratch paper; *option*: whiteboard)	150 minutes
Total Test Time	Success requires stamina; stamina improves with practice.	–	5 hours, 15 minutes

*MCQs: multiple-choice questions, 4 options per question with only 1 best answer. Note that the 'old' GAMSAT had a dedicated 'reading time' of 10 minutes for each of Section 1 and 3, and 5 minutes for Section 2. During that reading time, students were not permitted to write or mark their exam paper in any way. The new digital GAMSAT has added time for each of the 3 exam sections as a legacy to 'reading time'; however, in practice, you can use your exam time in any way that you see fit.

**It might be a good idea to allocate a whole day to sit the GAMSAT test to allow for any contingencies and/or technical issues that you might encounter. Safety measures and health protocols should be carefully anticipated when making travel arrangements and accommodations to and from the testing centre.

Common formula for acceptance:

GPA + GAMSAT score + Interview = Medical School Admissions

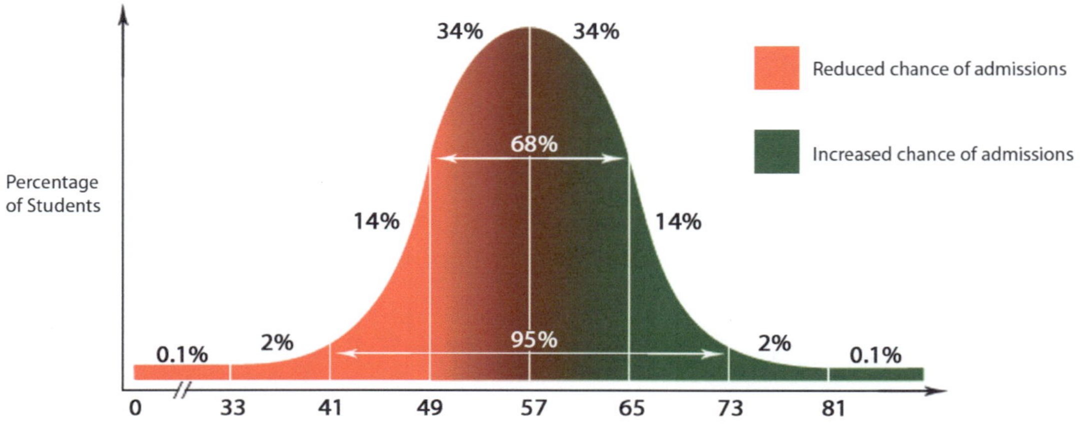

Typical Overall GAMSAT Score Distribution (Approx)

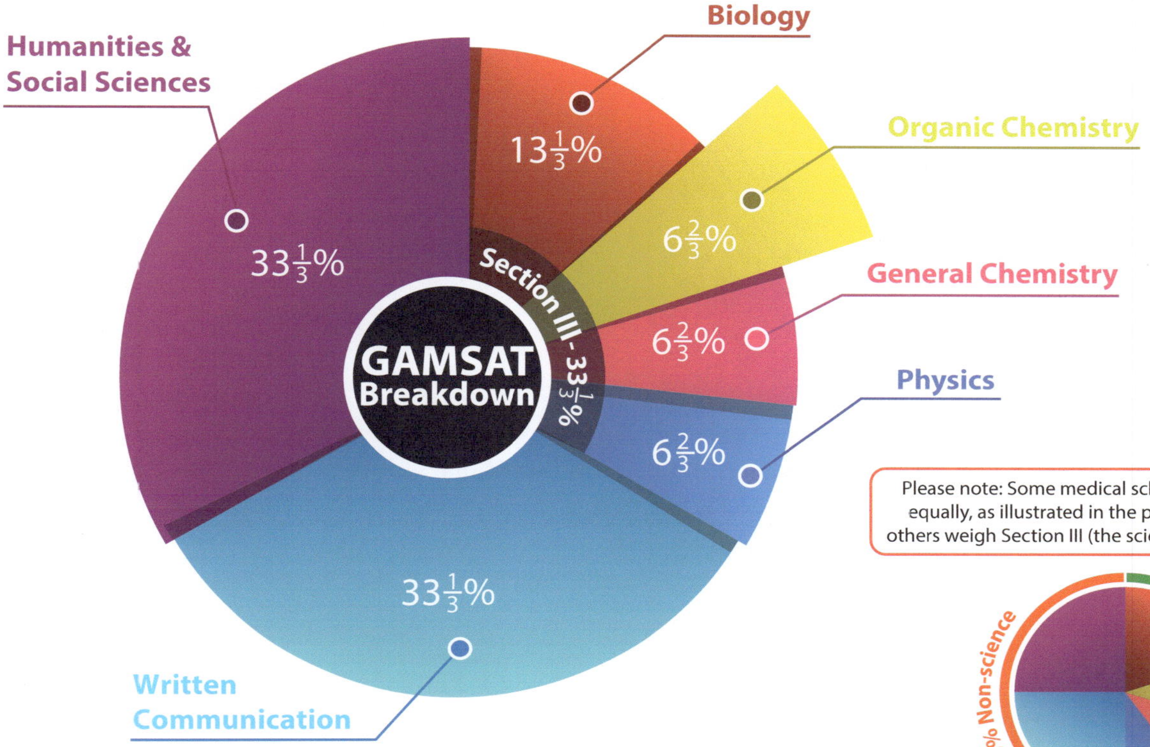

Please note: Some medical schools weigh all 3 sections equally, as illustrated in the pie chart to the left, while others weigh Section III (the sciences) twice as seen below.

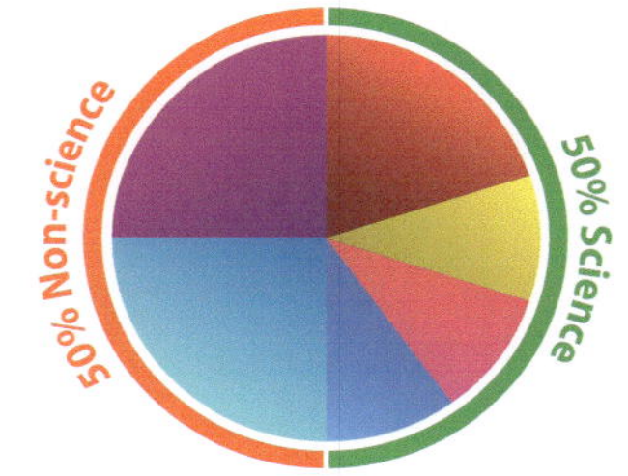

GAMSAT is challenging, get organised.

gamsat-prep.com/free-GAMSAT-study-schedule

1. How to study

- Learn, revise and practice using the GAMSAT Masters Series book(s) and/or videos.
- Complete all exercises and multiple-choice practice questions in this book.
- Consolidate: create and study from your personal summaries (= Gold Notes) daily. Create study cards or audio files from your Gold Notes to increase your study efficiency.

2. Once you have completed your studies

- Sit a full-length GAMSAT practice test.
- Analyse mistakes and all worked solutions.
- Consolidate: Revise all your Gold Notes and create more.

3. Sit multiple mock exams

- ACER GAMSAT practice exams with free Gold Standard worked solutions on YouTube
- Free full-length Gold Standard (GS) mock exam GS-Free with helpful, detailed worked solutions
- HEAPS: 15 full-length exams, 5 in the book and 10 online with the new, digital GAMSAT format

4. How much time do you need to study?

- On average, 3-6 hours per day for 3-6 months; depending on life experiences, 2 weeks may be enough and 8 months could be insufficient.
- Try to study full on for 1-2 weeks and then adjust your expectations for your personal, ideal study time.

5. Recommended GAMSAT Communities

- All countries (mainly Australia): pagingdr.net
- Mainly the UK: thestudentroom.co.uk (Medicine Community Discussion)
- Mainly Ireland: boards.ie (GAMSAT and GEM forum)

Is there something in the Masters Series that you did not understand? Don't get frustrated, get online:

gamsat-prep.com/forum

Table of Contents

Note that: H = High-level Importance; M = Medium-level Importance; L = Low-level Importance.

Note that: H = High-level Importance; M = Medium-level Importance; L = Low-level Importance.

Table of Contents

Note that: H = High-level Importance; M = Medium-level Importance; L = Low-level Importance.

Note that: H = High-level Importance; M = Medium-level Importance; L = Low-level Importance.

INTRODUCTION

GAMSAT Reasoning in Biological and Physical Sciences (i.e. GAMSAT Sciences, previously called: Section 3) is the final and longest of the 3 GAMSAT subtests. 'Biological Sciences' refers to Organic Chemistry and Biology. 'Physical Sciences' refers to Physics and General Chemistry. In our experience, most students with a non-science background (NSB) can successfully learn the assumed knowledge for GAMSAT independently, while a smaller number may need to enrol in a short tertiary-level science course.

Essentially, 20% of GAMSAT Sciences is Organic Chemistry. Officially, the level of assumed knowledge is first year university. However, the topics explored in the stimulus material during the exam can be quite advanced with the aim being to test your ability to learn on the spot and to apply your reasoning skills to novel scenarios.

What is GAMSAT Organic Chemistry?

Organic chemistry is the study of the structure, properties and reactions of **carbon-based compounds**. Organic compounds form the basis of life on Earth.

The simplest organic compounds are made up of only carbon and hydrogen atoms and thus, unsurprisingly, they are called *hydrocarbons*. The simplest hydrocarbon is **methane, CH_4**. Look at its structure: Although it may be a cartoonish representation of methane, its simplicity reminds us of the fact that *carbon is at the center*.

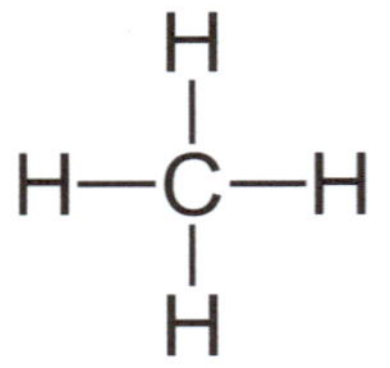

Methane

In more complex organic molecules, carbon can connect to other carbons in "circles" (*cyclic*) or one carbon after another (*chains*). Akin to a backbone (*spinal column or spine*), carbon in chains forms robust connections (*bonds*) central to the overall structure; for example, consider the following polyunsaturated omega-6 fatty acid (*yes, you will learn what each of those terms mean!*), linoleic acid (*note the central chain of carbons*):

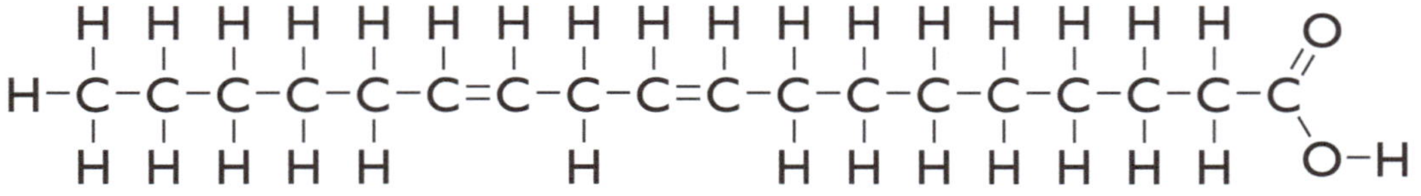

Linoleic acid: An essential fatty acid (thus it must be obtained through your diet)

GAMSAT Organic Chemistry is quite different from undergraduate, traditional organic chemistry. GAMSAT Organic Chemistry is little concerned with properties, aside from hydrogen bonding. GAMSAT Organic Chemistry appears to consider the memorisation of reactions to be strictly unnecessary, even though most university programs consider this important. However, the structure of molecules, following the story of a "brand new" reaction, seems quite important to ACER. In fact, **nomenclature** (*the naming of molecules*), **pattern recognition**, and **geometric reasoning** form a unique trio that spells success for GAMSAT Organic Chemistry.

Niacin is an organic compound and a form of vitamin B_3, an essential human nutrient. Its molecular formula is $C_6H_5NO_2$, which means 6 carbons (C), 5 hydrogens (H), 1 nitrogen (N) and 2 oxygens (O). Can you match the number and types of atoms in its molecular formula to the first structure below?

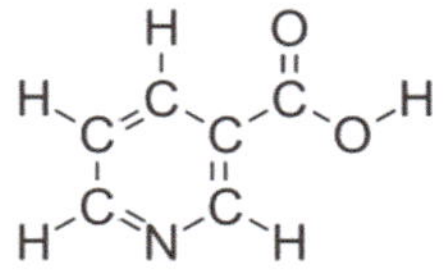
=
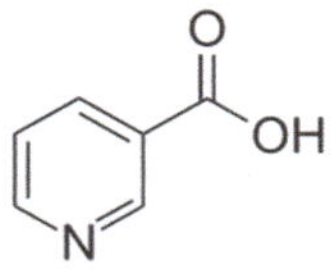
= $C_5H_4N\text{-}3\text{-}CO_2H$ = pyridine-3-carboxylic acid = niacin = vitamin B_3

Take a moment to consider the different representations above: They constitute the identical molecule, vitamin B_3.

And below, the cartoon of vitamin B_3 becomes a bit more realistic!

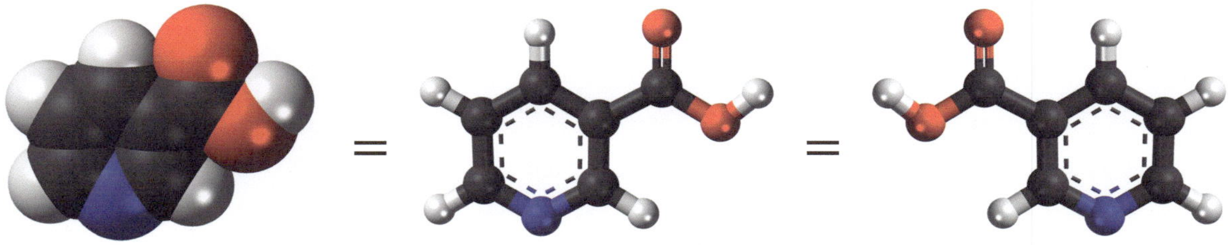

Marvel at the similarities and differences. Compare the structures in colour with those in black and white. What colour is carbon? What colour is hydrogen? Oxygen? Nitrogen? You are currently practicing pattern recognition and geometric reasoning (*albeit baby steps!*): 2 of the 3 keys for GAMSAT success.

We will see these 4 atoms again and again, throughout the entire textbook. Why? Because, despite there being over 100 atoms listed in the periodic table of the elements, only 4 atoms make up over 96% of the mass of your body: C (*black in the image above*), H (*white/silver*), O (*red*), and N (*blue*). Of course, it is still cartoonish since actual atoms are not colourised! However, adding colour to images is one of the many techniques that we will use throughout this textbook to follow atoms, or groups of atoms, during a chemical reaction.

How do I study GAMSAT Organic Chemistry?

We do not believe that it would be an efficient use of your time to plan to read all chapters in this textbook multiple times, nor to attempt to read straight through from the beginning to the end in one go. Ideally, you would plan to read each chapter once while taking very brief notes (less than 1 page per chapter = *Gold Notes*). Either before or after reading a chapter – where applicable – you may choose to watch some online videos at gamsat-prep.com relevant to that chapter while also taking very brief notes. Revise your notes often according to your GAMSAT study schedule which you can modify from the one we created (gamsat-prep.com/free-GAMSAT-study-schedule).

Practice Questions

We have 3 levels of multiple-choice practice questions, the first two are at the back of each chapter:

1) Foundational practice questions: Basic, understanding questions to ensure that you have read the chapter; if you have a NSB, if you do not know the answer, it would be better to treat these questions as 'open-book' questions rather than just looking at the worked solutions in your online account;

2) GAMSAT-level practice questions: Reasoning, application questions with the normal GAMSAT dosage of nomenclature, pattern recognition, and geometric reasoning;

3) Full-length practice tests which span the depth and breadth of a simulation of the real exam. Be warned: We do not replicate real-exam questions, we replicate real-exam reasoning. You can start with GS-Free which is a full-length GAMSAT mock exam with the new digital format, with free answers and worked solutions at gamsat-prep.com. GS-Free is one of 15 GS/HEAPS full-length mock exams.

For GAMSAT Sciences, "Study, practice, then full-length testing" should be your mantra for success!

Note for NSB students: If you read poems for months, you will increase your comfort reading poems. Reading science chapters is quite similar. It will feel bewildering at times, but less so as you progress. The real GAMSAT will have some articles that even the best science students do not fully grasp during the exam. However, they can still manage to obtain top GAMSAT scores by focusing on the minimum required in order to answer the questions correctly. This is a skill you can develop but it will not always feel comfortable.

What is so *new* about the new GAMSAT Masters Series?

As compared to all pre-pandemic Gold Standard GAMSAT paperback and hardback book editions since 2010, the new Masters Series launched a trifecta. We introduced 3 new tools to increase your study efficiency: Percent Importance, Spoiler Alerts and Chapter Checklists.

Percent Importance

'Importance' deals with the classic-student conundrum: How much effort should I invest in studying this or that chapter? How relevant is it to the GAMSAT?

After an exhaustive analysis of ACER's materials, we converted our previous Importance boxes to reveal percentages so students are better informed as to what they should emphasize when studying.

Here is the data-driven summary of the 'Importance' for the 14 GAMSAT Organic Chemistry chapters in this book:

Chapter	1	2	3	4	5	6	7	8	9	10	11	12	13	14
Percent Importance	7%	20%	0%	6%	2%	10%	15%	6%	6%	1%	2%	15%	5%	5%
Relative Importance	M	H	L	M	L	H	H	M	M	L	L	H	M	M

HIGH H (≥ 10%)   MEDIUM M (3% to 10%)   LOW L (< 3%)

The data is clear. The labels representing 'relative importance' is, of course, subjective. We will always remind you of the percentages on the first page of each chapter so that you do not have to accept our judgement as to the level of importance, you can decide for yourself. Note that 60% of GAMSAT Organic Chemistry lies within just 4 of the 14 chapters: 2, 6, 7 and 12.

Spoiler Alert!

And for those who only believe if they can see for themselves: Spoiler Alert! This feature is at the end of each chapter and provides specific cross-references to ACER official practice materials. This way, you may choose to either check our work through specific examples from official ACER GAMSAT content or continue your studies for that particular chapter. Please note: 1-2% of official ACER practice questions either change or are moved every year.

Chapter Checklists

Part 3 of the trifecta to improve your study efficiency: At the end of each chapter, we encourage you to participate in a reassessment of your understanding based on the learning objectives for that chapter, to take appropriate notes, to engage in multimedia learning, and more.

More Changes?

In addition to the trifecta, for the first time, this book contains many other features with the sole aim of increasing your study efficiency and understanding: *Need for Speed* exercises at the beginning of most chapters; improved quality and quantity of practice questions; detailed worked solutions; re-editing of each and every page; and finally, more online discussion boards to ensure that you have access to resolve any question you may have regarding the content in this book.

A word about your online access . . .

The GS Online Access has saved thousands of trees and have reduced the cost of this book to you. It is not just the hundreds of online answers and worked solutions that you get access to with your gamsat-prep.com account, it is the fact that we do not have to limit the length of our worked solutions because of printing cost restrictions. It permits this textbook to sell for less than most with the same production value, while at the same time, providing you with more detailed worked solutions than any other GAMSAT publication, ever. You will also be able to access dozens of hours of topical videos with clear teaching which help to convert a static book into a dynamic multimedia experience.

Cross-references!

Wherever possible, we will identify another chapter, section or subsection of the book where you can find more information regarding a particular topic. For the most part, each book is self-contained but there are some exceptional cases where we cross-reference between different Masters Series books. The following table contains a summary of the abbreviations used throughout the Masters Series.

Cross-references to the Masters Series books, videos, apps, etc.

Abbreviation	Subject	Theme, Book
RHSS	Reasoning in Humanities & Social Sciences	Book 1
WC	Written Communication	Book 2
GM	GAMSAT Maths	Physical Sciences, Book 3
PHY	Physics	Physical Sciences, Book 3
CHM	General Chemistry	Physical Sciences, Book 4
ORG	Organic Chemistry	Biological Sciences, Book 5
BIO	Biology	Biological Sciences, Book 6

For example, CHM 2.4 means that you will find more information by looking at the Masters Series textbook, Chapter 2 General Chemistry, in the section 2.4. After a few chapters, you will find the system to be quite straightforward and, often, helpful.

Note: Despite the many new additions throughout this textbook, it remains 99% error-free. Should you have any doubts, join us at gamsat-prep.com/forum.

And so, the adventure begins.

Good luck!

- BF, MD

GAMSAT ORGANIC CHEMISTRY

5 Sections • 14 Chapters

01
Bonds and Shapes of Carbon-based Molecules

Chapter 1: Molecular Structure of Organic Compounds
Chapter 2: Stereochemistry

C

02
Hydrogen meets Carbon: The Hydrocarbons

Chapter 3: Alkanes
Chapter 4: Alkenes
Chapter 5: Aromatics

C — H

03
Oxygen-containing Organic Molecules

Chapter 6: Alcohols
Chapter 7: Aldehydes and Ketones
Chapter 8: Carboxylic Acids
Chapter 9: Carboxylic Acid Derivatives
Chapter 10: Ethers and Phenols

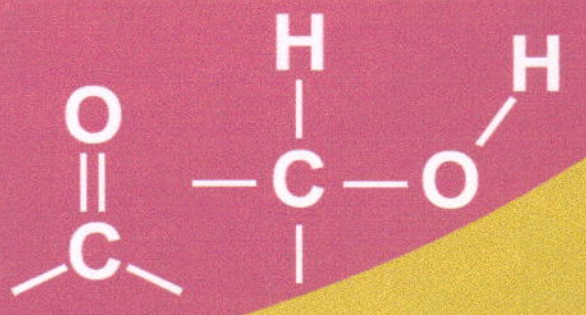

04
Nitrogen- and Complex Oxygen-containing Organic Molecules

Chapter 11: Amines
Chapter 12: Biological Molecules

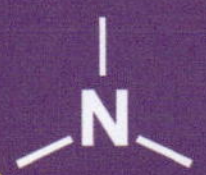

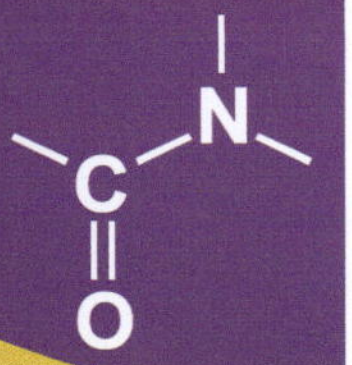

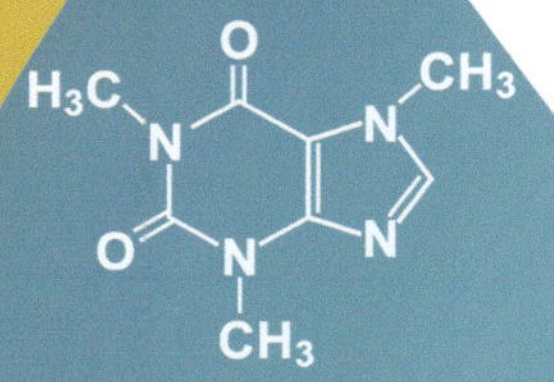

05
Isolating and Identifying Organic Molecules

Chapter 13: Separations and Purifications
Chapter 14: Spectroscopy

GAMSAT-prep.com

MOLECULAR STRUCTURE OF ORGANIC COMPOUNDS
Chapter 1

Memorise

* Periodic table trends
* Define: Lewis, dipole moments
* Ground rules for structures, resonance

Understand

* Pattern recognition, geometric reasoning
* Comparing resonance structures
* Hybrid orbitals, multiple bonds
* Structures and basic stereochemistry

Importance

Medium level: 7% of GAMSAT Organic Chemistry questions released by ACER are related to content in this chapter (in our estimation).
* Note that approximately 60% of the questions in GAMSAT Organic Chemistry are related to just 4 chapters: 2, 6, 7 and 12.

Introduction

Organic chemistry is the study of the structure, properties, composition, reactions, and preparation (i.e. synthesis) of chemical compounds containing carbon. Such compounds may contain hydrogen, nitrogen, oxygen, the halogens as well as phosphorus, silicon and sulfur. To give some perspective, it is interesting to note that almost 99% of the mass of the human body is made up of just six elements: carbon, hydrogen, oxygen, nitrogen, phosphorus, and calcium. If you master the basic rules in this chapter, you will be able to conquer GAMSAT Organic Chemistry with little further memorisation.

GAMSAT Maths, in one way or the other, is related to most GAMSAT Physics, General Chemistry and Biology questions on the real exam. GAMSAT Organic Chemistry has a very different, three-part foundation: Nomenclature, pattern recognition, and geometric reasoning. **Nomenclature** usually uses a standard system, which is easy to learn, that provides names for molecules (ORG 3.1, 4.1, 5.1, etc.). **Pattern recognition** and **geometric reasoning** both have little to do with memory: These are skills that you might already have (with or without your knowledge of it!), or that you can develop whereby you notice differences and similarities within images. This skill is specific to GAMSAT and is not often rewarded in undergraduate studies.

* The real GAMSAT may have advanced-level information presented (i.e. in a passage) but previous knowledge of said information is not required to answer the questions that would follow. Practice questions at the end of this chapter, as well as ACER and GS (HEAPS) practice GAMSATs can help you clarify this point.

1.0 GAMSAT has a *Need for Speed*!

Please draw!

If you do not have enough space, please use some A4 scratch paper (*to simulate the real digital GAMSAT!*). Why draw? Because of muscle memory: GAMSAT Organic Chemistry is the only one of the four GAMSAT sciences where maths rarely matters. Of course, it is important to learn the basic rules but then, after that, it is mostly pattern recognition and geometric (*shapes*) reasoning.

Need for Speed exercises are NOT GAMSAT-style practice questions! At the end of every chapter, as with other Masters Series books, you will find GAMSAT-level practice questions. *Need for Speed* are exercises in GAMSAT Organic Chemistry to help you remember, and actively experience, key themes within chapters.

For some students, this is the cart before the horse! If it has been a long time or if you have never studied organic chemistry, do what you can or just scan the exercises, and then begin studying Chapter 1 sequentially. After completing this chapter, return to the table below to ensure that you can complete all entries. Then you can proceed to answer the additional multiple-choice questions at the end of this chapter.

For those of you who are able to answer quickly but get stuck at some point, take note of the section number associated with the problem, and then you can skip forward to that particular section. We used a pink highlighter throughout the chapter so that you can quickly identify the practice questions from the table in order to check your answers and find the worked solutions.

Section	GAMSAT Organic Chemistry *Need for Speed* Exercises	
1.1	Below are two water molecules. Identify the partially positive (δ^+) and partially negative (δ^-) atoms, as well as the likely placement of the hydrogen bond.	What is the maximum number of atoms that carbon can bond to?

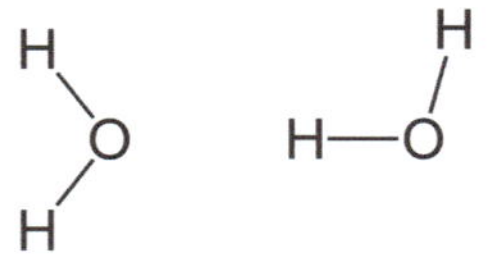

Draw the structures and charges for the missing entries in the table below. Assume that each atom only possesses single bonds, and is in a molecule.

Atom	Neutral	Cationic	Anionic
C			
N			
O			

Do not be concerned with lone pair electrons (dots).

Medium-level Importance

1.1

	Pentane, C_5H_{12}
Skeletal structure Do not worry about the 3D shape. Instead, draw this linear molecule while including all carbons (C) and hydrogens (H).	
Shorthand Draw the entire molecule using only lines and no overt C's or H's.	
Molecular formula Do not be concerned with the structure; but rather, expand the molecular formula for pentane, C_5H_{12}.	

Draw a simple, skeletal-line representation (shorthand) of the following molecules either below the structure or on some A4 scratch paper.

1)

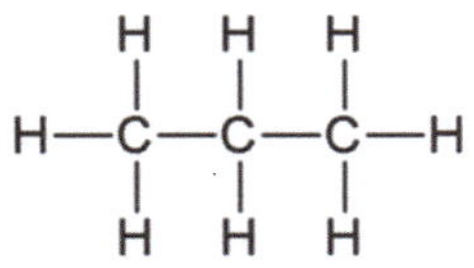

2)

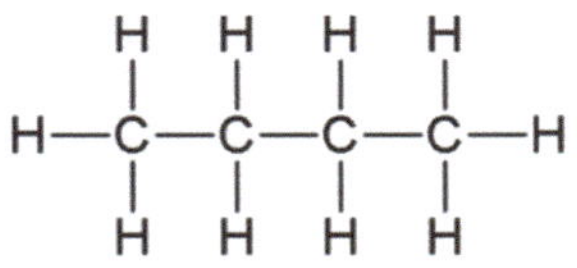

3)

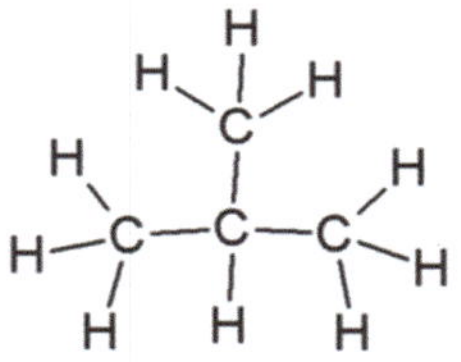

4)

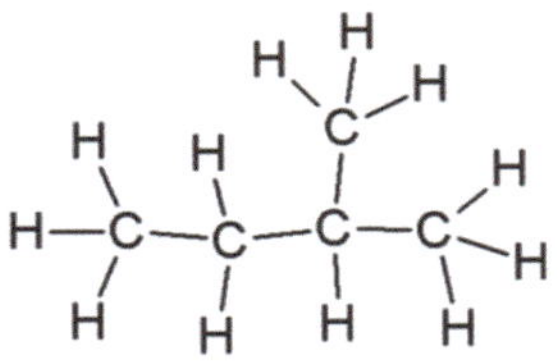

5)

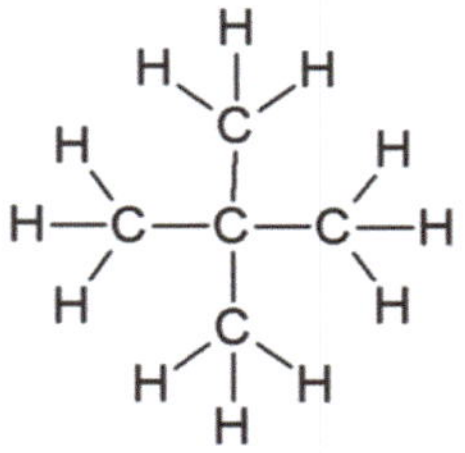

Medium-level Importance

1.1

6)

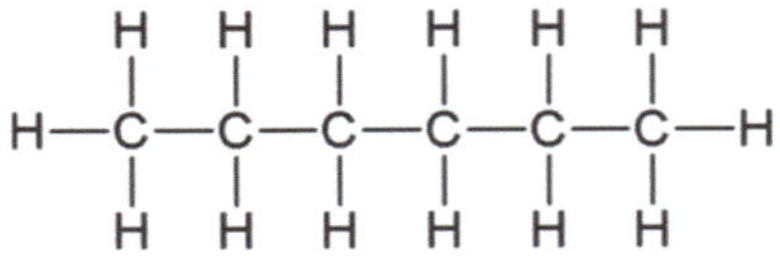

7)

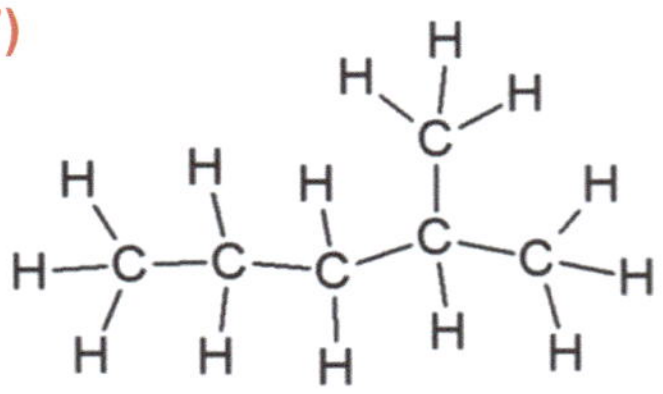

8)

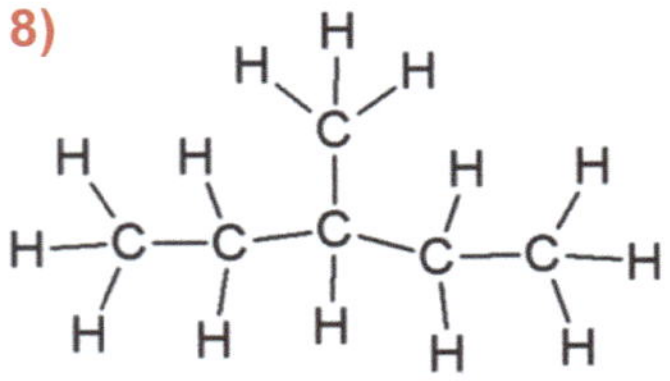

9)

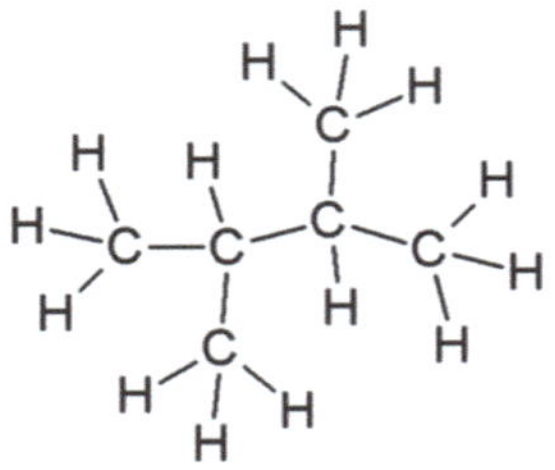

10)

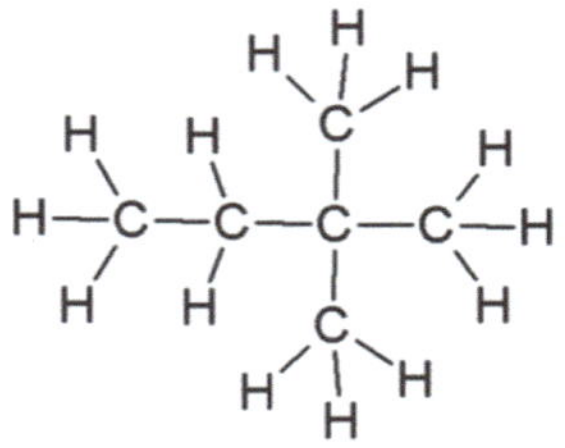

Answers (skeletal-line drawings) for exercises 1-10 can be found at the end of this chapter, just before Spoiler Alert.

1.1.1

Complete the statements below:

- Hydrogen is neutral when bonded __________ time(s).
- Oxygen is neutral when bonded __________ time(s).
- Nitrogen is neutral when bonded __________ time(s).
- Carbon is neutral when bonded __________ time(s).

1.4

Consider the following resonance structures. Annotate the two carbons missing negative charges with the "-" symbol.

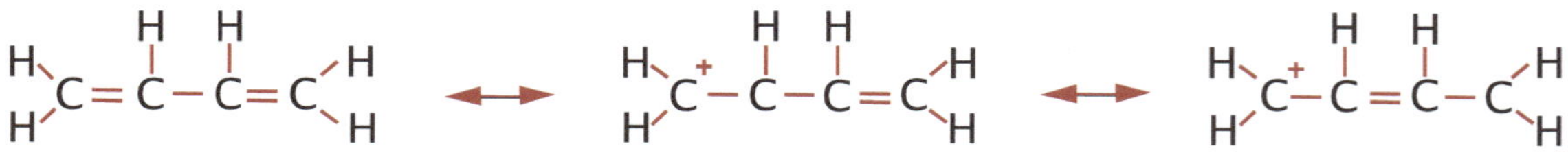

1.5 Carbon has four valence electrons and oxygen has six. Use dots to show how carbon dioxide follows the octet rule (8 dots surrounding each atom):

O C O

Draw bond vectors (*arrows, from positive to negative*) for any of the following bonds that would be considered dipoles. If any of the molecules have a non-zero dipole moment, also draw that vector.

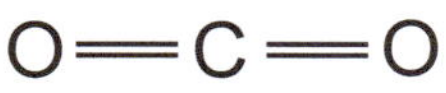

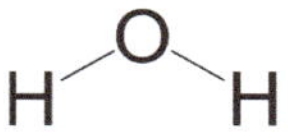

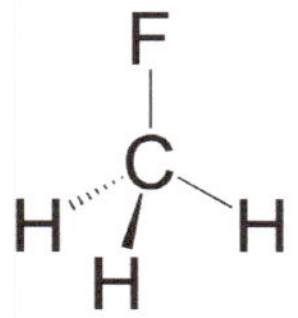

1.6.1 Classify the carbons in the structure below as either primary, secondary, tertiary, or quaternary.

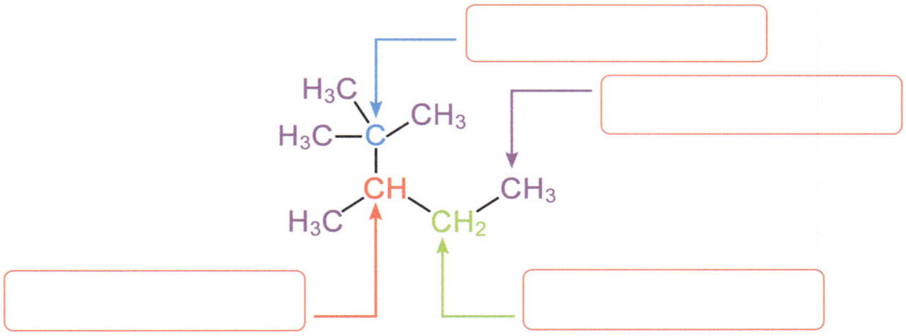

1.7 Do not worry about the 3D shape. In the empty boxes below, re-draw the molecule while including all carbons (C), hydrogens (H), oxygens (O), nitrogens (N), and bonds between atoms.

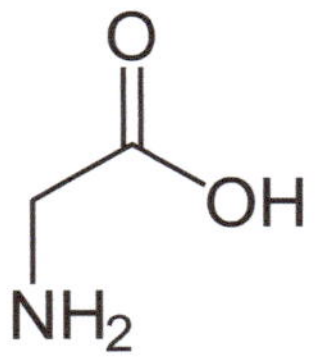

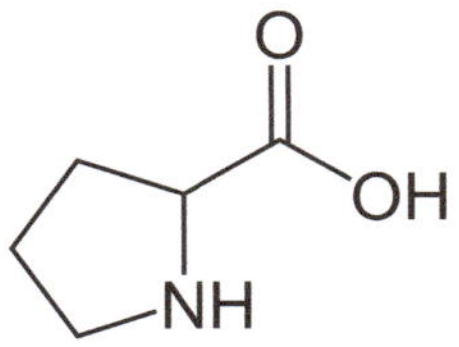

Consider the neutral carbon atom. Complete the missing entries in the table below.

When bonded to...	Hybridisation	Shape
2 atoms		
3 atoms		
4 atoms		

1.1 Carbon: The Centre of our World

Medium-level Importance

You have never heard of a 'helium tax' or an 'oxygen tax', etc., but you have likely heard of a 'carbon tax'. There are more than 100 elements in the periodic table, but one is the focus of international diplomacy and global climate change. This is related to the fact that the chemistry of carbon, organic chemistry, is the chemistry of life itself.

That 'carbon tax' is mostly due to the fact that hydrocarbon (hydrogen + carbon) fuels (coal, petroleum, and natural gas) are largely converted (by burning = *combustion*; ORG 3.2.1) to water (H_2O) and carbon dioxide (CO_2). We do not complain about the water, but even the media has identified excess carbon dioxide as a heat-trapping 'greenhouse' gas responsible for climate change. You may also have heard that fuels, 'fossil fuels', are not just hydrocarbons, but they are formed from the fossilised remains of ancient plants and animals - hundreds of millions of years old - and are thus limited in supply. Thus we can deduce that plants and animals make complex molecules involving carbon, hydrogen and oxygen and that is why, when burnt, molecules such as CO_2 and H_2O can be released.

And so, irrespective of your academic background, you have been exposed to many notions related to organic chemistry just by being informed and aware.

Fuels include a category of organic chemicals called 'alkanes' and, we will see later (Chapter 3), when naming alkanes, the suffix -*ane* is used. There tends to be public awareness of many alkanes: methane (the simplest alkane), propane (a fuel for barbecue grills), butane (lighter fuel for cigarettes), octane (used to improve engine performance and, when high, has entered English vernacular for 'intensity'!). Like acetone (think: nail polish remover, paint thinner), these alkanes evaporate quickly (= *volatile*) because the molecules in the liquid cannot hold each other together. Their volatility relates to that strong smell of acetone or propane, but why? Why isn't water turning to steam at room temperature?

The ability of molecules to interact and the impact that has on a substance's volatility (and therefore boiling point; CHM 4.4), will be discussed every time we present a new category of compounds. Hopefully, you recall from your General Chemistry studies, that hydrogen bonds (CHM 4.2) are the key and water is unusually efficient at H-bonding, while hydrocarbons are incapable since they do not have the necessary components, for example, –OH.

Due to differences in electronegativity (CHM 3.1.1, 3.3, 4.2; ORG 1.5), the attraction of the partially positive (= δ^+) hydrogen from one molecule to the partially negative (= δ^-) oxygen of another forms the basis for water's H-bonding (*dashed line*):

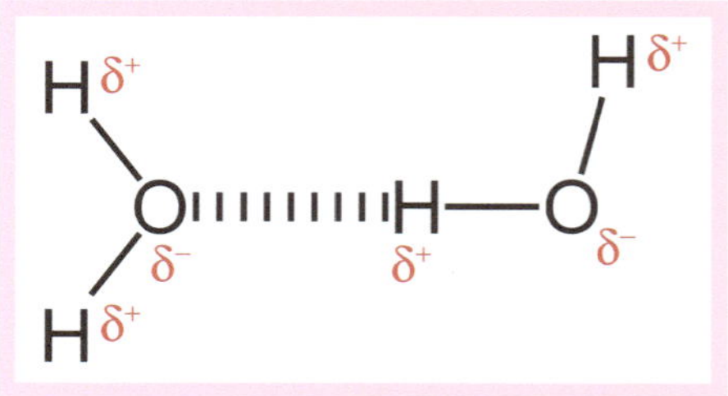

The human body is about two-thirds water. Thus water is the solvent that permits most of life's chemistry to take place.

PERIODIC TABLE OF THE ELEMENTS

96% of the mass of the human body is composed of: H, C, N, and O

Period ↓ / Group →	1	2	3	4	5	6	7	8	9	10	11	12	13	14	15	16	17	18
1	1 H																	2 He
2	3 Li	4 Be											5 B	6 C	7 N	8 O	9 F	10 Ne
3	11 Na	12 Mg											13 Al	14 Si	15 P	16 S	17 Cl	18 Ar
4	19 K	20 Ca	21 Sc	22 Ti	23 V	24 Cr	25 Mn	26 Fe	27 Co	28 Ni	29 Cu	30 Zn	31 Ga	32 Ge	33 As	34 Se	35 Br	36 Kr
5	37 Rb	38 Sr	39 Y	40 Zr	41 Nb	42 Mo	43 Tc	44 Ru	45 Rh	46 Pd	47 Ag	48 Cd	49 In	50 Sn	51 Sb	52 Te	53 I	54 Xe
6	55 Cs	56 Ba		72 Hf	73 Ta	74 W	75 Re	76 Os	77 Ir	78 Pt	79 Au	80 Hg	81 Tl	82 Pb	83 Bi	84 Po	85 At	86 Rn
7	87 Fr	88 Ra		104 Rf	105 Db	106 Sg	107 Bh	108 Hs	109 Mt	110 Ds	111 Rg	112 Cn	113 Nh	114 Fl	115 Ms	116 Lv	117 Ts	118 Og

Lanthanides	57 La	58 Ce	59 Pr	60 Nd	61 Pm	62 Sm	63 Eu	64 Gd	65 Tb	66 Dy	67 Ho	68 Er	69 Tm	70 Yb	71 Lu
Actinides	89 Ac	90 Th	91 Pa	92 U	93 Np	94 Pu	95 Am	96 Cm	97 Bk	98 Cf	99 Es	100 Fm	101 Md	102 No	103 Lr

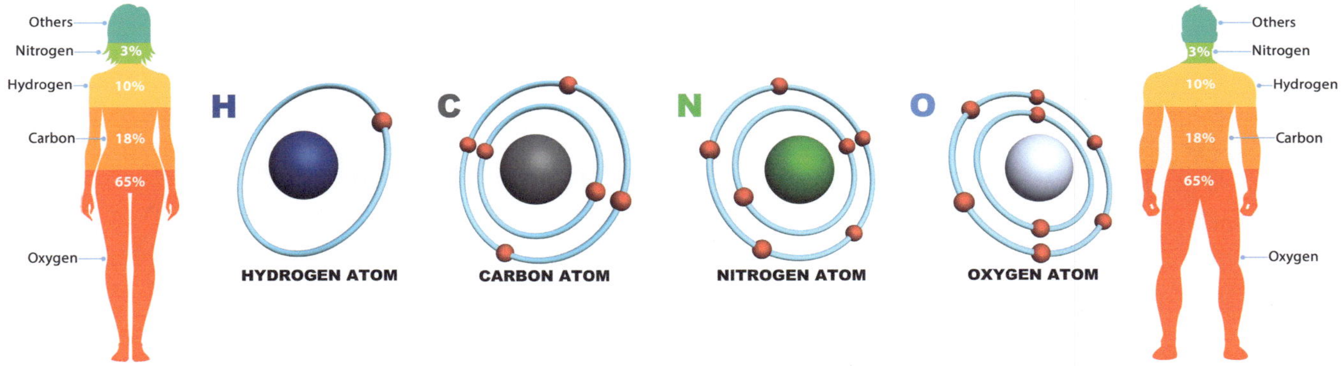

Figure IV.B.1.0: The periodic table (CHM 2.4) and the most important atoms in organic chemistry. (1) Group 1: alkali metals, red; Group 2: alkaline metals, beige; Groups 3-12 transition metals, peach; olive: metalloids; bright green: nonmetals; other nonmetals include the halogens in yellow (AKA 'halides' as anions), and noble gases in the last group (relatively unreactive, inert). For GAMSAT purposes, since a periodic table is NOT provided, you should be familiar with the location of the first 20 elements + the halogens Br and I. (2) Models (cartoons!) of H, C, N and O with red electrons in orbit around a central nucleus: Notice that the number of electrons matches the atomic number in the periodic table since the atoms are neutral (PHY 12.1; CHM 2.1; i.e. the negatively charged electrons = the number of positively charged protons = the atomic number in the periodic table). Chemical reactions/bonding do not include the nucleus - nor the inner ring of electrons - but rather the outer ring or *valence* electrons. Despite the cartoon, atoms are not like the solar system, as previously thought, where there is a nucleus like the sun and outer electrons like planets revolving in predictable orbits. Instead, electrons are described as probability distributions (ORG 1.2; CHM 2.1, 2.2). Verify the number of electrons in the outer rings: H, 1; C, 4; N, 5; O, 6. When these atoms bond together, we can represent the entirety of each atom as a sphere.

Medium-level Importance

Medium-level Importance

You are the stuff of stars and diamonds! Let's talk about carbon. What is so special about carbon? Why is it that all life, as we currently understand, must use carbon as the backbone for molecules?

Carbon, like other atoms, was forged in the heart of stars billions of years ago and blasted throughout space. All the atoms in your body are billions of years old and originate from another galaxy. On our planet, natural forms of carbon include graphite (*the main component of 'lead' in pencils*) and diamonds (= *graphite under high pressure*).

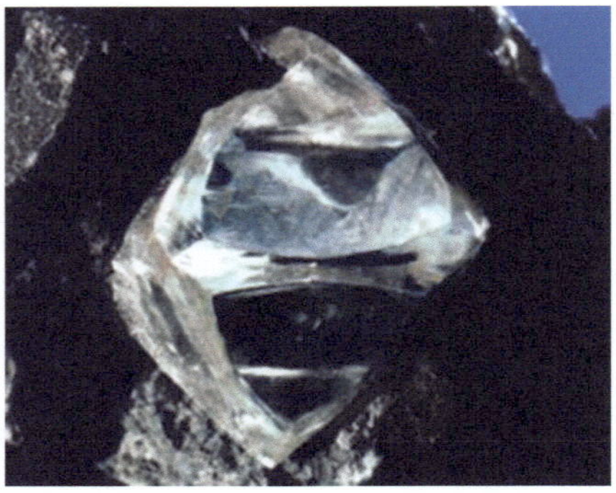

Rough diamond surrounded by graphite rock

Bonds between carbon atoms are strong and versatile. Carbon has 4 valence electrons (= *outer shell electrons, where all the bonding action takes place*). Since every bond - symbolised by a line between 2 atoms - contains 2 electrons, and atoms tend to share electrons in bonds, that means that carbon can bond with a maximum of 4 other atoms (= *saturated*). Keeping this simple fact straight and using your eagle eyes to notice when and how the rule is applied, is the source of several straightforward GAMSAT questions every year.

Part of your training includes, throughout this chapter and those to come, identifying carbons and ensuring that every neutral carbon has 4 bonds. In fact, the following table summarises different, common states for important atoms. After reading a few chapters, you should come back to this table to ensure your understanding.

Atom	Neutral	Cationic	Anionic
C	–C– (4 bonds)	–C⁺ (3 bonds)	–C:⁻ (3 bonds, 1 lone pair)
N	–N: (3 bonds, 1 lone pair)	–N⁺– (4 bonds)	N⁻ (2 bonds, 2 lone pairs)
O	O (2 bonds, 2 lone pairs)	–O:⁺ (3 bonds, 1 lone pair)	–O:⁻ (1 bond, 3 lone pairs)
X	–X: (1 bond, 3 lone pairs)	–X⁺– (2 bonds, 2 lone pairs)	:X:⁻ (4 lone pairs)

X = halogens (i.e. F, Cl, Br, I)

How strong is a carbon bond? Despite what you may have heard in a comic-book based movie, the hardest material known to humanity is still diamond: pure carbon. Diamond is so strong that it is used on the tips of machines to drill through metals, rock and concrete.

Why so strong? The bond between carbon atoms is very strong and the shape, the *tetrahedron*, creates both added strength and the ability to form an incredible array of chains and branches. Not only is the tetrahedron key to the strength of diamonds, it is the most common shape carbon takes in the molecules of life (*consider spending a few minutes looking at the pictures - from simple to complex structures - in Chapter 12, Biological Molecules*).

The tetrahedron is a pyramid (3D) with a triangular base, and carbon is right in the middle! Whenever carbon is bonded 4 times, which is often the case, each carbon is at the centre of a tetrahedron. Consider the following image of methane, CH_4.

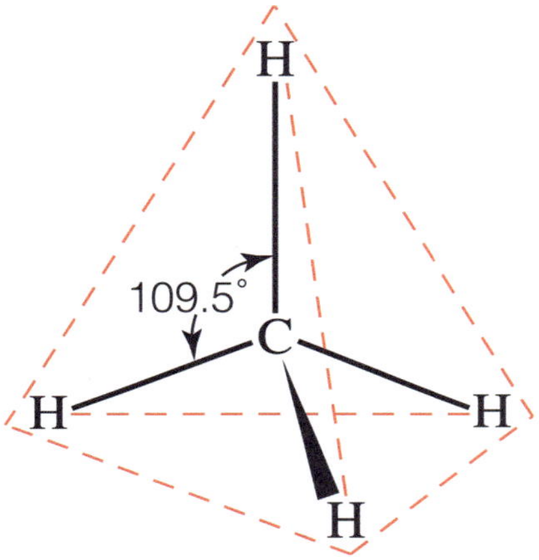

Note: in organic chemistry, a dark triangle means that the bond is coming towards you (i.e. it is coming OUT of the page), a straight line means that the bond is in the same plane as the page, and a dashed triangle means that the bond is going away from you. However, as we will see, there are many shorthand ways to draw molecules that ignore these rules for the sake of expediency. Here are just a couple of such shorthand representations of methane:

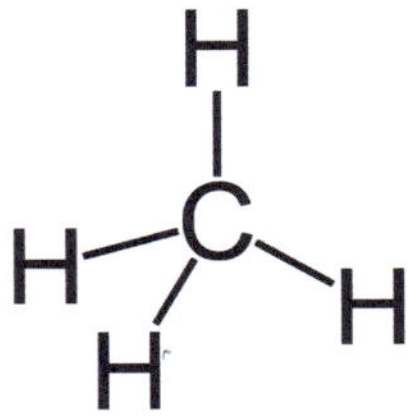

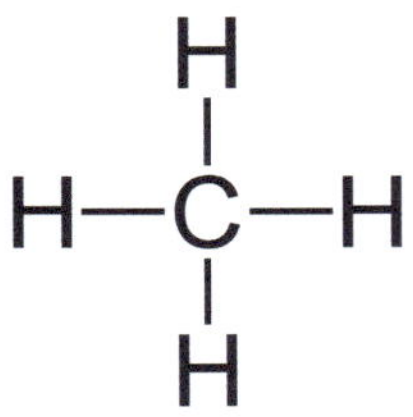

Organic chemistry requires a lot of imagination. Most students will be able to look at the hundreds of illustrations in this book without any difficulty. Some students prefer something more tangible: for example, either purchasing a molecular model set/kit, or making one with the help of YouTube, plasticine and/or Styrofoam. Here is tetrahedral methane using a molecular model set (notice that it is quite similar to the ball-and-stick model of the molecule, *see* Table IV.B.1.1 *au verso*):

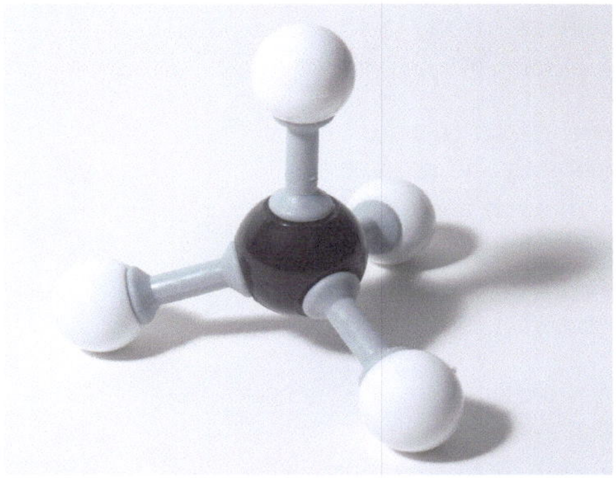

In considering real molecules, how representative are models, skeletal structures and other illustrations? Well, they are really cartoons. How much does Bugs Bunny represent rabbits? I suppose there are some basic features in common, but...

The illustrations of molecules are all simplified representations that, of course, share important characteristics with the real thing. Ideally, you will develop the flexibility to seamlessly go from one way to represent a molecule to another, while reflexively accounting for the key atoms and bonds. By developing your observational skills, as opposed to trying to commit details to memory, you will have a much easier time when faced with typical GAMSAT-exam questions.

Table IV.B.1.1: Various ways to represent simple hydrocarbons (*the structures are more or less the same 3D orientation, where possible*).

STRUCTURES OF COMMON HYDROCARBONS Hydrogen (H) + Carbon (C) = Hydrocarbons			
	Methane, CH_4	**Ethane, C_2H_6**	**Pentane, C_5H_{12}**
Space-filling model Most accurately represents real molecules - compared to other models - but least used since it is not easy to draw and not all atoms or bonds are visible; C: dark grey, H: white.	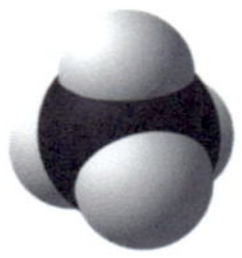	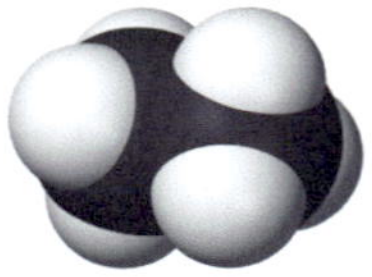	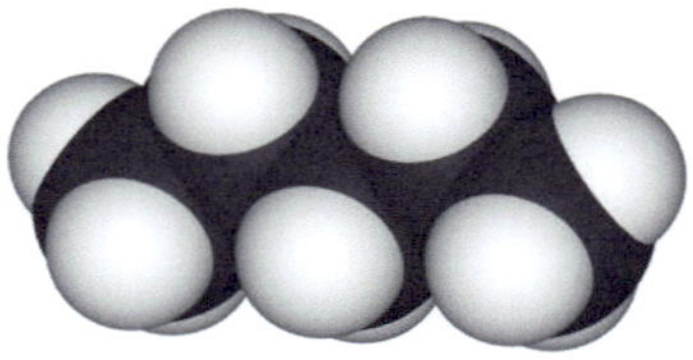
Ball-and-stick model Atoms, bonds and shapes are clearer (in each case, C is in the centre of a tetrahedron; C: dark grey, H: white); not any easier to draw!	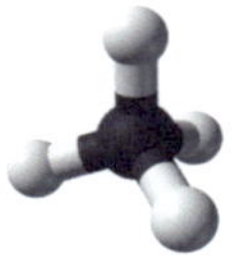	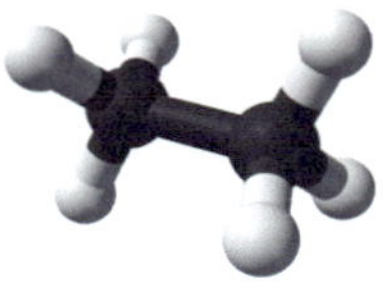	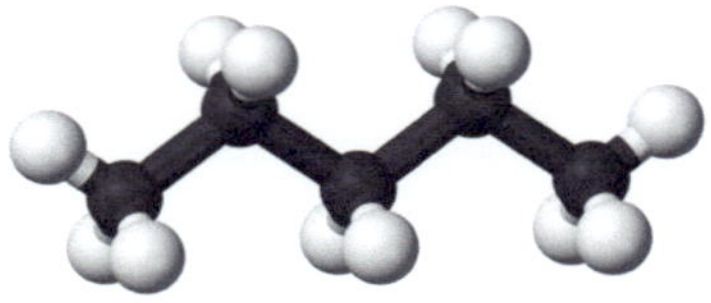
Skeletal structure AKA structural formula, line diagram, etc.; this form preserves the 3D shape with solid triangles (*towards you*) and dashed (*"broken"*) triangles (*away from you*).	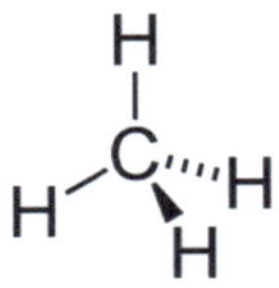	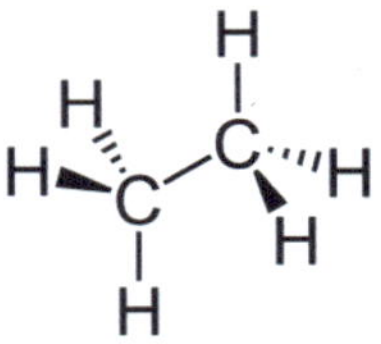	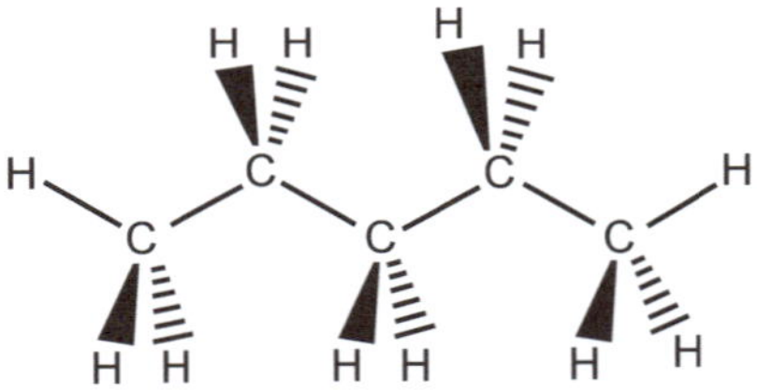
Skeletal structure During the real exam, you would usually use this form (+/– the H's) and/or the shorthand form below. 3D shape is not preserved.	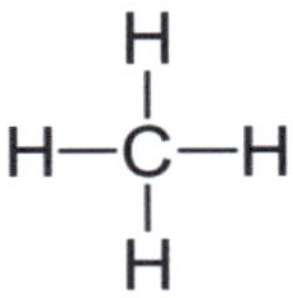	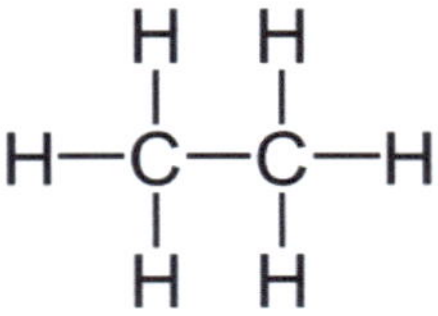	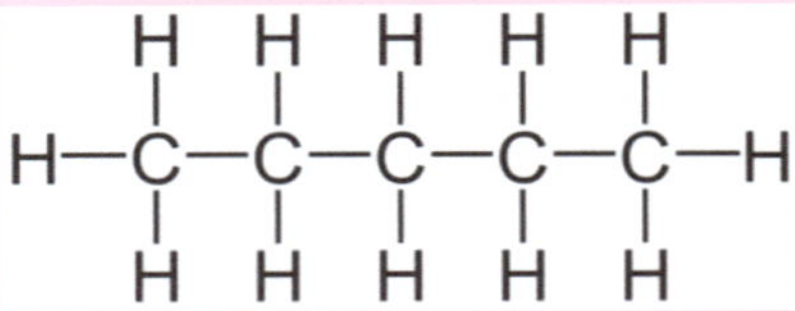
Shorthand Imagination and discipline: Every corner of a geometric figure is a carbon as well as the end of a line*. H's are assumed using the rule: 4 bonds to each C.	N/A		
Miscellaneous	CH_4	CH_3CH_3, CH_3-CH_3 H_3C-CH_3	$CH_3CH_2CH_2CH_2CH_3$ $CH_3(CH_2)_3CH_3$

*That is, as long as no other atom is present at the end of a line, then it can be assumed that carbon is present, and as many H's are bonded to that carbon so that neutral C has 4 bonds, i.e. the end of a single line must be $-CH_3$.

Medium-level Importance

1.1.1 Overview: A Closer Look at the Atoms of Organic Chemistry

Carbon (C), hydrogen (H), oxygen (O), nitrogen (N) and the halogens (i.e. fluorine – F, chlorine – Cl, bromine – Br, etc.) are common atoms found in organic compounds. The atoms in most organic compounds are held together by covalent bonds (*the sharing of an electron pair between two atoms*). Some ionic bonding (*the transfer of electrons from one atom to another*) does exist. Common to both types of chemical bonds is the fact that the atoms bond such that they can achieve the electron configuration of the nearest noble gas, usually eight electrons. This is known as the *octet rule*.

A **carbon** atom has one s and three p orbitals in its outermost shell, allowing it to form 4 single bonds. As well, a carbon atom may be involved in a double bond, where two electron pairs are shared, or a triple bond, where three electron pairs are shared. An **oxygen** atom may form 2 single bonds, or one double bond. It has 2 unshared (lone) electron pairs. A **hydrogen** atom will form only one single bond. A **nitrogen** atom may form 3 single bonds. As well, it is capable of double and triple bonds. It has one unshared electron pair. The **halogens** are all able to form only one (*single*) bond. Halogens all have three unshared electron pairs.

Throughout the following chapters we will be examining the structural formulas of molecules involving H, C, N, O, halides and phosphorus (P). However, it should be noted that less common atoms often have similar structural formulas within molecules as compared to common atoms. For example, silicon (Si) is found in the same group as carbon in the periodic table; thus they have similar properties. In fact, Si can also form 4 single bonds leading to a tetrahedral structure (i.e. SiH_4, SiO_4). Likewise sulfur (S) is found in the same group as oxygen. Though it can be found as a solid (S_8), it still has many properties similar to those of oxygen. For example, like O in H_2O, sulfur can form a bent, polar molecule (H_2S). We will later see that sulfur is an important component in the amino acid cysteine. {*To learn more about molecular structure, hybrid orbitals, polarity and bonding, see General Chemistry chapters 2 and 3* }

Medium-level Importance

Mnemonic: **HONC** increasing bonds for neutrality . . .

H requires 1 more electron in its outer shell to become stable: thus hydrogen is neutral when bonded once

O requires 2: thus oxygen is neutral when bonded twice

N requires 3: thus nitrogen is neutral when bonded 3 times

C requires 4: thus carbon is neutral when bonded 4 times

1.2 Hybrid Orbitals

In organic molecules, the orbitals of the atoms are combined to form **hybrid orbitals**, consisting of a mixture of the s and p orbitals. In a carbon atom, if the one s and three p orbitals are mixed, the result is four hybrid sp^3 orbitals. Three hybridised sp^2 orbitals result from the mixing of one s and two p orbitals, and two hybridised sp orbitals result from the mixing of one s and one p. The geometry of the hybridised orbitals is shown in Figure IV.B.1.1.

Take-home message regarding geometry and hybrids: When carbon is bonded 4 times, all 4 bonds are sp^3 and C is in the centre of a tetrahedron; when neutral carbon is bonded to 3 atoms, the 3 hybrids are sp^2 and C is in the centre of a flat triangle (= *trigonal planar*); when neutral carbon is bonded to 2 atoms, the 2 hybrids are sp and C is in the centre of a straight line (*linear*).

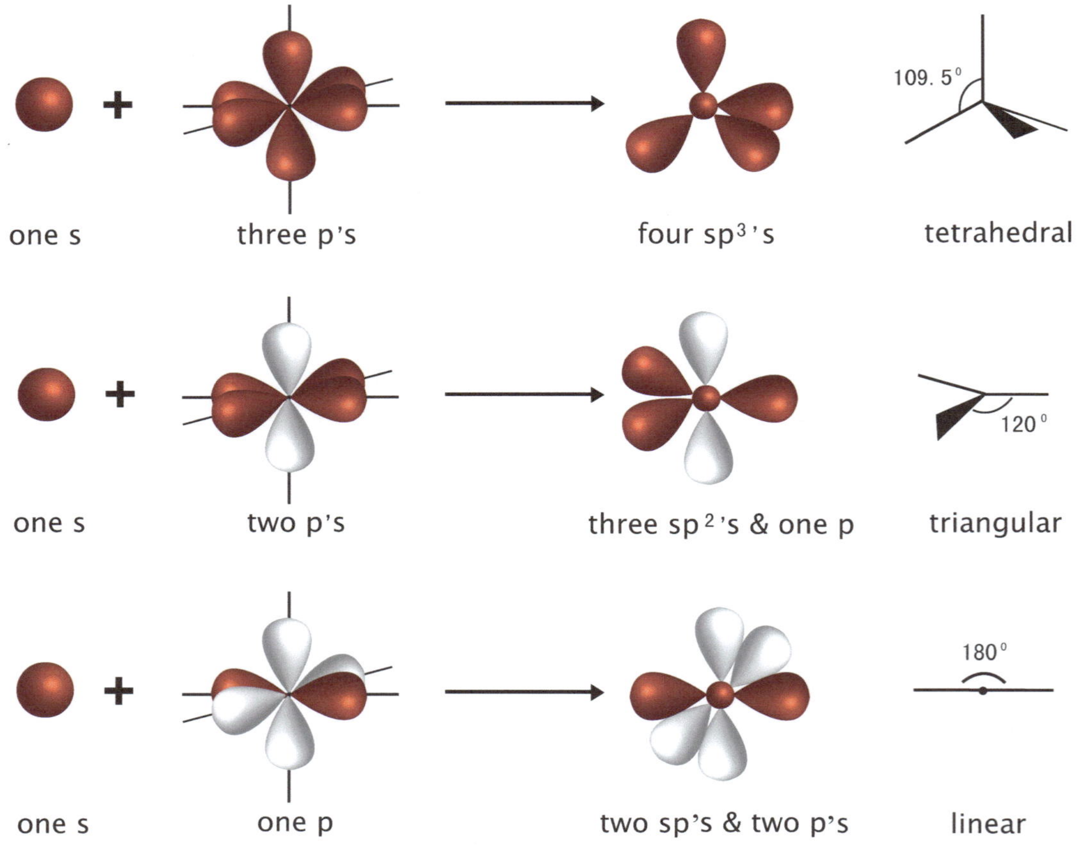

Figure IV.B.1.1: Hybrid orbital geometry

NOTE: For details regarding atomic structure and orbitals, *see* General Chemistry (CHM) sections 2.1, 2.2. For more details regarding hybridised bonds and bond angles (especially for carbon, nitrogen, oxygen and sulfur), *see* CHM 3.5. Notice in the first row of the image there are three p orbitals occupying the *x*, *y* and *z* axes (GM 3.6) thus p_x, p_y and p_z.

Medium-level Importance

Sigma (or single) bonds are those in which the electron density is between the nuclei. They are symmetric about the axis, can freely rotate, and are formed when orbitals (regular or hybridised) overlap directly. They are characterised by the fact that they are circular when a cross section is taken and the bond is viewed along the bond axis. The electron density in pi bonds overlaps both above and below the plane of the atoms. A single bond is a sigma bond (e.g. C-C); a double bond is one sigma and one pi bond (e.g. C=C); a triple bond is one sigma (σ) and two pi (π) bonds (e.g. C≡C).

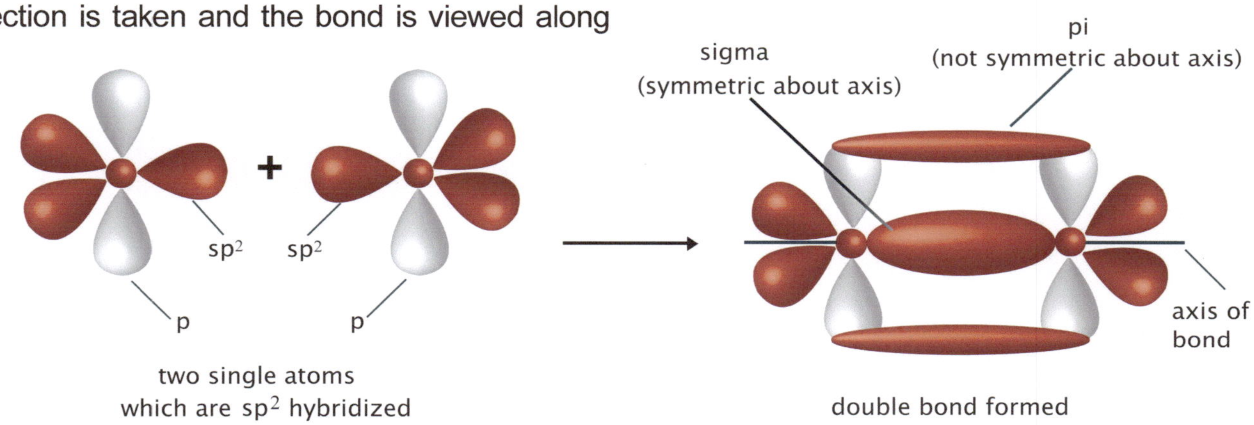

Figure IV.B.1.2a: Sigma and pi bonds. The sp^2 hybrids overlap between the nuclei to form a σ bond; the p orbitals overlap above and below the axis between the nuclei to form a π bond. The product above illustrates the probability distribution (i.e. the likely locations) for the electrons of 2 carbon atoms engaged in a double bond (e.g. the hydrocarbon *ethylene*).

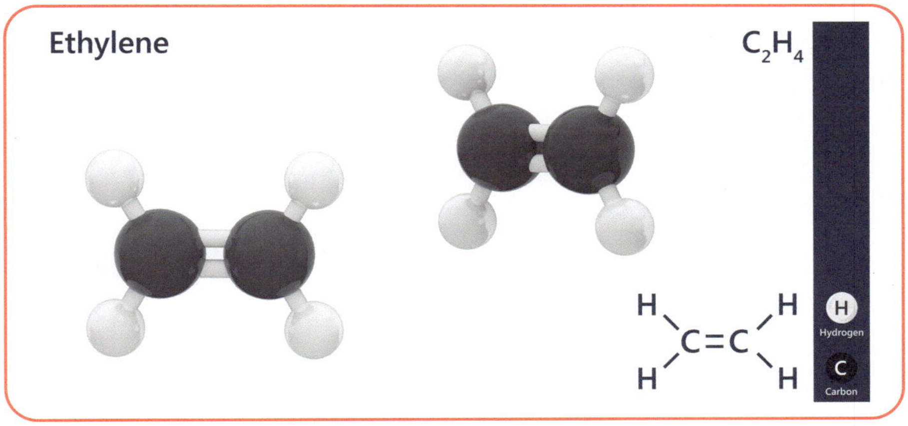

Figure IV.B.1.2b: Ethylene (AKA ethene, $H_2C{=}CH_2$). Note that each carbon is in the centre of a flat triangle: the corners of the triangle being 2 H's and the other C. The carbon-carbon double bond has 2 lines, C=C, one signifies the sigma bond (sp^2-sp^2) and the other is the pi bond (p-p). You may wonder: why does the pi bond only get 1 line when Fig. IV.B.1.2a shows p-p bonding above *and* below the sigma bond? Imagine each carbon like a block of wood with a big screw between the 2 blocks holding them together. The screw is 1 sigma bond. Imagine a very thick rubber band placed around the blocks, encompassing the two blocks thus reinforcing their bond. The rubber band, which goes above and below the screw, is just 1 bond, the pi bond. Side note: as a screw is stronger than a thick rubber band, sigma bonds are stronger than pi bonds.

1.3.1 The Effects of Multiple Bonds

The pi bonds in doubly and triply bonded molecules create a barrier to free rotation about the axis of the bond. Thus multiple bonds create molecules which are much more rigid than a molecule with only a single bond which can freely rotate about its axis.

As a rule, the length of a bond decreases with multiple bonds. For example, the carbon-carbon triple bond is shorter than the carbon-carbon double bond which is shorter than the carbon-carbon single bond.

Bond strength and thus the amount of energy required to break a bond (= *BE, the bond dissociation energy*) varies with the number of bonds. One σ bond has a BE $\approx$ 110 kcal/mole and one π bond has a BE $\approx$ 60 kcal/mole. Thus a single bond (one σ) has a BE $\approx$ 110 kcal/mole while a double bond (one σ + one π) has a BE $\approx$ 170 kcal/mole. Hence multiple bonds have greater bond strength than single bonds, although a sigma bond is clearly stronger than a pi bond.

Medium-level Importance

1.4 Delocalised Electrons and Resonance

Delocalisation happens when electrons spread over more than one atom. Delocalisation of charges in the pi bonds is possible when there are hybridised orbitals in adjacent atoms. This delocalisation may be represented in two different ways: the molecular orbital (MO) approach or the resonance (*valence bond*) approach. *See* Fig IV.B.1.3 and consider revising 'covalent bonds' (CHM 3.2).

The MO approach takes a linear combination of atomic orbitals to form molecular orbitals, in which electrons form the bonds. These molecular orbitals cover the whole molecule, and thus the delocalisation of electrons is depicted. In the resonance approach, there is a linear combination of different structures with localised pi bonds and electrons, which together depict the true molecule, or **resonance hybrid**. There is no single structure that represents the molecule.

For example, a 'diene' is a hydrocarbon (hydrogen + carbon) chain that has two double bonds that may or may not be adjacent to each other (ORG 4.1). Conjugated dienes (i.e. butadiene) have two double bonds separated by a

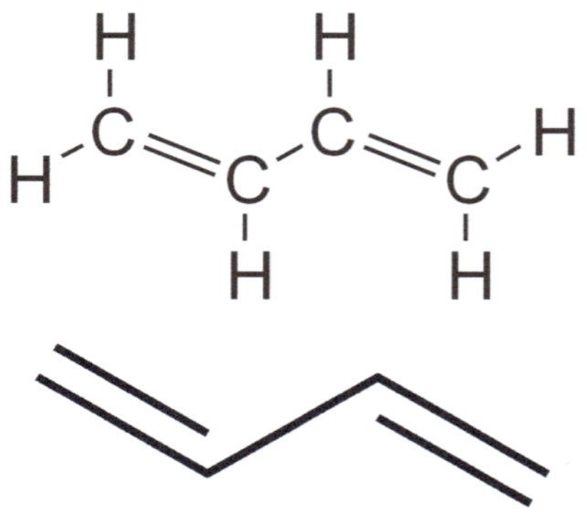

Representations of 1,3-butadiene, $H_2C=CH-CH=CH_2$

single bond and are more stable than nonconjugated dienes because: (1) the delocalisation of charge through resonance and (2) hybridisation energy. Basically, the positioning and overlap of the pi orbitals strengthen the single bond between the two double bonds.

Along with resonance, hybridisation energy affects the stability of the compound. For example in 1,3-butadiene (Fig IV.B.1.3), the carbons with the single bond are sp^2 hybridised, unlike in nonconjugated dienes where the carbons with single bonds are sp^3 hybridised. This difference in hybridisation shows that the conjugated dienes have more 's' character and draw in more of the pi electrons, thus making the single bond stronger and shorter than an ordinary alkane C-C bond. Questions on this concept would always be preceded by an explanatory passage so we will explore s character in the practice questions.

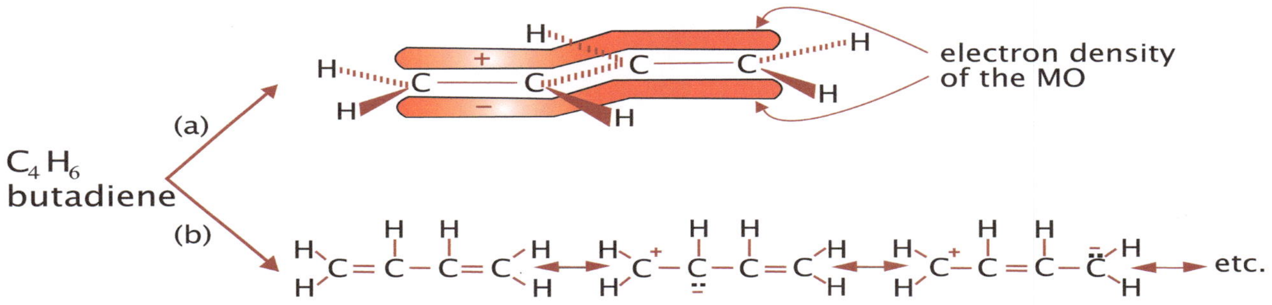

Figure IV.B.1.3: A comparison of MO and resonance approaches. (a) The electron density of the MO covers the entire molecule such that π bonds and p orbitals are not distinguishable. (b) No singular resonance structure accurately portrays butadiene; rather, the true molecule is a composite of all of its resonance structures. Notice that although the bonds can change, atoms do not move in resonance structures. We will be examining resonance structures repeatedly throughout the following chapters because they represent typical exam questions.

1.5 Lewis Structures, Charge Separation and Dipole Moments

The outer shell (or **valence**) electrons are those that form chemical bonds. **Lewis dot structures** are a method of showing the valence electrons and how they form bonds. These electrons, along with the octet rule (*which states that a maximum of eight electrons are allowed in the outermost shell of an atom*), hold only for the elements in the second row of the periodic table (e.g., C, N, O, F). The elements of the third row (e.g., Si, P, S, Cl) use d orbitals, and thus can have more than eight electrons in their outer shell.

Let us use CO_2 as an example. Carbon has four valence electrons and oxygen has six. By covalently bonding, electrons are shared and the octet rule is followed,

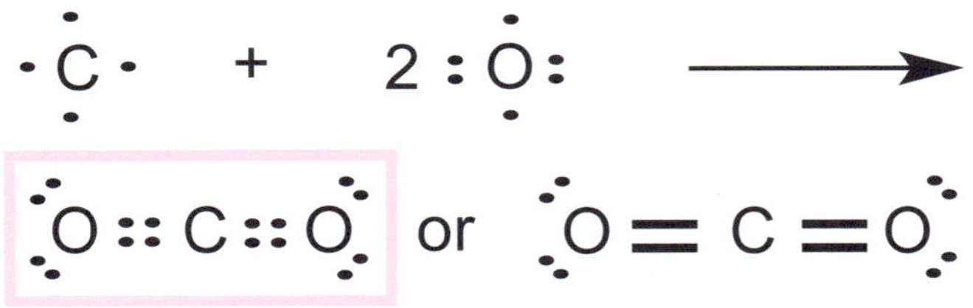

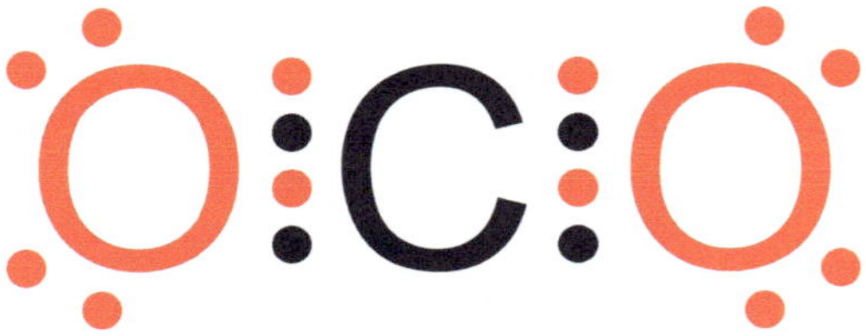

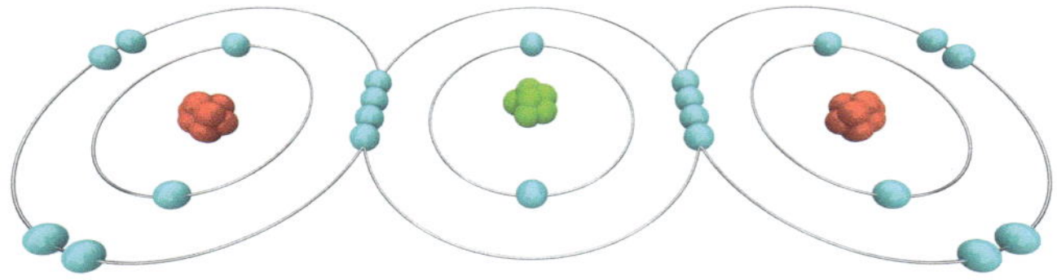

Carbon and oxygen can form resonance structures in the molecule CO_3^{-2}. The –2 denotes two extra electrons to place in the molecule. Once again the octet rule is followed,

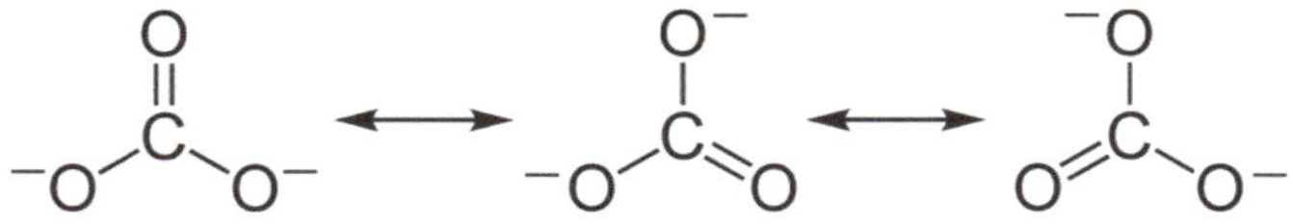

In the final structure, each element counts one half of the electrons in a bond as its own, and any unpaired electrons are counted as its own. The sum of these two quantities should equal the number of valence electrons that were originally around the atom.

If the chemical bond is made up of atoms of different electronegativity, there is a **charge separation:**

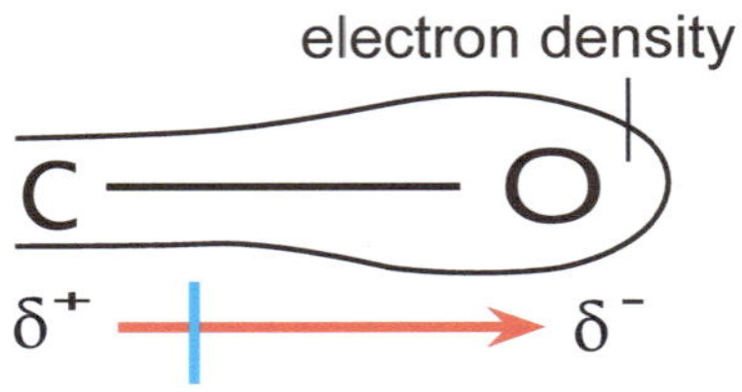

There is a slight pulling of electron density by the more electronegative atom (*oxygen in the preceding example*) from the less electronegative atom (*carbon in the preceding example*). This results in the C–O bond having **partial ionic character** (i.e. *a polar bond; see* CHM 3.3). The charge separation also causes an electrical dipole to be set up in the direction of the arrow. A dipole has a positive end (carbon) and a negative end (oxygen). A dipole will line up in an electric field (PHY 9.1, 10.4).

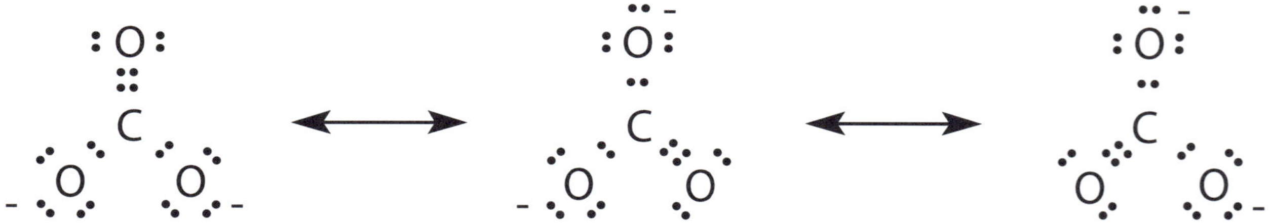

The most electronegative elements (in order, with electronegativities in brackets) are fluorine (4.0), oxygen (3.5), nitrogen (3.0), and chlorine (3.0). These elements will often be paired with hydrogen (2.1) and carbon (2.5), resulting in bonds with partial ionic character. The **dipole moment** is a measure of the charge separation and thus, the electronegativities of the elements that make up the bond; the larger the dipole moment, the larger the charge separation.

ELECTRONEGATIVITY

H 2.1																	He
Li 1.0	Be 1.6											B 2.0	C 2.5	N 3.0	O 3.5	F 4.0	Ne
Na 0.9	Mg 1.2											Al 1.5	Si 1.8	P 2.1	S 2.5	Cl 3.0	Ar
K 0.8	Ca 1.0	Sc 1.3	Ti 1.5	V 1.6	Cr 1.6	Mn 1.5	Fe 1.8	Co 1.9	Ni 1.9	Cu 1.9	Zn 1.6	Ga 1.6	Ge 1.8	As 2.0	Se 2.4	Br 2.8	Kr
Rb 0.8	Sr 1.0	Y 1.2	Zr 1.4	Nb 1.6	Mo 1.8	Tc 1.9	Ru 2.2	Rh 2.2	Pd 2.2	Ag 1.9	Cd 1.7	In 1.7	Sn 1.8	Sb 1.9	Te 2.1	I 2.5	Xe
Cs 0.7	Ba 0.9	La 1.0	Hf 1.3	Ta 1.5	W 1.7	Re 1.9	Os 2.2	Ir 2.2	Pt 2.2	Au 2.4	Hg 1.9	Tl 1.8	Pb 1.9	Bi 1.9	Po 2.0	At 2.1	Rn

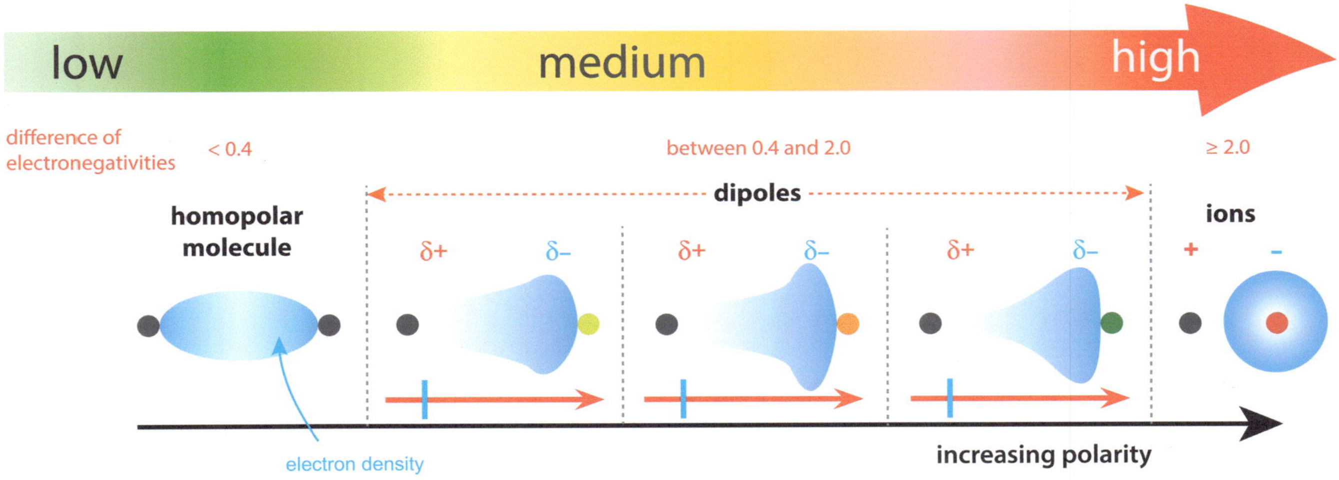

Figure IV.B.1.4: Periodic table showing Pauling's values for electronegativity (CHM 3.1.1) and their impact on bonding. Homopolar - little to no polarity - produces a nonpolar covalent bond whereby the electron density/distribution is symmetric meaning the bond is equally shared (e.g. C-C bond: 2.5 – 2.5 = 0). As described in General Chemistry (CHM 3.1.1, 3.2), a difference in electronegativity between 0.4 and 2.0 creates a separation of charge or dipole. These bonds can be described as polar covalent, or covalent with ionic character, thus the electron distribution is unequal (= asymmetric, not symmetric; e.g. C-O bond: 3.5 – 2.5 = 1.0). When the difference is greater than 2.0, complete electron transfer occurs which results in ionic bonding (e.g. table salt, Na-Cl: 3.0 – 0.9 = 2.1).

No dipole moment is found in molecules with no charge separation between atoms (i.e. Cl_2, Br_2), or, when the charge separation is symmetric resulting in a cancellation of bond polarity like vector addition in physics (i.e. CH_4, CO_2).

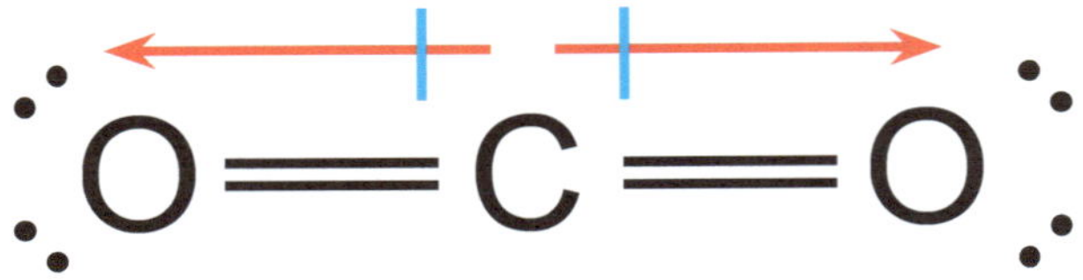

Figure IV.B.1.5: CO_2 - polar bonds but overall it is a non-polar molecule; therefore, CO_2 has a zero dipole moment. Notice that the arrows add to zero like typical vectors (PHY 1.1).

A molecule where the charge separation between atoms is not symmetric will have a non-zero dipole moment (e.g. H_2O, CH_3F: *see* below; NH_3 *see* ORG 11.1.2). It is important to note that lone pair electrons make large contributions to the overall dipole moment of a molecule.

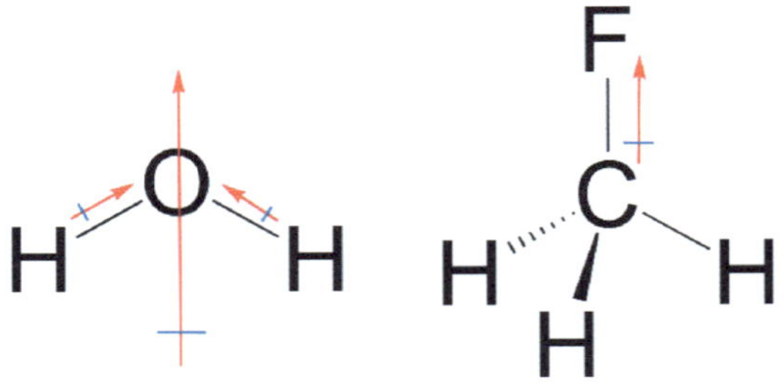

Note: Up to the time of publication, a periodic table has never been provided in a real GAMSAT. One of the purposes of completing the hundreds of chapter practice questions that are part of this textbook, is to increase your familiarity with the trends in the periodic table (CHM 2.3; ORG 1.1, 1.5) for the most frequently encountered atoms in GAMSAT Organic Chemistry.

1.5.1 Strength of Polar vs. Non-Polar Bonds

Non-polar bonds are generally stronger than polar covalent and ionic bonds, with ionic bonds being the weakest. However, in compounds with ionic bonding, there is generally a large number of bonds between molecules and this makes the compound as a whole very strong.

For instance, although the ionic bonds in one compound are weaker than the non-polar covalent bonds in another compound, the ionic compound's melting point will be higher than the melting point of the covalent compound.

Polar covalent bonds have a partial ionic character, and thus the bond strength is usually intermediate between that of ionic and that of non-polar covalent bonds. The strength of bonds generally decreases with increasing ionic character.

This section provides the ground rules to understand why two organic molecules react. Opposites attract. Like charges repel. Such simple statements are fundamental to understanding over 90% of organic reactions. Once you are comfortable with the basics - electronegativity, polarity and resonance - then reaction outcomes become play. You will be capable of quickly deducing the answer even when new scenarios are presented.

A substance which has a formal positive charge ($^+$) or a partial positive charge ("delta$^+$" or δ^+) is attracted to a substance with a formal negative charge ($^-$) or a partial negative charge (δ^-). In general, a substance with a formal charge would have a greater force of attraction than one with a partial charge when faced with an oppositely charged species. There is an important exception: spectator ions. Ions formed by elements in the first two groups of the periodic table (i.e. Na^+, K^+, Ca^{++}) do not actively engage in reactions in organic chemistry. They simply watch the reaction occur then at the very end they associate with the negatively charged product.

In most carbon-based compounds the carbon atom is bonded to a more electronegative atom. For example, in a carbon-oxygen bond the oxygen is δ^- resulting in a δ^+ carbon (*see* ORG 1.5). Because opposites attract, a δ^- carbon (*which is unusual*) could create a carbon-carbon bond with a δ^+ carbon (*which is common*). There are two important categories of compounds which can create a carbon-carbon bond; **a)** alkyl lithiums (RLi) and **b)** Grignard reagents (RMgBr), because they each have a δ^- carbon. Note that the carbon is δ^- since lithium is to the left of carbon on the periodic table (for electronegativity trends *see* ORG 1.5; CHM 2.3). {The letter R typically stands for any hydrocarbon group like alkyl (ORG 3.1), phenyl (ORG 5.1), etc.}

The expressions "like charges repel" and "opposites attract" are the basic rules of electrostatics (PHY 9.1). "Opposites attract" is translated in Organic Chemistry to mean "nucleophile attacks electrophile". The nucleophile is "nucleus loving" and so it is negatively charged or partially negative, and we follow its electrons using arrows in reaction mechanisms as it attacks the "electron loving" electrophile which is positively charged or partially positively charged. Sometimes we will use colour, or an asterix*, or a "prime" symbol on the letter R (i.e. R vs R' vs R'' vs R'''), or a superscript on the letter R (R^1, R^2, etc.), during reaction mechanisms to help you follow the movement of atoms or groups of atoms (the latter may be called *ligands* or *substituents*). Alternatively, an isotope of an atom is used (PHY 12.2). For example, instead of hydrogen, deuterium (^2H or D; PHY 12.2; ORG 14.2.1), or instead of 'normal' oxygen (O-16; ^{16}O), the stable isotope O-18 (^{18}O) is used. Any of the techniques above can be used on the GAMSAT (*except colour!*).

For nucleophiles, the general trend is that the stronger the nucleophile, the stronger the base it is. For example (do not memorise):

$$RO^- > HO^- \gg RCOO^- > ROH > H_2O$$

For information on the quality of leaving groups, *see* ORG 6.2.4.

Medium-level Importance

High-level Importance

In organic chemistry, functional groups are specific groups of atoms or bonds within molecules that are responsible for the characteristic chemical reactions of those molecules. The same functional group will undergo the same or similar chemical reaction(s) regardless of the size of the molecule that it is in.

You will find the most common functional groups illustrated below. Again, the shorthand for a carbon atom is each corner of a geometric figure as well as the end of a line. Hydrogens are presumed to be present such that each carbon is bonded 4 times (*see* ORG 1.1). We will be exploring the functional groups below and many others over the following chapters.

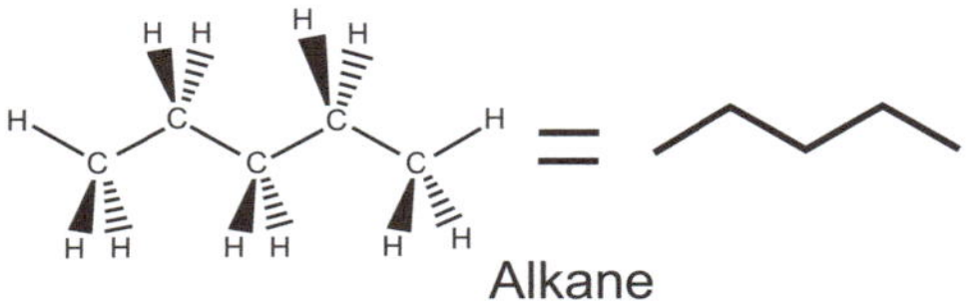

Alkane

Alkene

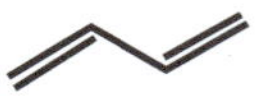

Conjugated Alkene

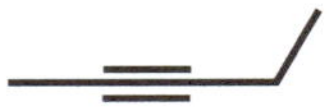

Alkyne

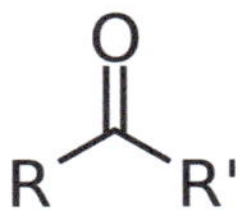

Ketone

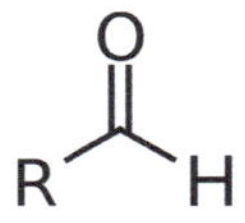

Aldehyde

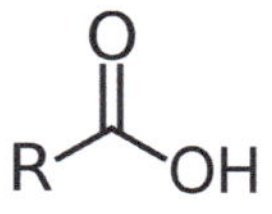

Carboxylic Acid

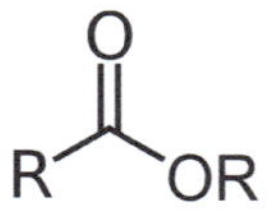

Ester

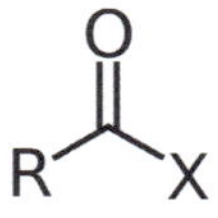

Acid Halide

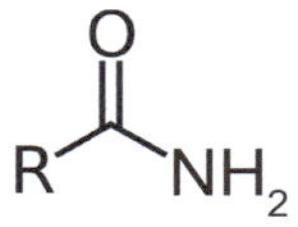

Amide

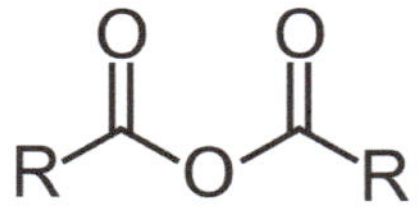

Anhydride

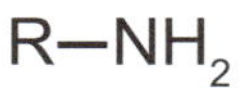

Primary Amine

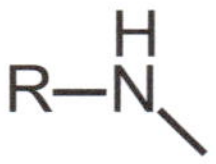

Secondary Amine

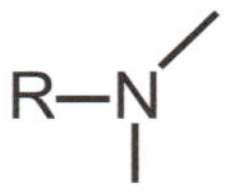

Tertiary Amine

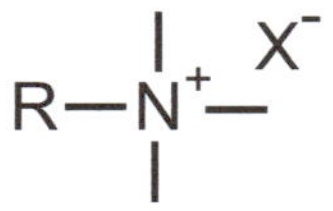

Quaternary Ammonium Salt

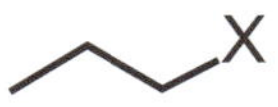

Primary (1°) Alkyl Halide

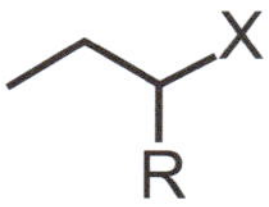

Secondary (2°) Alkyl Halide

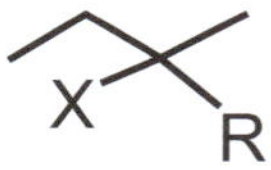

Tertiary (3°) Alkyl Halide

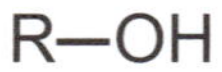

Alcohol (can be 1°, 2° or 3°)

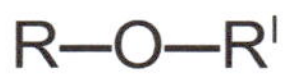

Ether

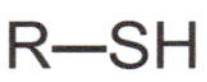

Thiol

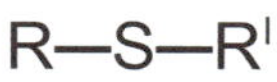

Thioether

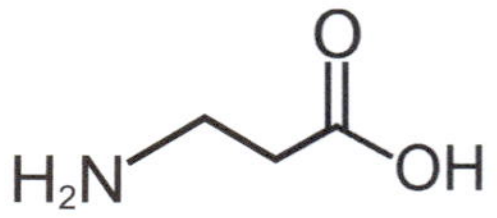

Amino Acid
(Two functional groups: amine + carboxylic acid)

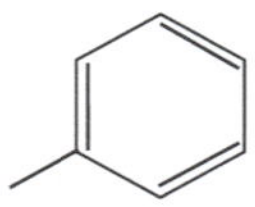

Benzene Ring
(benzene is just the ring; as an attachment: 'phenyl')

1.6.1 Primary, Secondary, Tertiary, and Quaternary Carbons and Molecules

Carbon atoms can be classified according to the number of other carbon atoms to which it is attached. In this classification, only carbon atoms are counted:

- **Primary (1°) carbon atom** – bonded to one other carbon atom;
- **Secondary (2°) carbon atom** – bonded to two other carbon atoms;
- **Tertiary (3°) carbon atom** – bonded to three other carbon atoms;
- **Quaternary (4°) carbon atom** – bonded to four other carbon atoms.

Note that the central carbon in methane, CH_4, is attached to no carbon and thus is neither primary, secondary, tertiary, nor quaternary. Also note that if any of the primary carbons, in the image below, had one or more hydrogens replaced with -Br, -Cl, -OH, or any other non-carbon attachment, it would still be a primary carbon.

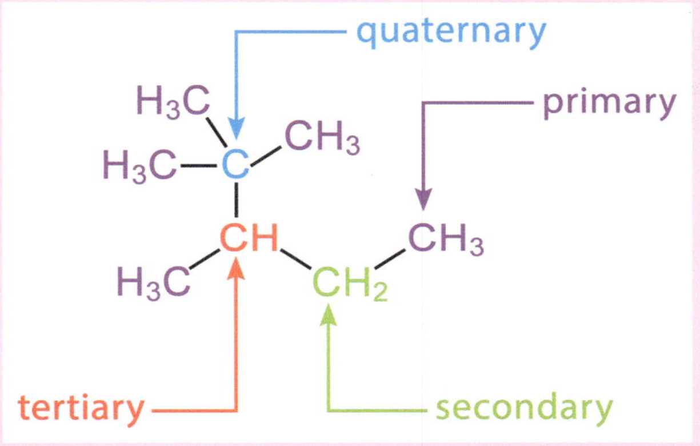

1.6.2 Exercise: Introduction to Identifying Functional Groups

Write the name of the functional group below the molecular structure or on your A4 scratch paper. If it is your first time, then please feel free to use the information on the facing page to guide you to the answer.

We will be re-exploring all GAMSAT-relevant functional groups in detail from chapters 3 to 12. The answers are upside down at the bottom of the next page. If you find it distracting, you can use paper to block the facing page.

1)

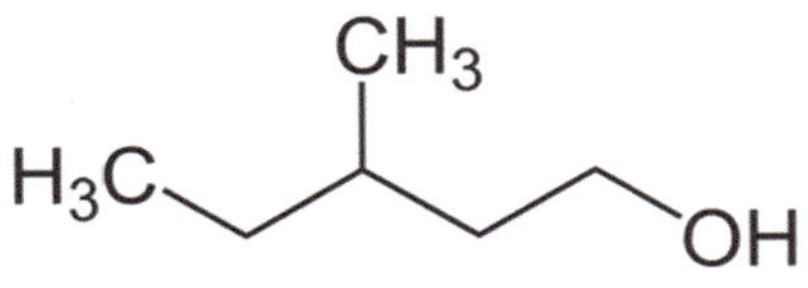

____

2)

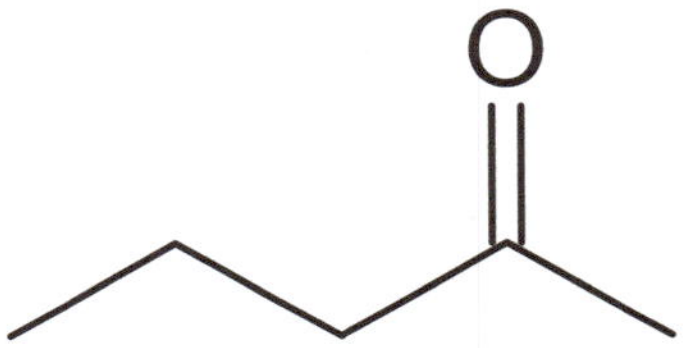

____

High-level Importance

3) 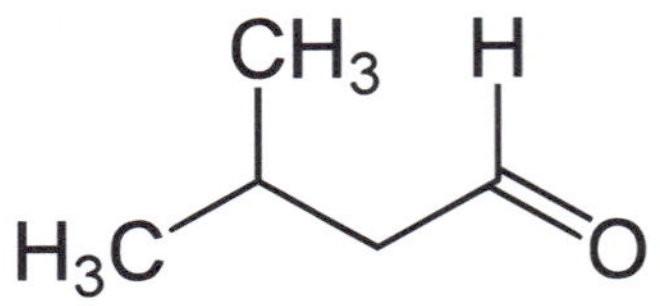

4) 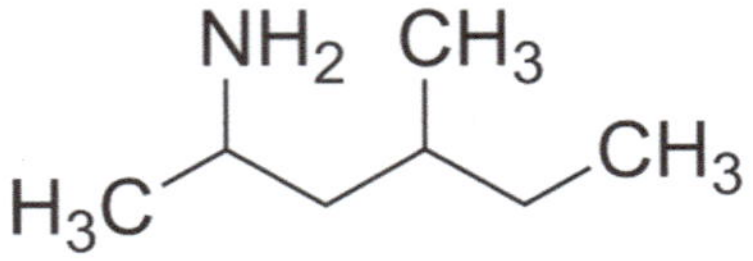

5) 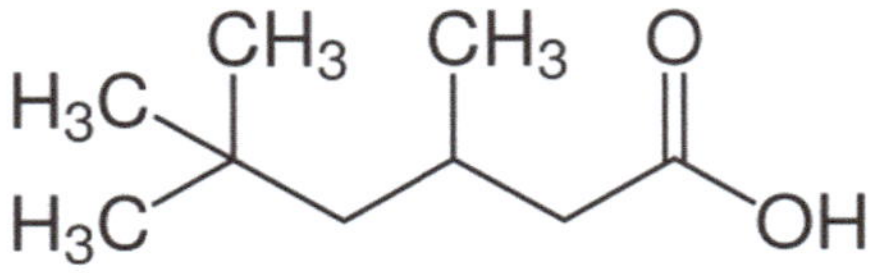

6) 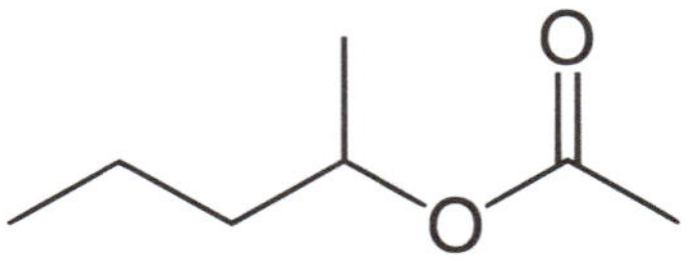

7) 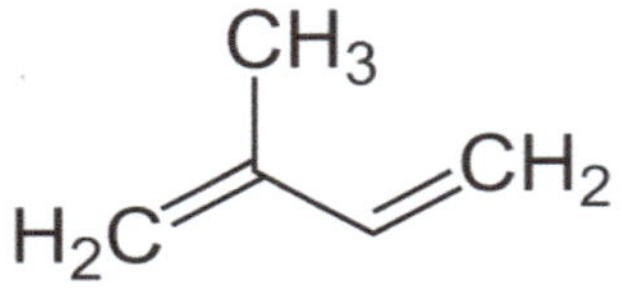

8) 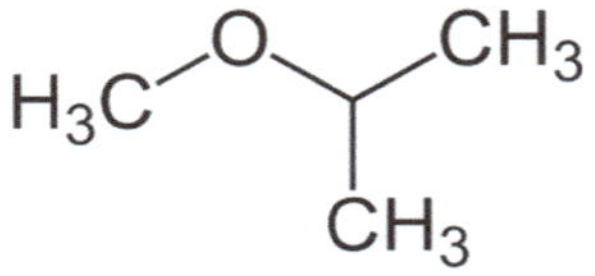

9) 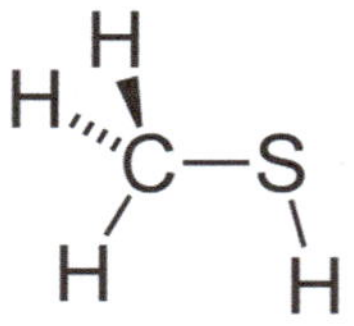

10) 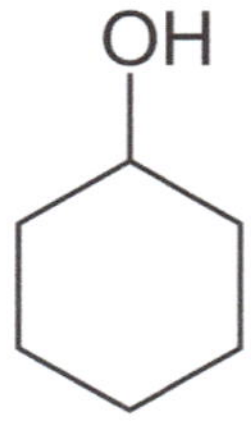

1) Alcohol (note that saturated hydrocarbons, *alkanes*, form the basic structure so if there is any functional group in addition to the hydrocarbon, in this case the alcohol -OH, then the molecule as a whole is considered to be based on that additional functional group, e.g., molecule 1 is an *alcohol*; also note that this is NOT a carboxylic acid because it is missing the C=O group; in fact, it is a *primary alcohol*); 2) ketone; 3) aldehyde; 4) amine (*primary*; the N is only connected to one C); 5) carboxylic acid; 6) ester; 7) alkene (*conjugated*); 8) ether; 9) thiol; 10) alcohol (*secondary*).

1.7 Drawing Molecular Structures of Organic Compounds

As part of GAMSAT Organic Chemistry problem-solving, being able to draw basic skeletal structures while maintaining an accurate inventory of all the atoms present in the molecule, is a very important skill. For this exercise, please consider using your carbon-based pencil just in case some erasing is needed! Also, if this is your first time, feel free to re-examine any of the previous sections in this chapter to find information to help you answer (esp. ORG 1.1, 1.1.1, 1.3, 1.4). It is far more valuable to experience the process of problem-solving, rather than simply glance at solutions. The worked answers follow the exercise.

For now, do not be concerned with the 3D shapes of the molecules in this exercise. We will be pursuing a detailed examination of molecular shapes in the next chapter on stereochemistry. For now, these skeletal, shorthand line-drawings do not respect spatial orientation, we are only concerned with which atoms are connected to which other atoms (i.e. *connectivity*).

In this exercise, all atoms are neutral so, as discussed at the beginning of this chapter, every H is bonded once, every O is bonded twice, every N is bonded 3 times, and every C is bonded 4 times. If the line diagram shows less than 4 bonds to a carbon, then we assume that H makes up the deficit. If you get tired of drawing every H, feel free to just write H_2 or H_3 when a multiple is present.

For each molecule, draw the expanded structure being sure to account for all atoms including hydrogens. Subsequently, you should also write the molecular formula. Do not worry about naming the molecules for now; however, once you have finished GAMSAT Organic Chemistry, consider coming back to this exercise to confirm that most, if not all, of the names make sense to you. We have started with 2 examples below: You can see the shorthand, skeletal formula followed by the expanded form of glycine on the left and proline on the right. They are both amino acids used by the body to produce proteins. Side note: You may notice by looking back at ORG 1.6 that both molecules have functional groups including alkanes, amines (primary for the former, secondary for the latter), and carboxylic acids.

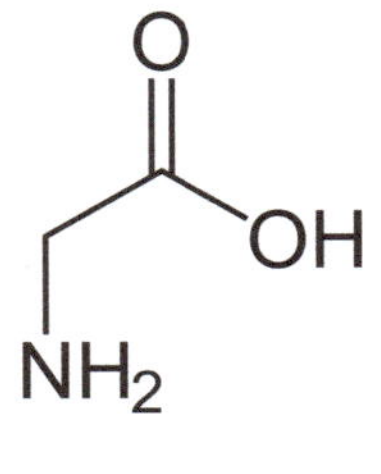

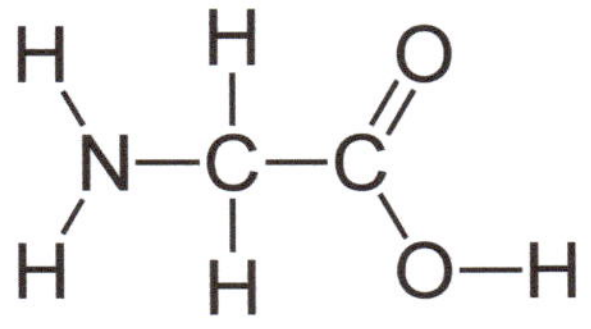

Molecular Formula: $C_2H_5NO_2$

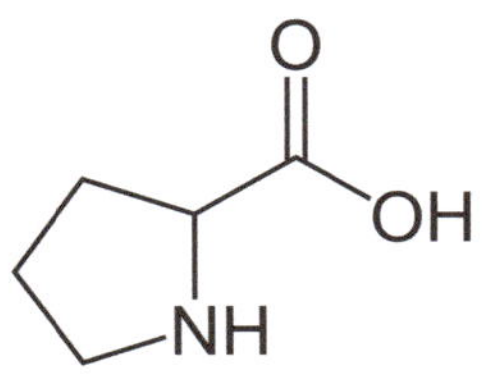

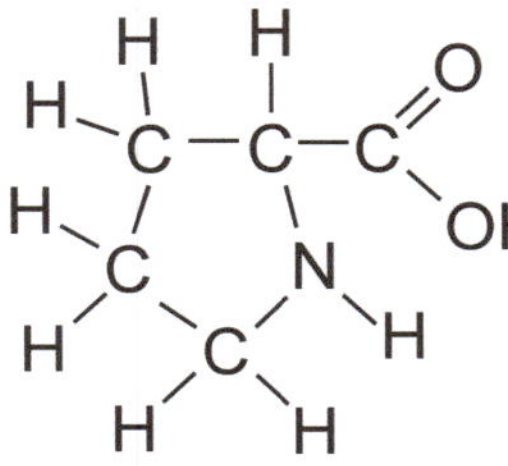

Molecular Formula: $C_5H_9NO_2$

High-level Importance

	1) Molecular Formula:	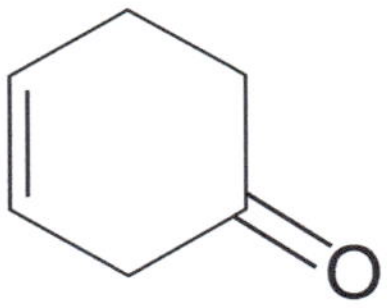	6) Molecular Formula:
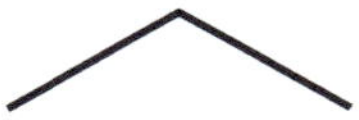	2) Molecular Formula:	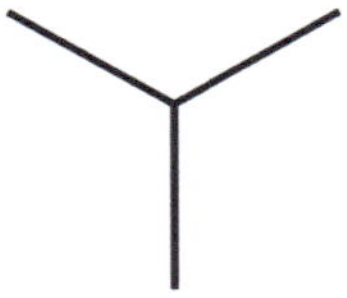	7) Molecular Formula:
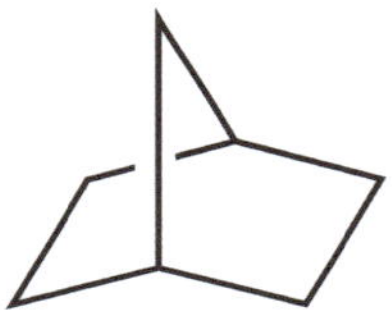	3) Molecular Formula:	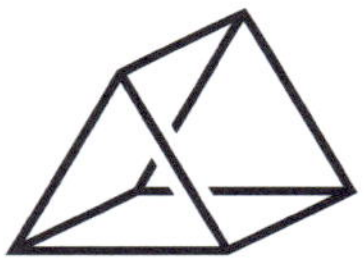	8) Molecular Formula:
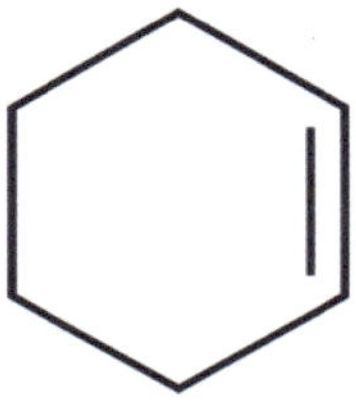	4) Molecular Formula:	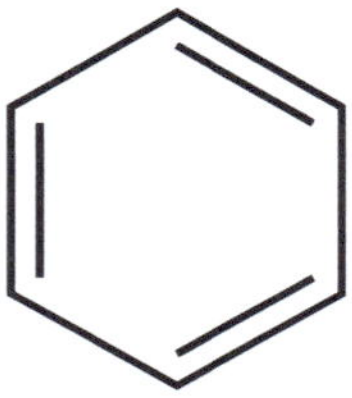	9) Molecular Formula:
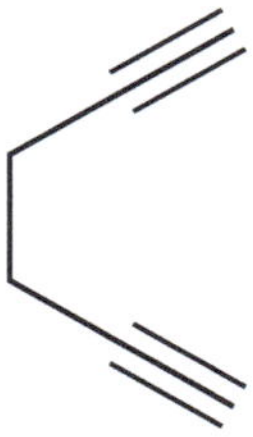	5) Molecular Formula:	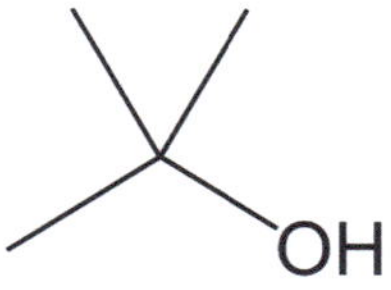	10) Molecular Formula:

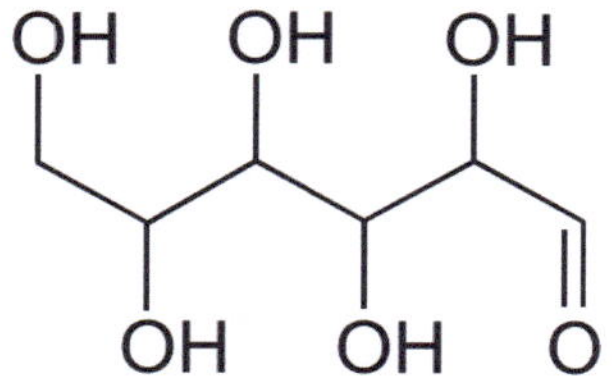

11)

Molecular Formula:

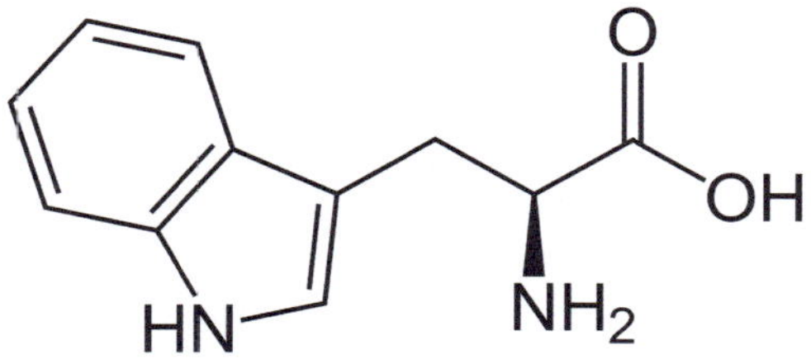

12)

Molecular Formula:

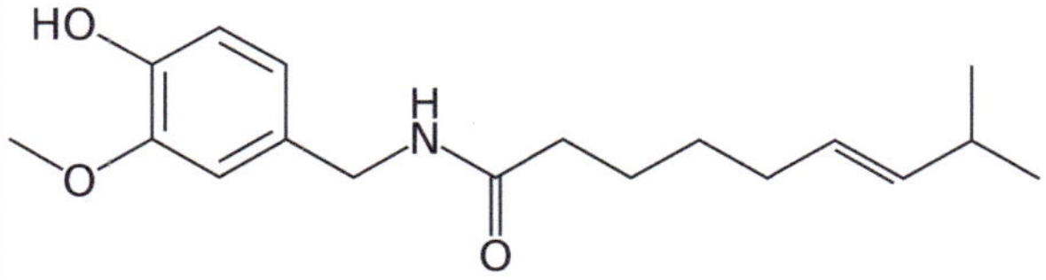

13)

Molecular Formula:

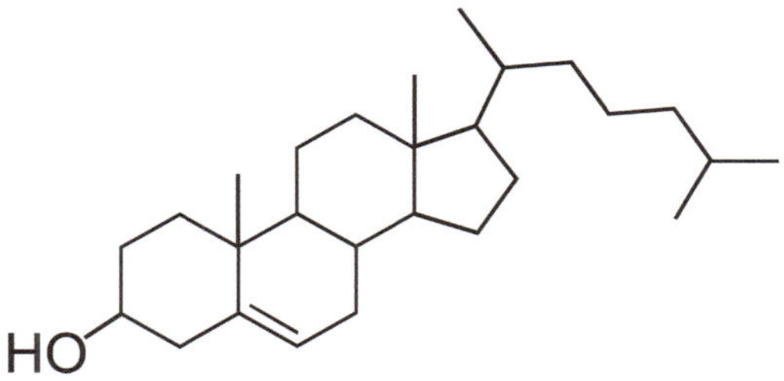

14)

Molecular Formula:

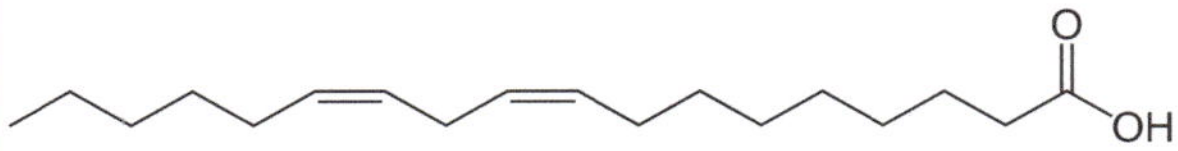

...which is the same as...

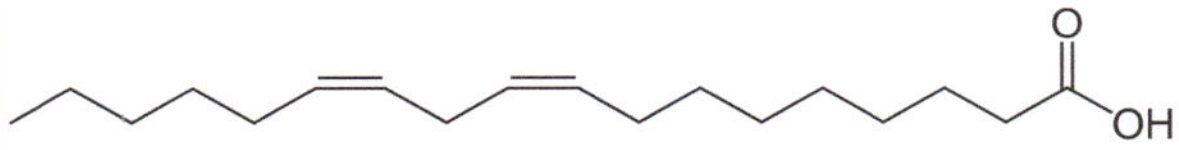

Note: It does not matter which side of the first bond that the second bond is placed.

15)

Molecular Formula:

High-level Importance

	1) 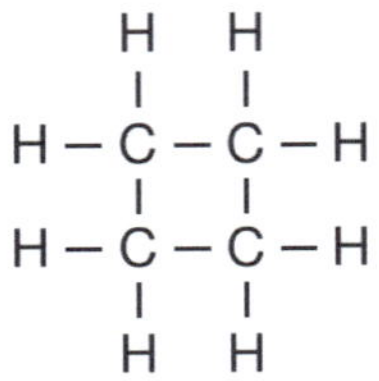 Molecular Formula: C_4H_8 Name: cyclobutane (notice that each C is bonded 4 times)	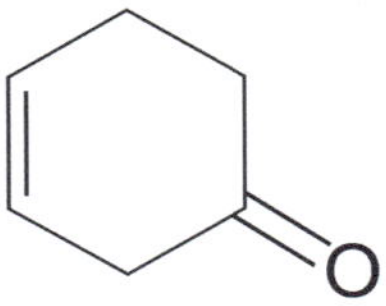	6) 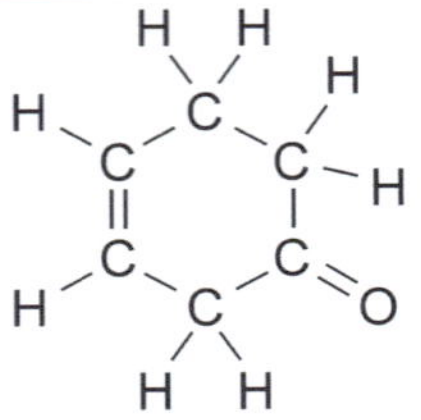 Molecular Formula: C_6H_8O Name: cyclohex-3-en-1-one (notice that O is bonded twice and each C is bonded 4 times)
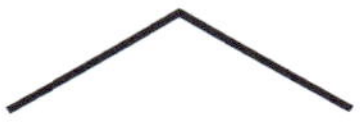	2) 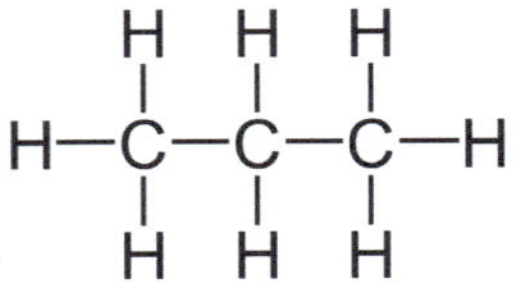 Molecular Formula: C_3H_8 Name: propane	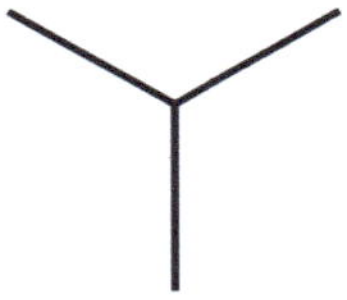	7) 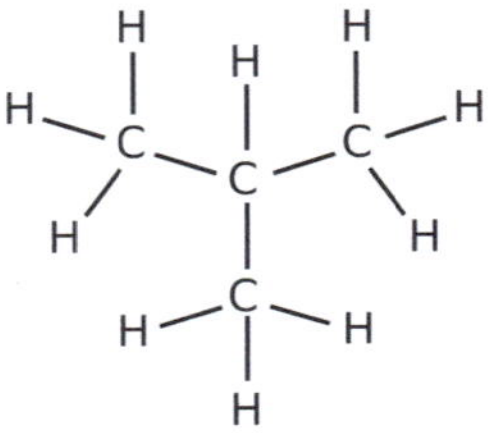 Molecular Formula: C_4H_{10} Name: 2-methylpropane (side note: an isomer of butane; ORG 2.1, 3.1)
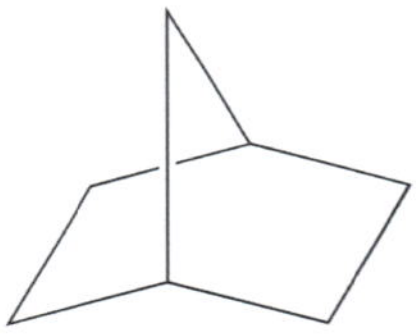	3) 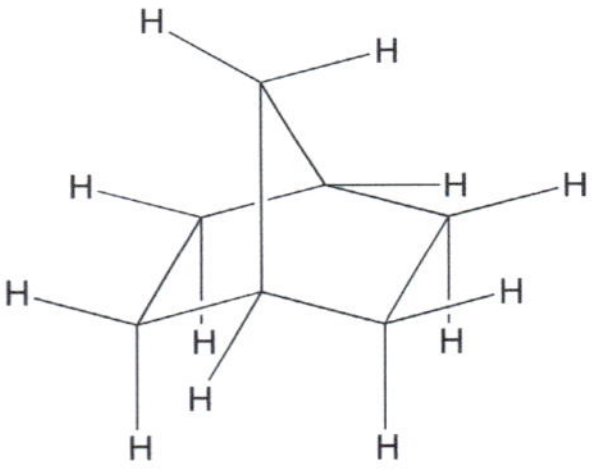 Molecular Formula: C_7H_{12} Name: bicyclo[2.2.1]heptane	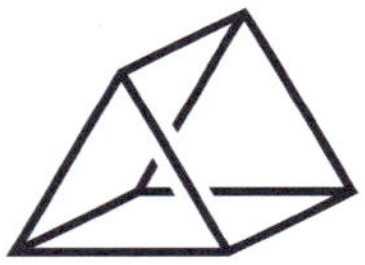	8) 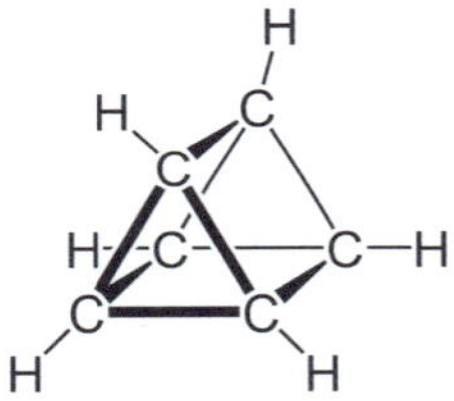 Molecular Formula: C_6H_6 Name: prismane (side note: it is a tetracyclohexane and a benzene isomer)
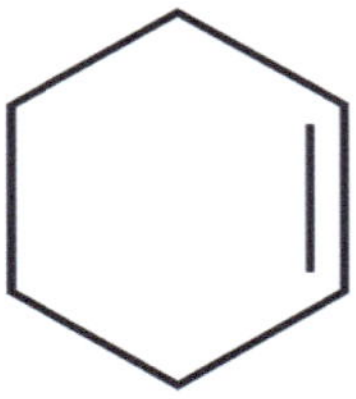	4) 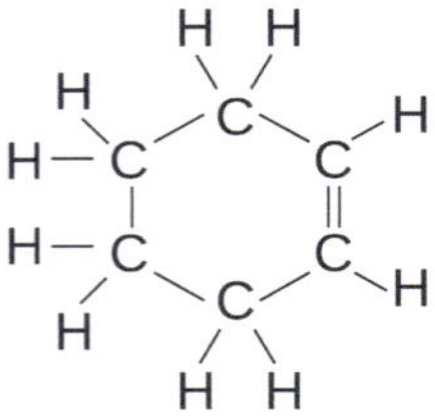 Molecular Formula: C_6H_{10} Name: cyclohexene	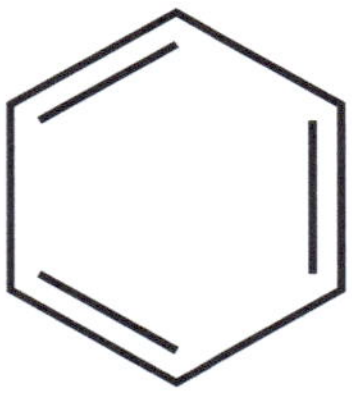	9) 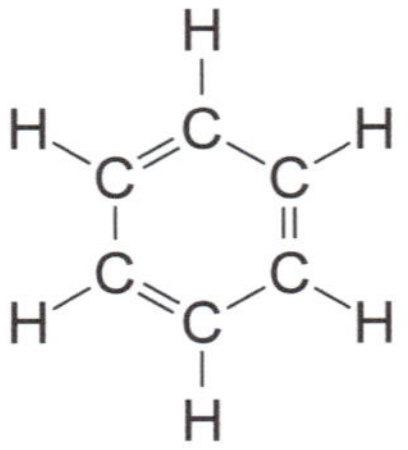 Molecular Formula: C_6H_6 Name: benzene (= the most famous aromatic; ORG 5.1)
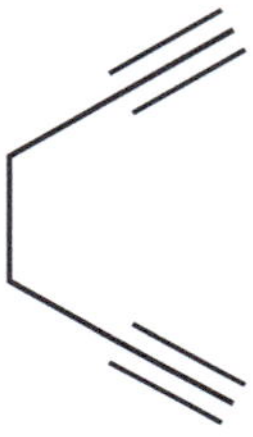	5) HC≡C-CH_2-CH_2-C≡CH Molecular Formula: C_6H_6 Name: hexa-1,5-diyne Reminder: As you look to the left and right of this cell, all focus should be on connectivity (*what is attached to what*) rather than shape.	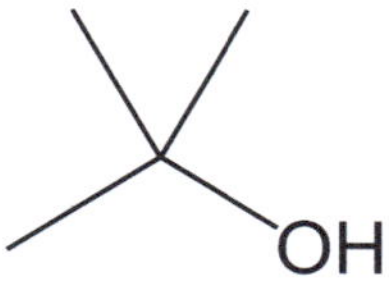	10) 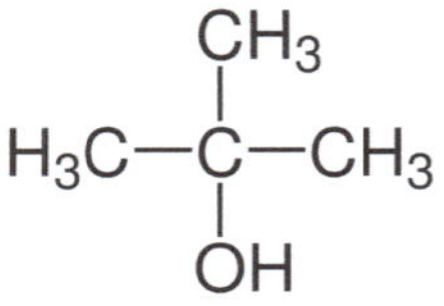 Molecular Formula: $C_4H_{10}O$ Name: 2-methylpropan-2-ol (= a tertiary alcohol, isomer of butanol)

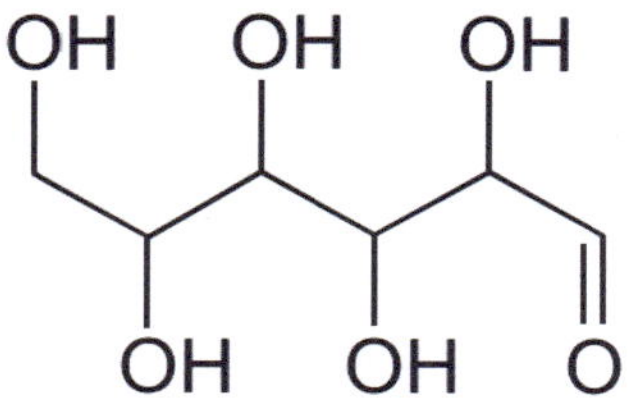

11)

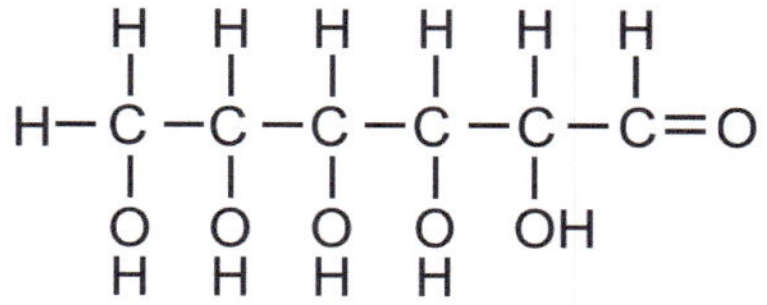

Molecular Formula: $C_6H_{12}O_6$
Name: Glucose (= 2,3,4,5,6-Pentahydroxyhexanal)

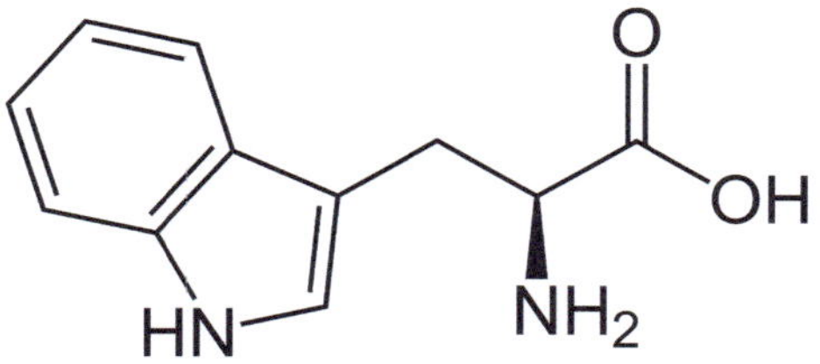

12)

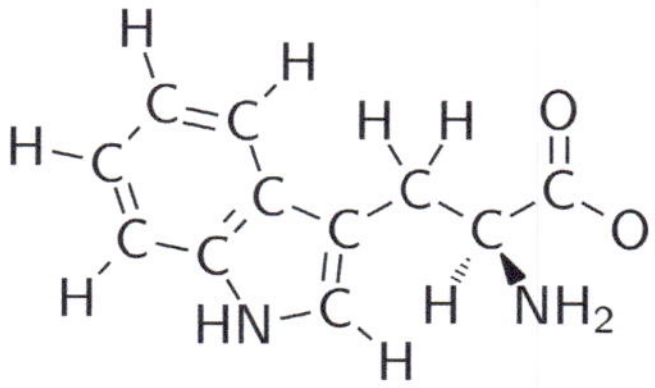

Molecular Formula: $C_{11}H_{12}N_2O_2$
Name: Tryptophan (= an aromatic amino acid essential for the production of proteins in humans; ORG 12.1, 12.2)

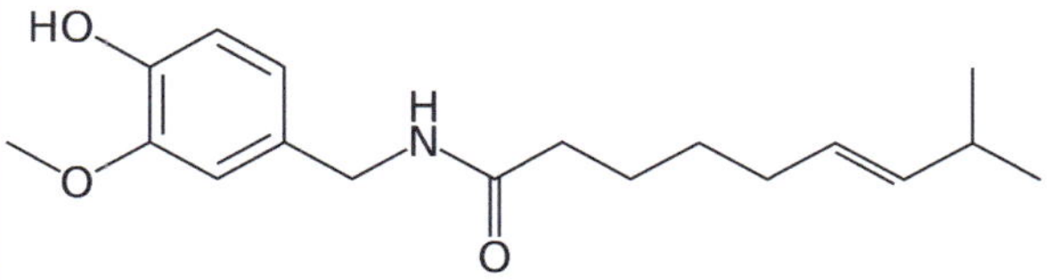

13)

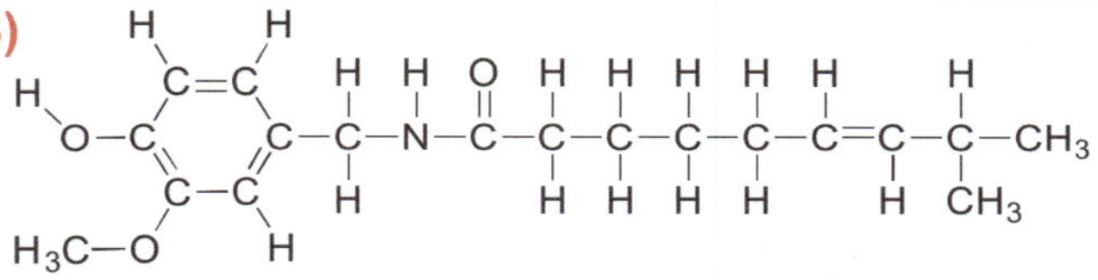

Molecular Formula: $C_{18}H_{27}NO_3$
Name: Capsaicin, AKA: (6*E*)-*N*-[(4-Hydroxy-3-methoxyphenyl)methyl]-8-methylnon-6-enamide (= the active ingredient in chili peppers!). Consider going back to ORG 1.6 to see if you can identify the many functional groups in capsaicin: for example, the phenyl alcohol (= *phenol*), amide, alkane, alkene, and the ether in the bottom left of the molecule. Of course, we will be examining all the preceding functional groups over the next 11 chapters, or so.

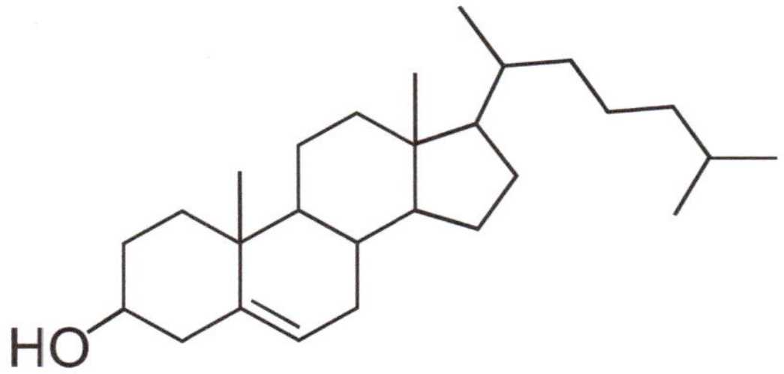

14)

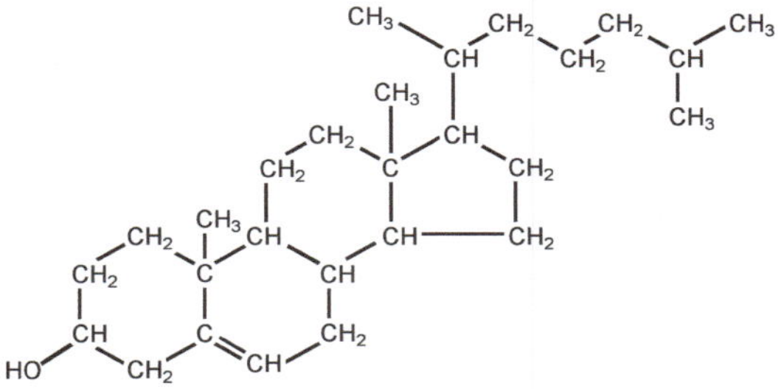

Molecular Formula: $C_{27}H_{46}O$
Name: Cholesterol (the most famous fat! More formerly: a lipid)

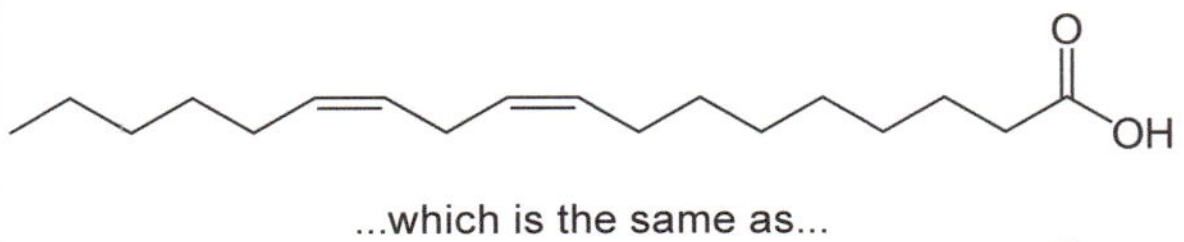

...which is the same as...

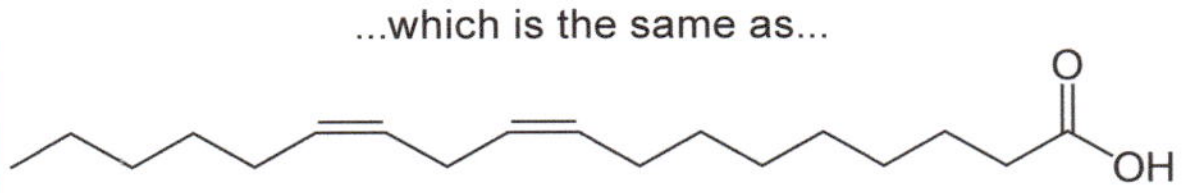

Note: It does not matter which side of the first bond that the second bond is placed.

15)

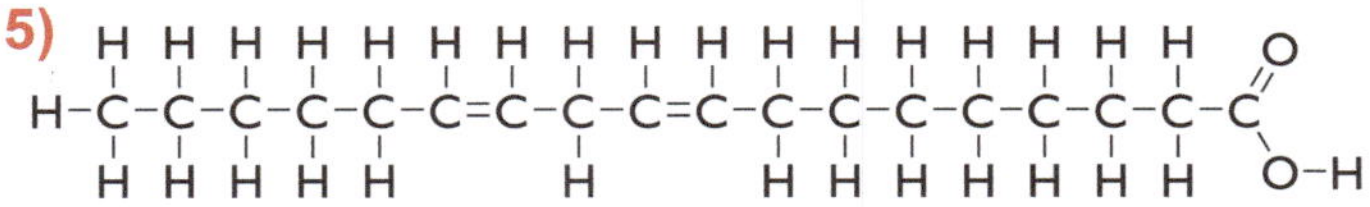

Molecular Formula: $C_{18}H_{32}O_2$
Name: Linoleic acid, AKA: *cis*, *cis* or (9*Z*,12*Z*)-octadeca-9,12-dienoic acid; an essential, polyunsaturated (= *more than 1 double bond*) fatty acid with functional groups: alkane, alkene, carboxylic acid.
You may wonder: 'Really, will I ever need to count that many atoms during an exam that provides 2 minutes per question in GAMSAT Sciences?' Short answer: Yes, sometimes!

To extend your exercise, consider going back and adding 1 lone pair of electrons on each nitrogen atom and 2 lone pairs on each oxygen atom (ORG 1.1, 1.1.1; for examples: ORG 1.5, 11.1.1, 11.2). Also, just keep in mind that every carbon bonded 4 times has $4sp^3$ hybrids and sits in the centre of a tetrahedron; when bonded to 3 atoms, there are $3sp^2$ hybrids and C is in the centre of a flat triangle; and finally, when bonded to 2 atoms, there are 2 sp hybrids and C is in the centre of a straight line (*see* ORG 1.2). Below is a table with a summary of neutral carbon's bond hybrids.

The selection of molecules that you have now seen foreshadows what you will see as you practice using GS and ACER materials. Of course, the reason for this is that the molecules that you have seen in Chapter 1 - and their derivatives - are frequently part of the real exam.

When bonded to...	Hybridisation	Shape	Bond angle
2 atoms	sp	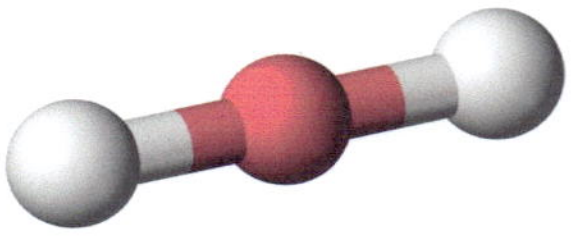 linear	180°
3 atoms	sp^2	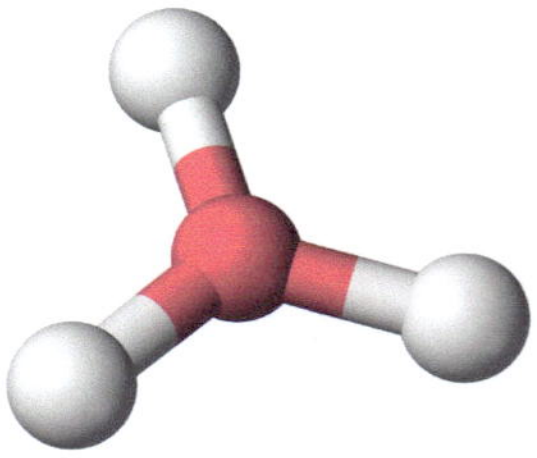 trigonal planar (= flat triangle)	120°
4 atoms	sp^3	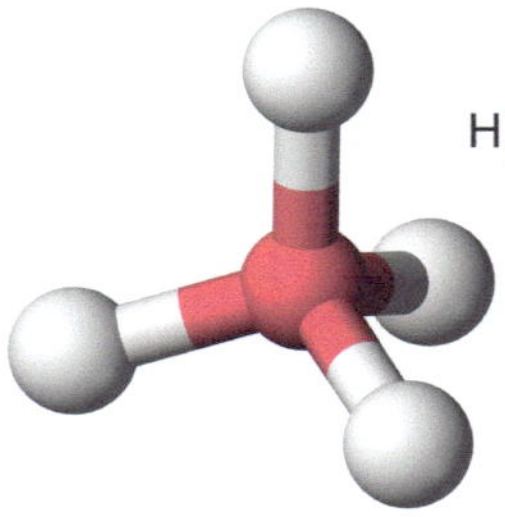 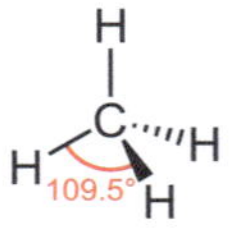 tetrahedral	109.5°

1.8 Pattern Recognition, Geometric Reasoning and Problem-based Learning

GAMSAT Organic Chemistry is unlike organic chemistry as taught at the introductory-university level, which ACER states is the basis of knowledge needed for the GAMSAT. At university, one learns how to name organic chemicals (*nomenclature*, which is monitored by a 'priesthood', *IUPAC*). Thereafter, one learns basic rules which allow students to reasonably understand *reaction mechanisms*: why molecules react together, how and where do they react, and what are the possible outcomes (*products*). Most students learn the reaction mechanisms, while some students are able to succeed by memorising the mechanisms and potential products.

GAMSAT views reaction mechanisms, the heart of 'uni' ORG, as a side show! They may present a mechanism during the exam, but the questions are only focused on your ability to recognise patterns and to use basic, general-reasoning skills based on shapes (*geometric reasoning*). We will practice both of these skills using problem-based learning in this section, and then again throughout this book.

The one priority that GAMSAT shares with uni ORG is nomenclature. You will need to learn how to name molecules in a logical, *systematic* way; but also, unfortunately, you will need to learn a few trivial names of molecules that have been handed down from history. We have already started flirting with the names of some molecules (e.g., methane, ethane, pentane; Table IV.B.1.1), but we will begin to take this more seriously in the very first section of most chapters in this book beginning with Chapter 3.

Get ready, we are about to take a deep dive into pattern recognition and geometric reasoning. Take the time that you need. Again, we understand that some of you may have little or no background for the following questions. If it gets to be too much, don't worry, stop and continue reading subsequent chapters and return after you have completed 5 or 6 chapters. But keep in mind: The real exam is designed to expose you to new content on the day of the exam to see if you can reason through to a solution. In keeping with 'learning is better by doing', let's begin.

GAMSAT-level Practice Questions: GAMSAT Organic Chemistry

Unit 1, Question 16

A polymer is composed of many simple molecules that are repeating structural units called monomers. Covalent bonds, often symbolised by black lines, hold the atoms in polymer molecules together. If A-B-C-A-B-C-A-B-C were a polymer, we can see that the smallest unit that continually repeats is A-B-C, which is therefore the monomer. Neither shorter segments (e.g. A-B), nor longer segments that are not multiples of the monomer (e.g. A-B-C-A), would accurately recreate the polymer by being repeated.

High-level Importance

Rubber, plastics, and many storage macromolecules for sugars such as glucose, are polymers. For example, amylose, a component of starch, is a polymer of glucose:

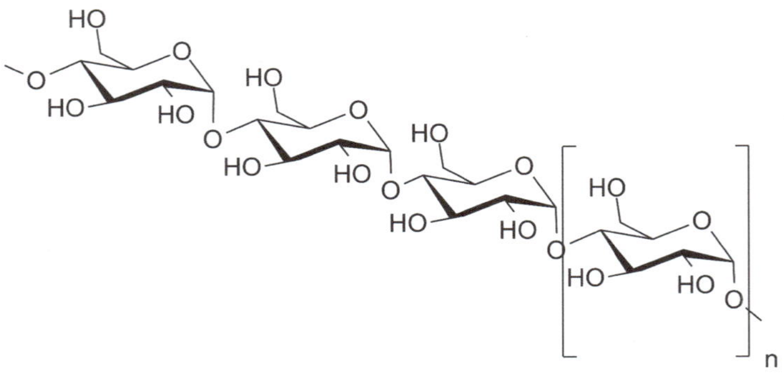

Of course, the molecular structure of amylose continues to the left and right. In fact, the smallest repeating unit, or 'building block', is identified within the square brackets and repeats in the polymer n times, where n can be between 300 and 3000 units. Note that anything smaller than the structure in square brackets would not represent a structure that could be repeated in order to reconstruct amylose.

Kevlar® is a plastic strong enough to stop bullets and knives. Consider the structure of Kevlar®.

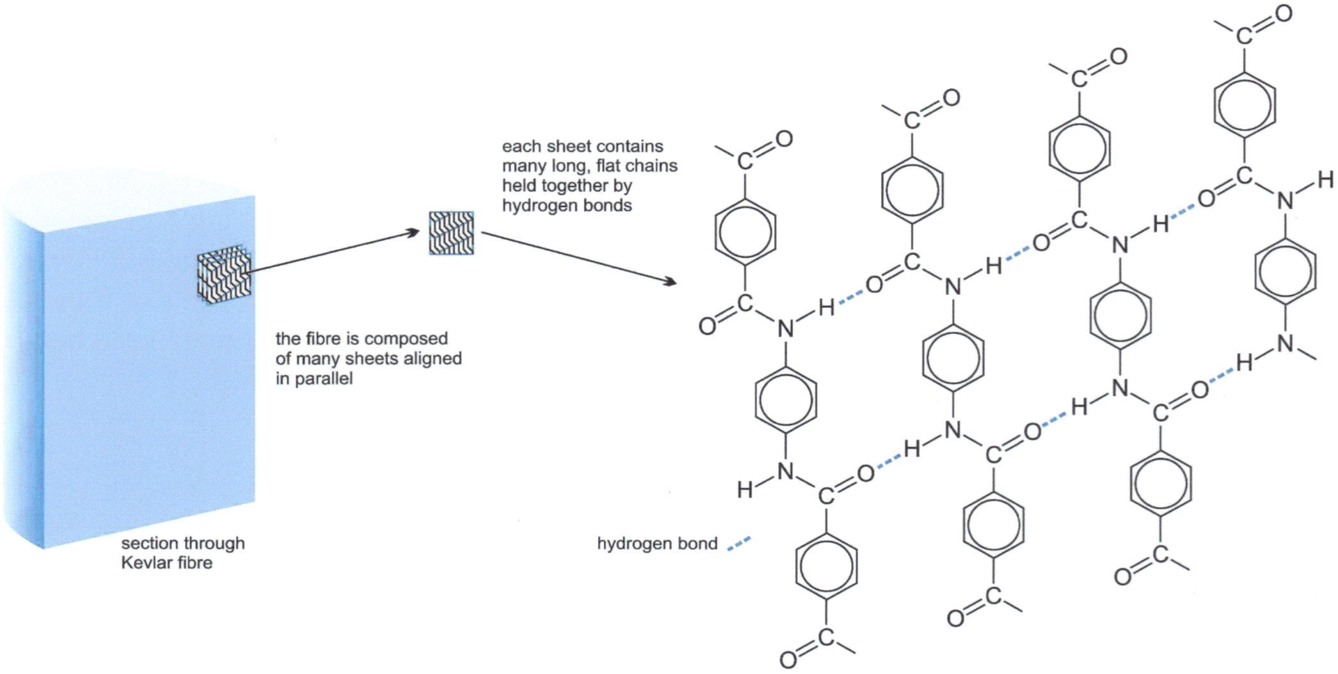

Figure 1: The structure of Kevlar®
essentialchemicalindustry.org (2016)

Note that: Though hydrogen bonds are instrumental to the function of Kevlar®, they are a form of non-covalent bonding.

16) Which of the following represents a monomer (the smallest repeating unit) in the polymer Kevlar®?

A.

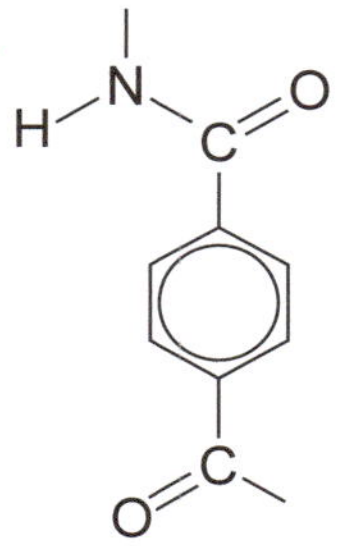

B.

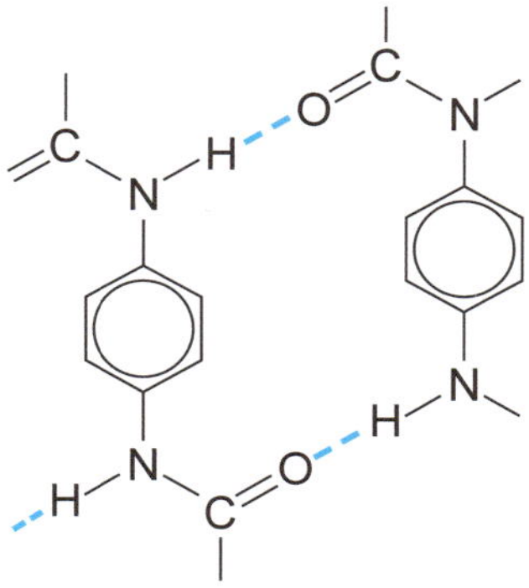

C.

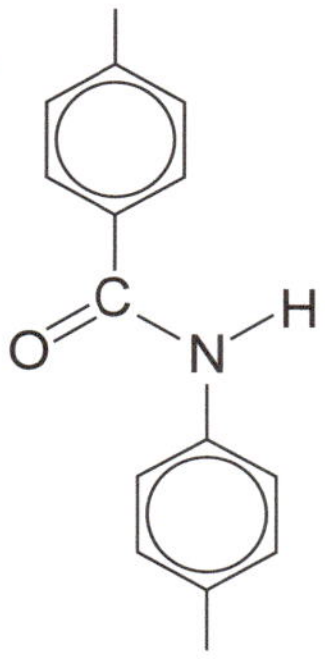

D.

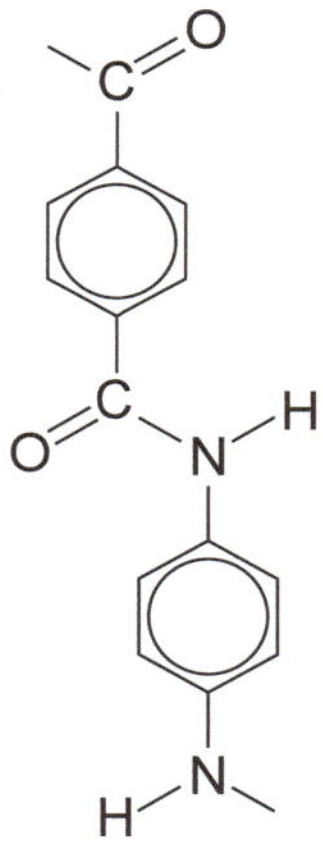

On the Surface: According to the preamble and examples, we are looking for the smallest repeating unit that can be used to recreate the entire structure. Also, according to the preamble, the smallest repeating unit is held together by covalent bonds whereas the blue 'hydrogen bonds', according to the "Note that" following the figure, are *not* covalent. So answer choice B cannot represent a monomer.

Now it becomes a matter of pattern recognition. Notice that each hexagon (6-sided figure) in Figure 1 has either of the following attachments: 2 N's are directly attached to it or 2 C's are directly attached to it, there are no other possibilities. So whatever the smallest repeating structure is, it cannot simply be a hexagon with 2 N's attached because that does not represent the polymer (i.e., if you kept repeating the hexagon with 2 N's you cannot make Kevlar® because you are missing a key component: the hexagon with the 2 C's attached). Only answer choice D fulfils both the preceding requirements and is thus the correct answer.

For NSB: Think of a gold chain that someone wears around their neck. If you look close enough, you can see a small link in the chain (a monomer) that repeats over and over to form the chain (the polymer). Figure 1 shows us a large, blue structure (section of a fibre) to the left and then we zoom in to take a close look at a very small portion of the whole, just to see a few links in 4 vertical chains. After all, Figure 1 tells us that "each sheet contains many long, flat chains." In other words, we assume that the molecules that we see represent all we need in order to deduce the repeating pattern which must extend upwards and downwards by covalent bonds (black lines), as well as to the left and to the right by hydrogen bonds (blue, dashed lines).

Going Deeper: Those hexagons represent the most famous aromatic compound in Organic Chemistry: benzene. We will explore benzene and aromatic chemistry in GAMSAT Organic Chemistry Chapter 5. Below are different representations of benzene.

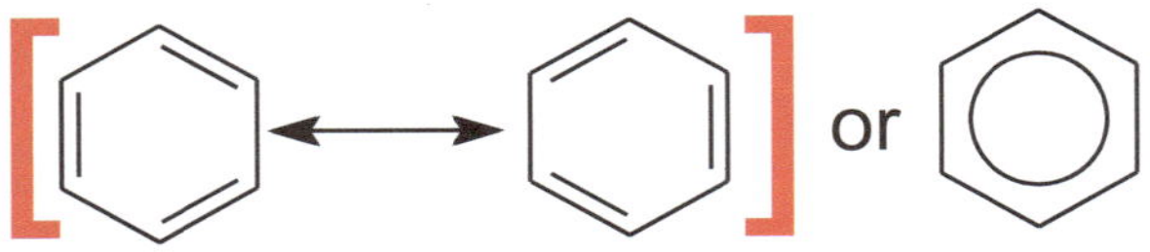

Figure 1 includes two types of bonds that would win any GAMSAT-bond-popularity contest (!!): the hydrogen bond, which is a weaker-than-covalent attraction between a partially positive hydrogen atom and, in this case, a partially negative oxygen atom; and the very covalent amide bond. You can identify the latter in the middle of answer choice D; notice this combination of atoms: O=C-N-H.

That identical arrangement (O=C-N-H), though labelled 'amide' generally, when present in proteins, it is called a 'peptide' bond. Identifying that combination of atoms was not necessary for Question 16 but it is a pattern-recognition skill that would have been of value for almost every past GAMSAT exam. Ideally, you will learn to identify such combinations upside-down, left-right and under a table! The following is a generic dipeptide (ORG Chapter 12) held together by a peptide (*amide*) bond highlighted in red.

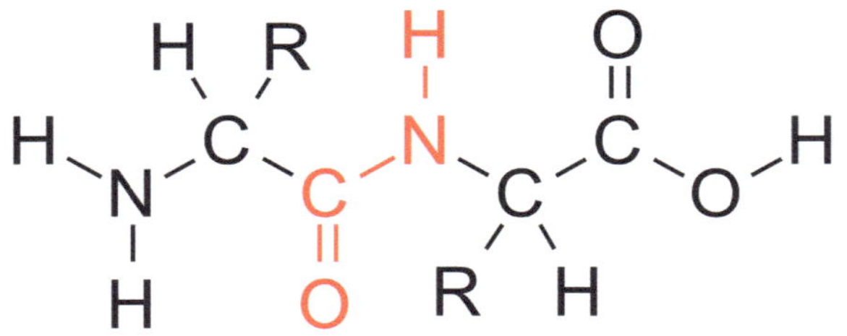

Unit 2, Questions 17 and 18

Carbocations are positively charged carbon ions. Carbocations can be imagined as the neutral alkane form minus 1 hydrogen. The positive charge is then left at a position which can be tertiary, secondary, or primary as represented below:

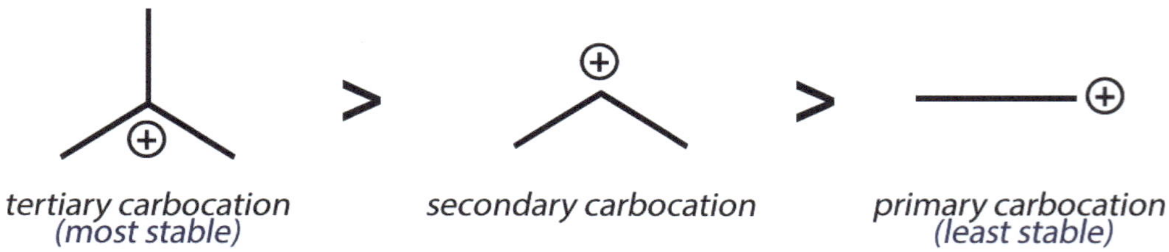

For NSB: There are 2 points for you to consider: 1) notice that the word 'primary' suggests 1; and so the primary position, where the '+' symbol is, has 1 incoming line; the secondary '+' sign has 2 incoming lines; the tertiary '+' has 3 incoming lines; 2) there is one small point that is assumed knowledge: if you were to add a line leading to the centre of the tertiary carbocation (the expression would be a 'quaternary' position which does NOT need to be committed to memory), then that position is full. There can never be more than 4 lines going to any position in these structures. As you know by now, each corner of a geometric figure represents carbon, and carbon cannot bond more than 4 times. Focus on the number of lines that come into each position (resulting in primary, secondary or tertiary) and the rule: more than 4 lines to carbon is impossible.

Consider the bicyclic molecule *norbornane* on the left, AKA bicyclo[2.2.1]heptane, and *camphor* on the right, AKA 1,7,7-trimethylbicyclo[2.2.1]heptan-2-one.

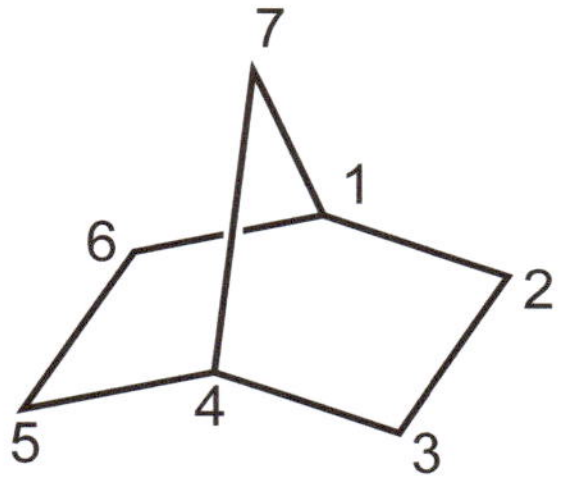

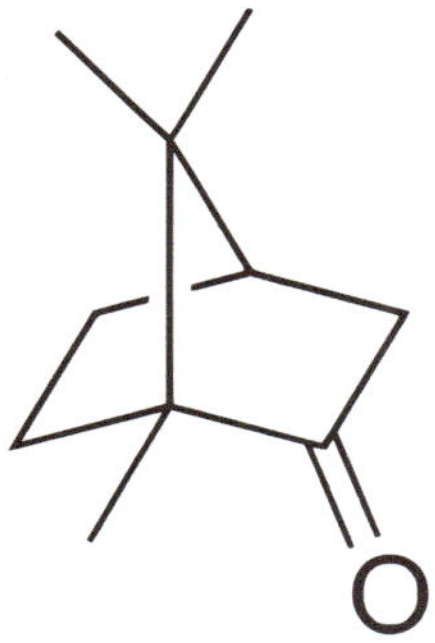

17) If one hydrogen is removed from each of the 7 positions on norbornane, how many of the carbocations would be considered primary, secondary, or tertiary carbocations, respectively?

A. 0 primary, 5 secondary, 2 tertiary
B. 0 primary, 4 secondary, 3 tertiary
C. 1 primary, 4 secondary, 2 tertiary
D. 1 primary, 2 secondary, 4 tertiary

18) As compared to norbornane, camphor has 3 additional carbon positions. How many carbon positions in camphor, if positively charged due to the removal of one hydrogen, would be considered primary, secondary, or tertiary carbocations, respectively?

A. 3 primary, 3 secondary, 1 tertiary
B. 3 primary, 3 secondary, 4 tertiary
C. 2 primary, 4 secondary, 4 tertiary
D. None of the above

On the Surface: Notice in norbornane, positions 2, 3, 5, 6, and 7, each has exactly 2 incoming lines. That represents a total of 5 secondary positions. If one hydrogen was removed from each of those positions, they would become 5 secondary carbocations. Note that positions 1 and 4 each has 3 lines coming into those positions meaning that they are both tertiary. Thus we have evaluated all 7 positions: 0 primary, 5 secondary, 2 tertiary. Answer choice A is correct.

If you did not get Question 17 correct but you can now understand the reasoning, you can try to reevaluate your answer for Question 18. You can always choose to discuss this or any of the subsequent questions on gamsat-prep.com/forum.

Now for camphor: Please apply the identical numbering system used on norbornane to camphor so the worked solution will be easier to follow. On camphor, positions 2, 5, and 6, each has exactly 2 incoming lines. Thus they represent a total of 3 secondary positions, if one hydrogen is removed from each of those positions, there would be 3 secondary carbocations. Note that position 1 has 3 lines coming into that position meaning that it is tertiary. Notice that positions 3, 4 and 7, all have 4 lines coming in to those positions: that's not tertiary! The name does not matter (= *quaternary!*) but the point is that carbon is bonded to its maximum extent and so it could not have a hydrogen at the position that could be removed. The question does not ask about quaternary positions, and we have already determined: 3 secondary, 1 tertiary, which thus far makes answer choice A appealing.

In comparing the 2 structures provided, notice the 3 single lines added to norbornane to create camphor produced 3 primary positions. Because, if we were to remove one hydrogen and thus add a positive charge at the end of each of those lines, just like the example in the preamble, those 3 positions would be primary carbocations.

By the way, yes, ACER infrequently uses “None of the above” or a similar expression and, no, there is no reliable pattern for guessing based on ACER's use of such statements.

Going Deeper: If you complete all your end-of-chapter practice questions, you will learn how to name norbornane and camphor systematically. This is not assumed knowledge; however, it is the kind of question that can come up on the real exam only if the rules are provided first.

Before we go further, let's formalise a point that has been alluded to already: when using 'stick' shorthand drawings, every corner of a geometric figure, and the end of a line with no other atom, is a carbon; carbon is bonded a maximum of 4 times; hydrogen - H - is not always drawn in the shorthand form of molecules but we must assume their presence such that each carbon is bonded 4 times. And so, as an example, the following represents the shorthand skeletal structure and its long form, respectively, for the 6-carbon hydrocarbon *hexane*:

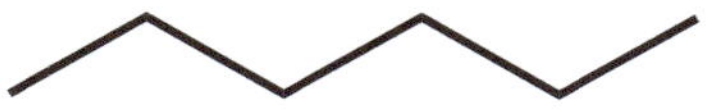

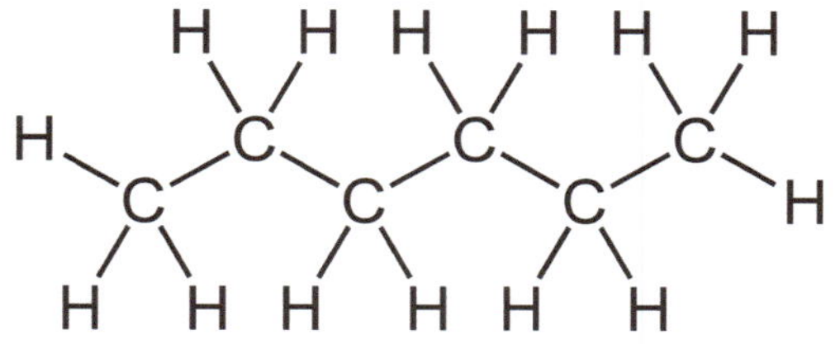

Unit 3, Questions 19–22

'Aldol condensation' is a base catalysed reaction of aldehydes that have α-hydrogens. The intermediate, an *aldol*, is both an <u>al</u>dehyde and an alcoh<u>ol</u>. The aldol undergoes a dehydration reaction producing a carbon-carbon bond in the condensation product, an *enal* (= alk<u>en</u>e + <u>al</u>dehyde). If the same reaction begins with a ketone, then an *enol* is the intermediate, and an *enone* is the condensation product. Reactions beginning with either aldehydes or ketones are still generally referred to as 'aldol condensation'.

Aldol condensation may be summarised as follows:

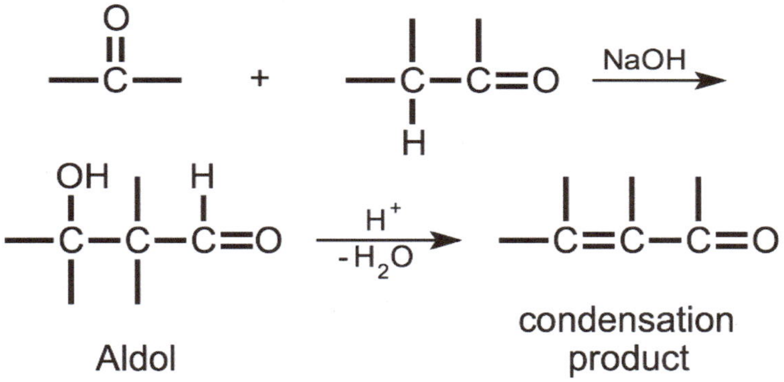

Note: The α-hydrogen is the hydrogen attached to the carbon (e.g., the α-carbon) next to the carbonyl group (C=O).

Consider the following 5 structures ('Me' represents the methyl group; 'Ph' represents the phenyl group).

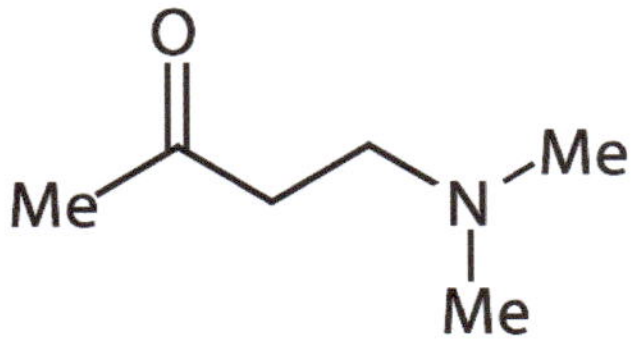

I

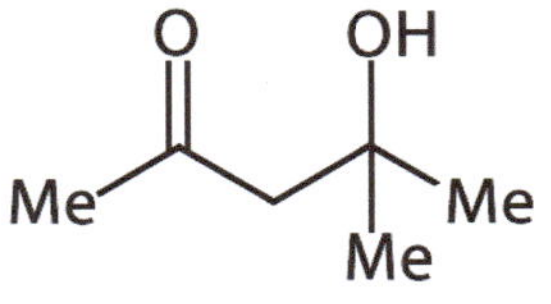

II

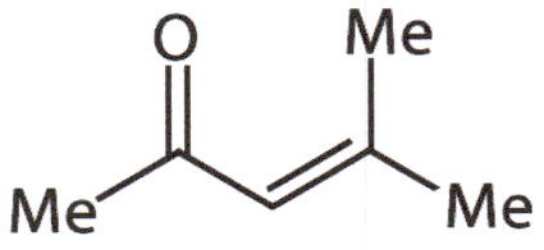

III

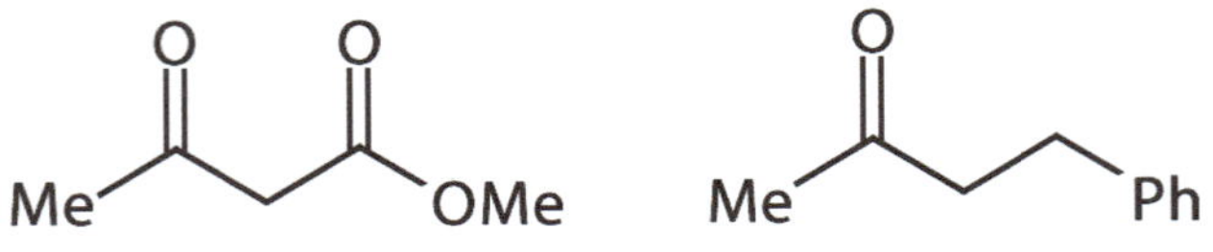

IV V

19) Which of the structures provided would be consistent with the condensation product and the intermediate (aldol), respectively?

A. I & IV **B.** II & III **C.** II & V **D.** III & II

20) For the following reaction, choose the condensation product **Z**:

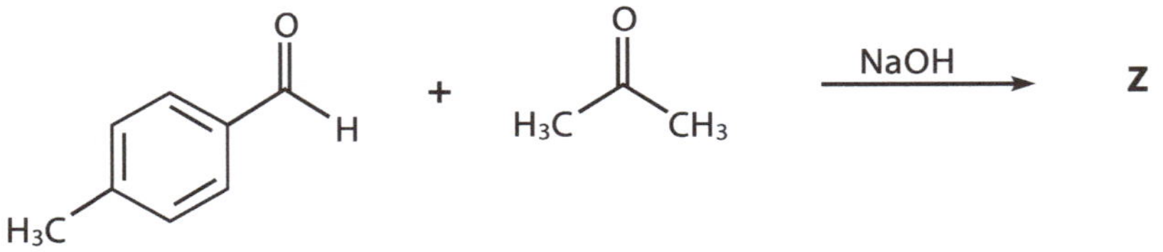

A.
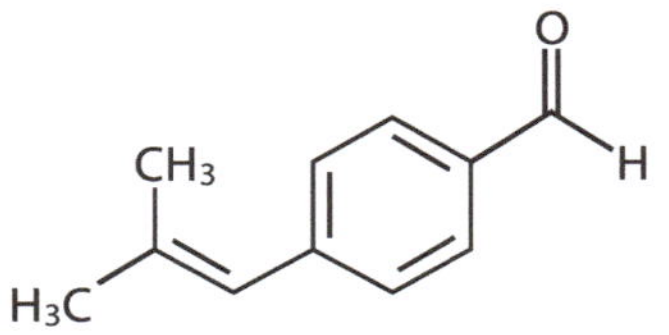

C.
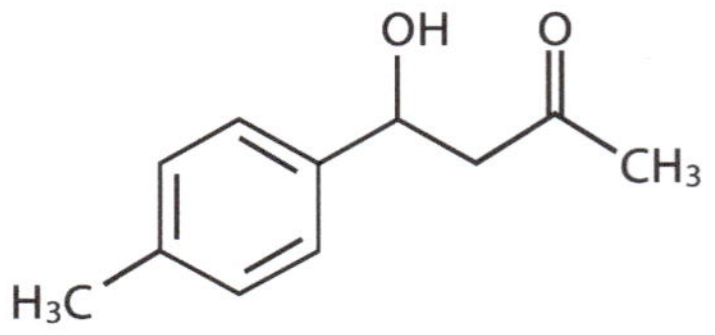

B.
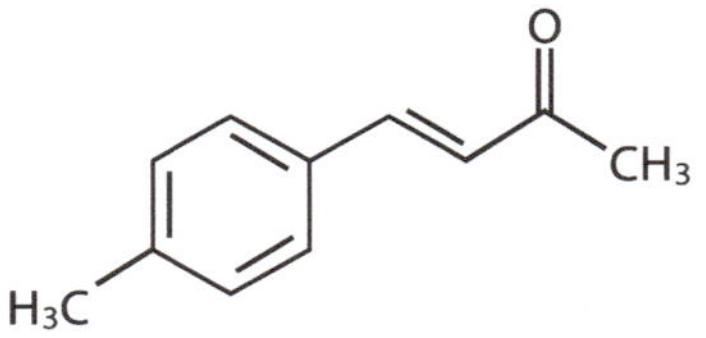

D.
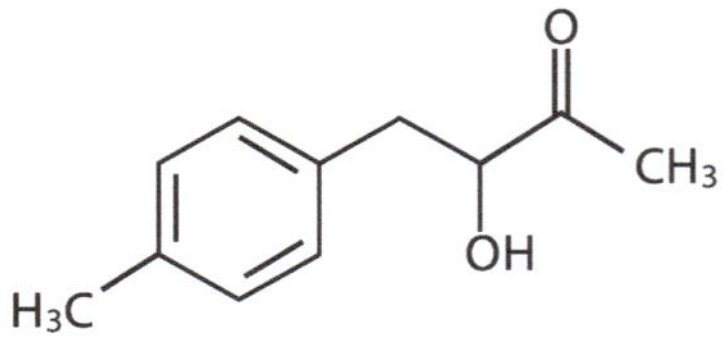

21) For the following reaction, the ketone reacts with PhCHO. Identify the condensation product **Z**:

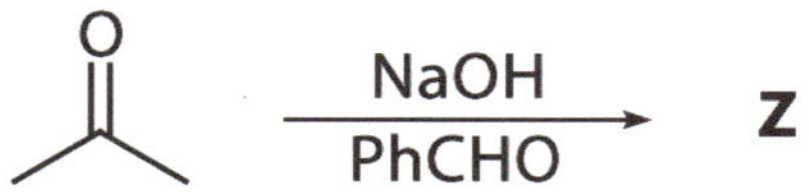

A.
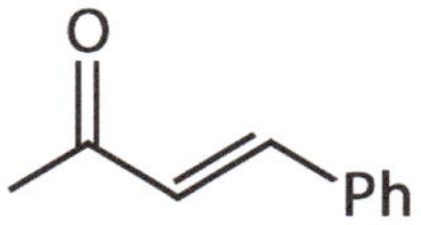

B.
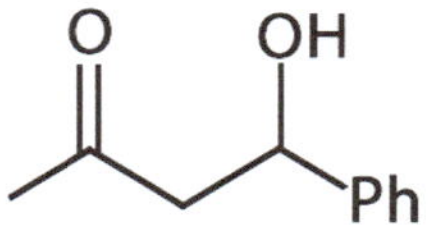

C.
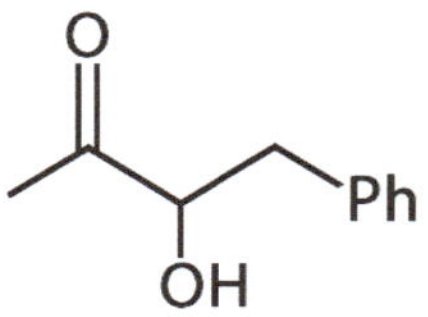

D.
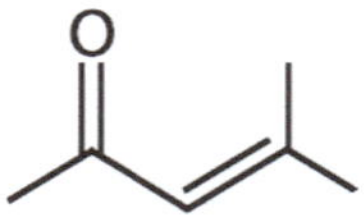

22) The condensation product from an aldol reaction can also occur in the presence of an acid catalyst in aqueous conditions. For the following reaction, identify the condensation product **Z**:

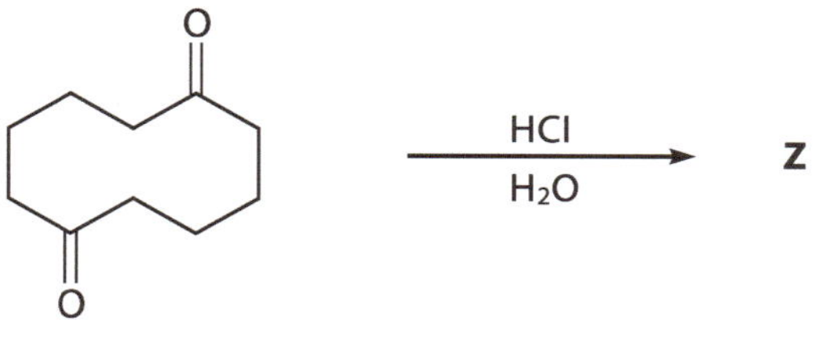

A. 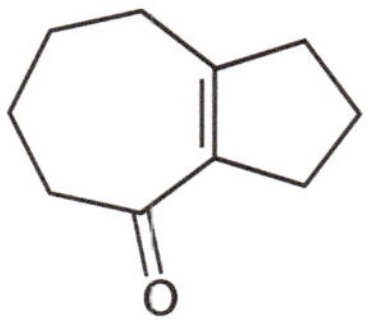

B. 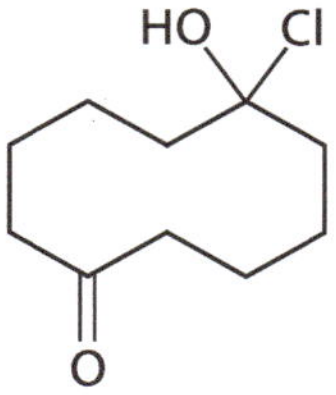

C. 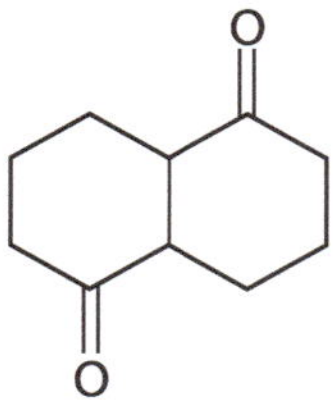

D. 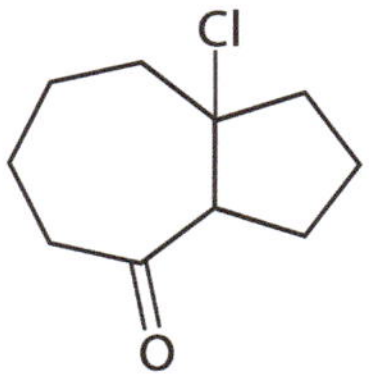

You may have felt that this unit was written in a foreign language! Well, it is our hope to show you that despite the "blah blah blah," the questions can be distilled down to basic pattern recognition and geometric reasoning. Have you ever seen the comics where the illustrator changes a few details from one image to the other as a challenge for you to observe the differences and similarities? If you find those comics easy, then you have already developed an important skill for GAMSAT Organic Chemistry!

In the reaction summary provided in the preamble, here is the pattern (*if it remains unclear to you, please see the string of letters/atoms encircled in red on the next page*):

- in the sample reaction provided in the preamble, the final product is called the 'condensation product' and has this arrangement: C=C-C=O (*look carefully at the reaction and confirm that you can identify that string of letters and bonds in the condensation product*).
- ½ way to the final product must be the intermediate and it is labelled 'Aldol' and has this arrangement: (OH)-C-C-C=O (side note: we put the OH in brackets because it could be written either HO or OH and it has the same meaning; however, 'OH' is simpler to identify in the preamble and questions. If you have a science background then you know that it is the O that must be in between the H and the C, which should be very clear after ORG Chapter 1).

Look back at the reaction provided in the preamble and confirm that you agree with the 2 patterns as described. If you are only now seeing the pattern, consider re-evaluating your answers for Questions 19–22 based on your recognition of the pattern.

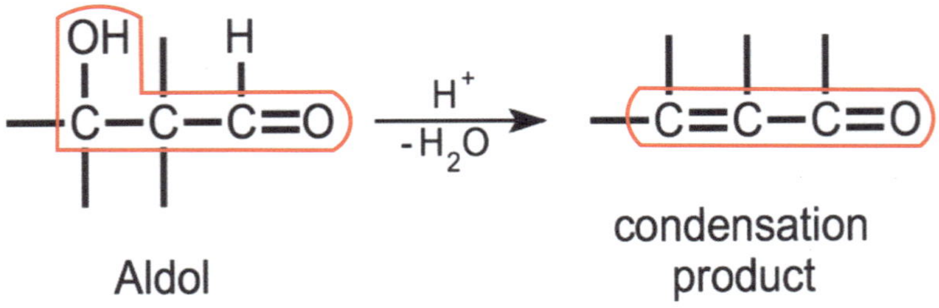

Question 19 asks for “the condensation product and the intermediate (aldol), respectively.” Of course, ‘respectively’ means ‘*in the order already mentioned*’ so we must first identify the condensation product.

Thus we look at all 5 structures to find the condensation product with this pattern: C=C-C=O. All 5 structures have 2 lines going to an O (i.e., C=O which is called the ‘carbonyl group’), so now we only need to identify C=C. Only structure **III** has a double line (=) that is NOT associated with O, so **III** is the condensation product. Also, for your interest, notice that structure **III** has 1 single line between the 2 double lines just like our pattern: C=C-C=O.

Looking for the aldol (OH)-C-C-C=O in Question 19, notice that there is only one structure, **II**, that has an OH group! So the answer for Question 19 must be D (meaning, the structures are **III** and **II**, in that order).

Also for your interest, notice that for structure **II**, (OH)-C-C-C=O, between the OH group and the carbonyl group, you should be able to count 3 straight, single lines (bonds) consistent with our identified pattern.

If it is ‘clicking’ now, consider reassessing your other answer choices before continuing.

From this point forward, it only gets easier! Question 20 is looking for the condensation product C=C-C=O which basically means the structure to the right.

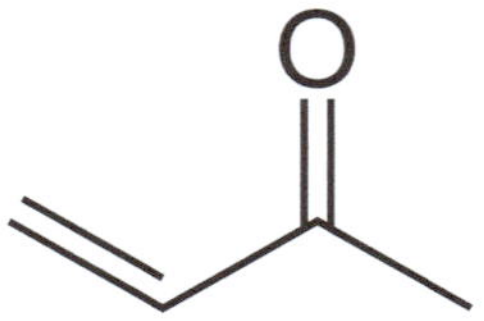

Only answer choice B has a double bond between 2 carbons (C=C) which is then single bonded to a carbonyl group (C=O), and so B is correct. We must maintain the correct order consistent with the pattern that we were provided.

Question 21 is also looking for the condensation product C=C-C=O. There are only 2 options that have the correct pattern, answer choices A and D. So we must identify how they are different from each other and see if we can justify either answer. Answer choice A has ‘Ph’ attached. We can see ‘Ph’ under the arrow as part of PhCHO (and the question stem stated that the reaction was with PhCHO making it a good candidate). Answer choice D has 2 separate lines attached (i.e. 2 primary carbons) but how can we justify that? The reactant to the left of the arrow, which has 2 primary carbons, would have had to react with itself. We know the latter did not occur since the question stem stated that the reaction was with PhCHO. Thus answer choice A is correct.

Going Deeper: Just for your interest, answer choice B would be the intermediate of the reaction that would lead to the final condensation product, answer choice A. Later, in ORG chapters, you will learn that the reaction that goes from answer choice B to A occurs as 3 atoms are lost: H + OH = H_2O. When water is lost from a reactant, just like when water is lost from your body, it is called *dehydration*.

The reaction was described in the preamble as 'base catalysed' which refers to the sodium hydroxide (NaOH, a powerful base) above the arrow.

In Question 21, the reactants are (do not worry about nomenclature for now, we will learn how to name these and more complex molecules later):

1) To the left of the arrow is the ketone called 'acetone' (propan-2-one, the active ingredient in nail polish remover and paint thinner; can be smelled on the breath of a diabetic with poorly regulated insulin levels). Among the many ways that the molecular formula for acetone can be presented, here are a few: $(CH_3)_2CO$, $(CH_3)_2C{=}O$, $CH_3(CO)CH_3$, CH_3-(C=O)-CH_3, H_3C-(C=O)-CH_3, and so of course, C_3H_6O.

2) Below the arrow is PhCHO. In the preamble, 'Ph' was identified as a phenyl group. Phenyl refers to the benzene ring as an attachment (*see* ORG 1.6). PhCHO is shorthand for Ph-(C=O)-H, benzaldehyde (the image to the right). Of course, the preceding information was not necessary to correctly answer the question.

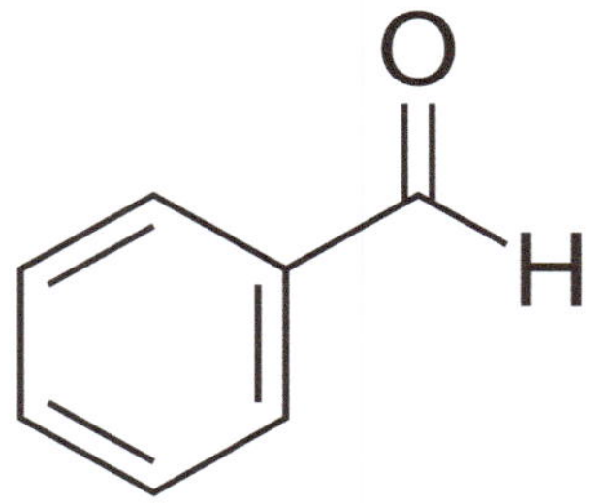

And finally, Question 22 is also looking for the condensation product C=C-C=O: this one has to be the easiest question because only 1 option has a C=C, and so answer choice A is correct. The introduction of the fact that the same reaction can occur in the presence of acid (e.g. HCl) catalyst is simply a distractor. After all, a catalyst increases the rate of a chemical reaction but it is not used up in the process (CHM 9.7), so there can be no Cl attached to the products (i.e. answer choices B and D are impossible for that reason alone).

High-level Importance

High-level Importance

Going Deeper: Though it was not necessary to notice in order to identify the correct pattern among the answer choices, it is interesting to note that Question 22 presents the only case in this unit where both reactants were in the same molecule! The other reactions were between different molecules, *intermolecular*, while Question 22 had the two necessary components for the reaction within the same molecule, *intramolecular*. The reactant's name is cyclodecane-1,6-dione.

For those of you who want to go even deeper (nomenclature for reactant and product, as well as the overall mechanism that leads to answer choice A): Login to your gamsat-prep.com account, click on Videos in the top Menu, then Organic Chemistry, then "**New: Adjacent to Carbonyl, Practice Problem II with Bicyclic Compound**".

Organic Chemistry at university requires that you recite the names of chemicals used in mixtures (*reagents*), and that you commit to memory what can be added to what to make another what and why (!!) - all of which is largely irrelevant for GAMSAT Organic Chemistry. Although geometric reasoning and pattern recognition are most important, you will hopefully develop other important skills that apply to this exam: the basic rules to name compounds - nomenclature, functional groups, stereochemistry, counting carbons and/or hydrogens to ensure that the reaction makes sense, following the groups in the reactants to see where they end up in the products, etc.

Again, you must largely restrain yourself from trying to commit outcomes to memory (which is a basic requirement in tertiary-level courses) but rather to develop an awareness as to the change in bonding patterns and locations of atoms or groups as the reaction takes place. So, during the real exam, when you are presented with reactions that you are not expected to have seen before, as long as an adequate example is provided, you would have already honed your skills to prepare you to successfully reason the outcomes of novel reactions.

Unit 4, Questions 23–25

Consider the following table which is a summary of neutral carbon's bond hybrids and molecular shapes.

When bonded to…	Hybridisation	Shape	Bond angle
2 atoms	sp	linear	180°
3 atoms	sp^2	trigonal planar (= flat triangle)	120°
4 atoms	sp^3	tetrahedral	109.5°

Table 1

23) The molecule ethylene (IUPAC name: ethene) is illustrated below. Based on the information in Table 1, what is the hybridisation of each carbon in ethylene?

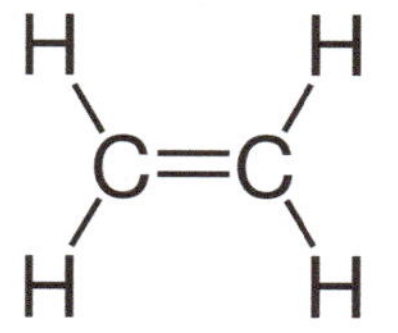

A. sp **B.** sp^2 **C.** sp^3 **D.** sp^2 and sp^3

24) Consider the structure of 2-methylpropane.

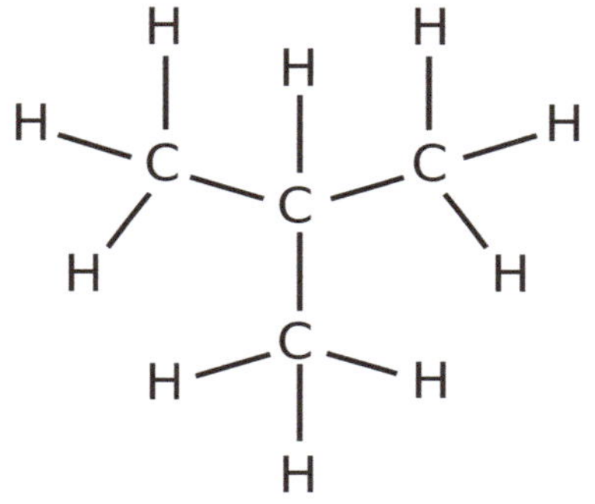

Based on the information in Table 1, what is the percentage p-character in the carbon-atom hybrids?

A. 25% **B.** 50% **C.** 66.67% **D.** 75%

25) A carbon to carbon bond may be composed of 2 different hybrids depending on the hybridisation status of the two carbons involved in the bond. The bond between the second carbon (C-2) and the third carbon (C-3) is indicated by an arrow in the image below.

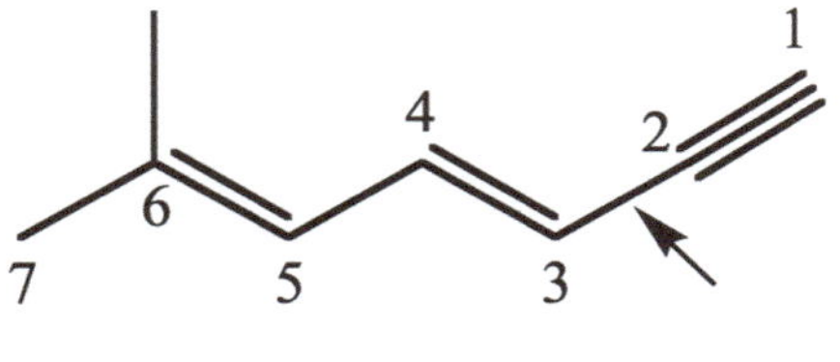

Which of the following represents the atomic-orbital hybrids in the bond between C-2 and C-3, respectively?

A. sp and sp^2 **B.** sp and sp **C.** sp^2 and sp **D.** sp^3 and sp^3

Question 23: In the illustration provided of ethylene, we can see that each carbon is connected to 3 other atoms (2 hydrogens and the other carbon). According to Table 1, 3 atoms ONLY corresponds to a carbon that is a sp^2 hybridised. Thus the answer is B.

Note that a *substituent* is a group or atom attached to carbon (it may *substitute* for hydrogen). Table 1 is simplified by considering the attachment as being to other atoms. We could replace the word "atoms" in Table 1 with the more 'professional' Organic Chemistry expression, *substituents*. And so, from Table 1, we can confirm that when carbon has 4 substituents, it is sp^3 and tetrahedral (109.5°); 3 substituents: sp^2 and trigonal planar (120°); and 2 substituents: sp and linear (180°).

Question 24: Each carbon atom is clearly attached to 4 other atoms. From Table 1, we can confirm that the hybridisation of carbon must be sp^3 (and the shape tetrahedral!). Yes, at this point, it is as intuitive as you would imagine . . . sp^3 means that: 1 s and 3 p combine which is a total of 4 orbitals, thus ¼ s and ¾ p. And so, in sp^3 hybridisation, s-character is 25% and p-character is 75%. Thus, the answer is D. Of course, sp^2 is 33% s-character, and sp is 50% s-character.

Note that the statement "sp^3 means that: 1 s and 3 p combine which is a total of 4 orbitals" directly converts to the idea of 4 sp^3 bonds when carbon is bonded to 4 atoms.

Question 25: After reading about alkynes (*the end of Chapter 4*), come back to ensure that you can name the molecule in this question (*nomenclature*). Of course, if you have named molecules before, try naming it before continuing. Its name is at the end of this worked solution.

Table 1 relates the hybridisation to the number of atoms bonded to carbon. Before tallying up the atoms, we must account for the hydrogens since they are not drawn in the skeletal structure as presented in the question. Thus, the first step is to add hydrogens to the molecule provided so that each carbon is clearly bonded 4 times. That is basic assumed knowledge.

The easiest way to add the hydrogens is to just add the additional bonds to the molecule as provided, or you can expand the molecule on your scratch paper as we have done below. If you have not considered this before, then please try to answer the question using Table 1 before continuing with the worked solution.

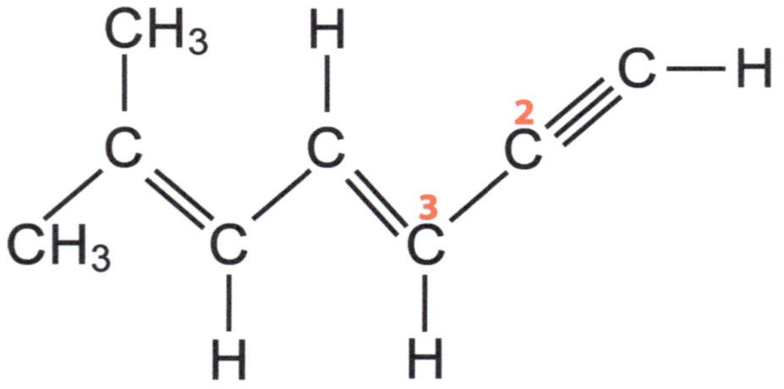

Be sure that you can see that every carbon is now bonded 4 times. We have added the number of hydrogens necessary to fulfill this basic requirement for the bonding of the neutral carbon atom.

Now we can see that the C-2 is bonded to only 2 atoms (2 carbons), which Table 1 indicates must be sp hybridisation. We can see that C-3 is bonded to 3 atoms (2 carbons and 1 hydrogen), and Table 1 indicates that must be sp^2 hybridisation. Since "respectively" means *in the order mentioned*, C-2 is mentioned first in the question stem, and then C-3, sp and sp^2. Thus the answer is A.

Notice the carbons at the far left of the image comprise *methyl* groups (CH_3), each bonded to a carbon (*thus 4 bonds in total*), and thus each methyl carbon must possess the famous 4 sp^3 hybrids. According to Table 1, those methyl carbons are in the centre of the most famous shape in Organic Chemistry, the tetrahedron. That structure is called: *tetrahedral molecular geometry.* And, btw (!!), the name of the molecule is: 6-methylhepta-3,5-dien-1-yne. And yes, if you do not know yet, you will learn how to name such lovely structures beginning with Chapter 3.

This is the first and last chapter with worked solutions in the physical book. From Chapter 2, all answers and worked solutions will be waiting for you in your online account, and sometimes with accompanying video.

Answers (skeletal-line drawings) for the additional *Need for Speed* exercises for 1.0 can be found below. Please note, in each instance, it would not matter if you drew the image 'upside down' or 'left-right inverted' because it would represent the same molecule. These images do not respect the 3D aspect of molecules. We are only looking at the connectivity (i.e. *how the carbon atoms are connected to each other*).

1) 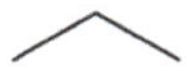

2) 

3) 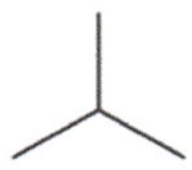

4) 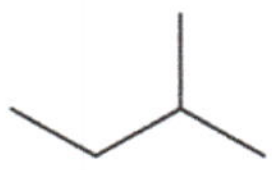

5) 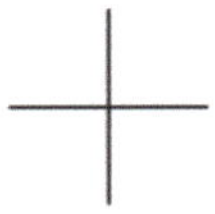

6) 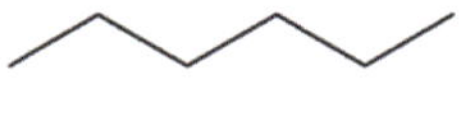

7) 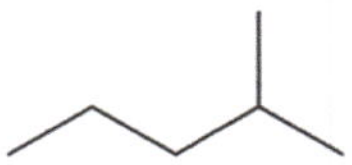

8) 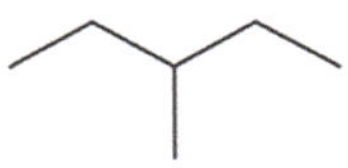

9) 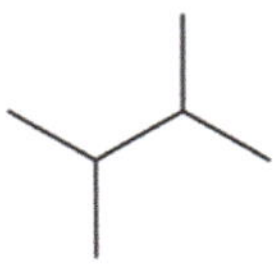

10) 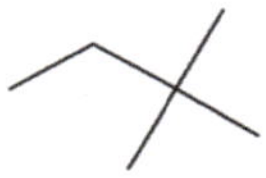

Questions or concerns? gamsat-prep.com/forum

High-level Importance

SPOILER ALERT

Gold Standard has cross-referenced the content in this chapter to examples from ACER's official GAMSAT practice materials (note that only ACER sells their eBooks brand new). It is for you to decide when you want to explore these questions since you may want to preserve some of ACER's materials for timed mock-exam practice.

Number	1	2	3	4	5
Title	GAMSAT Practice Questions	GAMSAT Sample Questions	GAMSAT Practice Test 1	GAMSAT Practice Test 2	GAMSAT Practice Test 3

Examples – Identifying s and p orbital hybrids in the context of s-character and electronegativity: Q8 of 1; resonance structures (*we will revisit resonance in chapters 4 to 11*): Q72-74 of 3; functional groups and conjugated bonds (*we will revisit conjugation in chapters 4 and 5*): Q82-84 of 5. Note that "Q" is followed by the question number, and, for example, "of 1" refers to booklet number 1 in the table above. Also note that your gamsat-prep.com Masters Series online account has direct links to the step-by-step worked solutions for all of ACER's GAMSAT Sciences practice questions (the solutions can also be found in the Gold Standard GAMSAT YouTube Channel). The 15 full-length GAMSAT practice tests by Gold Standard, HEAPS-1 through HEAPS-15, contain specific cross-references to this chapter within the worked solutions.

Chapter Checklist

- ☐ Access your free online account at www.gamsat-prep.com/gamsat-organic-chemistry to view answers, worked solutions and discussion boards for chapter-ending practice questions.
- ☐ Reassess your 'learning objectives' for this chapter: Go back to the first page of this chapter and re-evaluate the top 3 boxes and the Introduction.
    - ☐ Please be sure that you have completed the *Need for Speed* exercises at the beginning of this chapter.
- ☐ Complete a maximum of 1 page of notes using symbols/abbreviations to represent the entire chapter based on your learning objectives. These are your Gold Notes.
- ☐ Consider your multimedia options based on your optimal way of learning:
    - ☐ Download the free Gold Standard GAMSAT app for your Android device or iPhone.
    - ☐ Create your own, tangible study cards or try the free app: Anki.
    - ☐ Record your voice reading your Gold Notes onto your smartphone (audio files, e.g., *memo* or MP3s) and listen during exercise, transportation, etc.
    - ☐ Try out the Gold Standard GAMSAT online videos at gamsat-prep.com, or you can try other options on YouTube like Khan Academy or Crash Course Organic Chemistry.
- ☐ Schedule your full-length GAMSAT practice tests: ACER and/or HEAPS exams. Schedule one full day to complete a practice test and 1-2 days for a thorough assessment of worked solutions while adding to your abbreviated Gold Notes.
- ☐ Schedule and/or evaluate stress reduction techniques such as regular exercise (sports), yoga, meditation and/or mindfulness exercises (*see* YouTube for suggestions).

High-level Importance

Memorise
* Categories of stereoisomers
* Define isomers, chiral (stereocentre)

Understand
* Basic stereochemistry
* Identify meso compounds
* Assign R/S/E/Z (cis/trans)
* Fischer projections

Importance

High level: 20% of GAMSAT Organic Chemistry questions released by ACER are related to content in this chapter (in our estimation).

* Note that approximately 60% of the questions in GAMSAT Organic Chemistry are related to just 4 chapters: 2, 6, 7 and 12.

Introduction

Stereochemistry is the study of the relative spatial (3-D) arrangement of atoms within molecules. An important branch of stereochemistry, and most relevant to the GAMSAT (*and to optimise the effectiveness of medications*), is the study of chiral molecules.

This chapter requires pattern recognition and geometric reasoning. Clearly, the percent importance of this chapter is significant. Of course, this does not guarantee the balance of questions on your upcoming exam, but it underlines the relative importance of this chapter. Normally, but not always, ACER will reiterate - in the exam's stimulus material - the rules for assigning R/S/E/Z configuration ("stimulus material" refers to the passage, article, graphs, tables or diagrams that precede multiple-choice questions).

Multimedia Resources at GAMSAT-Prep.com

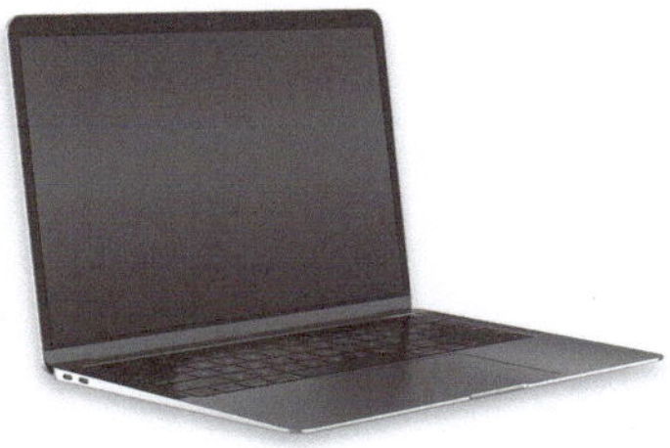

Open Discussion Boards
(*gamsat-prep.com/forum*)

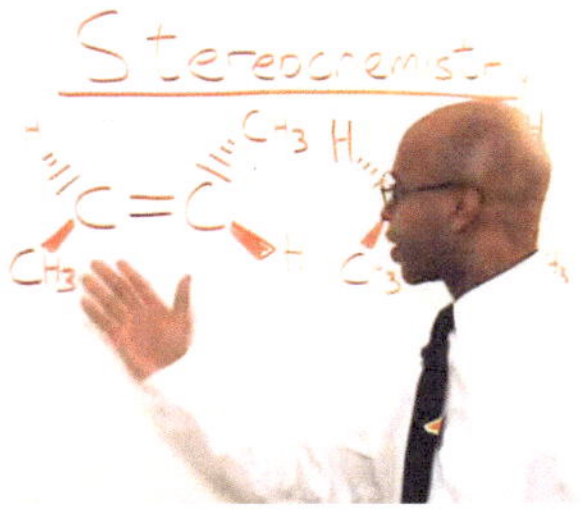

Science Preparation Videos

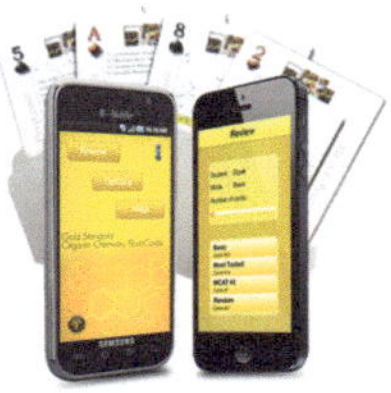

Flashcards

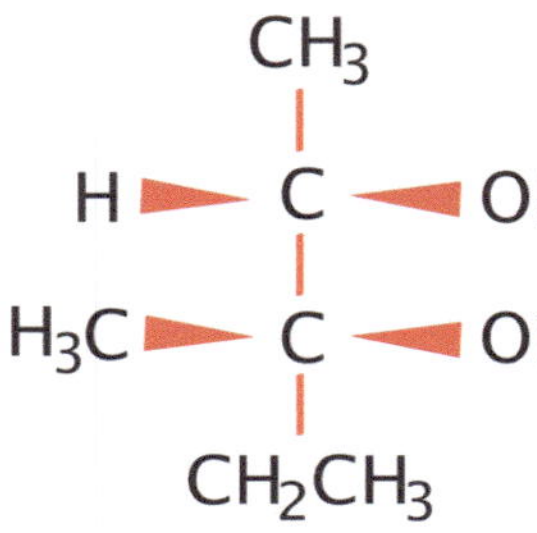

Special Guest

* The real GAMSAT may have advanced-level information presented (i.e. in a passage) but previous knowledge of said information is not required to answer the questions that would follow. Practice questions at the end of this chapter, as well as ACER and GS (HEAPS) practice GAMSATs can help you clarify this point.

2.0 GAMSAT has a *Need for Speed*!

High-level Importance

Section	GAMSAT Organic Chemistry *Need for Speed* Exercises
2.1	Two *different molecules* with the same number and type of atoms (= *the same molecular formula*) are called ____________________.
2.2.1	Consider the two structures below and circle the correct label. The molecule on the left is (*cis* / *trans*) and the molecule on the right is (*cis* / *trans*). 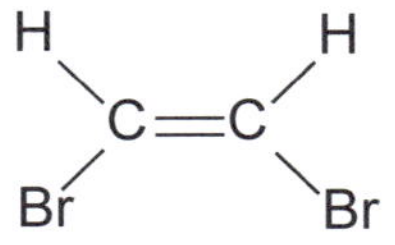 and 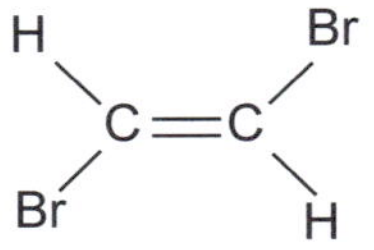
2.2.2	Does the structure below have a line of symmetry? If so, draw the line of symmetry. 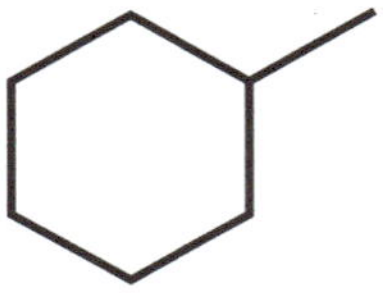
	Add the missing atoms to the structures on the right in order to complete the mirror images of the structures on the left. 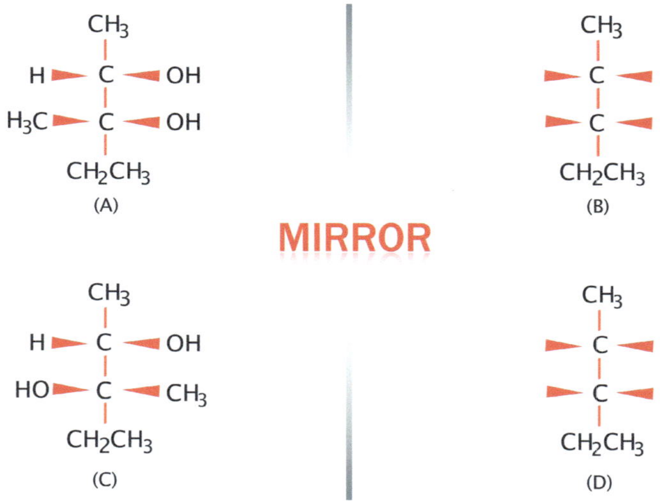
2.3.1	Is the absolute configuration of the structure below *R* or *S*? 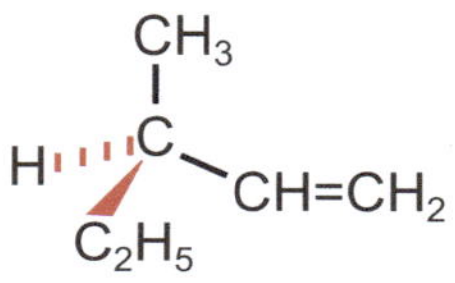

2.3.3

1) Add the missing atoms to the structure on the right in order to complete the mirror image of the structure on the left.

2) Do the structures below have a line of symmetry? *yes / no*
If so, draw those lines of symmetry.

3) Are the two structures superposable (i.e. *meso*)? *yes / no*

4) Each structure below has 2 stereocentres (*chiral carbons*). Label each stereocentre either *R* or *S* (*be careful: currently the lowest priority group, H, is pointing towards you*).

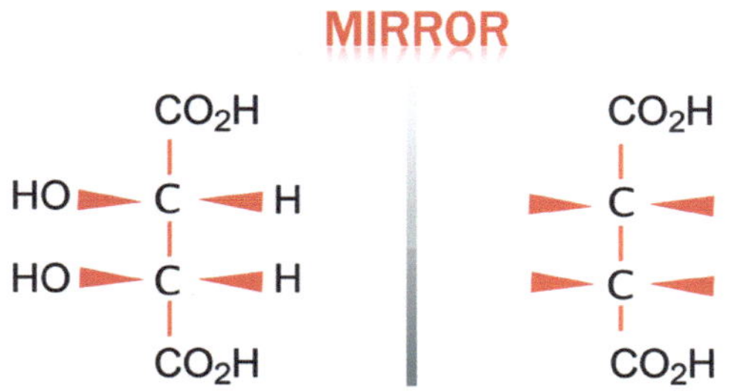

2.4

There are 3 incomplete Newman projections of butane conformers in the rightmost column below. Add the missing atoms in the correct positions.

anti conformation

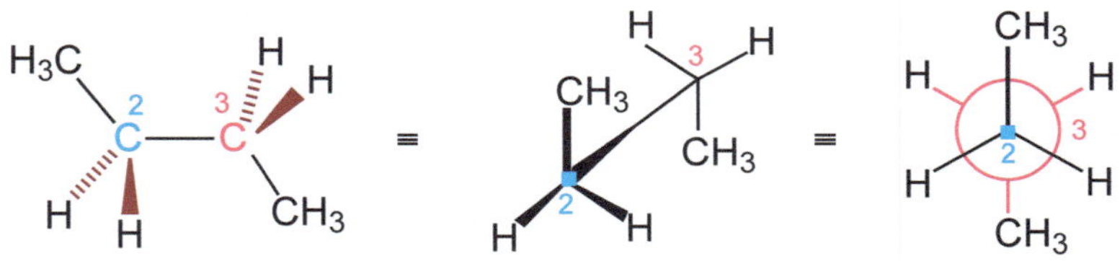

eclipsed conformation

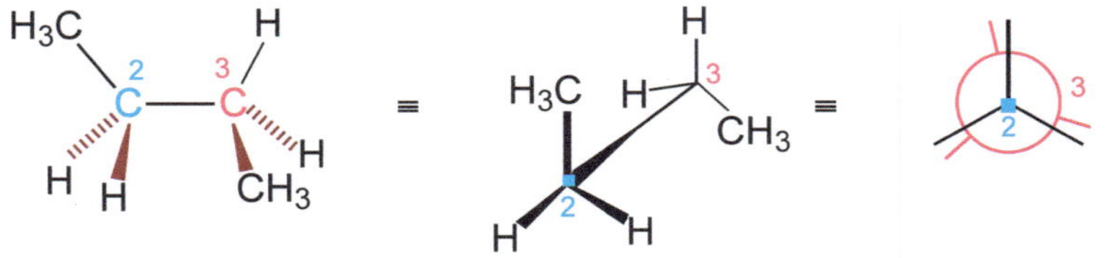

gauche conformation

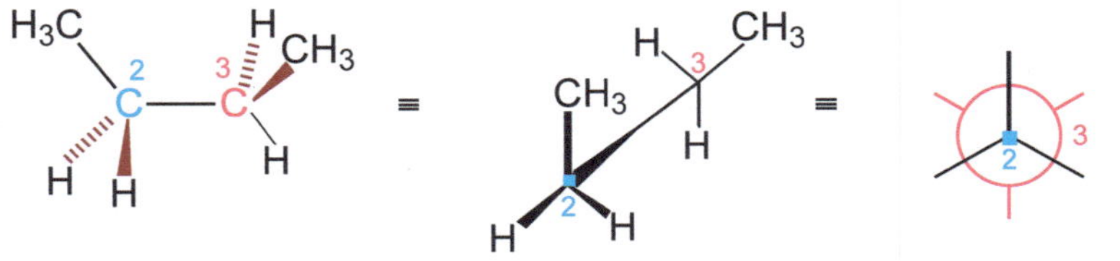

eclipsed conformation

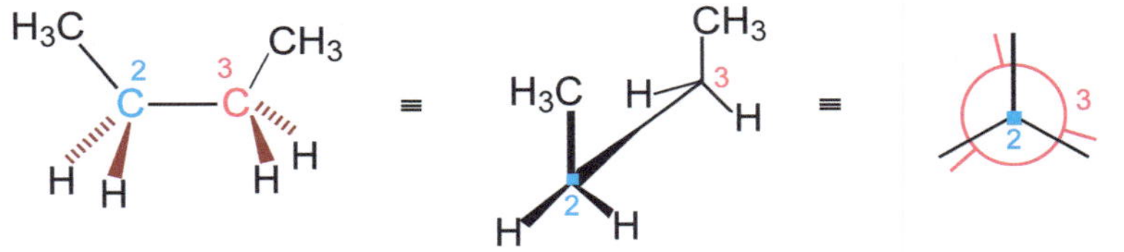

2.1 Isomers

High-level Importance

Stereochemistry is the study of the arrangement of atoms in a molecule, in three dimensions. Two *different molecules* with the same number and type of atoms (= *the same molecular formula*) are called isomers. Isomers fall into two main categories: *structural* (constitutional) isomers and *stereoisomers* (spatial isomers). Structural isomers differ by connectivity (= the order and/or kinds of bonds), and stereoisomers differ in the way their atoms are arranged in space (enantiomers and diastereomers; *see* Fig. IV.B.2.1.1).

2.1.1 Structural (Constitutional) Isomers

Structural isomers have different atoms and/or bonding patterns in relation to each other like the following *chain* or *skeletal* isomers of hexane, C_6H_{14}:

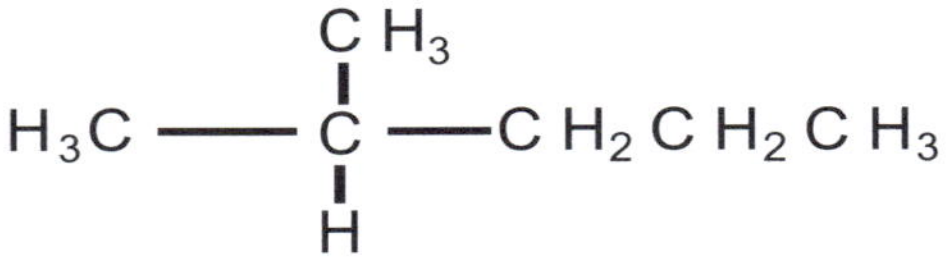

and

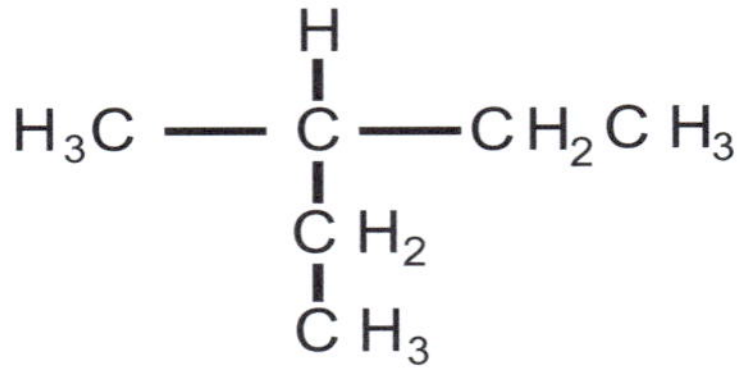

Functional isomers are structural isomers that have the same molecular formula but have different functional groups (ORG 1.6) or *moieties*. For example, the following alcohol (ORG 6.1) and ether (ORG 10.1), $C_4H_{10}O$:

IUPAC: butan-1-ol
(n-butanol)

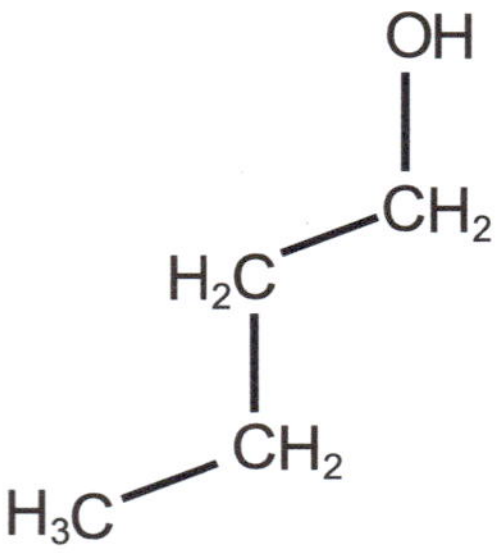

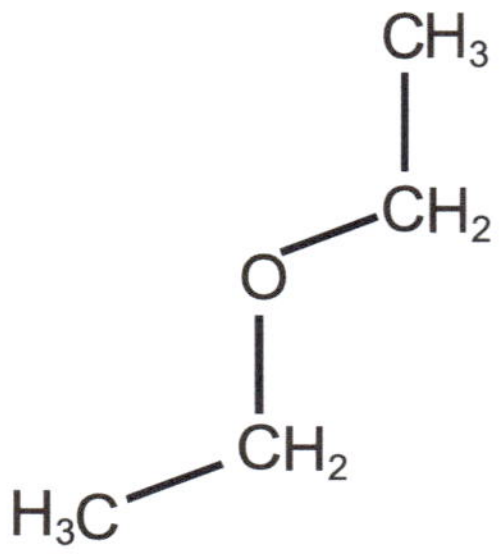

IUPAC: ethoxyethane
(diethyl ether)

Positional or regioisomers are structural isomers where the functional group changes position on the parent structure. For example, the hydroxyl group (-OH) occupying 3 different positions on the n-pentane (= normal, non-branched alkane with 5 carbons) chain resulting in 3 different compounds, $C_5H_{12}O$:

IUPAC: pentan-1-ol
(1-pentanol)

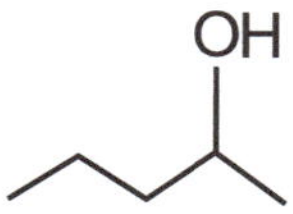

IUPAC: pentan-2-ol
(2-pentanol)

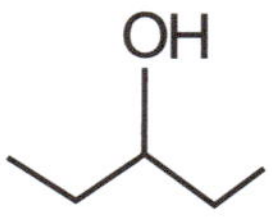

IUPAC: pentan-3-ol
(3-pentanol)

2.2.1 Geometric Isomers *cis/trans*, E/Z

Geometric isomers occur because carbons that are in a ring or double bond structure are *unable* to freely rotate (*see* conformation of cycloalkane; ORG 3.3, 3.3.1). This results in *cis* and *trans* compounds. When the substituents (e.g., Br) are on the same side of the ring or double bond, it is designated cis. When they are on opposite sides, it is designated trans. The *trans* isomer is more stable since the substituents are further apart, thus electron shell repulsion is minimised (ORG 2.4).

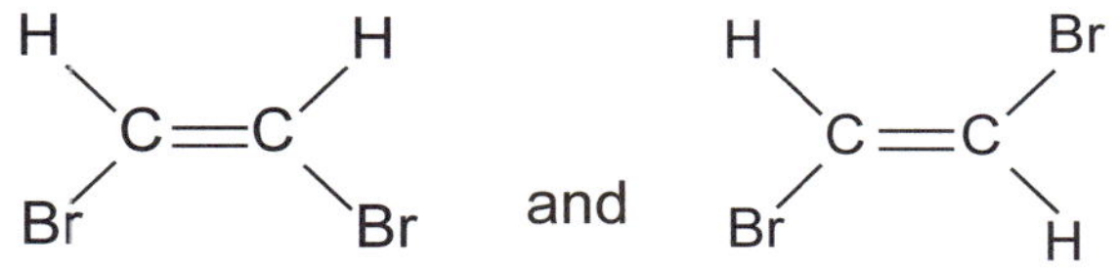

cis-dibromoethene   *trans*-dibromoethene

In general, structural and geometric isomers have different reactivity, spectra and physical properties (i.e. boiling points, melting points, etc.). Geometric isomers may have different physical properties but, in general, tend to have similar chemical reactivity.

The E, Z notation is the IUPAC preferred method for designating the stereochemistry of double bonds. E, Z is particularly used for isomeric compounds with 4 different substituent groups bonded to the two *ethenyl* or *vinyl* carbons (i.e. C=C which are sp^2 hybridised carbon atoms). We have just reviewed how to use *cis/trans*. The E, Z notation is used on more complex molecules and, as described, on situations were 4 different substituents are present.

To begin with, each substituent at the double bond is assigned a priority (*see* 2.3.1 for rules). If the two groups of higher priority are on opposite sides of the double bond, the bond is assigned the configuration E, (from *entgegen*, the German word for "opposite"). If the two groups of higher priority are on the same side of the double bond, the bond is assigned the configuration Z, (from *zusammen,* the German word for "together"). {Generally speaking, learning German is NOT required for the GAMSAT!}

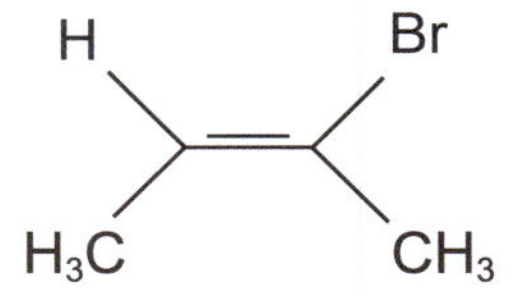

cis-2-bromobut-2-ene
(2 methyl groups on the same side)

BUT

(*E*)-2-bromobut-2-ene
(Br is higher priority than methyl)

Mnemonic: Z = Zame Zide; E = Epposites.

Note: From ORG 2.1.1 onwards, until you are in the habit of doing so quickly and efficiently, always make sure that there are 4 bonds to each, neutral carbon (ORG 1.1). When you do not see 4 bonds, like the positional isomers in ORG 2.1.1 or the functional groups presented in ORG 1.6, take the time to work out how many hydrogens – which are not being shown – must be attached to each carbon to complete the rule: '4 bonds to each, neutral carbon'. Similarly, always try to make sure that the number of carbons being presented is correct: either because it matches its isomer (ORG 2.1.1, 2.2) or, if presented, its molecular formula or name (if it is your first time seeing the name of organic molecules, please return to ORG 2.1.1 once you have learned nomenclature in subsequent chapters). Perceiving the correct number of H's and/or C's is a basic requirement for the real GAMSAT.

2.2.2 Enantiomers and Diastereomers

High-level Importance

Stereoisomers are different compounds with the same structure (= *connectivity*), differing only in the spatial orientation of the atoms (= *configuration*). Stereoisomers may be further divided into enantiomers and diastereomers. Enantiomers must have opposite, absolute configurations at each and every chiral carbon.

We will soon highlight the easy way to remember the meaning of a *chiral molecule*; however, the formal definition of chirality is of an object that is not identical with its mirror image and thus exists in two enantiomeric forms. A molecule cannot be chiral if it contains a plane of symmetry. A molecule that has a plane of symmetry must be superposable on its mirror image and thus must be *achiral.* The most common chirality encountered in organic chemistry is when the carbon atom is bonded to four different groups. Such a carbon lacks a plane of symmetry and is referred to as a *chiral centre*. When a carbon atom has only three different substituents, such as the central carbon in methylcyclohexane, it has a plane of symmetry and is therefore achiral.

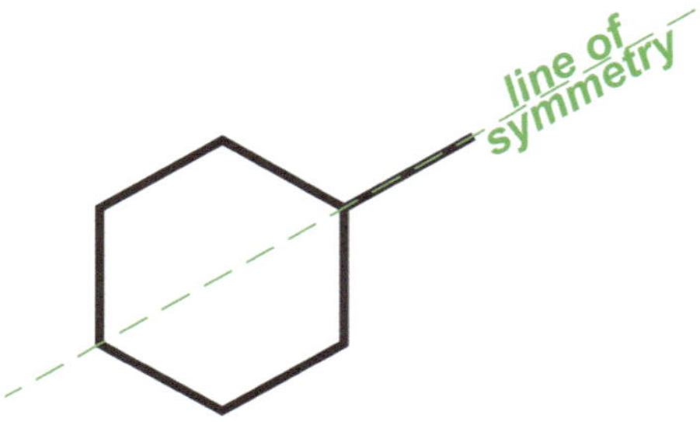

methylcyclohexane

A stereocentre (= stereogenic centre) is an atom bearing attachments such that interchanging any two groups produces a stereoisomer. If a molecule has n stereocentres, then it can have up to 2^n different non-superimposable (non-superposable) structures (= enantiomers).

Enantiomers come in pairs. They are two non-superposable molecules, which are mirror images of each other. In order to have an enantiomer, a molecule must be chiral. Chiral molecules contain at least one chiral carbon which is a carbon atom that has four different substituents attached. For the purposes of the GAMSAT, the concepts of a chiral carbon, asymmetric carbon and stereocentre are interchangeable.

Enantiomers have the same chemical and physical properties. The only difference is with their interactions with other chiral molecules, and their rotation of plane-polarised light.

Conversely, diastereomers are any pair of stereoisomers that are not enantiomers. Diastereomers are both chemically and physically different from each other.

Superimposable vs Superposable: Most exams and many textbooks use these terms interchangeably. On the real GAMSAT, unless the question is preceded by their definitions, then the 2 words have the same meaning. Technically, "superimposable" is to lay or place (something, i.e. a molecule) on or over something else (i.e. another molecule). If the preceding proves that the 2 molecules are identical, then they are "superposable".

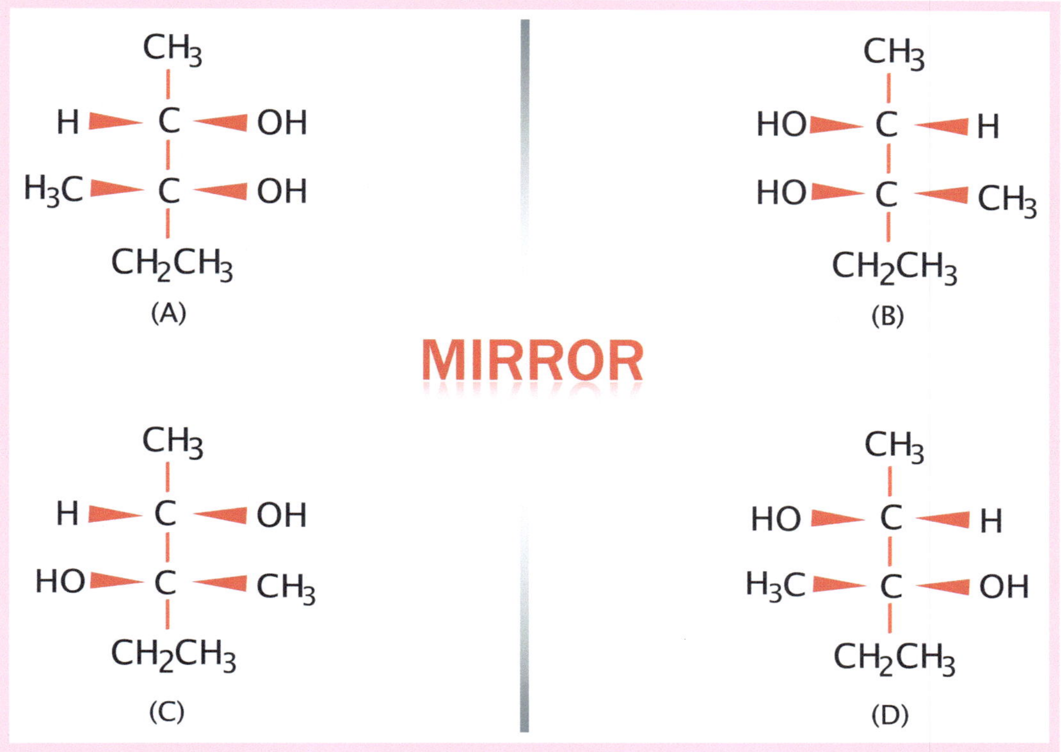

Figure IV.B.2.1: Enantiomers and diastereomers. The enantiomers are A & B, C & D. The diastereomers are A & C, A & D, B & D, B & C. Thus there are 2 pairs of enantiomers. This is consistent with the 2^n equation since each of the structures above have exactly 2 chiral carbons (stereocentres) and thus $2^2 = 4$ enantiomers.

2.3 Absolute and Relative Configuration

Absolute configuration uses the R, S system of naming compounds (*nomenclature;* ORG 2.3.1) and relative configuration uses the D, L system.

Before 1951, the absolute three-dimensional arrangement or configuration of chiral molecules was not known. Instead chiral molecules were compared to an arbitrary standard (*glyceraldehyde*). A molecule was determined to be in its D-form if it has the same relative configuration as D-glyceraldehyde, and its L-form if it has the same relative configuration as L-glyceraldehyde. Thus the *relative* configuration could be determined.

Once the actual spatial arrangements of groups in molecules were finally determined, the *absolute* configuration could be known (ORG 2.3.1).

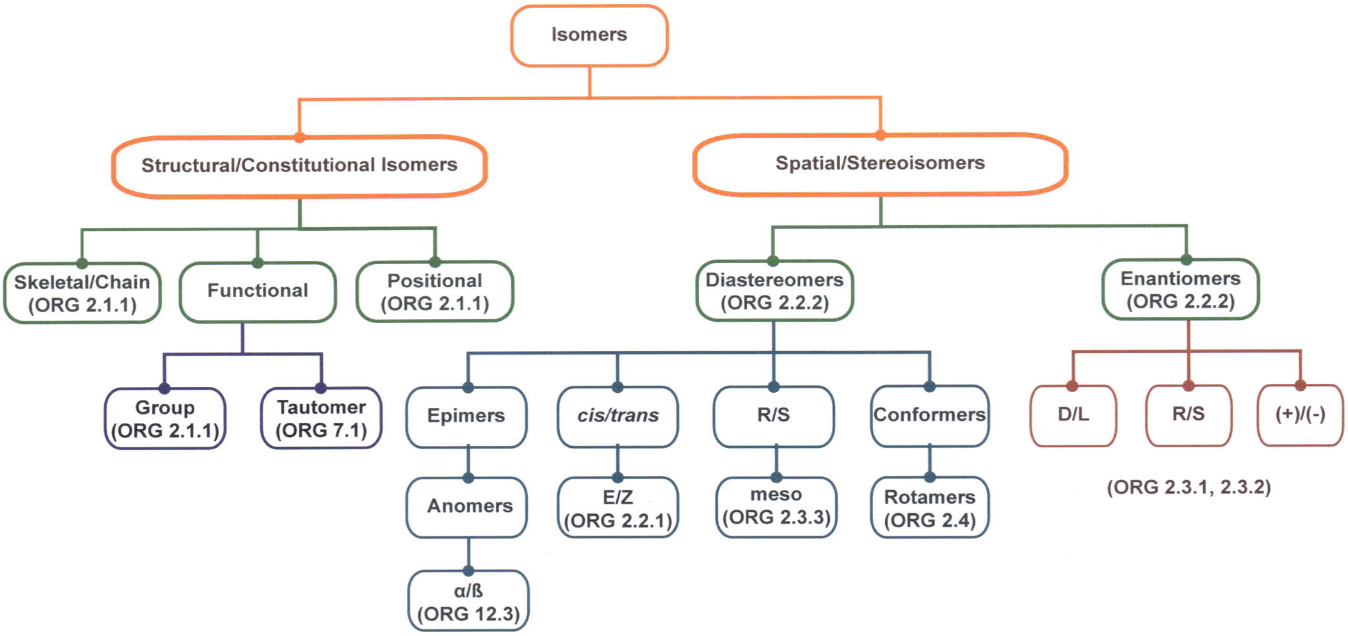

Figure IV.B.2.1.1: Categories of isomers relevant to the GAMSAT.

2.3.1 The R, S System and Fischer Projections

One consequence of the existence of enantiomers, is a special system of nomenclature: the R, S system. This system provides information about the absolute configuration of a molecule. This is done by assigning a stereochemical configuration at each asymmetric (*chiral*) carbon in the molecule by using the following steps:

1. Identify an asymmetric carbon, and the four attached groups.

2. Assign priorities to the four groups, using the following rules (Cahn–Ingold–Prelog priority rules = CIP system):

   i. Atoms of higher atomic number have higher priority.
   ii. An isotope of higher atomic mass receives higher priority.
   iii. The higher priority is assigned to the group with the atom of higher atomic number or mass at the first point of difference.
   iv. If the difference between the two groups is due to the number of otherwise identical atoms, the higher priority is assigned to the group with the greater number of atoms of higher atomic number or mass.

v. To assign priority of double or triple bonded groups, multiple-bonded atoms are considered as equivalent number of single bonded atoms:

–CH=CH is taken as 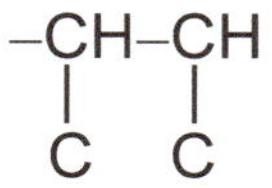

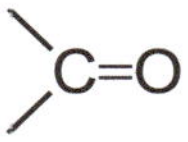 is taken as 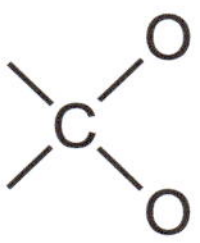

–C≡C is taken as 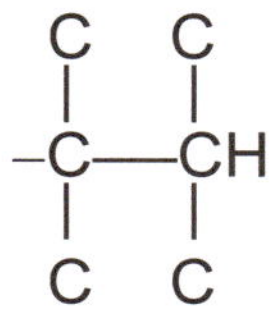

3. You must reorient the molecule in space so that the group of lowest priority is pointing directly back, away from you. The remaining three substituents with higher priority should radiate from the asymmetric carbon atom like the spokes on a steering wheel.

4. Consider the clockwise or counterclockwise order of the priorities of the remaining groups. If they increase in a clockwise direction, the asymmetric carbon is said to have the R configuration. If they decrease in a clockwise direction, the asymmetric carbon is said to have the S configuration {Mnemonic: Clockwise means that when you get to the top of the molecule, you must turn to the Right = R}.

A stereoisomer is named by indicating the configurations of each of the asymmetric carbons.

A Fischer projection is a 2-D way of looking at 3-D structures. All horizontal bonds project toward the viewer, while vertical bonds project away from the viewer. In organic chemistry, Fischer projections are used mostly for carbohydrates (*see* ORG 12.3.1, 12.3.2). To determine if 2 Fischer projections are superposable (i.e. identical), you can: (1) rotate one projection 180° or (2) keep one substituent in a fixed position and then you can rotate the other 3 groups either clockwise or counterclockwise (3-D configuration preserved):

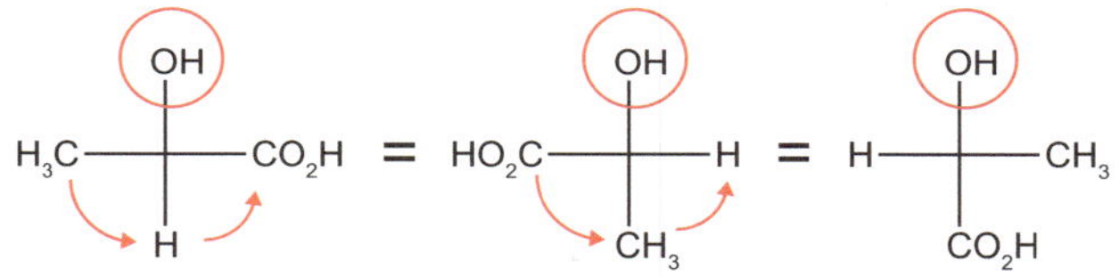

(3) interchange (switch) the positions of all 4 substituents, in any direction, <u>at the same time:</u>

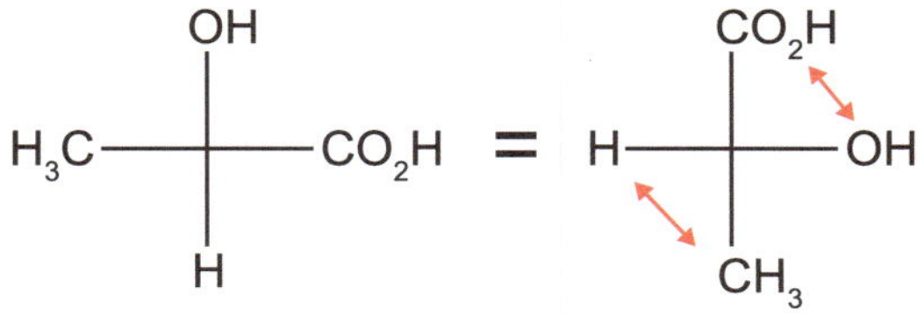

Assigning R, S configurations to Fischer projections:

1. Assign priorities to the four substituents.

2. If the lowest priority group is on the vertical axis, determine the direction of rotation by going from priority 1 to 2 to 3, and then assign R or S configuration.

3. If the lowest priority group is on the horizontal axis, determine the direction of rotation by going from priority 1 to 2 to 3, obtain the R or S configuration, now the TRUE configuration will be the <u>opposite</u> of what you have just obtained.

High-level Importance

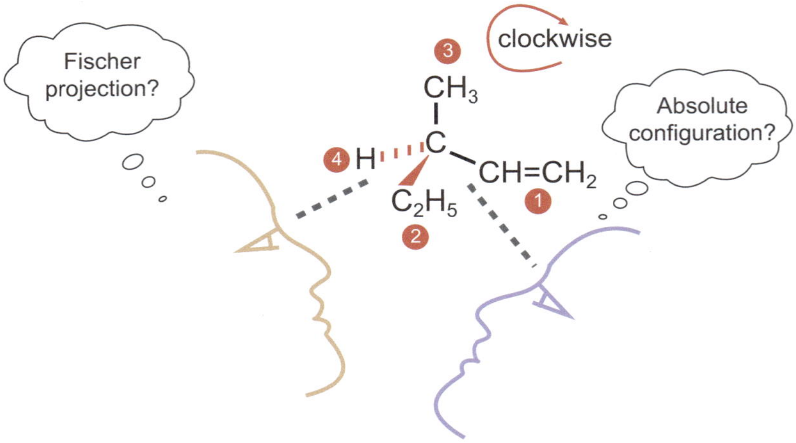

(*R*)-3-methylpent-1-ene

Figure IV.B.2.2(a): Assigning absolute configuration. In organic chemistry, the directions of the bonds are symbolised as follows: a broken line extends away from the viewer (i.e. INTO the page), a solid triangle projects towards the viewer, and a straight line extends in the plane of the paper. According to rule #3, we must imagine that the lowest priority group (H) points away from the viewer. Note: The 'gold' person and the 'blue' person are looking at the same molecule from different perspectives. As long as they both use the same, official rules for assigning the absolute configuration, naturally they will arrive at the same conclusion.

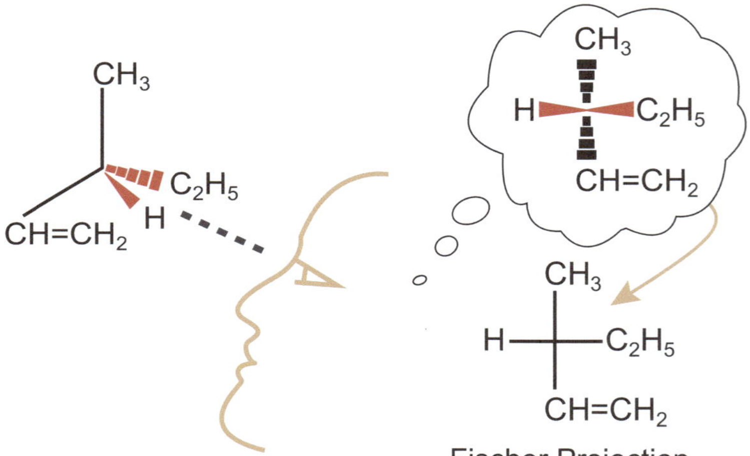

Fischer Projection

Figure IV.B.2.2(b): Creating the Fischer projection of (*R*)-3-methyl-1-pentene. Notice that the perspective of the viewer in the image is the identical perspective of the viewer on the left of Figure IV.B.2.2(a). In either case, a perspective is chosen so that the horizontal groups project towards the viewer. Note: Although the 'gold' person's perspective appears to be *S*, notice that the position of the lowest priority group (H) points *towards* the viewer. Whenever this is the case, the absolute configuration must be the *opposite*, thus *R*.

Note: For the GAMSAT, it is not normally expected that you have memorised the rules to assign *R*, *S* configurations. They would normally provide the rules and an example before asking questions to confirm that you know how to apply the rules. However, it is normally expected that you know the rules to compare different Fischer projections (ORG 2.3.1). Consider watching the stereochemistry videos at gamsat-prep.com.

2.3.2 Optical Isomers

Optical isomers are enantiomers and thus are stereoisomers that differ by different spatial orientations about a chiral carbon atom. Light is an electromagnetic wave that contains oscillating fields. In ordinary light, the electric field oscillates in all directions. However, it is possible to obtain light with an electric field that oscillates in only one plane. This type of light is known as **plane-polarised light**. When plane-polarised light is passed through a sample of a chiral substance, it will emerge vibrating in a different plane than it started. Optical isomers differ only in this rotation. If the light is rotated in a clockwise direction, the compound is dextrorotary, and is designated by a *d*– or (+). If the light is rotated in a counterclockwise direction, the compound is levrorotary, and is designated by an *l*– or (–). Note that these "d-" and "l-" prefixes are distinct from the uppercase "D" and "L" prefixes (relative configuration, ORG 2.3) and there is no direct correlation between the two systems of nomenclature.

A racemic mixture will show no rotation of plane-polarised light. This is a consequence of the fact that a racemate is a mixture with equal amounts of the (+) and (–) forms of a substance.

Specific rotation (α) is an inherent physical property of a molecule. It is defined as follows:

$$\alpha = \frac{\text{Observed rotation in degrees}}{(\text{tube length in dm})\ (\text{concentration in g/mL})}$$

The observed rotation is the rotation of the light passed through the substance. The tube length is the length of the tube that contains the sample in question. The specific rotation is dependent on the solvent used,

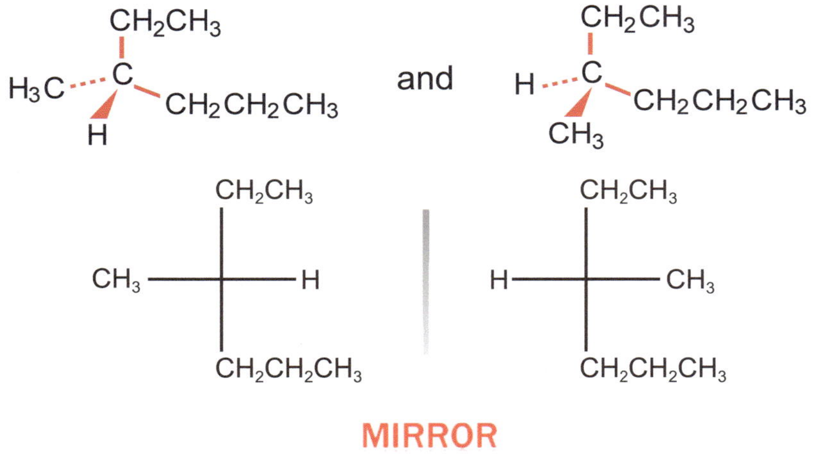

Figure IV.B.2.3: Optical isomers and their Fischer projections: on the left, (R)-(-)-3-methylhexane; on the right: (S)-(+)-3-methylhexane. To prove to yourself that the 2 molecules are non-superposable mirror images (enantiomers), review the rules for Fischer projections (ORG 2.3.1) and compare.

the temperature of the sample, and the wavelength of the light.

It should be noted that there is no clear correlation between the absolute configuration (i.e. *R*, *S*) and the direction of rotation of plane-polarised light, designated by (+) or (-). Therefore, the direction of optical rotation cannot be determined from the structure of a molecule and must be determined experimentally. Also note, with the aim to reduce side effects, the stereochemistry of drugs has been increasing in importance over the past few years.

2.3.3 Meso Compounds

Tartaric acid (= 2,3-dihydroxybutanedioic acid which, in the chapters to come, is a compound that you will be able to name systematically = using IUPAC rules) has two chiral centres that have the same four substituents and are equivalent. As a result, two of the four possible stereoisomers of this compound are identical due to a plane of symmetry. Thus there are only three stereoisomeric tartaric acids. Two of these stereoisomers are enantiomers and the third is an achiral diastereomer, called a meso compound. Meso compounds are achiral (optically inactive) diastereomers of chiral stereoisomers.

In a *meso compound*, an internal plane of symmetry exists by drawing a line that will cut the molecule in half. For example, notice that in *meso*-tartaric acid, you can draw a line perpendicular to the vertical carbon chain creating 2 symmetric halves {**M**e**S**o = **M**irror of **S**ymmetry}.

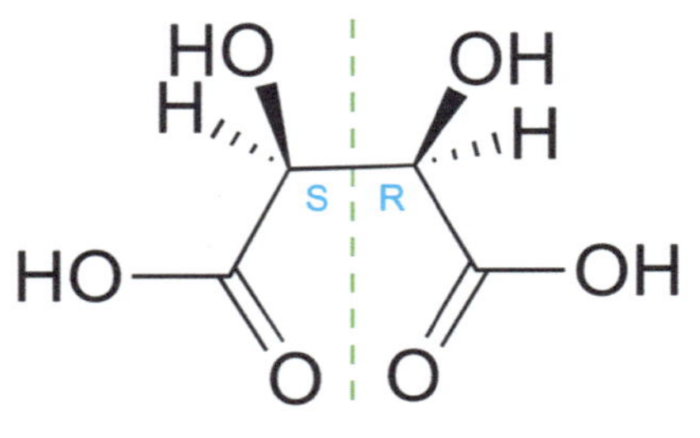

meso-tartaric acid

Perspective with the lowest priority group (H) pointing away.

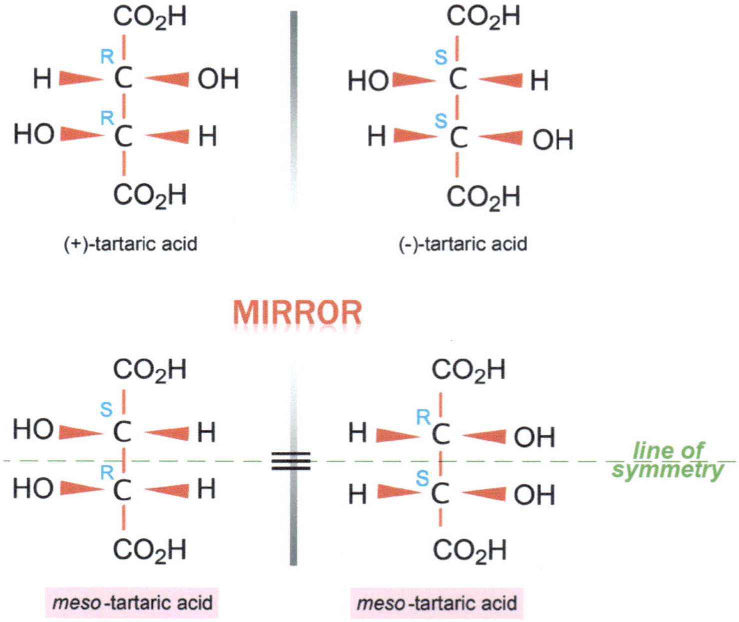

2.4 Conformational Isomers

Conformational isomers are isomers which differ only by the rotation about single bonds. As a result, substituents (= *ligands* = *attached atoms or groups*) can be maximally close (*eclipsed conformation*), maximally apart (*anti or staggered conformation*) or anywhere in between (i.e. *gauche conformation*).

Though all conformations occur at room temperature, anti is most stable since it minimises electron shell repulsion. Conformational isomers (= *conformers*, Fig. IV.B.2.1.1) are not true isomers since they are really just different spatial orientations of the same molecules.

Different conformations can be seen when a molecule is depicted from above and from the right, sawhorse projection, or where the line of sight extends along a carbon-carbon bond axis, a Newman projection. The different conformations occur as the molecule is rotated about its axis.

Example 1: Ethane

The lowest energy, most stable conformation, of ethane is the one in which all six carbon-hydrogen bonds are as far away from each other as possible: *staggered*. The reason, of course, is that atoms are surrounded by an outer shell of negatively charged electrons and, the basic rule of electrostatics is that, like charges repel (= electron shell repulsion = **ESR**).

The highest energy, or least stable conformation, of ethane is the one in which all six carbon-hydrogen bonds are as close as possible: *eclipsed*. In between these two extremes are an infinite number of possibilities. As we have previously reviewed, when carbon is bonded to four atoms (i.e. ethane), its bonds are sp^3 hybridised and the carbon atom sits in the centre of a tetrahedron (ORG 1.2, CHM 3.5).

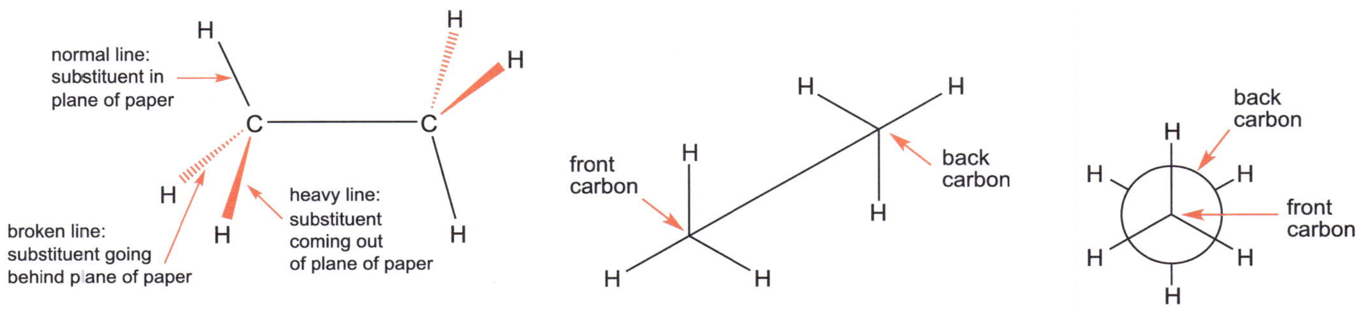

skeletal formula (structure) sawhorse projection Newman projection

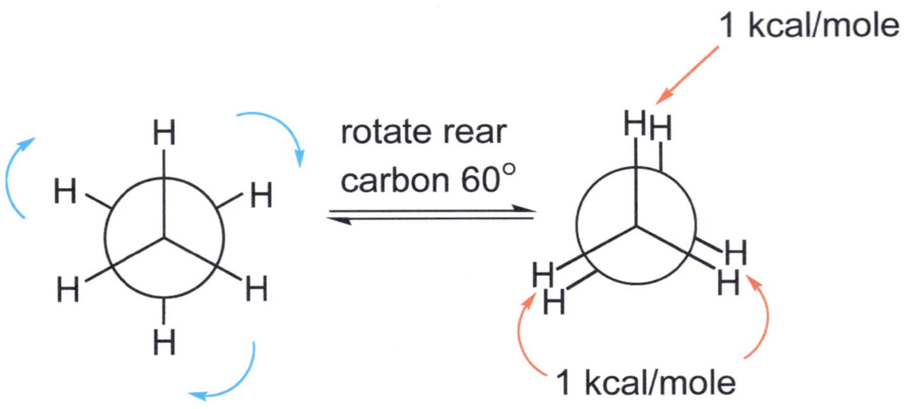
rotate rear
carbon 60°
1 kcal/mole
1 kcal/mole

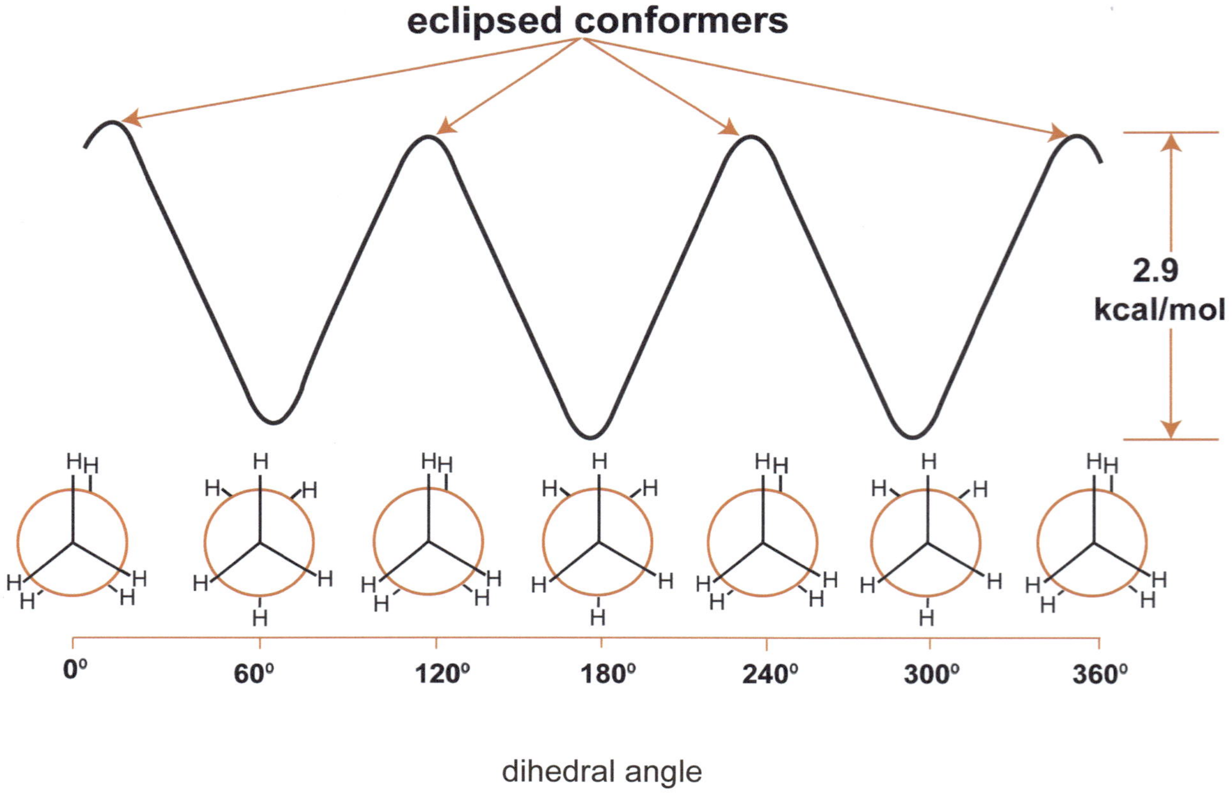
eclipsed conformers
2.9
kcal/mol
0°
60°
120°
180°
240°
300°
360°
dihedral angle

Example 2: Butane

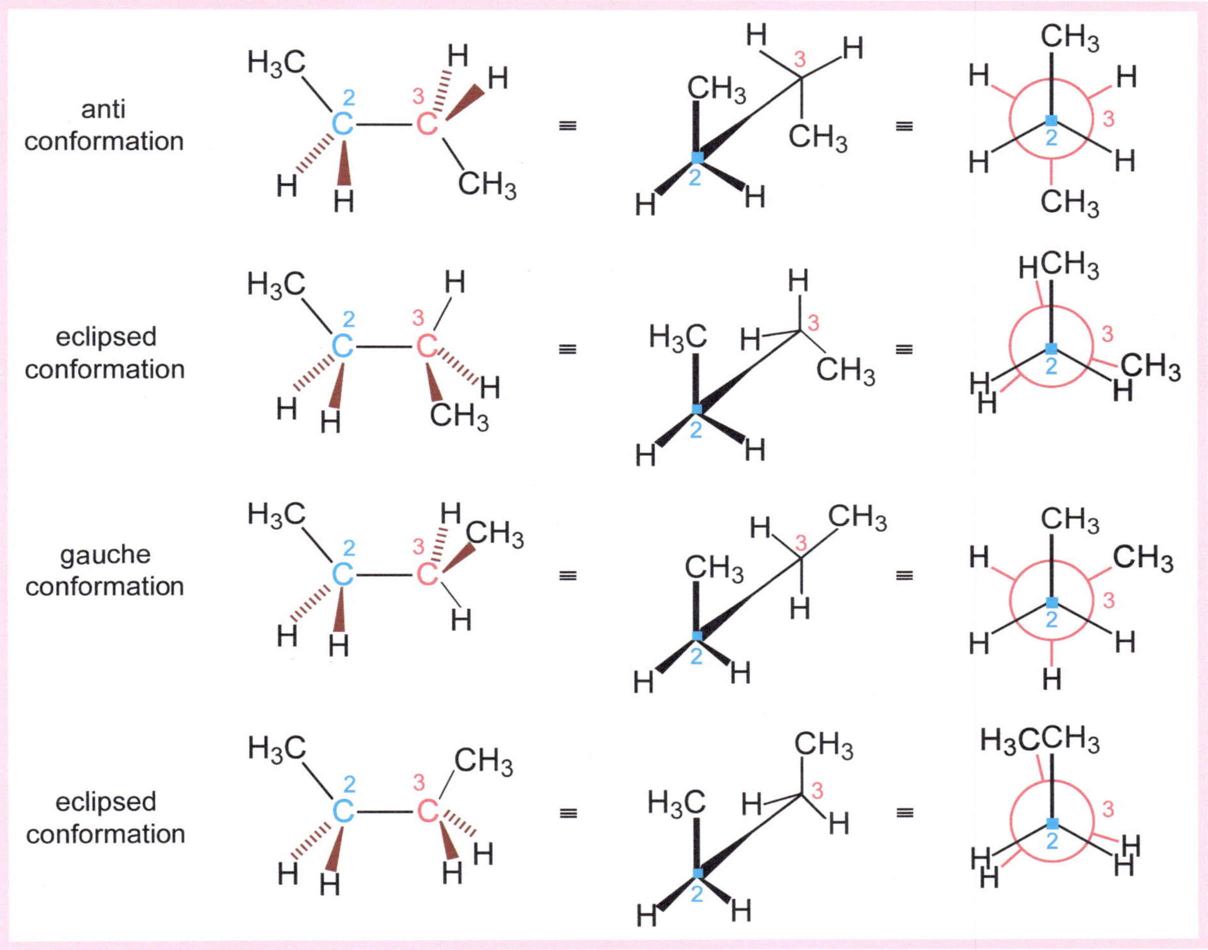

The illustration on the next page (*au verso*) is a plot of potential energy versus rotation about the C2-C3 bond of butane.

The lowest energy arrangement, the anti conformation, is the one in which two methyl groups (C1 and C4) are as far apart as possible, that is, 180 degrees from each other. When two substituents (i.e. the two methyl groups) are anti and in the same plane, they are *antiperiplanar* to each other.

As rotation around the C2-C3 bond occurs, an eclipsed conformation is reached when there are two methyl-hydrogen interactions and one hydrogen-hydrogen interaction. When the rotation continues, the two methyl groups are 60 degrees apart, thus the gauche conformation. It is still higher in energy than the anti conformation even though it has no eclipsing interactions. The reason, again, is ESR. Because ESR is occurring due to the relative bulkiness

High-level Importance

(i.e. big size) of the methyl group compared to hydrogens in this molecule, we say that *steric strain* exists between the two close methyl groups.

When two methyl groups completely overlap with each other, the molecule is said to be totally eclipsed and is in its highest energy state (least stable).

At room temperature, these forms easily interconvert: all forms are present to some degree, though the most stable forms dominate.

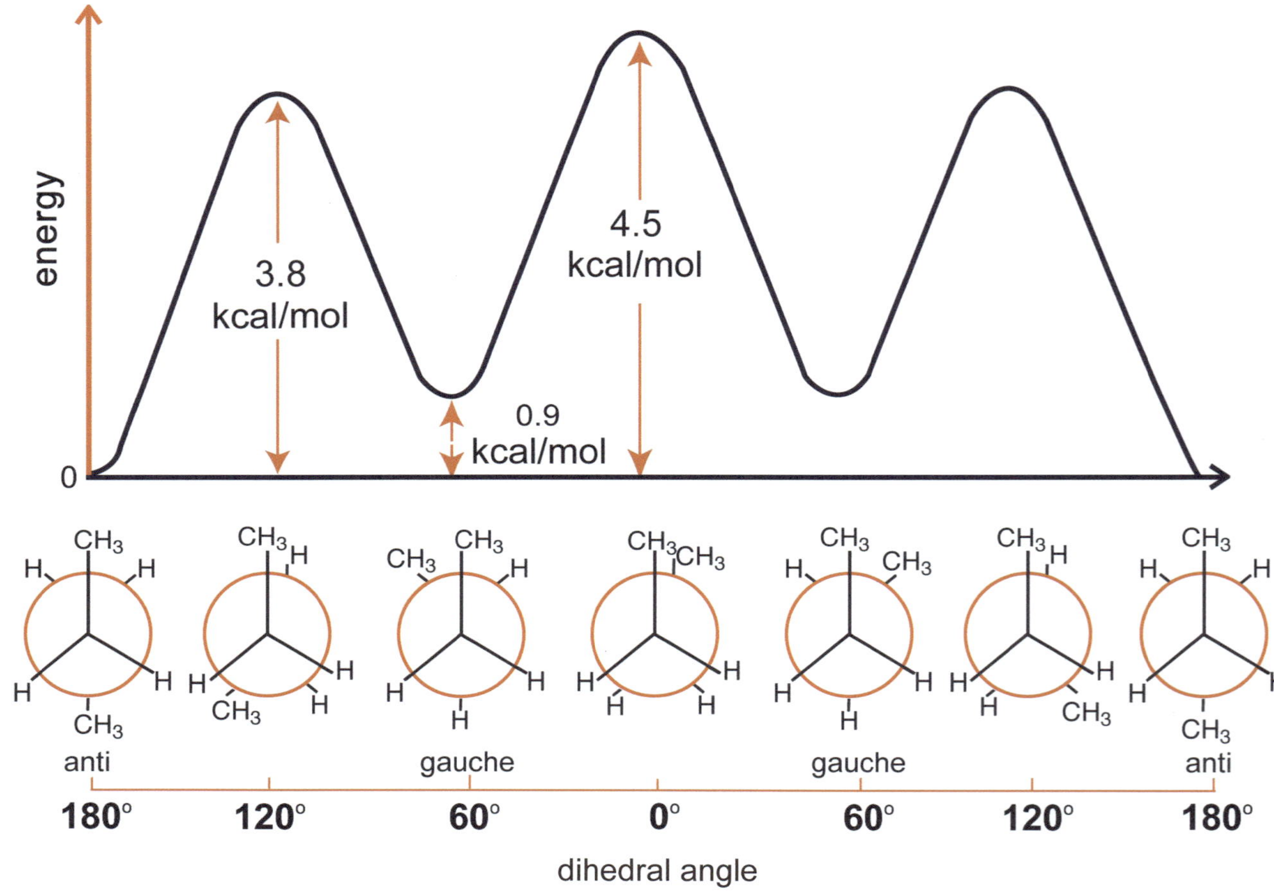

We have seen that conformers rotate about their single bonds. The rotational barrier, or barrier to rotation, is the activation energy (CHM 9.5) required to interconvert a subset of the possible conformations called rotamers. Butane has three rotamers: two gauche conformers and an anti conformer, where the four carbon centres are coplanar. The three eclipsed conformations with angles between the planes (= dihedral angles) of 120°, 0°, and 120° (which is 240° from the first), are not considered to be rotamers, but are instead transition states.

Common Terms

- dihedral angle: torsion (turn/twist) angle
- gauche: skew, synclinal
- **anti**: *trans*, antiperiplanar
- eclipsed: **syn**, *cis*, synperiplanar, torsion angle = 0°

"anti" and "syn" are IUPAC preferred descriptors.

There is no need to try to memorise the terms above. If they are required during the exam, the term(s) will be repeated with some context (image or explanatory text). The key is to understand the ideas behind these terms which have been described in this section (ORG 2.4). Again, chapter review practice questions and/or videos will help clarify any doubts and, thereafter, we also have the free forum.

CHAPTER 2: Stereochemistry

GOLD STANDARD FOUNDATIONAL GAMSAT PRACTICE QUESTIONS

Questions 1–2

Consider the following molecules.

I. $CH_3CH_2CH{=}CHCH_2CH_3$
II. $CH_3CH_2CH_2CH_2CH{=}CH_2$
III. $CH_3CH{=}CHCH_2CH_2CH_3$
IV. $CH_2{=}CHCH_2CH_2CH_2CH_3$

1) Which of the structures represent the same compound?

A. **I** and **II**
B. **II** and **III**
C. **I** and **III**
D. **II** and **IV**

2) Which of the structures can have cis/trans (E/Z) isomers?

A. **I** and **III**
B. **II** and **IV**
C. **III** only
D. **IV** only

3) Consider the 2 structures below:

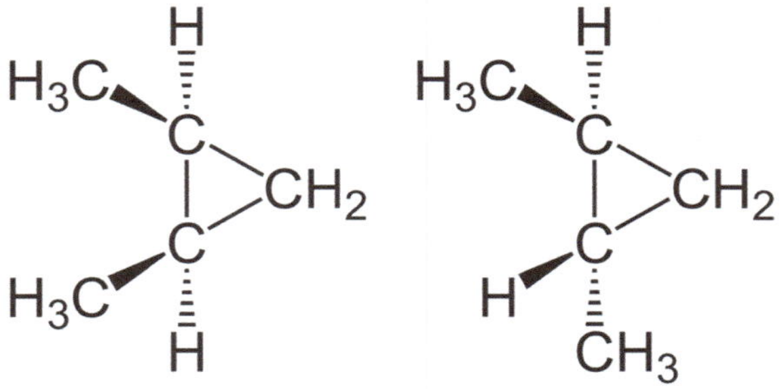

I **II**

A. Structure **I** is *cis* and Structure **II** is *trans*.
B. Structure **I** is *trans* and Structure **II** is *cis*.
C. The two structures are identical.
D. Neither structure has a plane of symmetry.

High-level Importance

GOLD STANDARD GAMSAT-LEVEL PRACTICE QUESTIONS

Questions 4–9

An isomer is each of two or more compounds with the same formula but with a different arrangement of atoms in the molecule. There are two main categories of isomers: 1) structural isomers; and 2) stereoisomers.

Structural (*constitutional*) isomers have different atoms and/or bonding patterns in relation to each other. There are many different kinds of structural isomers including:

- Functional isomers which have the same molecular formula but have different functional groups (ORG 1.6) or *moieties*;
- Positional or *regioisomers* where the functional group changes position on the parent structure.

Stereoisomers are molecules having the same molecular formula and atomic arrangement, but different spatial arrangements. Geometric isomers, a subcategory of stereoisomers, occur because carbons that are in a ring or double bond structure are unable to freely rotate. This results in *cis* and *trans* compounds.

Consider the following molecules.

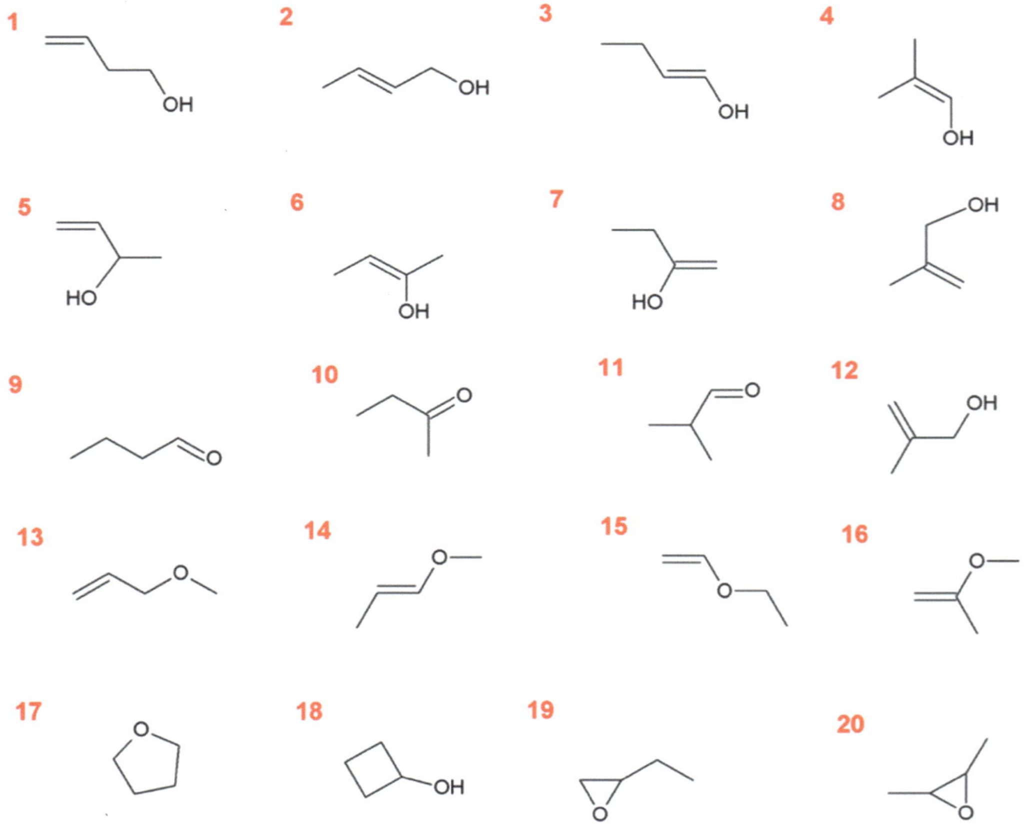

Figure 1

4) Structures 2 and 6 are related to each other as:

A. functional isomers.
B. regioisomers.
C. geometric isomers.
D. More than one of the above is correct.

5) Among the structures 1, 5, 10, and 14, pairs of which of the following can be identified?

A. Functional isomers
B. Regioisomers
C. Geometric isomers
D. More than one of the above is correct.

6) Are structures 7 and 17 isomers?

A. No, they differ in terms of the number and/or types of atoms in the structures.
B. No, they are completely different molecules.
C. Yes, they have the same molecular formula.
D. Yes, they have the same number of carbon atoms.

7) How many possible structural isomers are there for C_4H_8?

A. 2
B. 4
C. 5
D. More than 5

Question 8 is based on the following new information.

8) Consider three standard ways to represent benzene.

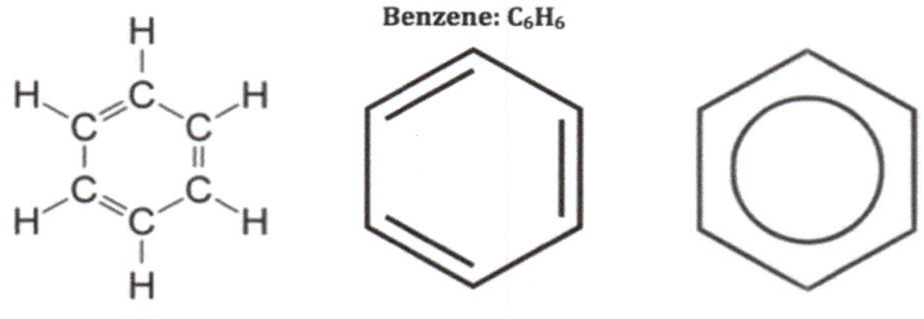

(1) (2) (3)

How many of the following 5 structures are constitutional isomers of benzene?

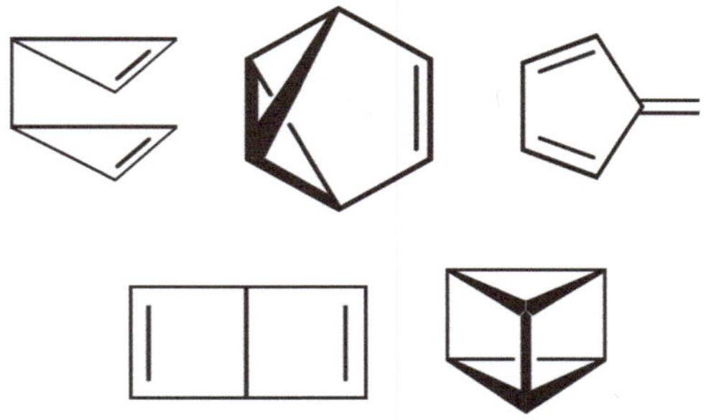

A. Less than 3
B. 3
C. 4
D. 5

9) Which of the following is in the *trans* configuration?

A.
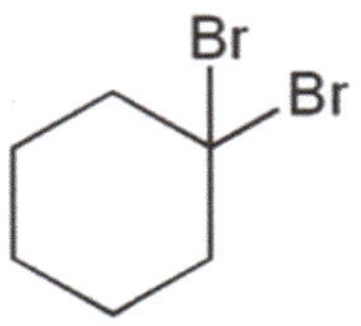

C.
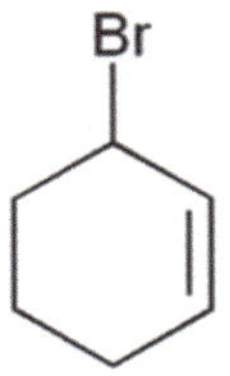

B.
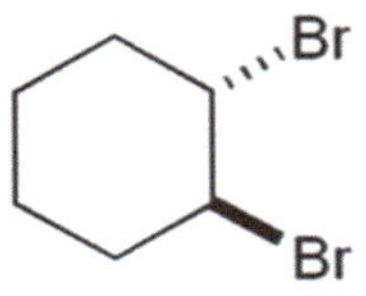

D.
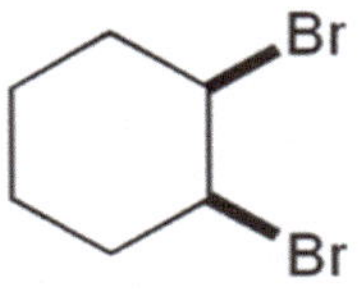

High-level Importance

Questions 10–12

Because of the symmetry of the benzene ring, if a monosubstituted benzene is evaluated, there could only be one such molecule. The one substituent, or ligand, replaces hydrogen at a carbon which would then be referred to as carbon-1.

However, when the benzene ring already has a substituent then substituted isomers are possible. Consider the following structure of methylbenzene.

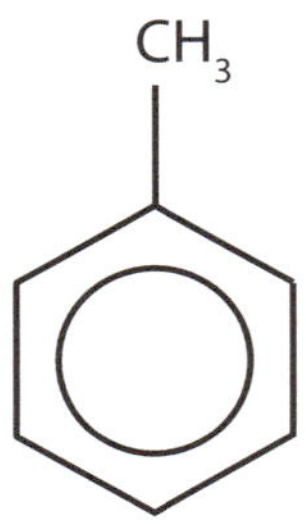

Any single hydrogen - whether from the ring or from the substituent - on methylbenzene can be replaced (monosubstituted) but that does not always result in a different isomer. For example, there are 3 hydrogens on the methyl substituent, but replacing any one of them with another atom (e.g. fluorine) would produce three identical molecules because the connectivity would not have changed. Whereas, substituting non-equivalent hydrogens like a methyl hydrogen vs. one of the ring hydrogens would produce 2 different isomers. Occasionally, the number of disubstituted or trisubstituted isomers must be determined.

For each of the following three questions, assess the substitution of any hydrogen in methylbenzene by fluorine and then determine if the products created are different from one another.

10) How many different monosubstituted isomers of methylbenzene are possible?

A. 2
B. 4
C. 5
D. 7

11) How many different disubstituted isomers of methylbenzene are possible?

A. 4
B. 6
C. 8
D. 10

12) As compared to disubstituted isomers of methylbenzene, how many trisubstituted isomers of methylbenzene are possible?

A. Fewer
B. Same
C. An increase of 50%
D. An increase greater than 50%

---

13) For which of the compounds below are *cis-trans* isomers possible?

I. $CH_3CH{=}CHCH_3$
II. $CH_3CH{=}CHCH_2CH_3$
III. $CH_3CH{=}CH_2$

A. **I** only
B. **I** and **II** only
C. **II** and **III** only
D. **I**, **II** and **III**

14) Consider the following conversion of one form of Vitamin A into another.

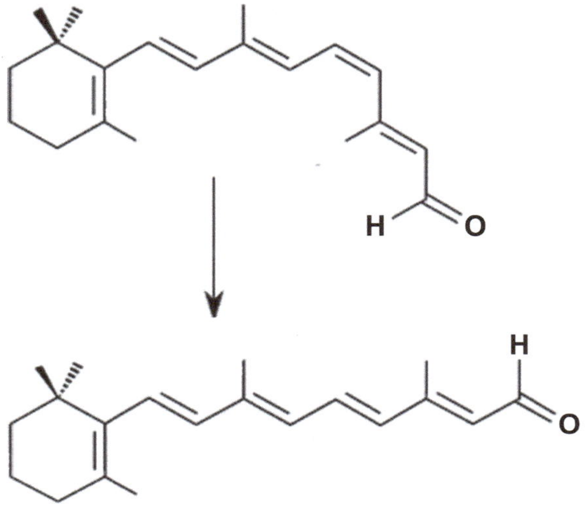

What is the difference between the 2 structures above?

A. Different number of carbons

B. Different number of hydrogens

C. Different *cis/trans* isomers at one double bond

D. Different *cis/trans* isomers at two double bonds

Questions 15–16

Tamoxifen, is a selective estrogen receptor modulator used to prevent breast cancer in high-risk women and to treat breast cancer in select women and men. Consider the molecular structure of tamoxifen below.

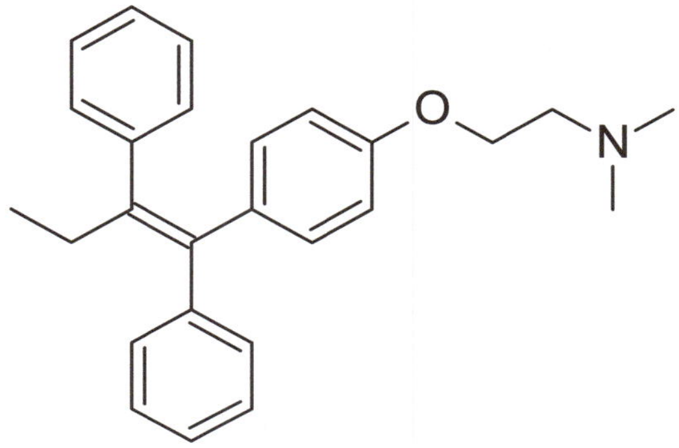

15) All carbon-carbon double bonds in tamoxifen are in which configuration?

A. *Z*

B. *E*

C. Most are *Z* but one is *E*.

D. Neither **A**, nor **B**, nor **C** is correct.

16) A molecule of tamoxifen has how many carbons?

A. Less than 25

B. 25

C. 26

D. More than 26

High-level Importance

Questions 17–24

A Newman projection, useful in alkane stereochemistry, visualises the conformation of a chemical bond from front to back, with the front atom represented by a dot (*where 3 lines meet*) and the back carbon as a circle. The front carbon atom is called *proximal*, while the back atom is called *distal*. This type of representation clearly illustrates the specific *dihedral angle* between the groups attached to the proximal and distal atoms. The Newman projection is an alternative to a sawhorse projection, which views a carbon-carbon bond from an oblique angle.

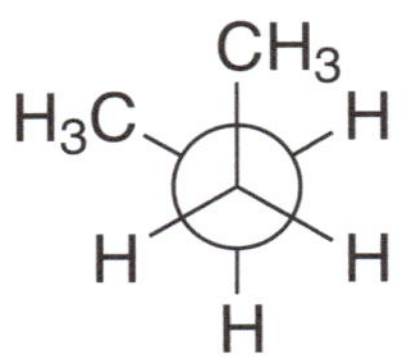

Newman projection: butane in the gauche conformation

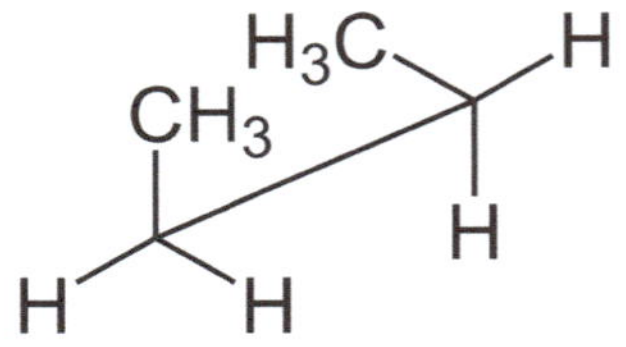

Sawhorse projection with the left side forward: butane in the gauche conformation

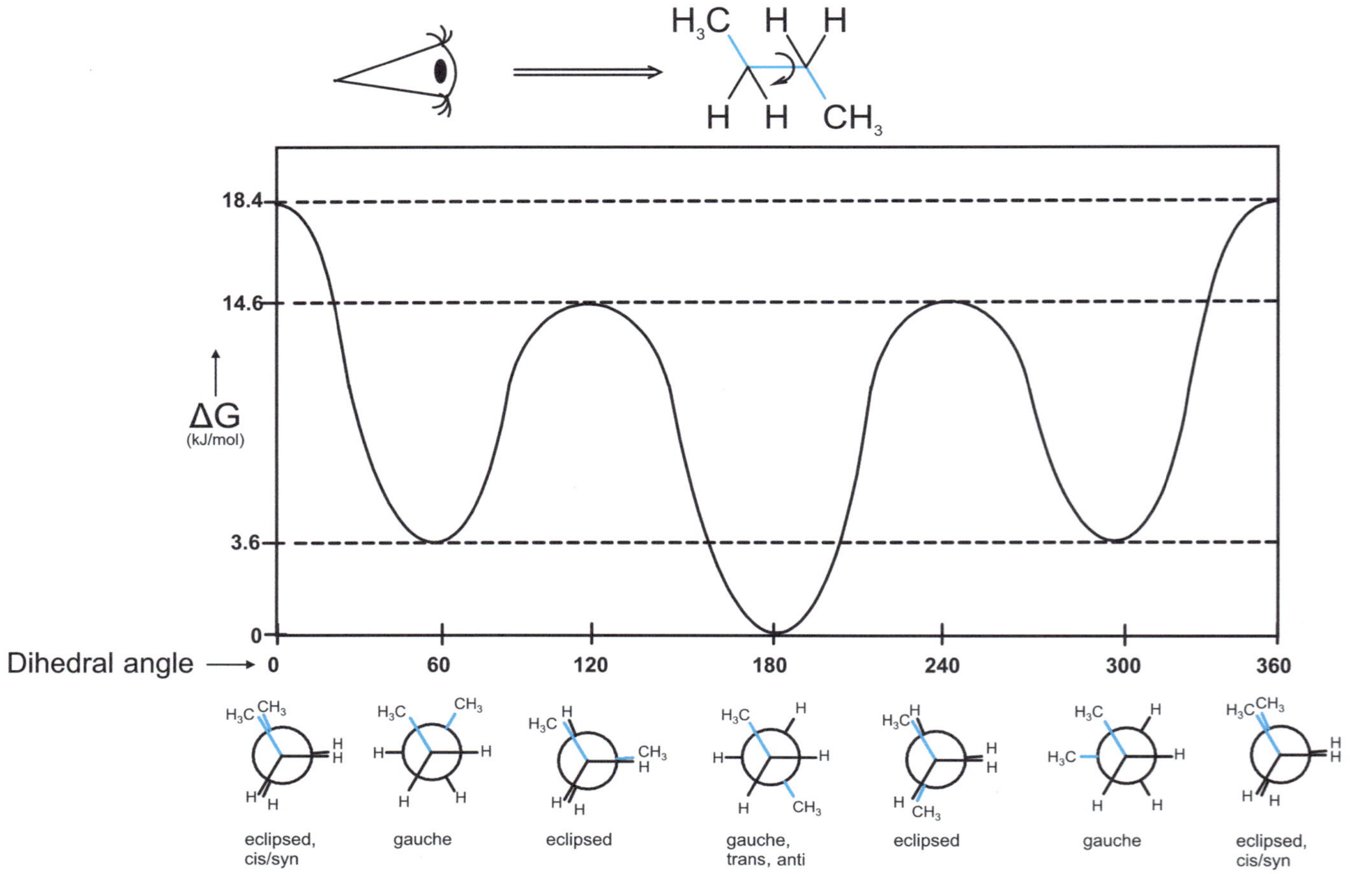

Figure 1: Free energy diagram of n-butane as a function of the dihedral angle in degrees (modified from Roland Mattern with anti/gauche corrections and axis labels; Wikimedia Commons 2021)

17) According to Figure 1, which of the following conformations has a dihedral angle approximately midway between 60° and 180°?

A. 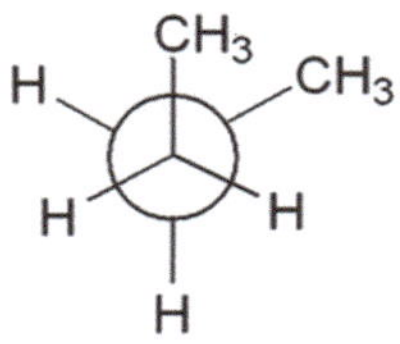

C. 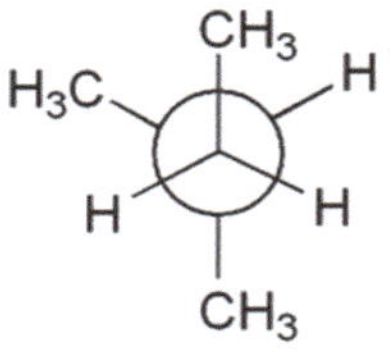

B. 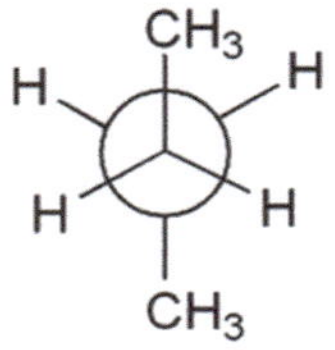

D. 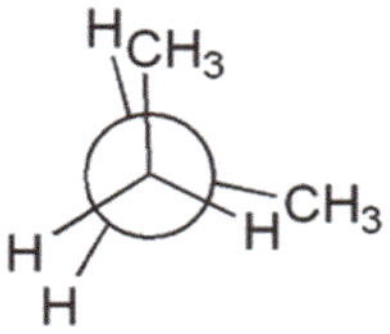

18) According to Figure 1, which of the following conformations of butane has a free energy of less that 14 kJ/mol?

Note that:

1) Me represents the methyl group, CH_3;

2) a darkened line projects towards you and a broken line projects away from you.

A. 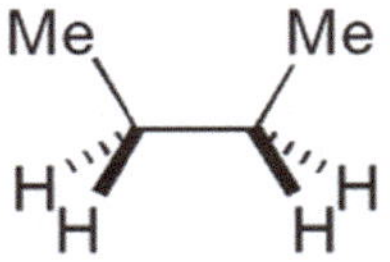

C. 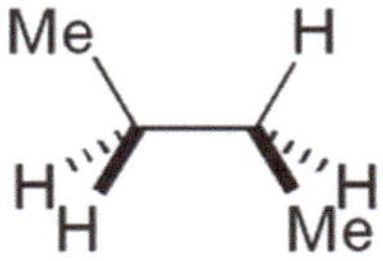

B. 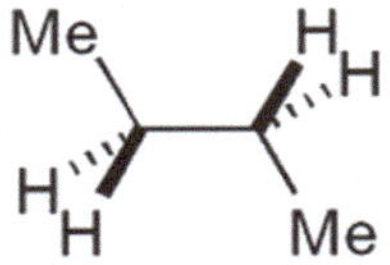

D. 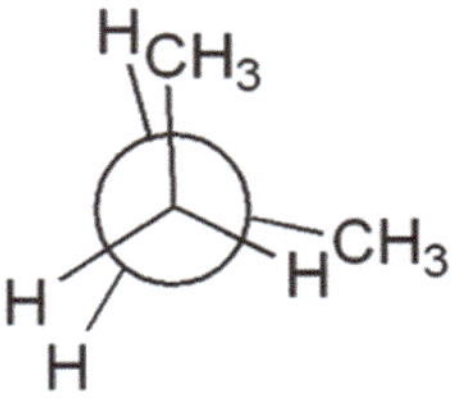

19) What is the minimum dihedral angle of rotation to convert the gauche conformation of butane to the anti conformation?

A. 30 degrees
B. 60 degrees
C. 90 degrees
D. 120 degrees

20) The phenyl group, or phenyl ring, is a cyclic group of atoms with the formula C_6H_5 which serves as an attachment to another atom or group of atoms. It is sometimes symbolised as Ph.

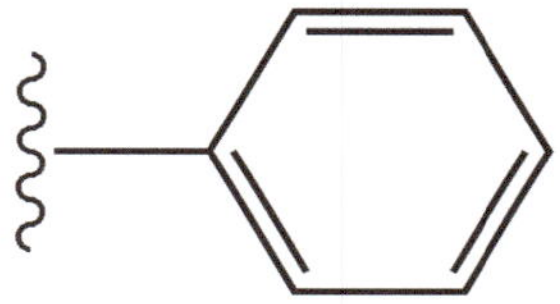

According to Figure 1, which of the following conformations of 1,2-diphenylethane is likely to have a free energy of approximately 0 kJ/mol?

A. 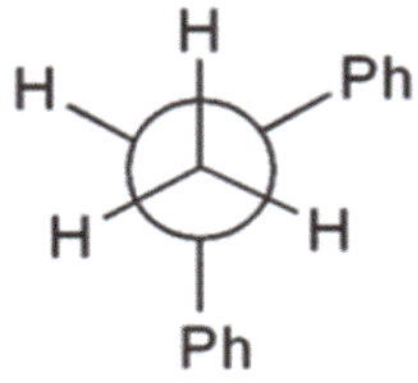

C. 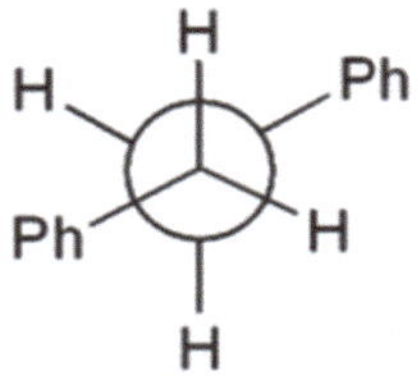

B. 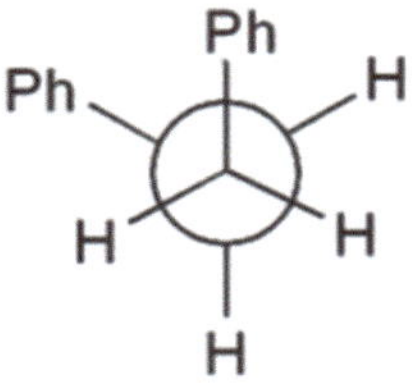

D. 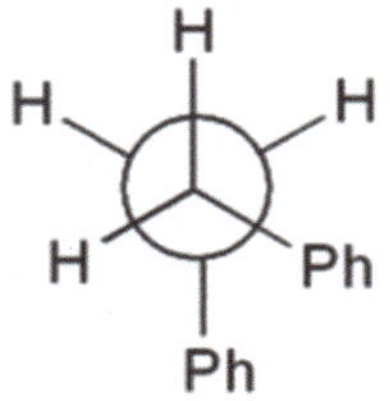

High-level Importance

21) Identify accurate representations for the linear structure **Z**.

$CH_3CH_2CH_2CH(CH_3)Cl$

Z

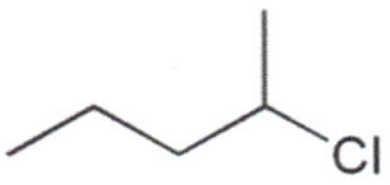

I

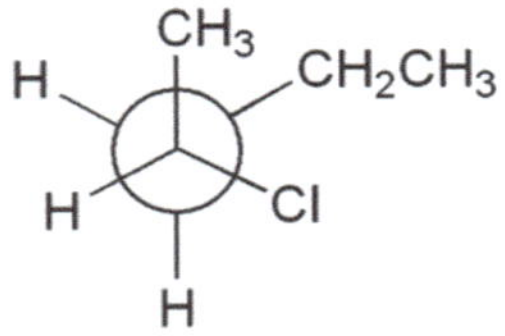

III

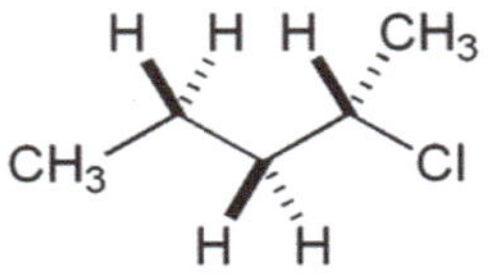

II

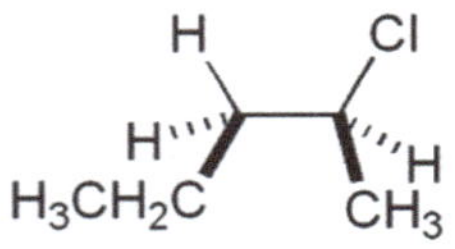

IV

A. **I** and **III** only
B. **II** and **IV** only
C. **I**, **II** and **III** only
D. **I**, **II**, **III** and **IV**

22) For the following sawhorse projection **Z**, choose its Newman projection viewed along the C_2-C_3 bond from the right-hand side:

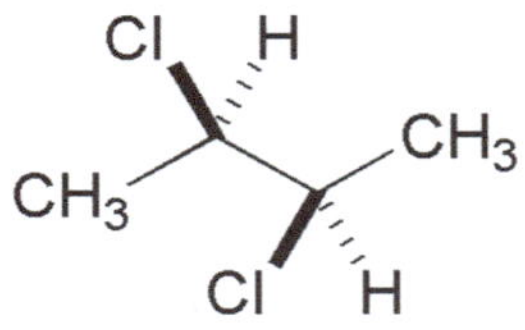

Z

A.
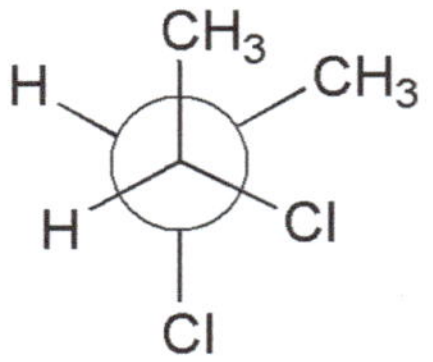

C.
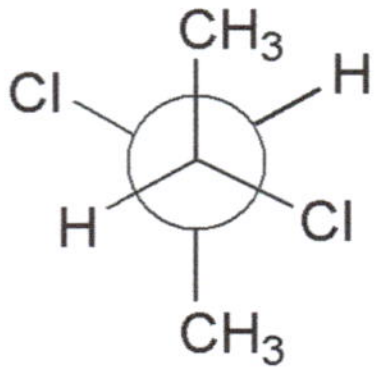

B.
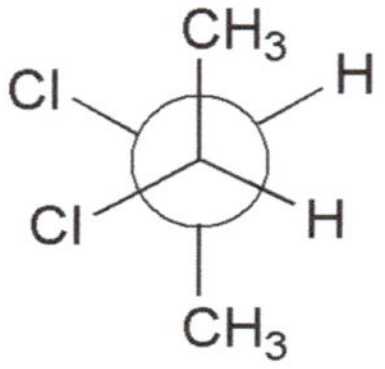

D.
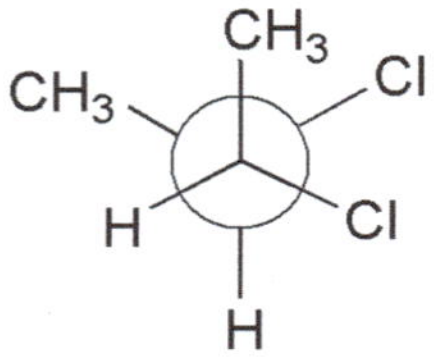

23) For the following sawhorse projection **Z**, choose its Newman projection (viewed along the C_2-C_3 bond from the right-hand side):

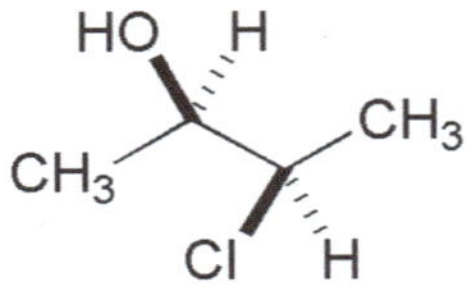

Z

A.
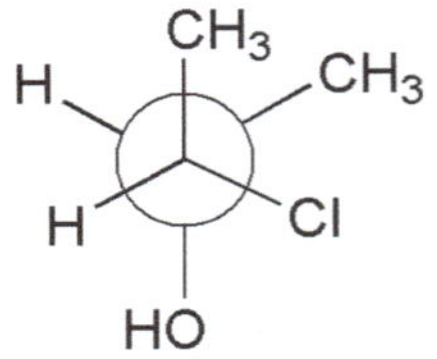

C.
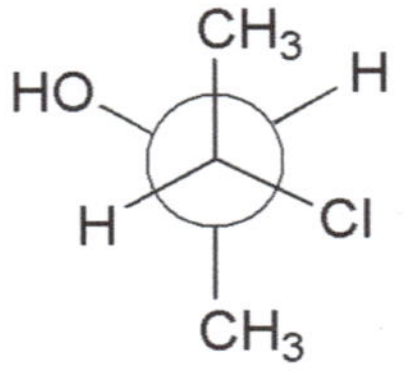

B.
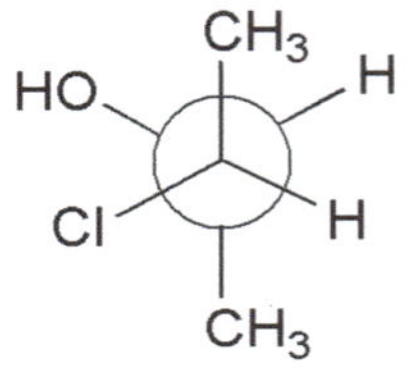

D.
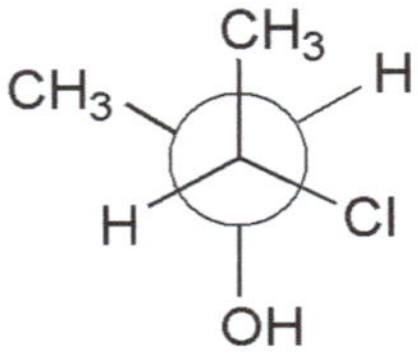

24) Note: If you have no experience naming organic compounds, skip this question and do not look at the worked solution; instead, try this question after you have read ORG 3.1.

Consider the following Newman projection for 2,2-dimethylbutane.

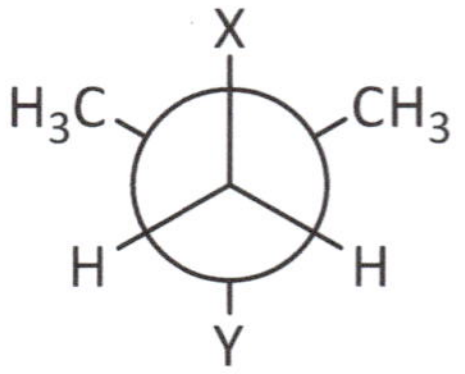

The letters X and Y, respectively, must represent which of the following?

A. H and H
B. H and CH_3
C. CH_3 and H
D. CH_3 and CH_3

Questions 25–31

An asymmetric carbon atom (i.e. a stereocentre, or *chiral* carbon) is attached to four different types of atoms or groups of atoms. Le Bel-van't Hoff rule states that the number of stereoisomers of an organic compound is 2^n, where n represents the number of chiral carbon atoms (*unless there is an internal plane of symmetry*).

Assigning a stereochemical configuration at each chiral carbon in a molecule can be done by using the following CIP priority rules:

1. Identify the chiral carbon, and the four attached groups.
2. Assign priorities to the four groups, using the following rules:
   i. Atoms of higher atomic number have higher priority.
   ii. The higher priority is assigned to the group with the atom of higher atomic number or mass at the first point of difference.
   iii. If the difference between the two groups is due to the number of otherwise identical atoms, the higher priority is assigned to the group with the greater number of atoms of higher atomic number or mass.
   iv. To assign priority of double or triple bonded groups, multiple-bonded atoms are considered as equivalent number of single bonded atoms, thus:

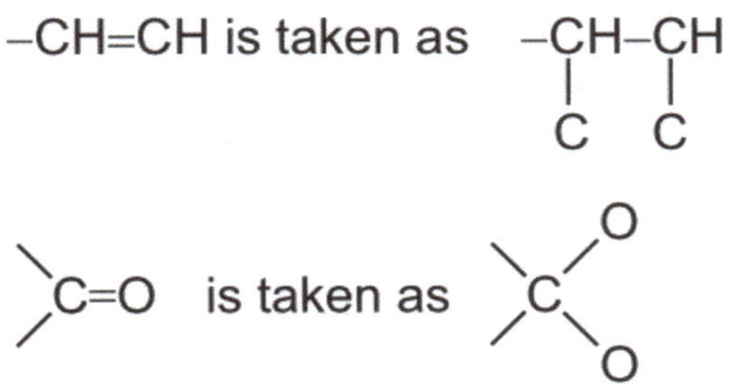

3. The chiral carbon is then evaluated from the side opposite the atom or group with the lowest priority. If the order of the other three atoms or groups in decreasing priorities is clockwise, the arrangement is designated *R*; if counterclockwise, the arrangement is designated *S*.

If two groups with the higher priorities are on opposite sides of a double bond, then it is an *E*-isomer, and if on the same side of the double bond, then it is a *Z*-isomer.

25) Which of the following molecules are chiral?

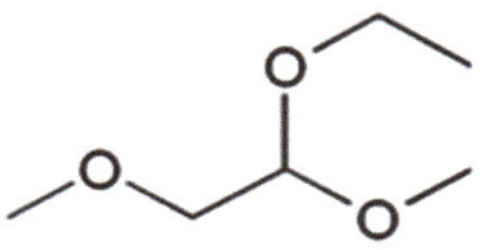

I

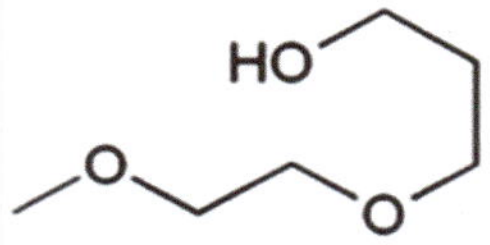

II

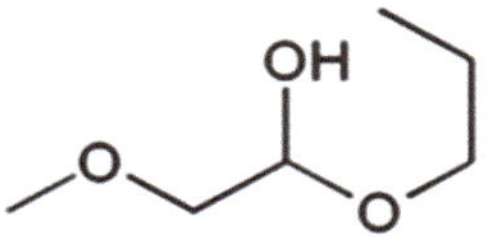

III

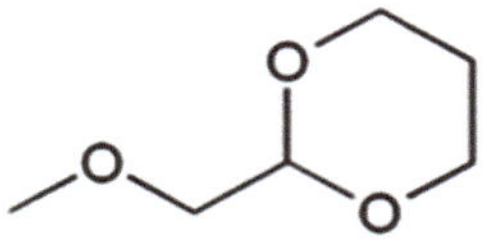

IV

A. **I** and **III**
B. **II** and **III**
C. **III** and **IV**
D. **I** and **II**

26) Predict the number of stereoisomers for molecule **A** (note: Me = methyl; Et = ethyl):

EtCH(OH)CH(Cl)Me

A

A. 0
B. 1
C. 2
D. 4

27) Assign the configuration of molecule **A**:

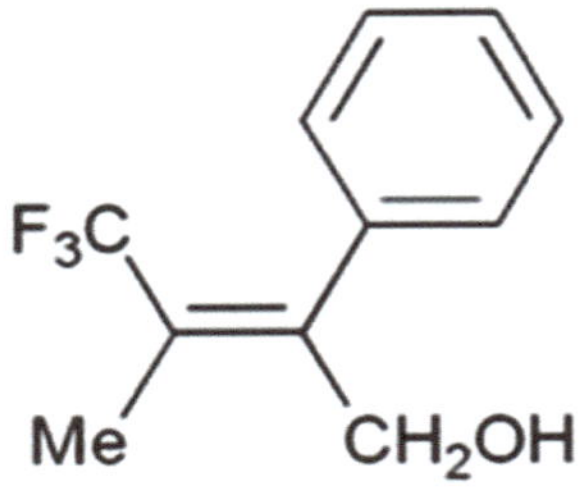

A

A. (*R*)-
B. (*S*)-
C. (*E*)-
D. (*Z*)-

28) Identify the (*S*)-configuration among the following molecules.

Note that the broken line indicates the direction of the attached group is away from you; whereas, the bold (dark) line indicates the direction of the attached group is towards you.

A. 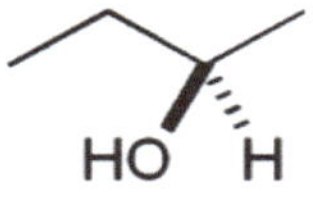

C. 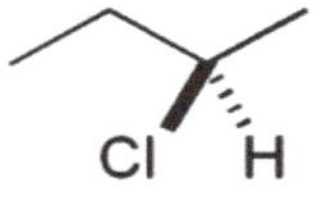

B. 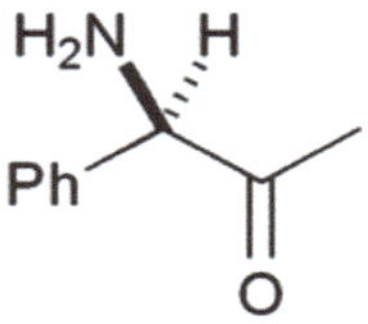

D. 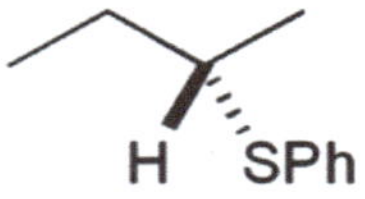

29) Meso compounds are achiral (*not* chiral) compounds that have multiple chiral centres (*stereocentres*). A meso compound can be "superposed" on its mirror image, and is optically inactive despite its stereocentres.

Identify the meso compound.

A. 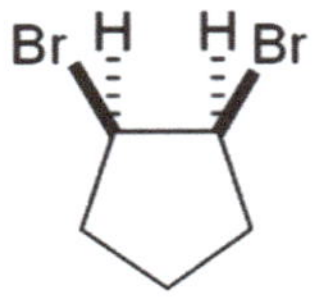

C. 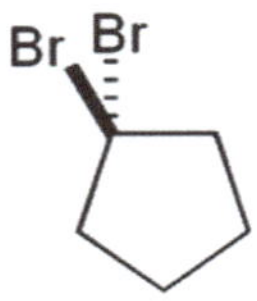

B. 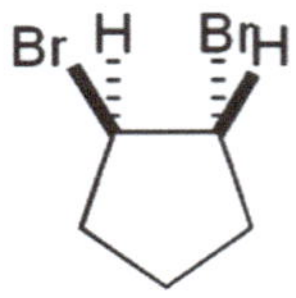

D. 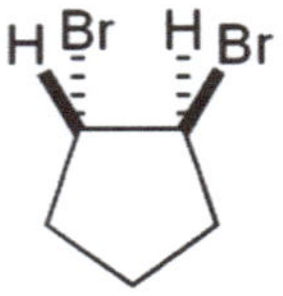

30) Which of the following molecules have the same configurations as molecule **Z**?

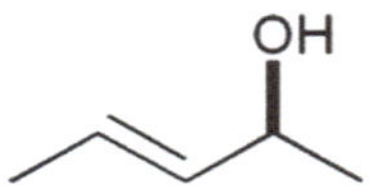

Z

I: 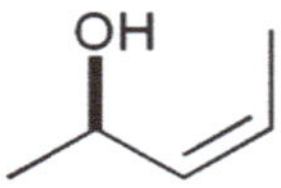

III: 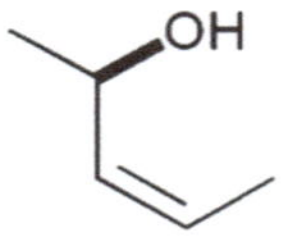

II: 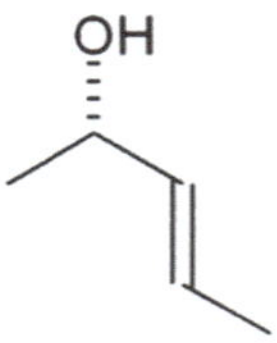

IV: 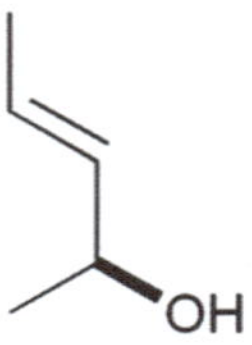

A. **I** and **III**
B. **II** and **IV**
C. **III** and **IV**
D. **I** and **II**

High-level Importance

31) Vitamin B_{12} is illustrated below with the moiety (*portion of the molecule*) containing the corrin ring within the blue box.

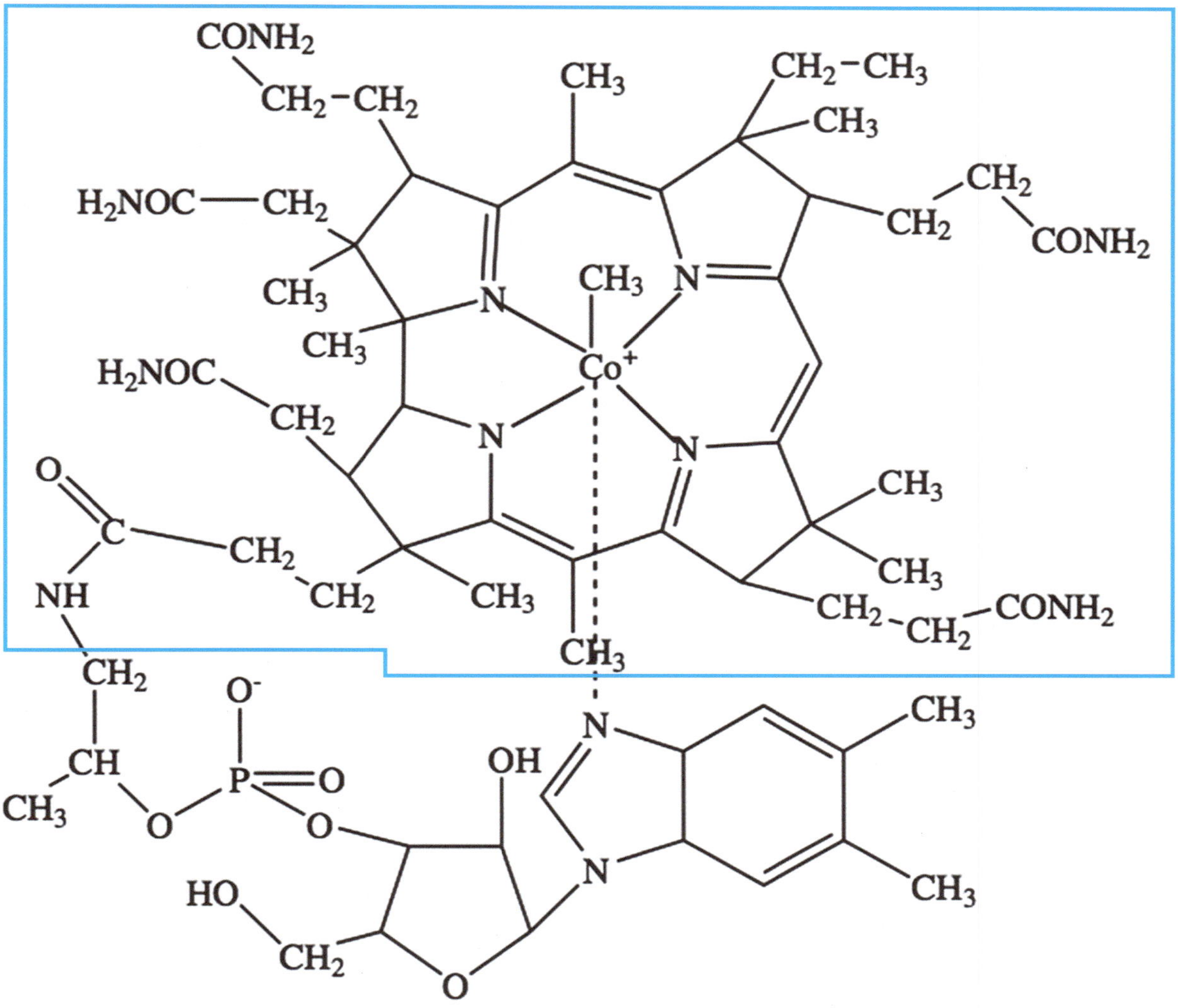

How many stereocentres (chiral carbons) are there in the moiety of Vitamin B_{12} within the blue box?

A. Less than 8

B. 8

C. 9

D. More than 9

Question 32

Stereoisomers may be divided into enantiomers and diastereomers. Enantiomers must have opposite, absolute configurations at each and every chiral carbon.

Conversely, diastereomers are any pair of stereoisomers that are not enantiomers. Diastereomers are both chemically and physically different from each other.

Stereoisomers *always* have the same connectivity. Among molecules with the same connectivity:

- Molecules that are mirror images but *non*-superposable are **enantiomers**.
- If they are not superposable, and they are not mirror images, then they are **diastereomers**.

Consider the following structures.

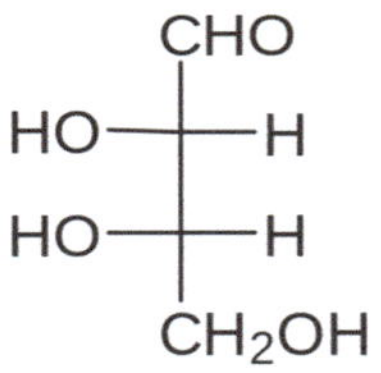

I

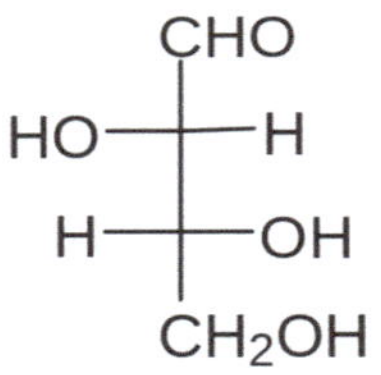

II

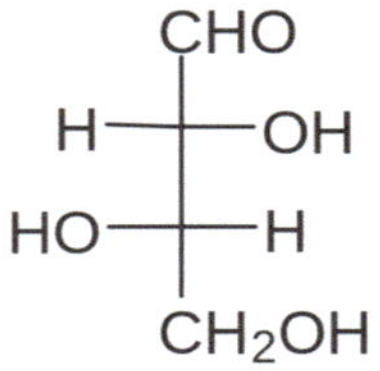

III

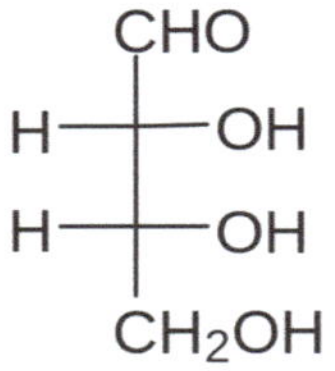

IV

32) Structure **IV** is the enantiomer of which of the following structures?

A. **I**
B. **II**
C. **III**
D. Neither **I**, nor **II**, nor **III**

Questions 33–35

Optical isomers are enantiomers, and thus are stereoisomers that differ by different spatial orientations about a chiral carbon atom (*stereocentre*). An optical isomer exhibits *optical activity* which means that the isomer can rotate the plane of plane-polarised light to some non-zero degree.

Optical activity is a useful way to classify the identity of a substance.

A group of students performed an exercise to determine the specific rotation $[\alpha_D]$ of the poison coniine, using the formula:

$$[\alpha_D] = \frac{\text{observed rotation, } \alpha \text{ (degrees)}}{\text{path length, } l \text{ (dm)} \times \text{concentration, } C \text{ (g/ml)}}$$

The students carefully dissolved 3.00 g of coniine in 20.0 ml ethanol. It was then placed in a sample cell with a 5.00 cm path length. They then observed a rotation which was +1.51°.

33) Approximate the specific rotation of coniine.

A. +10.9°
B. +20.1°
C. –10.1°
D. –20.9°

34) A mixture of compound A ($[\alpha]_D^{25}$ = +20.00) and its enantiomer B ($[\alpha]_D^{25}$ = –20.00) has a specific rotation of +10.00. What is the composition of the mixture?

A. 25% A, 75% B
B. 50% A, 50% B
C. 75% A, 25% B
D. 50% A, 0% B

Question 35 is based on the following additional information.

Meso compounds are achiral (*not* chiral) compounds that have multiple chiral centres (*stereocentres*). A meso compound can have an internal plane of symmetry and/or be superposed on its mirror image. Meso compounds are optically **inactive** despite its stereocentres.

35) Identify which of the following molecules do **not** rotate the plane of plane-polarised light.

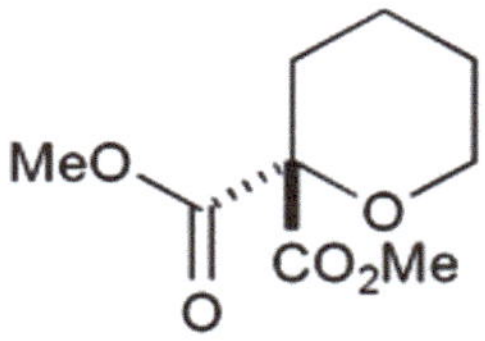

I

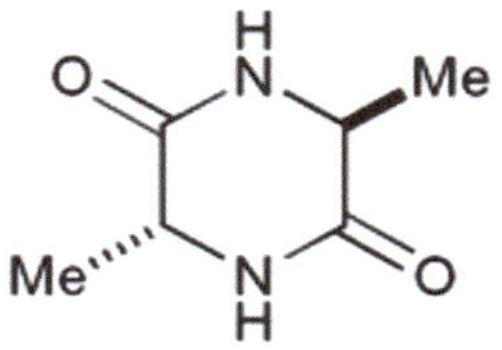

II

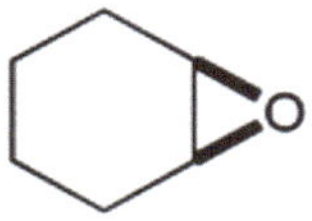

III

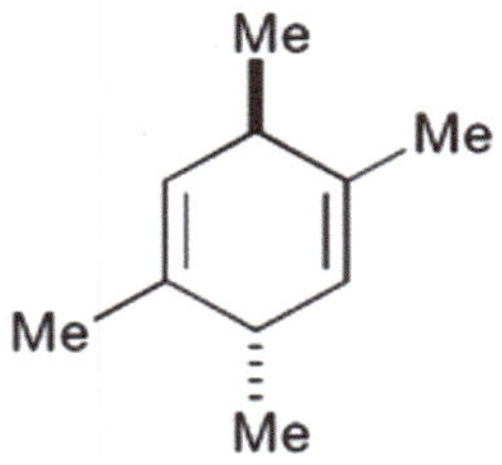

IV

A. **I** and **II** **B.** **II** and **III** **C.** **II** and **IV** **D.** **I**, **II**, **III** and **IV**

SPOILER ALERT

Gold Standard has cross-referenced the content in this chapter to examples from ACER's official GAMSAT practice materials. It is for you to decide when you want to explore these questions since you may want to preserve some of ACER's materials for timed mock-exam practice.

Examples – Identifying structural isomers: Q36 of 1; comparing different stereoisomers (*'superimposable' or not, able to produce stereoisomers or not + basic nomenclature*): Q40-41 of 2; chiral carbons, 3D vs Fischer projections (*'superimposable' or not; R or S*): Q83-86 of 3; challenge unit with substitutions of benzene isomers: Q18-23 of 4; would ACER force you to count over half-dozen chiral centres in a large molecule? Yes, cholesterol; this unit also includes meso compounds (*note: some versions are missing structures in Q60; you can find the structures using Google Images*): Q59-62 of 4; constitutional (*structural*) isomers, but very basic nomenclature is needed: Q93-94 of 4; count the number of stereocentres in carbohydrates: Q76-78 of 5. Note that "Q" is followed by the question number, and, for example, "of 1" refers to booklet number 1 which is referenced in the Spoiler Alert table at the end of Chapter 1. The 15 full-length GAMSAT practice tests by Gold Standard, HEAPS-1 through HEAPS-15, contain specific cross-references to this chapter within the worked solutions. Note that the preamble (set up) for the unit with *R/S*, *E/Z* configurations is from HEAPS-3, but all of the questions are novel; the mono and disubstitution of benzene isomers is from HEAPS-6.

High-level Importance

Chapter Checklist

- ☐ Access your online account to view answers, worked solutions and discussion boards.
- ☐ Reassess your 'learning objectives' for this chapter: Go back to the first page of this chapter and re-evaluate the top 3 boxes and the Introduction.
  - ☐ Please be sure that you have completed the *Need for Speed* exercises at the beginning of this chapter.
- ☐ Complete a maximum of 1 page of notes using symbols/abbreviations to represent the entire chapter based on your learning objectives. These are your Gold Notes.
- ☐ Consider your multimedia options based on your optimal way of learning:
  - ☐ Download the free Gold Standard GAMSAT app for your Android device or iPhone.
  - ☐ Create your own, tangible study cards or try the free app: Anki.
  - ☐ Record your voice reading your Gold Notes onto your smartphone (audio files, e.g., *memo* or MP3s) and listen during exercise, transportation, etc.
  - ☐ Try out the Gold Standard GAMSAT online videos at gamsat-prep.com, or you can try other options on YouTube like Khan Academy or Crash Course Organic Chemistry.
- ☐ Reassess your schedule for your full-length GAMSAT practice tests: ACER and/or HEAPS exams. Ensure that you have scheduled one full day to complete a practice test and 1-2 days for a thorough assessment of worked solutions while adding to your abbreviated Gold Notes.
- ☐ Reassess your progress in scheduling and/or evaluating stress reduction techniques such as regular exercise (sports), yoga, meditation and/or mindfulness exercises (*see* YouTube for suggestions).

Chapter 3

Memorise

* IUPAC nomenclature

Understand

* Trends based on length, branching
* Ring strain, ESR
* Complete combustion
* Free radicals

Importance

Low level: 0% of GAMSAT Organic Chemistry questions released by ACER are related to content in this chapter (in our estimation).
* Note that approximately 60% of the questions in GAMSAT Organic Chemistry are related to just 4 chapters: 2, 6, 7 and 12.

GAMSAT-Prep.com

Introduction

Alkanes (a.k.a. paraffins) are compounds that consist only of the elements carbon (C) and hydrogen (H) (i.e. hydrocarbons). In addition, C and H are linked together exclusively by single bonds (i.e. they are *saturated* compounds). Methane is the simplest possible alkane while saturated oils and fats are much larger.

Alkanes are used primarily as fuels (i.e. burned to produce heat or energy), but their derivatives can be found in paints, plastics, cosmetics, cleaners and pharmaceuticals. They are highly combustible and form carbon dioxide and water as they burn. The main components of natural gas are methane and ethane. Propane and butane are used as liquefied petroleum gas. Propane is also used in a propane gas burner (barbecue), butane in disposable cigarette lighters. Other alkanes with more carbons are components in different types of fuels and lubricating oils.

Although it is unlikely that this chapter will provide you with direct, assumed knowledge that will be required for your test, Chapter 3 is the first chapter to lay down the **rules for nomenclature which is an essential component for GAMSAT**, though usually related to oxygen and nitrogen-containing molecules, which we will learn about in later chapters. As always, the **GAMSAT-level practice questions in this chapter** *definitely* require the type of reasoning that you could be exposed to during your upcoming digital GAMSAT.

Multimedia Resources at GAMSAT-Prep.com

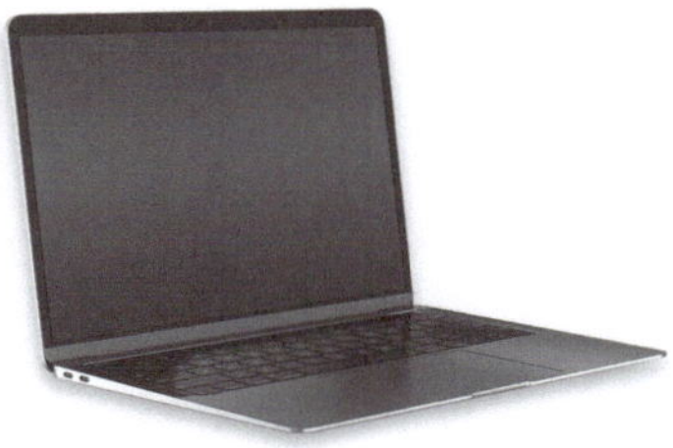

Open Discussion Boards
(*gamsat-prep.com/forum*)

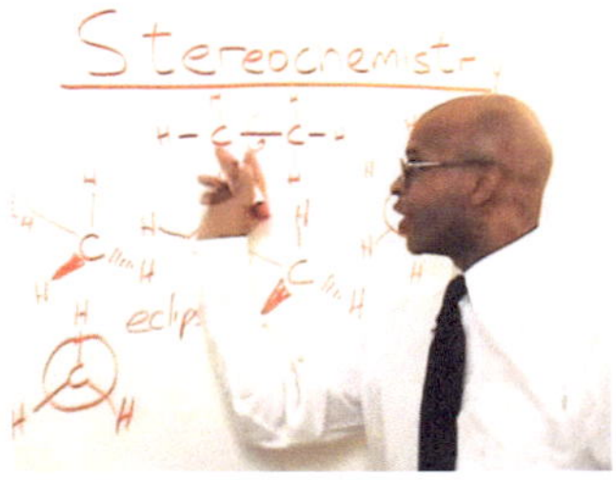

Science Preparation Videos

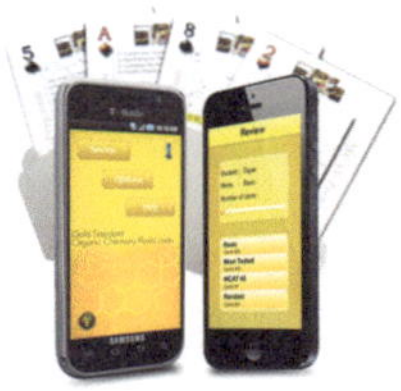

Flashcards

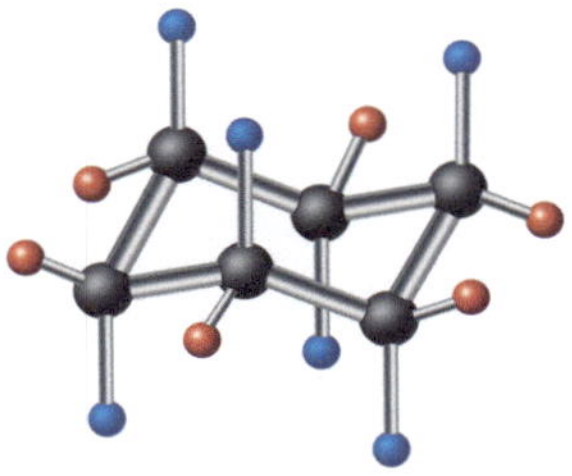

Special Guest

* The real GAMSAT may have advanced-level information presented (i.e. in a passage) but previous knowledge of said information is not required to answer the questions that would follow. Practice questions at the end of this chapter, as well as ACER and GS (HEAPS) practice GAMSATs can help you clarify this point.

3.0 GAMSAT has a *Need for Speed*!

Section	GAMSAT Organic Chemistry *Need for Speed* Exercises

3.1

Indicate the IUPAC-approved prefixes based on the number of carbons in the longest carbon chain:

C_1 = ____________ C_5 = ____________ C_8 = ____________

C_2 = ____________ C_6 = ____________ C_9 = ____________

C_3 = ____________ C_7 = ____________ C_{10} = ____________

C_4 = ____________

Label the indicated carbons as follows: primary carbon atom (1°); secondary carbon atom (2°); tertiary carbon atom (3°); quaternary carbon atom (4°).

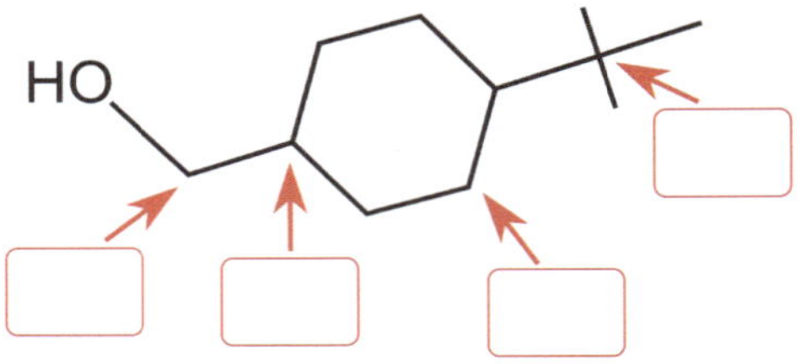

3.2.1

What are the two final chemical products of the complete combustion of hydrocarbons?

____

{Side note: this is true whether it be from a car's internal combustion engine, an animal's cellular respiration, or even a forest fire.}

3.2.2

The following is a radical substitution reaction (*involving free radicals*). Indicate the missing reactant or product in each case (*naturally, all reactions must be balanced*).

i. Initiation:

$Cl\!:\!Cl$ + UV light or heat $\rightarrow 2Cl\cdot$

ii. Propagation:

$CH_4 + Cl\cdot \rightarrow \cdot CH_3 + \boxed{}$

$\boxed{} + Cl_2 \rightarrow CH_3Cl + Cl\cdot$

iii. Termination:

$\boxed{} + \cdot CH_3 \rightarrow CH_3Cl$

$\cdot CH_3 + \boxed{} \rightarrow CH_3CH_3$

$Cl\cdot + Cl\cdot \rightarrow \boxed{}$

3.3

Circle either axial or equatorial.

axial / equatorial hydrogen (blue)
axial / equatorial hydrogen (red)
carbon (black)

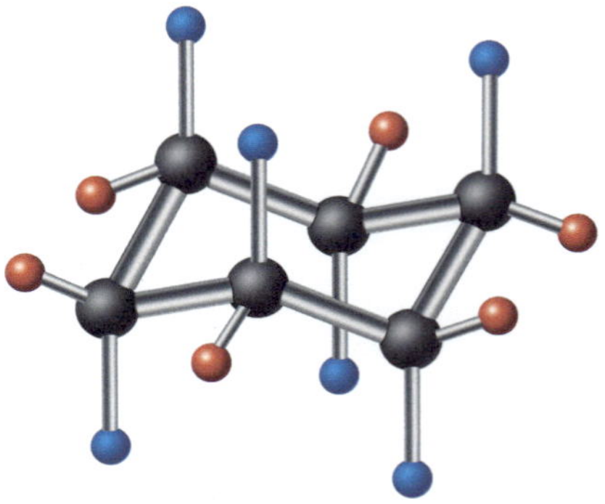

Low-level Importance

<u>Alkanes</u> are hydrocarbon molecules containing only sp^3 hybridised carbon atoms (*single bonds*). They may be unbranched, branched or cyclic. Their general formula is C_nH_{2n+2} for a straight chain molecule; 2 hydrogen (H) atoms are subtracted for each ring. They contain no functional groups and are fully-saturated molecules (= *no double or triple bonds*). As a result, they are chemically unreactive except when exposed to heat or light.

Systematic naming of compounds (= *nomenclature*) has evolved from the International Union of Pure and Applied Chemistry (IUPAC). **The nomenclature of alkanes is the basis of that for many other organic molecules.** The root of the compound is named according to the number of carbons in the longest carbon chain:

C_1 = meth	C_5 = pent	C_8 = oct
C_2 = eth	C_6 = hex	C_9 = non
C_3 = prop	C_7 = hept	C_{10} = dec
C_4 = but		

When naming these as fragments, (alkyl fragments: *the alkane minus one H atom*, symbol: R), the suffix '–yl' is used. When naming an alkane, the suffix '-ane' is used. Some prefixes result from the fact that a carbon with *one* R group attached is a *primary* (normal or n –) carbon, *two* R groups is *secondary* (sec), and with *three* R groups it is a *tertiary* (tert or t –) carbon. Some alkyl groups have special names:

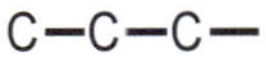

n-propyl
(= propyl)

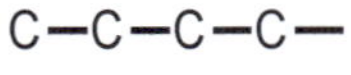

n-butyl
(= butyl)

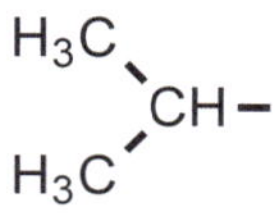
isopropyl
(= 2-propyl or propan-2-yl)

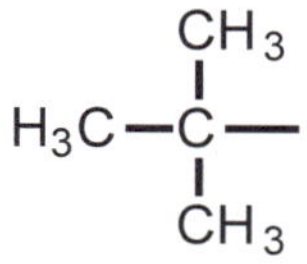
tert-butyl
(= 1,1-dimethylethyl)

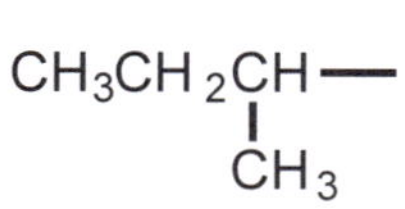
sec-butyl
(= 1-methylpropyl)

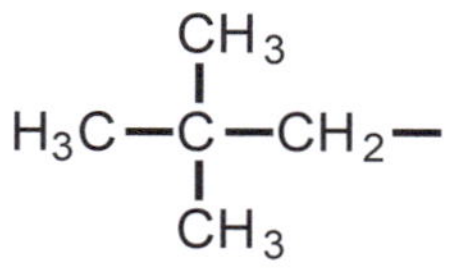
neopentyl
(= dimethylpropyl)

Cyclic alkanes are named in the same way (*according to the number of carbons*), but the prefix 'cyclo' is added. The shorthand for organic compounds is a geometric figure where each corner represents a carbon; hydrogens need not be written, though it should be remembered that the number of hydrogens would exist such that the number of bonds at each carbon is four (ORG 1.1, 1.6).

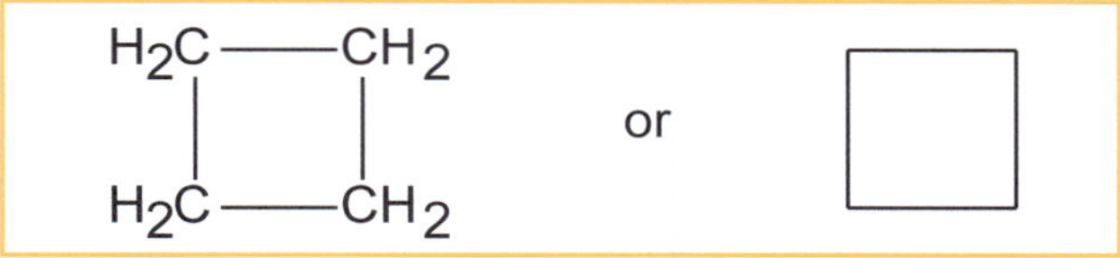
cyclobutane

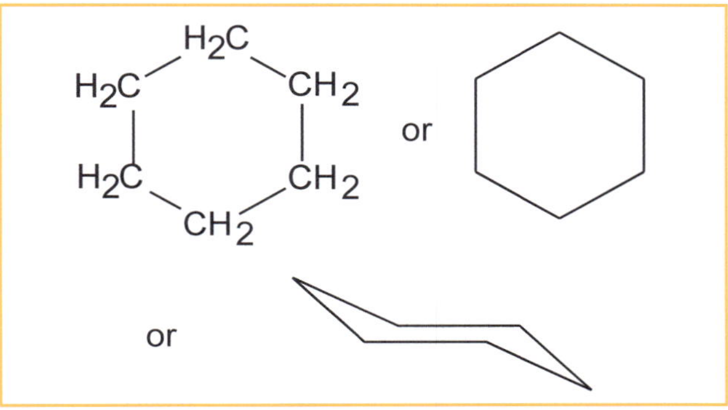
cyclohexane

As mentioned, carbon atoms can be characterised by the number of other carbon atoms to which they are directly bonded. It is very important for you to train your eyes to quickly identify a primary carbon atom (**1°**), which is bonded to only one other carbon; a secondary carbon atom (**2°**), which is bonded to two other carbons; a tertiary carbon atom (**3°**), which is bonded to three other carbons; and a quaternary carbon atom (**4°**), which is bonded to four other carbons.

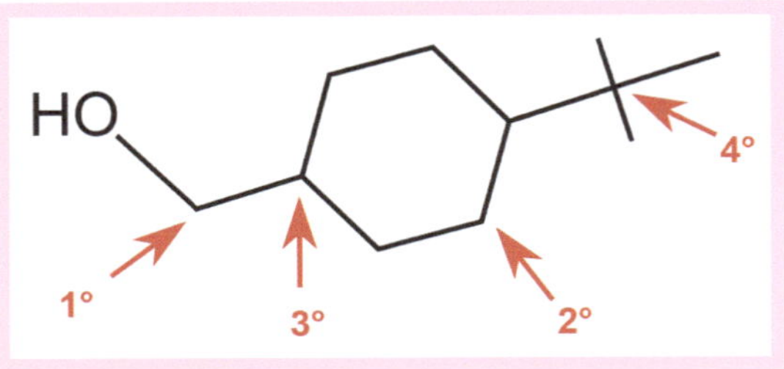

The nomenclature for branched-chain alkanes begins by determining the longest straight chain (i.e. *the highest number of carbons attached in a row*). The groups attached to the straight or *main* chain are numbered so as to achieve the lowest set of numbers. Groups are cited in alphabetical order. If a group appears more than once, the prefixes di-(2), tri-(3), tetra-(4) are used.

Prefixes such as di-, tri-, tetra- as well as tert-, sec-, n- are not used for alphabetising purposes. However, cyclo-, iso-, and neo- are considered part of the group name and are used for alphabetising purposes. If two chains of equal length compete for selection as the main chain, choose the chain with the most substituents.

For example:

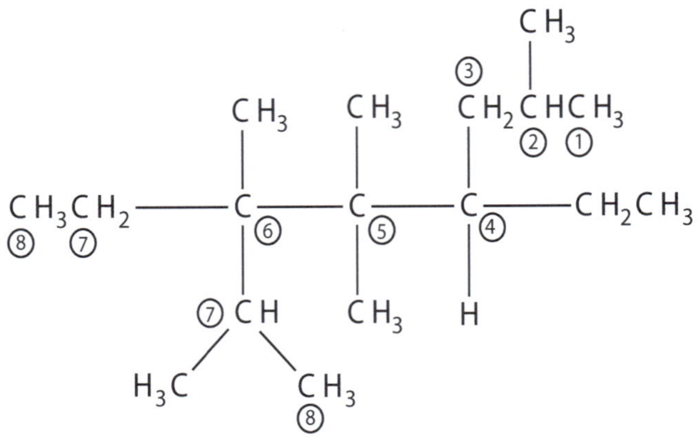

3,5-Diethyl-2,3,4,4,7-pentamethyloctane (7 substituents), NOT 4,6-Diethyl-2,5,5,6,7-pentamethyloctane (7 substituents but larger numbers)

Naming cycloalkanes:

1. Use the cycloalkane name as the parent name. The only exception is when the alkyl side chain contains a larger number of carbons than the ring. In that case, the ring is considered as a substituent to the parent alkane.

2. Number the substituents on the ring to arrive at the lowest sum. When two or more different alkyl groups are present, they are numbered by alphabetical order.

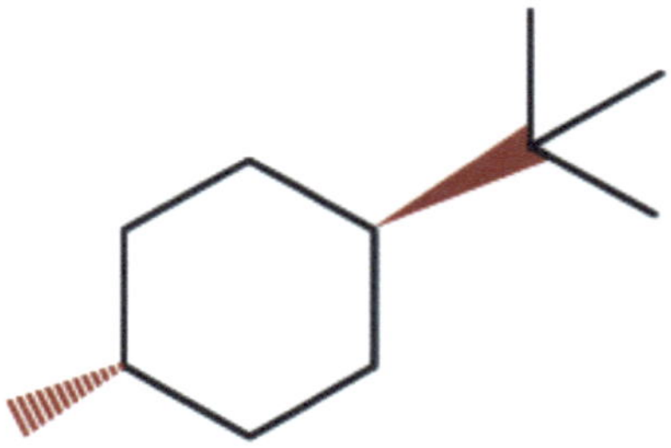

trans-1-tert-butyl-4-methylcyclohexane

3.1.1 Bicycloalkanes: Examples of Isomeric C_8H_{14}

Consider the following table which provides a summary of the main categories of saturated hydrocarbons with two rings (i.e. *bicycloalkanes*). The 10 structures represent 8 different constitutional isomers of C_8H_{14}. At this point you should be reasonably efficient at confirming that all of the structures in the table are indeed isomers.

Isolated Rings	**Spiro Rings**	**Fused Rings**	**Bridged Rings**
No common atoms	One common atom	One common bond	2^+ common atoms
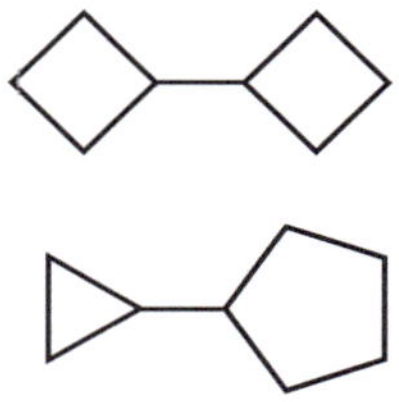	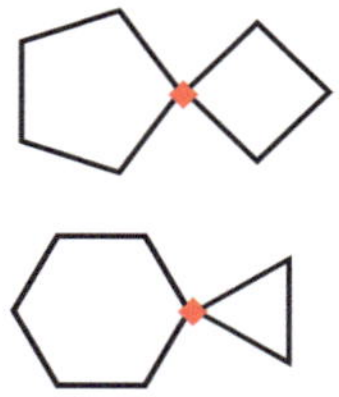	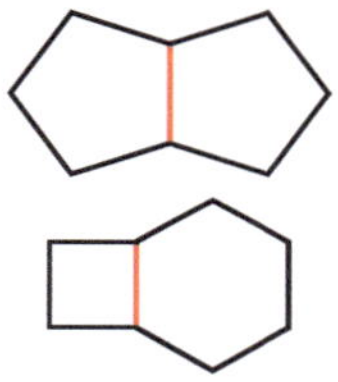	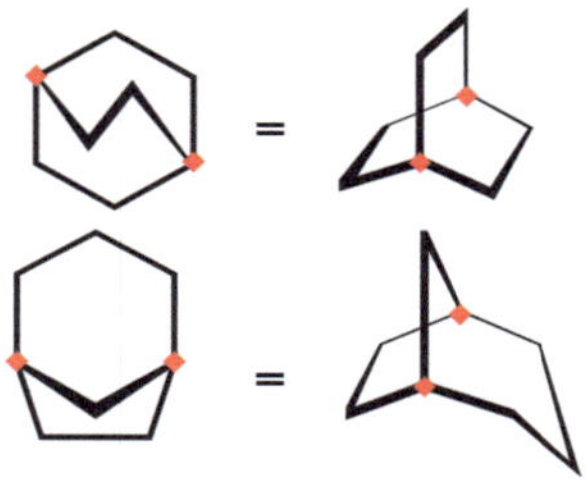

We will have some fun naming some of the lovely structures above in the GAMSAT-level practice questions!

3.1.2 Foundational Nomenclature Exercises: Alkanes

Name the following ten compounds. If it is your first time, feel free to keep consulting the nomenclature rules from ORG 3.1. The answers are at the end of this chapter.

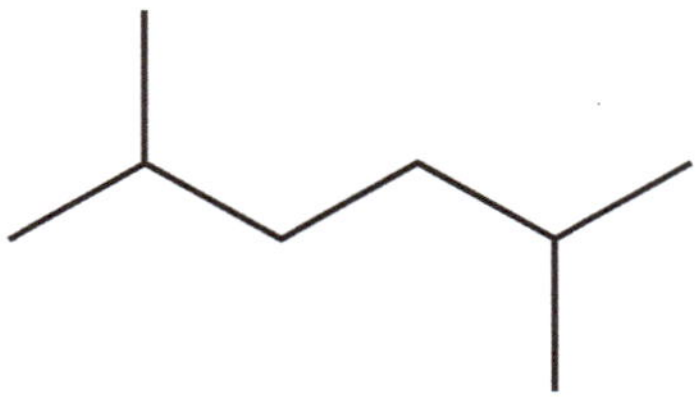 **1)** ______________________	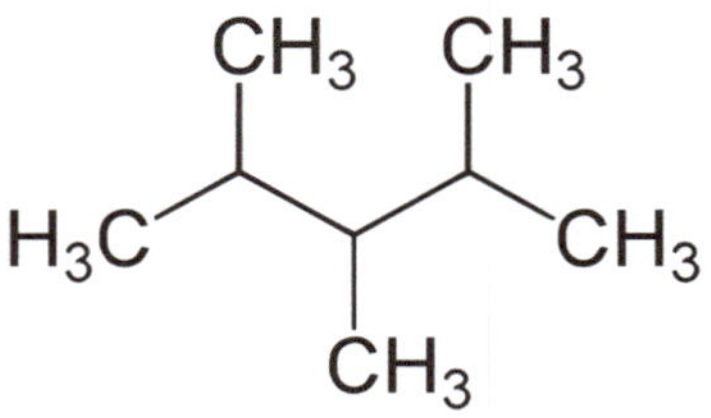 **2)** ______________________

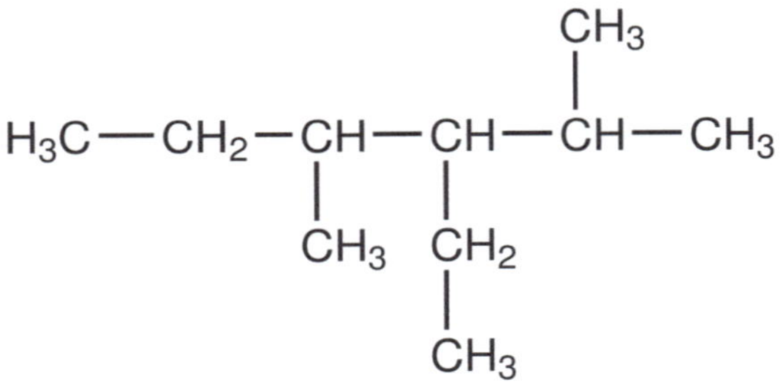

3) ______________________

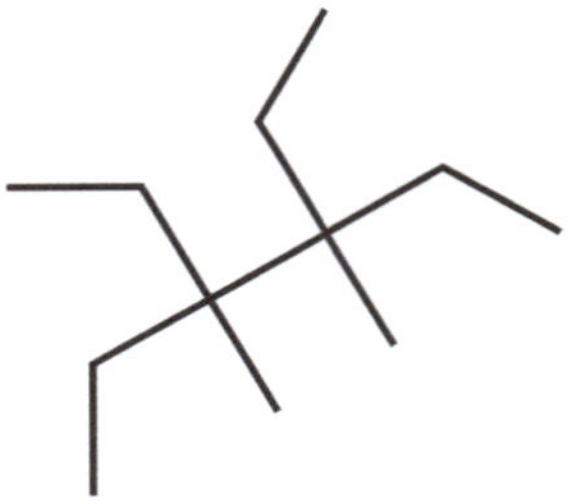

4) ______________________

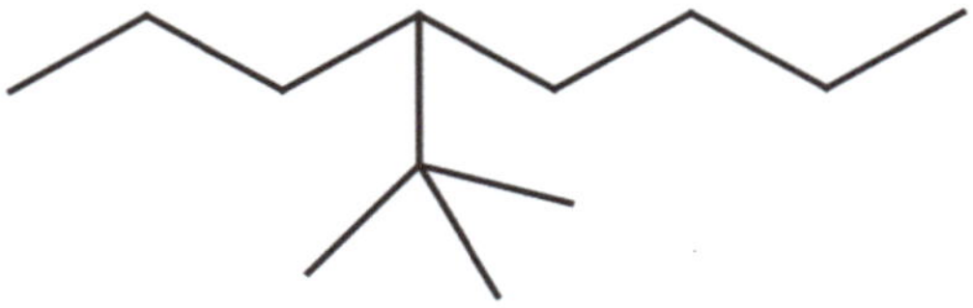

5) ______________________

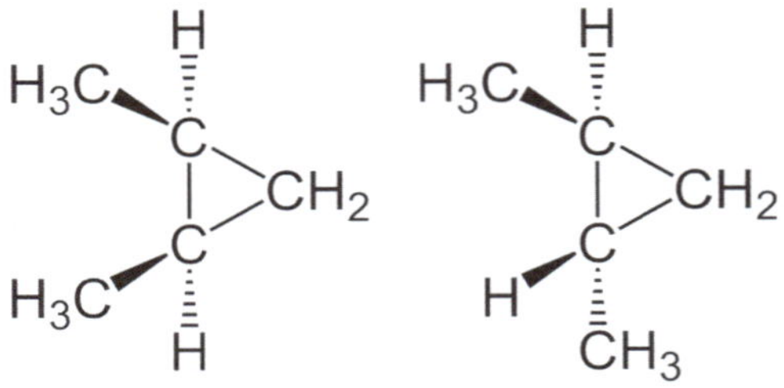

6) ______________________

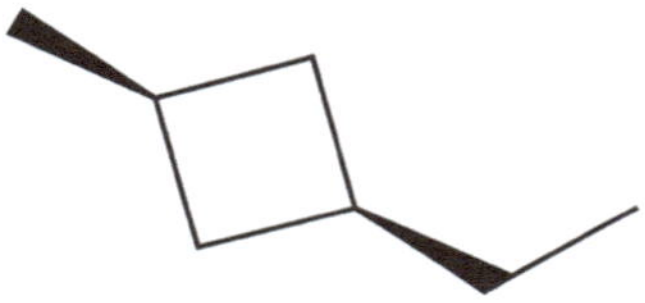

7) ______________________

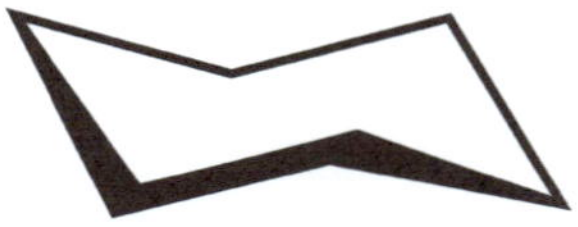

8) ______________________

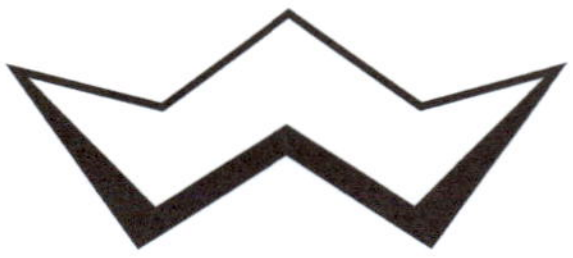

9) ______________________

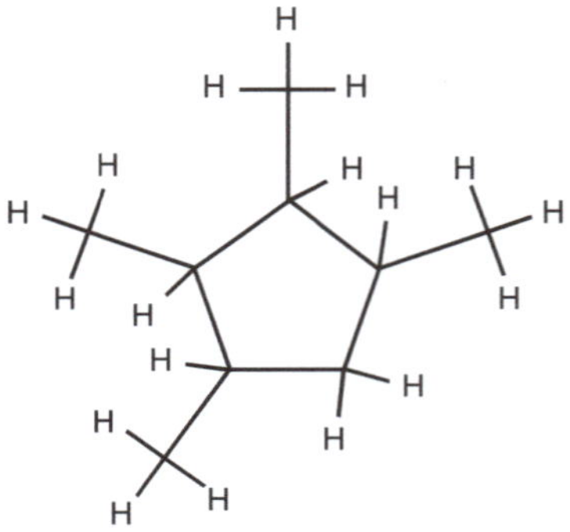

10) ______________________

Low-level Importance

3.1.3 Physical Properties of Alkanes

At room temperature and one atmosphere of pressure, straight chain alkanes with 1 to 4 carbons are gases (i.e. CH_4 – methane, CH_3CH_3 – ethane, etc.), 5 to 17 carbons are liquids (e.g. oils), and more than 17 carbons are solid (e.g. wax). Boiling points of straight chain alkanes (= *aliphatic*) show a regular increase with increasing number of carbons. This is because they are nonpolar molecules, and have weak intermolecular forces. Branching of alkanes leads to a dramatic decrease in the boiling point. As a rule, as the number of carbons increase the melting points also increase.

Alkanes are soluble in nonpolar solvents (i.e. benzene, CCl_4 – carbon tetrachloride, etc.), and not in aqueous solvents (= *hydrophobic*). They are insoluble in water because of their low polarity and their inability to hydrogen bond. Alkanes are the least dense of all classes of organic compounds ($\ll \rho_{water}$, 1 g/ml). Thus petroleum, a mixture of hydrocarbons rich in alkanes, floats on water.

3.2 Important Reactions of Alkanes

3.2.1 Combustion

Combustion (CHM 1.4) is typically when a substance reacts with oxygen, releasing energy in the form of heat and light. Combustion includes the burning of hydrocarbons found in fossil fuels like gasoline (i.e. octane and other alkanes for internal combustion engines) and natural gas (i.e. methane and other alkanes for heating, cooking, and electricity generation).

Note that the "heat of combustion" is the change in enthalpy of a combustion reaction. Therefore, the higher the heat of combustion, the higher the energy level of the molecule, the less stable the molecule was prior to combustion.

Combustion may be either complete or incomplete. In complete combustion, the hydrocarbon is converted to carbon dioxide (CO_2) and water (H_2O). If there is insufficient oxygen for complete combustion, the reaction gives other products, such as carbon monoxide (CO) and soot (molecular C). This strongly exothermic reaction may be summarised:

$$C_nH_{2n+2} + \text{excess } O_2 \rightarrow nCO_2 + (n+1)H_2O.$$

Low-level Importance

3.2.2 Radical Substitution Reactions

Radical substitution reactions with halogens may be summarised (recall E = hf, *see* PHY 9.2.4; also *see* CHM 9.4):

$$RH + X_2 + \text{UV light } (hf) \text{ or heat} \rightarrow RX + HF$$

The halogen X_2, may be F_2, Cl_2, or Br_2. I_2 does not react. The concept of this reaction is that a halogen will replace a hydrogen from the hydrocarbon (*replacement* = ***substitution**, a common type of reaction in chemistry*). The mechanism of *halogenation* may be explained and summarised by example:

i. Initiation: This step involves the formation of *free radicals* (highly reactive substances which contain an unpaired electron, which is symbolised by a single dot):

$$Cl{:}Cl + \text{UV light or heat} \rightarrow 2Cl\bullet$$

ii. Propagation: In this step, the chlorine free radical begins a series of reactions that form new free radicals:

$$CH_4 + Cl\bullet \rightarrow \bullet CH_3 + HCl$$

$$\bullet CH_3 + Cl_2 \rightarrow CH_3Cl + Cl\bullet$$

iii. Termination: These reactions end the radical propagation steps. Termination reactions destroy the free radicals (*coupling*).

$$Cl\bullet + \bullet CH_3 \rightarrow CH_3Cl$$

$$\bullet CH_3 + \bullet CH_3 \rightarrow CH_3CH_3$$

$$Cl\bullet + Cl\bullet \rightarrow Cl_2$$

Radical substitution reactions can also occur with hydrogen halides (i.e. HCl, HBr) and peroxides (i.e. HOOH – hydrogen peroxide). Chain propagation (step ii) can destroy many organic compounds fairly quick. This step can be inhibited by using a resonance stabilised free radical to "mop up" (*termination*) other destructive free radicals in the medium. For example, BHT is a resonance stabilised free radical added to the packaging of many breakfast cereals in order to inhibit free radical destruction of the cereal (= *spoiling*).

The stability of a free radical depends on the ability of the compound to stabilise the unpaired electron. This is analogous to stabilising a positively charged carbon (= *carbocation*). Thus, in both cases, a tertiary compound is more stable than secondary which, in turn, is more stable than a primary compound.

Low-level Importance

Also in both cases, the reason for the trend is the same: the charge on the carbon is stabilised by the electron donating effect of the presence of alkyl groups. Alkyl groups are not strongly electron donating, they are normally described as "somewhat" electron donating; however, the combined effect of multiple R groups has an important stabilising effect that we will see as a critical feature in many reaction types.

$$\bullet CR_3 > \bullet CR_2H > \bullet CRH_2 > \bullet CH_3$$
$$3^o > 2^o > 1^o > \text{methyl}$$

Pyrolysis occurs when a molecule is broken down by heat (*pyro* = fire, *lysis* = separate). C-C bonds are cleaved and smaller chain alkyl radicals often recombine in termination steps creating a variety of alkanes.

Please note that the rate law for free radical substitution reactions was discussed in CHM 9.4.

3.3 Ring Strain in Cyclic Alkanes

Cyclic alkanes are strained compounds. This **ring strain** results from the bending of the bond angles in greater amounts than normal. This strain causes cyclic compounds of 3 and 4 carbons to be unstable, and thus not often found in nature. The usual angle between bonds in an sp^3 hybridised carbon is 109.5° (= *the normal tetrahedral angle*).

The expected angles in some cyclic compounds can be determined geometrically: 60° in cyclopropane; 90° in cyclobutane and 108° in cyclopentane. Cyclohexane, in the chair conformation, has normal bond angles of 109.5°. The closer the angle is to the normal tetrahedral angle of 109.5°, the more stable the compound. In fact, cyclohexane can be found in a chair or boat conformation or any conformation in between; however, at any given moment, 99% of the cyclohexane molecules would be found in the chair conformation because it is the most stable (lower energy).

It is important to have a clear understanding of electron shell repulsion (ESR). Essentially all atoms and molecules are surrounded by an electron shell (CHM 2.1, ORG 1.2) which is more like a cloud of electrons. Because like charges repel, when there are options, atoms and molecules assume the conformation which minimises ESR.

For example, when substituents are added to a cyclic compound (i.e. *see* ORG 12.3.1, Fig. IV.B.12.1 Part II) the most stable position is equatorial (equivalent to the anti conformation, ORG 2.1) which minimises ESR. This conformation is most pronounced when the substituent is bulky (i.e. isopropyl, t-butyl, phenyl, etc.). In other words, a large substituent takes up more space thus ESR has a more prominent effect.

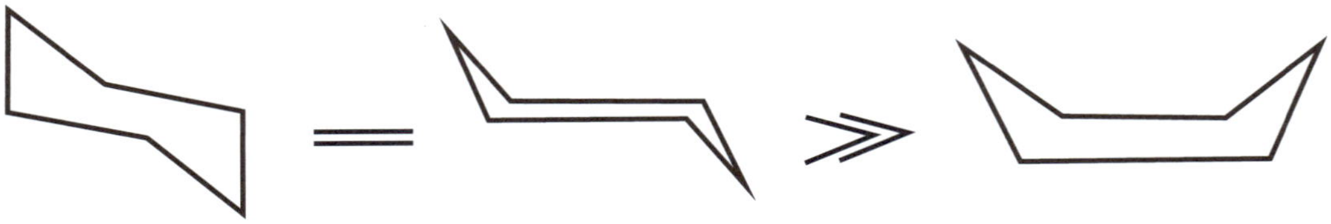

Figure IV.B.3.1: The chair and boat conformations of cyclohexane. Some students like to remember that you sit in a chair because a chair is stable. However, a boat can be tippy and so it's less stable.

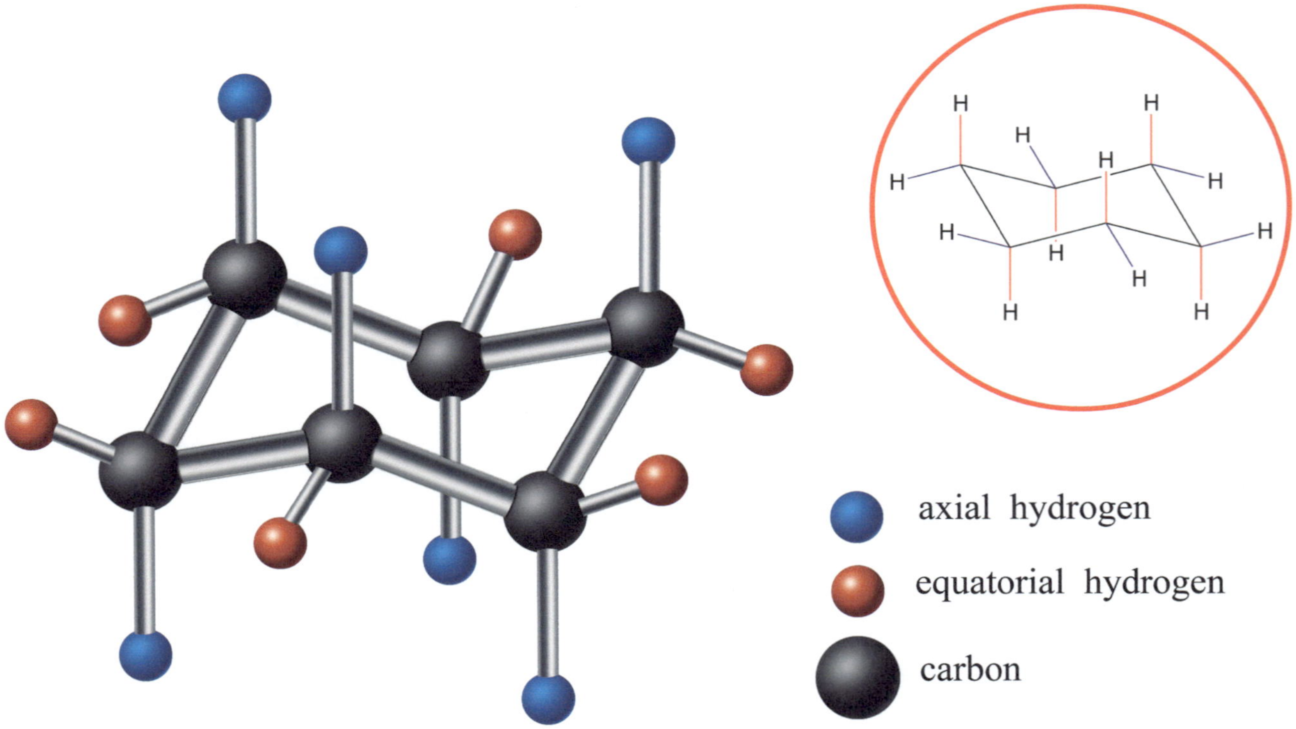

Figure IV.B.3.2: The chair conformation of cyclohexane. The hydrogens which are generally in the same plane as the ring are equatorial. The hydrogens which are generally perpendicular to the ring are axial. The hydrogen atoms are maximally separated and staggered to minimise electron shell repulsion. Note that the inset (in the circle) shows another way to present a chair conformer: the red bond indicates axial and the blue indicates equatorial. Note that cyclohexane can be presented in all the different ways seen on this page, as well as ORG 3.1.

Low-level Importance

Solutions to Foundational Nomenclature Exercises: Alkanes

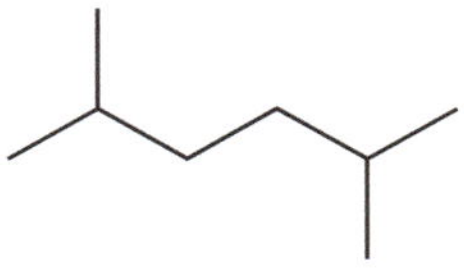

1) 2,5-dimethylhexane

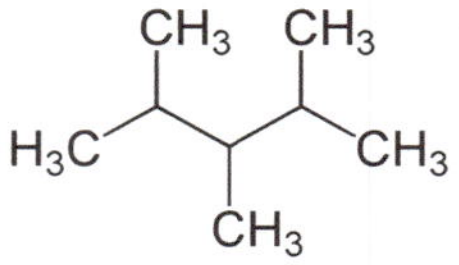

2) 2,3,4-trimethylpentane

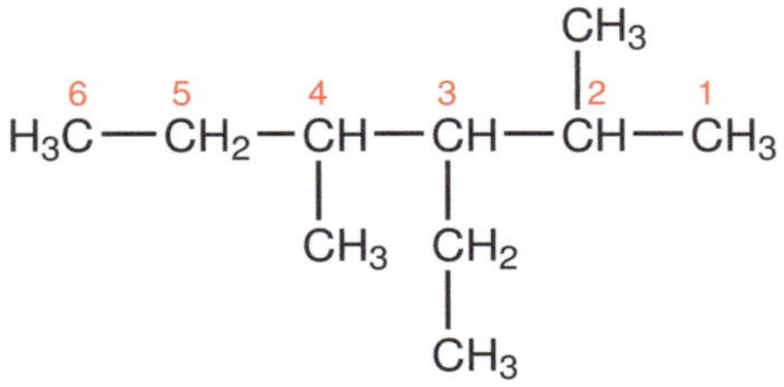

3) 3-ethyl-2,4-dimethylhexane

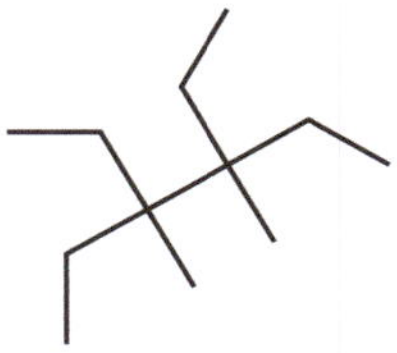

4) 3,4-diethyl-3,4-dimethylhexane

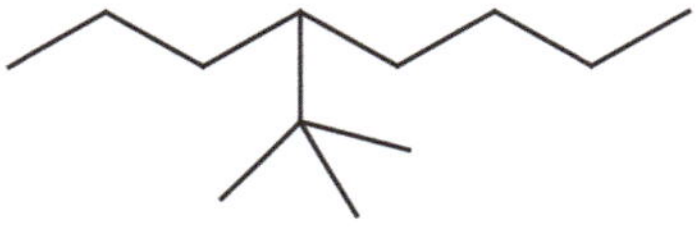

5) 4-tert-butyloctane [note: only if you were given guidance in the passage, 4-(1,1-dimethylethyl)octane]

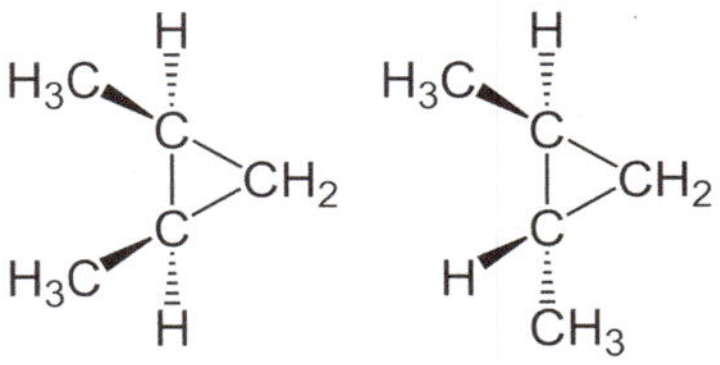

6) *cis*- and *trans*-1,2-dimethylcyclopropane

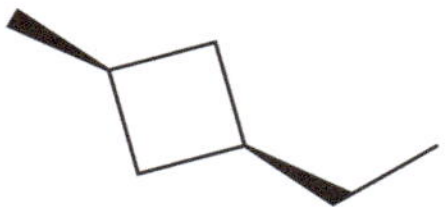

7) *cis*-1-ethyl-3-methylcyclobutane

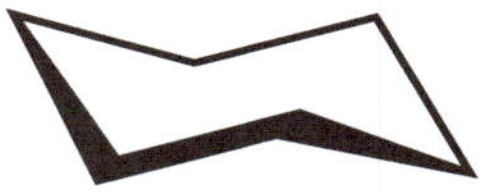

8) cyclohexane (side note: chair conformation)

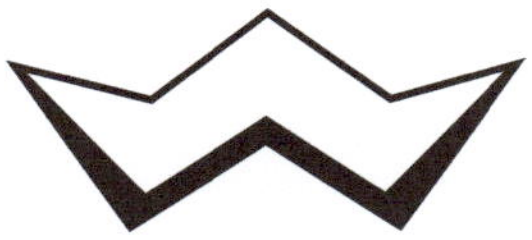

9) Cyclooctane (for the curious only: the crown conformation)

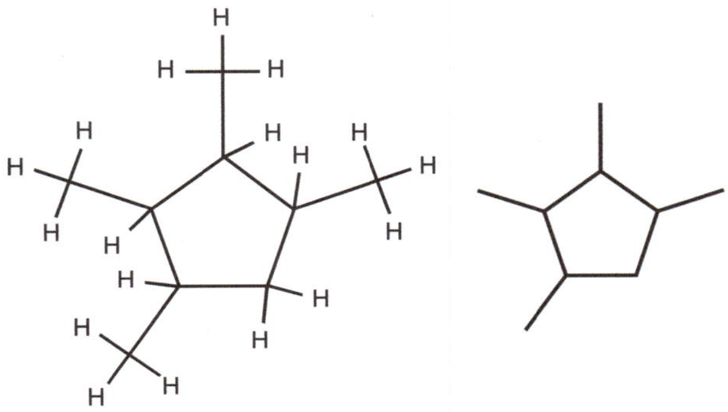

10) 1,2,3,4-tetramethylcyclopentane

Questions or concerns? gamsat-prep.com/forum

CHAPTER 3: Alkanes

GOLD STANDARD GAMSAT-LEVEL PRACTICE QUESTIONS

Questions 11–12

Combustion may be either complete or incomplete. In complete combustion, the hydrocarbon is converted to carbon dioxide (CO_2) and water (H_2O). If there is insufficient oxygen for complete combustion, the reaction gives other products, such as carbon monoxide (CO) and soot (molecular C). This strongly exothermic reaction may be summarised:

$$C_nH_{2n+2} + \text{excess } O_2 \rightarrow nCO_2 + (n+1)H_2O.$$

11) The complete combustion of 2 moles of pure octane is likely to produce how many moles of water?

A. 2
B. 3
C. 9
D. 18

12) In a separate experiment, a barely detectable amount of soot was identified after the combustion of one mole of octane. How many moles of oxygen must have been present at the start of the reaction?

A. No moles of oxygen
B. Just above 12.5 moles of oxygen
C. Just below 12.5 moles of oxygen
D. An excess amount of oxygen

Questions 13–19

Compounds that contain two rings are called "bicyclic". Fused and bridged ring systems follow the same IUPAC rules of nomenclature and both systems use the prefix "bicyclo". If the 2 ring systems meet only at a single carbon, then instead the prefix "spiro" is used.

A fused ring is where two rings share two common atoms (i.e. "bridgehead" atoms). There are 3 paths between the bridgehead atoms: the longest path is counted first, then the shorter path, and finally the shortest path. To number the carbon atoms, always start at a bridgehead, continue around the larger ring, through the other bridgehead and around the shorter ring.

Consider the following 2 examples.

Note: the bridgeheads are marked with a black dot for emphasis.

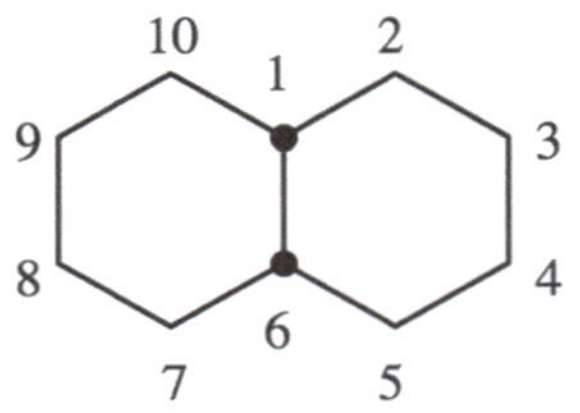

bicyclo[4.4.0]decane
(path of 4 atoms in each direction)

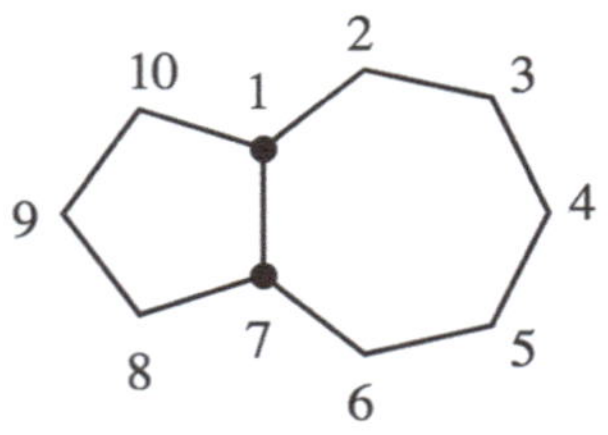

bicyclo[5.3.0]decane
(path of 5 atoms and path of 3 atoms)

A bridged ring is where two rings have more than two common atoms. Consider the following 2 examples.

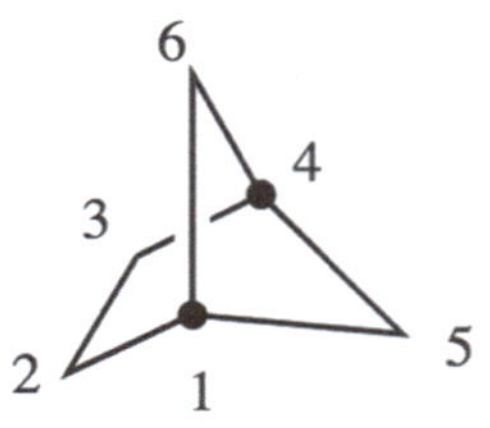

bicyclo[2.1.1]hexane
(paths of 2 atoms, 1 atom, and 1 atom)

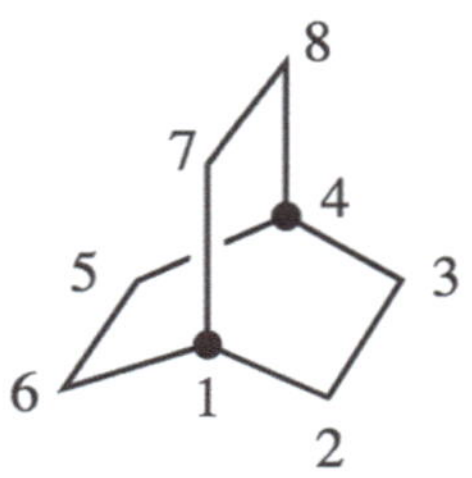

bicyclo[2.2.2]octane
(three paths of 2 atoms)

13) Which of the following molecules is a bicyclo-hexane?

A. 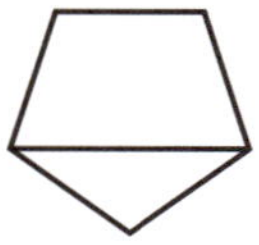

C. 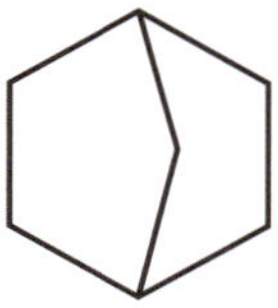

B. 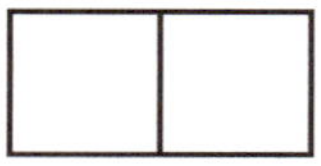

D. 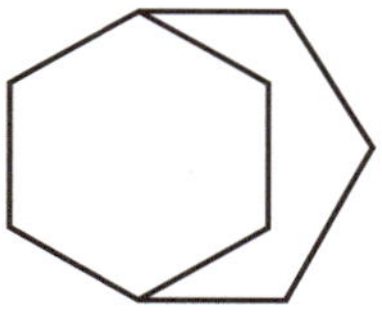

14) Name the following compound.

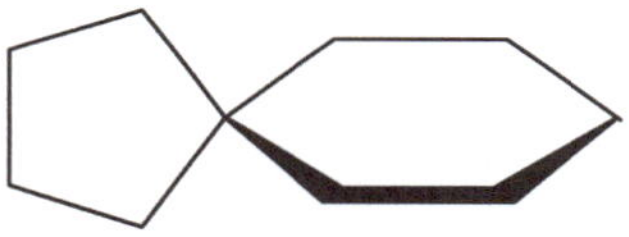

A. Bicyclo[5.4.0]decane
B. Bicyclo[6.5.0]decane
C. Spiro[5.4]decane
D. Spiro[6.5]decane

15) Name the following compound.

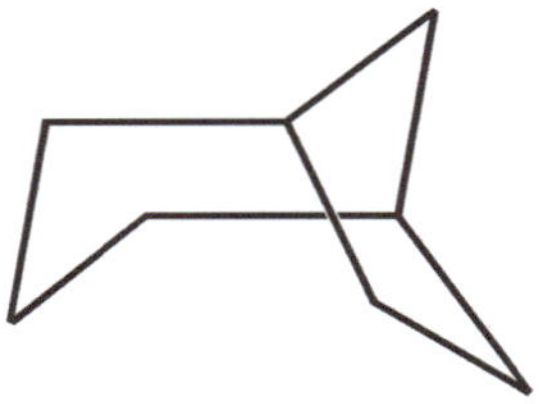

A. Bicyclo[3.2.1]octane
B. Bicyclo[5.4.1]octane
C. Bicyclo[3.2.1]nonane
D. Bicyclo[5.4.1]nonane

16) The suffix -ene is used to identify the position of a double bond. Which of the following structures represents bicyclo[4.1.0]hepta-2,4-diene?

A. 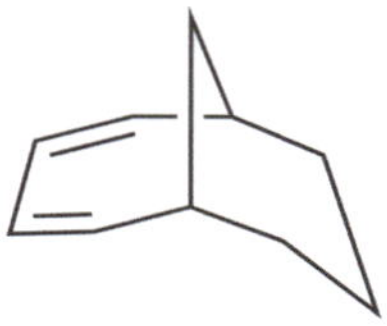

C. 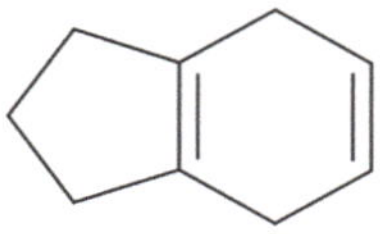

B. 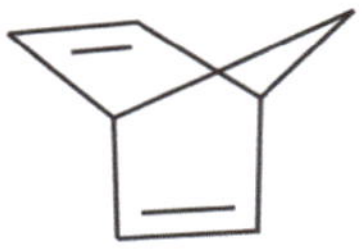

D. 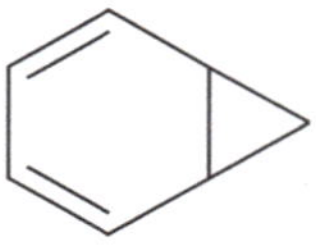

17) Which of the following accurately describes the structure of the molecule in the previous question (bicyclo[4.1.0]hepta-2,4-diene)?

A. Bridged bicyclic
B. Fused bicyclic
C. Spiro bicyclic
D. More than one of the above

18) Name the following compound.

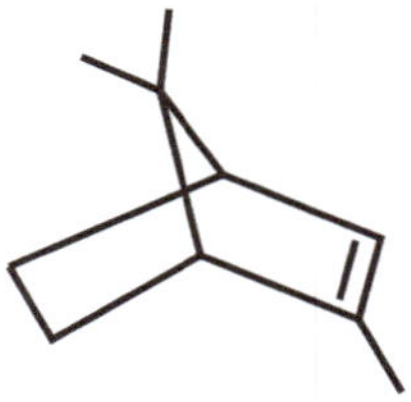

A. 2,7,7-trimethylbicyclo[2.2.1]hept-2-ene
B. 2,5,5-trimethylbicyclo[3.2.1]hept-2-ene
C. trimethylbenzene
D. bicylo[3.2.1]dec-2-ene

19) When naming bicyclic compounds, consider the relationship between the sum of the numbers within the square brackets [ ] and the total number n of carbons in the bicyclic component of the molecule. The sum of the numbers in the square brackets is equivalent to which of the following?

A. $n-2$
B. n
C. $n+2$
D. The relationship is exponential.

Questions 20–25

Cyclohexane conformations are any of several three-dimensional shapes adopted by molecules of cyclohexane. Because many compounds feature structurally similar six-membered rings, the structure and dynamics of cyclohexane are important prototypes of a wide range of compounds.

Consider the major conformations of cyclohexane in Figure 1 and their relative energy differences in Figure 2.

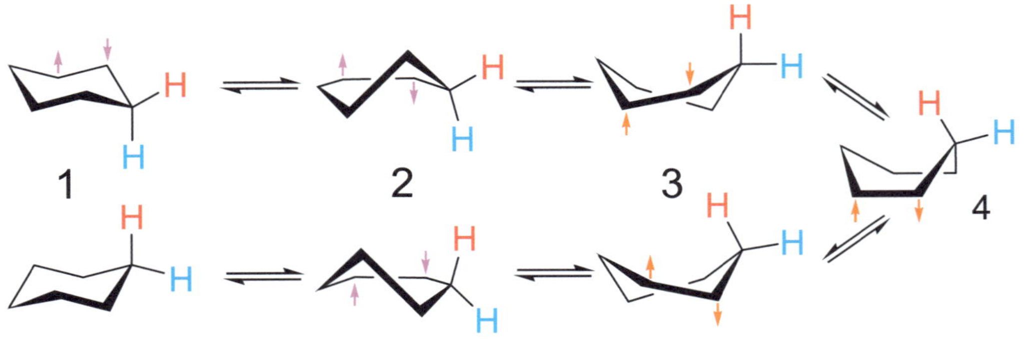

Figure 1: Cyclohexane chair flip (ring inversion) reaction via boat conformation (**4**). Structures of the significant conformations of cyclohexane are shown: chair (**1**), half-chair (**2**), twist-boat (**3**) and boat (**4**). When ring flip happens completely from chair-to-chair, hydrogens that were previously axial (blue H in upper-left structure) turn equatorial, and equatorial ones (red H in upper-left structure) turn axial. When hydrogen is replaced by a substituent, the equatorial position is more stable since it minimises electron-shell repulsion.

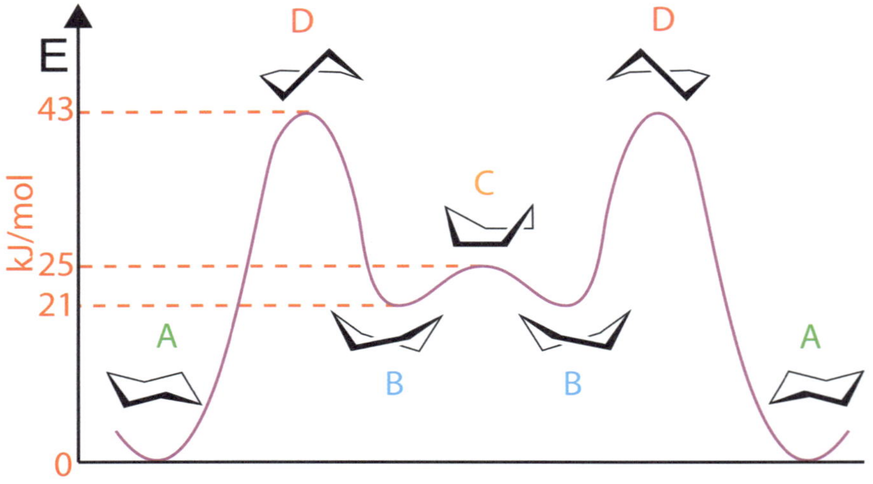

Figure 2: Cyclohexane chair flip (ring inversion) reaction. Structures of the significant conformations (A, B, C and D) of the reaction are shown and plotted against their energy differences (*not* total energies). Inversion happens quickly and constantly at room temperature.

20) Based on the information provided, the most stable conformation of cyclohexane is represented by which of the following?

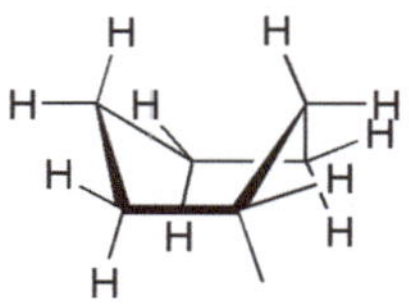
I
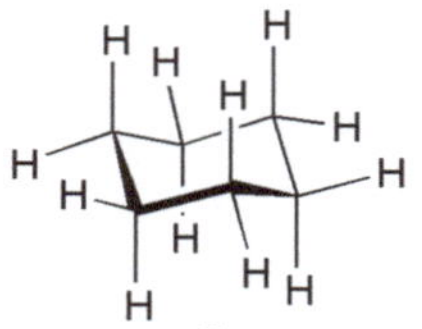
II
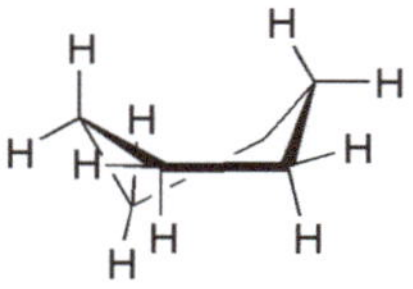
III
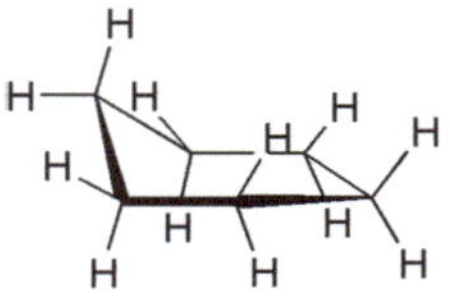
IV
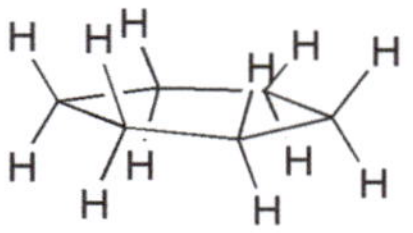
V

A. **II** only
B. **IV** only
C. **I**, **II** and **V** only
D. **I**, **III**, **IV** and **V** only

21) What structure represents the most stable conformation of *cis*-1,3-difluorocyclohexane?

A.
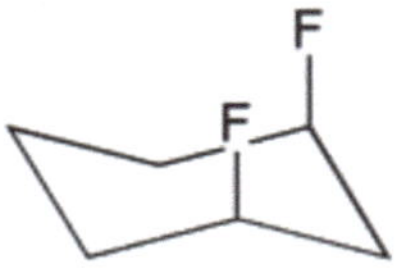
C.
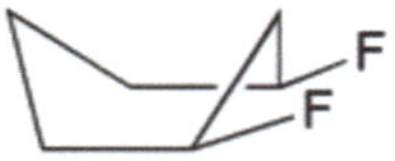
B.
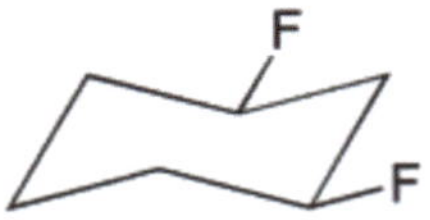
D.
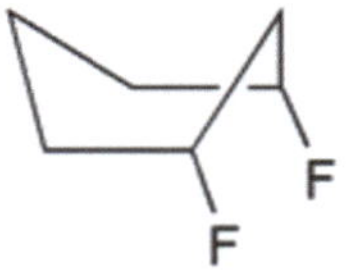

22) According to the information provided, the preferred conformation of *cis*-1-tert-butyl-3-methylcyclohexane is the one in which:

A. the tert-butyl group is axial and the methyl group is equatorial.
B. the methyl group is axial and the tert-butyl group is equatorial.
C. both groups are axial.
D. both groups are equatorial.

23) What structure represents the most stable conformation of compound **Z**?

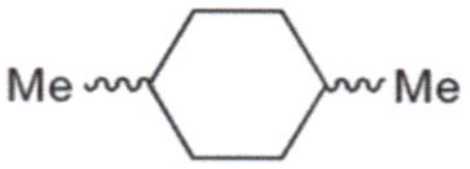
Z

A.
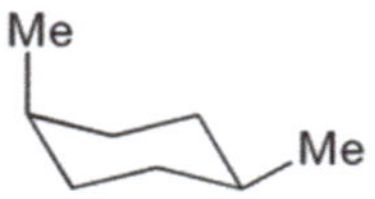
C.
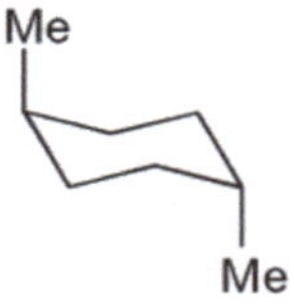
B.
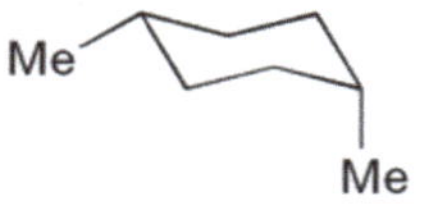
D.
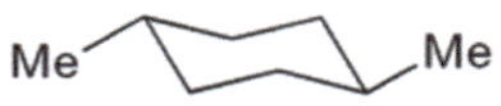

24) Which structures represent the most stable conformations of compound **Z**?

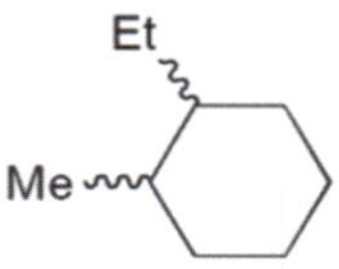
Z

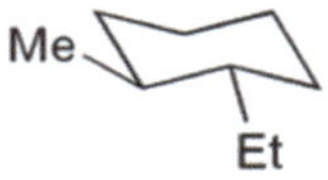
I
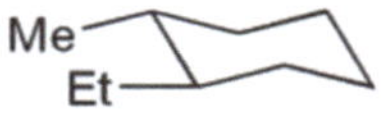
II
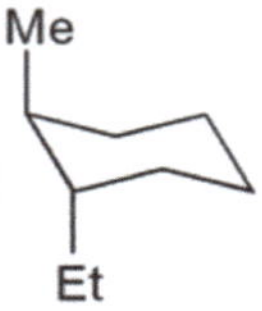
III
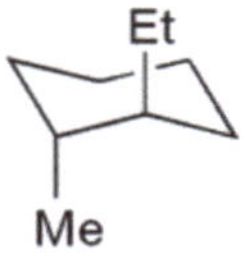
IV

A. **I** and **II**
C. **III** and **IV**
B. **II** and **III**
D. **I** and **IV**

25) Based on the information provided, which of the following structures has the least difference in energy?

A. Chair and twist-boat
B. Chair and boat
C. Twist-boat and half-chair
D. Boat and half-chair

High-level Importance

High-level Importance

SPOILER ALERT

Gold Standard has cross-referenced the content in this chapter to examples from ACER's official GAMSAT practice materials. It is for you to decide when you want to explore these questions since you may want to preserve some of ACER's materials for timed mock-exam practice.

Examples – None that directly point to assumed knowledge from Chapter 3. Note that the unit with bicyclic compound naming, which has been a useful skill from time to time as publicly reported, is a composite from HEAPS-8 with additional novel questions.

Chapter Checklist

- ☐ Access your online account to view answers, worked solutions and discussion boards.
- ☐ Reassess your 'learning objectives' for this chapter: Go back to the first page of this chapter and re-evaluate the top 3 boxes and the Introduction.
  - ☐ Please be sure that you have completed the *Need for Speed* exercises at the beginning of this chapter.
- ☐ Complete a maximum of 1 page of notes using symbols/abbreviations to represent the entire chapter based on your learning objectives. These are your Gold Notes.
- ☐ Consider your multimedia options based on your optimal way of learning:
  - ☐ Download the free Gold Standard GAMSAT app for your Android device or iPhone.
  - ☐ Create your own, tangible study cards or try the free app: Anki.
  - ☐ Record your voice reading your Gold Notes onto your smartphone (audio files, e.g., *memo* or MP3s) and listen during exercise, transportation, etc.
  - ☐ Try out the Gold Standard GAMSAT online videos at gamsat-prep.com, or you can try other options on YouTube like Khan Academy or Crash Course Organic Chemistry.
- ☐ Reassess your schedule for your full-length GAMSAT practice tests: ACER and/or HEAPS exams. Ensure that you have scheduled one full day to complete a practice test and 1-2 days for a thorough assessment of worked solutions while adding to your abbreviated Gold Notes.
- ☐ Reassess your progress in scheduling and/or evaluating stress reduction techniques such as regular exercise (sports), yoga, meditation and/or mindfulness exercises (*see* YouTube for suggestions).

ALKENES

Chapter 4

Memorise	Understand	Importance
* Basic nomenclature	* Electrophilic addition, hydrogenation, Markovnikov's rule, oxidation	**Medium level: 6% of GAMSAT Organic Chemistry** questions released by ACER are related to content in this chapter (in our estimation). * Note that approximately 60% of the questions in GAMSAT Organic Chemistry are related to just 4 chapters: 2, 6, 7 and 12.

GAMSAT-Prep.com

Introduction

Unsaturated hydrocarbons are hydrocarbons that have double or triple bonds between adjacent carbon atoms. The expression *unsaturated* means that more hydrogen atoms may be added to the hydrocarbon to make it *saturated*, thus consisting of all single bonds. An alkene (a.k.a. olefin) is an unsaturated hydrocarbon containing at least one carbon-to-carbon double bond, while its close cousin, an alkyne, contains at least one carbon-to-carbon triple bond.

The breadth of topics and reasoning for the practice questions in this chapter is incredible: sigma/pi bonds, resonance, conjugation, substitutions, Markovnikov's rule, Diels–Alder, ozonolysis, sigmatropic reactions, and electrocyclic reactions. It would be unusual if your exam did not touch on one or more of these topics, though certainly the reasoning needed to solve many of the problems in this chapter will be on your exam.

Multimedia Resources at GAMSAT-Prep.com

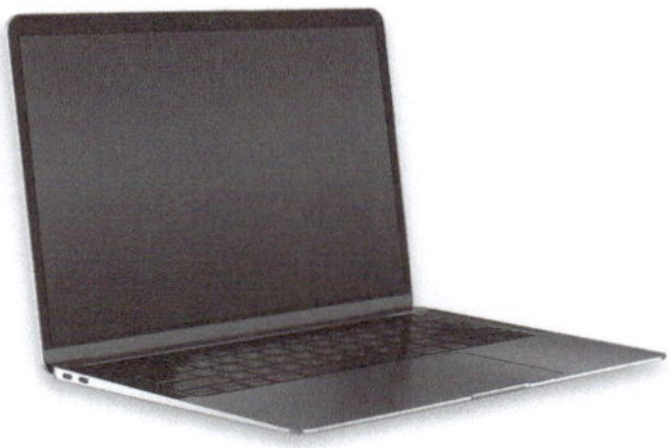

Open Discussion Boards
(*gamsat-prep.com/forum*)

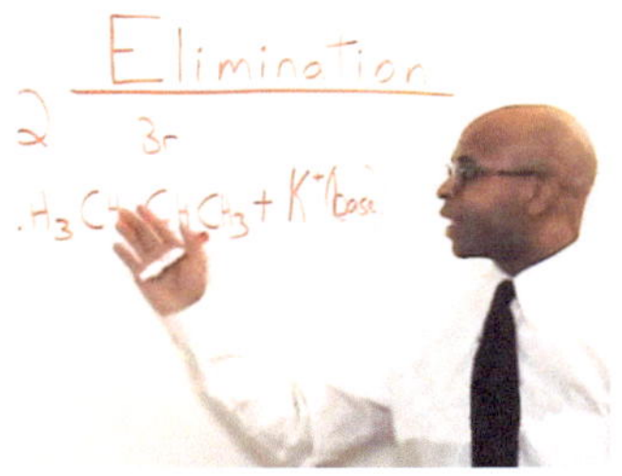

Science Preparation Videos

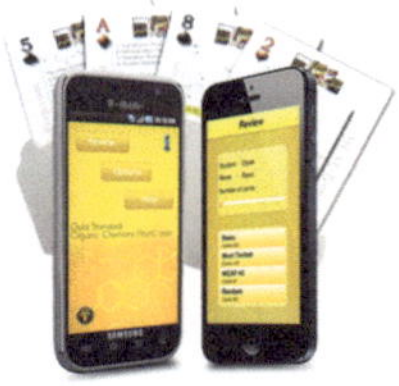

Flashcards

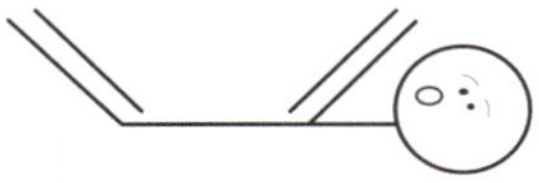

Special Guest

* The real GAMSAT may have advanced-level information presented (i.e. in a passage) but previous knowledge of said information is not required to answer the questions that would follow. Practice questions at the end of this chapter, as well as ACER and GS (HEAPS) practice GAMSATs can help you clarify this point.

4.0 GAMSAT has a *Need for Speed*!

Medium-level Importance

Section	GAMSAT Organic Chemistry *Need for Speed* Exercises
4.1	Consider the molecular structure of beta-carotene below. 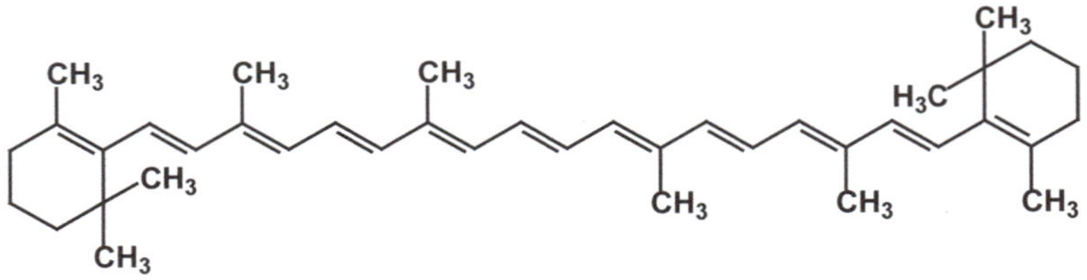 1) How many conjugated double bonds are there? ______________ 2) How many double bonds are in the *cis* configuration? ______________
	What must the missing inorganic product be in order to maintain balance? 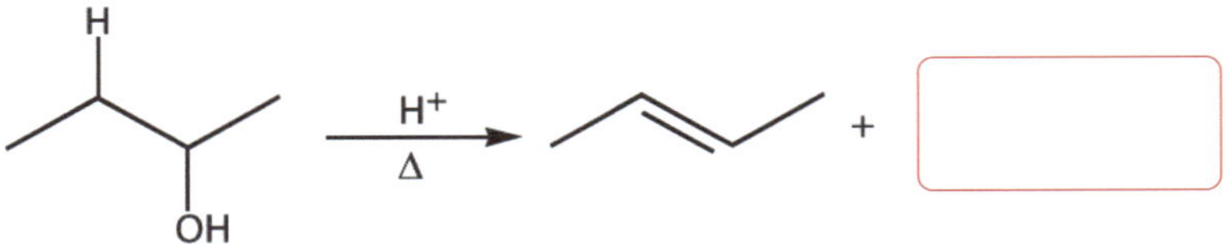
4.2.1	The carbon that is the *most* substituted is numbered: _____ ; the *least* substituted carbon: _____ 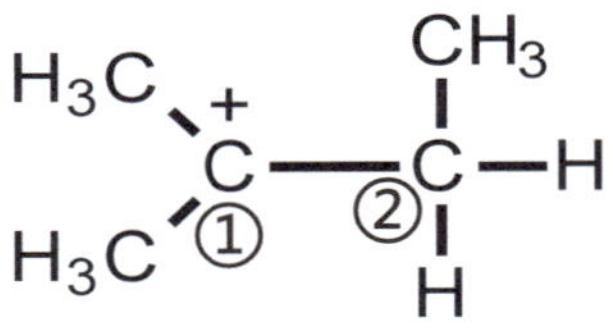 Write a number in the box for each case to indicate if the carbocation is primary (**1°**), secondary (**2°**) or tertiary (**3°**). 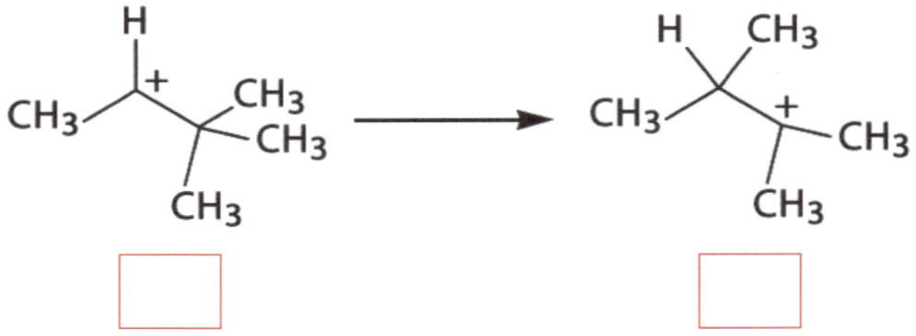
4.2.5	Identify the 2 carbons (*using arrows*) in the resonance forms below that must have a formal charge (ORG 1.1). 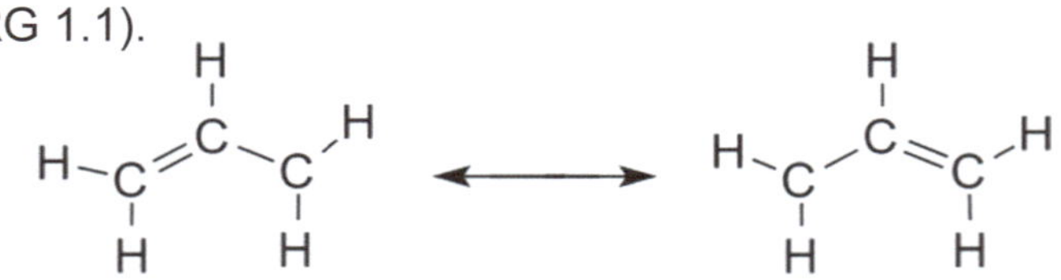
4.3	Consider the following transformation. 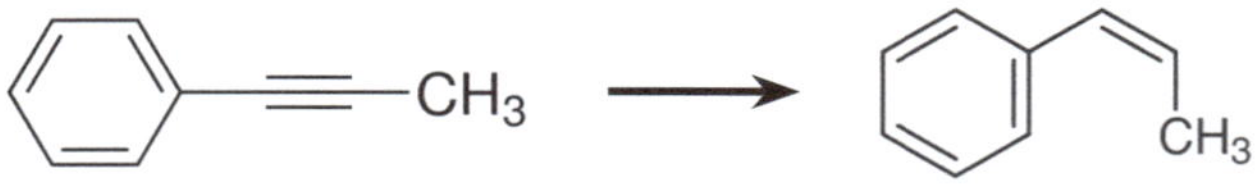 Complete this sentence: Alkynes can be partially hydrogenated yielding alkenes with just one equivalent of __________.

4.1 Description and Nomenclature

Alkenes *(olefins)* are unsaturated hydrocarbon molecules containing carbon-carbon double bonds. Their general formula is C_nH_{2n} for a straight chain molecule; 2 hydrogen (H) atoms are subtracted for each ring. The *functional group* in these molecules is the double bond which determines the chemical properties of alkenes. Double bonds are sp^2 hybridised (*see* ORG 1.2, 1.3).

The nomenclature is the same as that for alkanes, except: **i)** the suffix 'ene' replaces 'ane' and **ii)** the double bond is (are) numbered in the molecule, trying to get the smallest number for the double bond(s). Always select the longest chain that contains the double bond or the greatest number of double bonds as the parent hydrocarbon. For cycloalkenes, the carbons of the double bond are given the 1– and 2– positions.

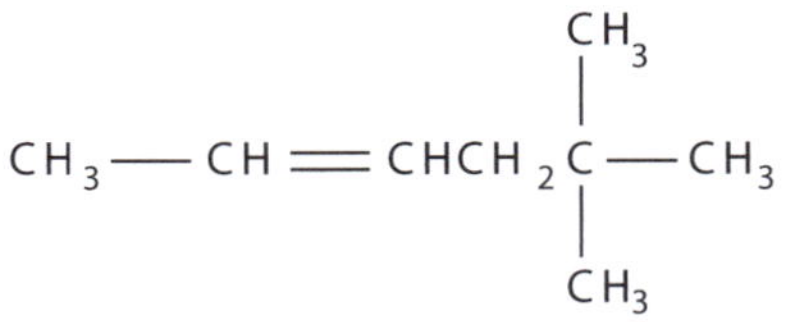

5,5 - Dimethyl - 2 - hexene

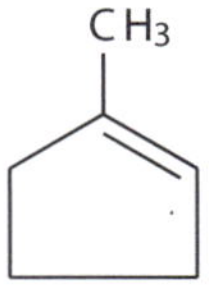

1 - methylcyclopentene

Two frequently encountered groups are sometimes named as if they were substituents.

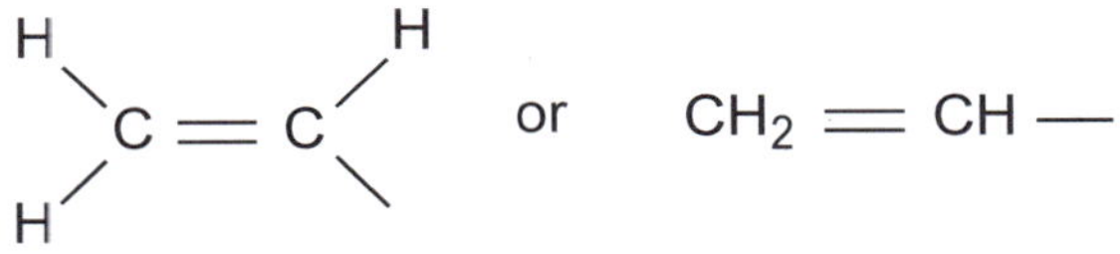

the vinyl group

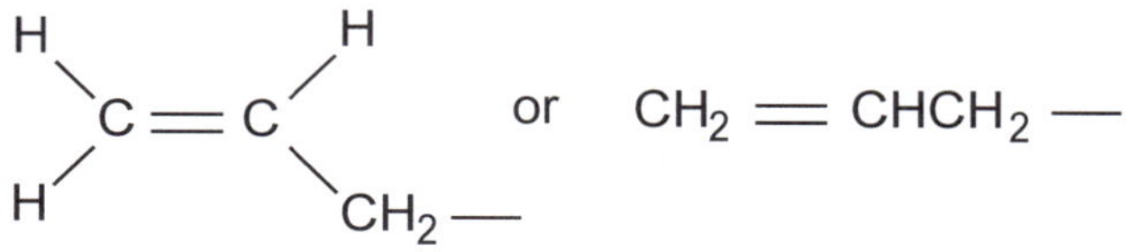

the allyl group

Alkenes have similar physical properties to alkanes. *Trans* compounds tend to have higher melting points (due to better symmetry), and lower boiling points (due to less polarity) than its corresponding *cis* isomer. Alkenes, however, due to the nature of the double bond may be polar. The dipole moment is oriented from the electropositive alkyl group toward the electronegative alkene.

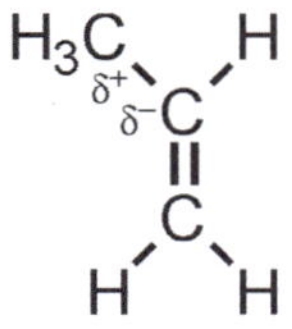

has a small dipole moment

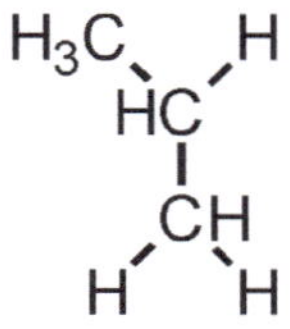

has no dipole moment

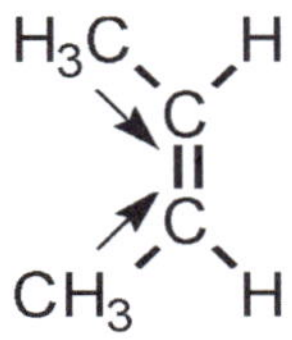

(cis) small dipole moment

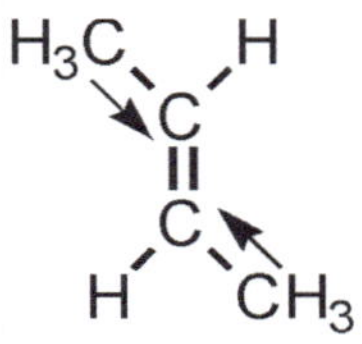

(trans) no dipole moment

The greater the number of attached alkyl groups (i.e. *the more highly substituted the double bond*), the greater is the alkene's stability. The reason is that alkyl groups are somewhat electron donating, thus they stabilise the double bond.

An alkene with 2 double bonds is a diene, 3 is a triene. A diene with one single bond in between is a conjugated diene. Conjugated dienes are more stable than non-conjugated dienes primarily due to resonance stabilisation. We first saw the resonance-stabilised, conjugated molecule *1,3-butadiene* in ORG 1.4. You can see a few of its many resonance forms below including a symbolic cartoon which is closer to reality: the pi electrons are not simply located between any 2 carbons, but rather they are spread out over the molecule (*delocalised, which affords greater stability*).

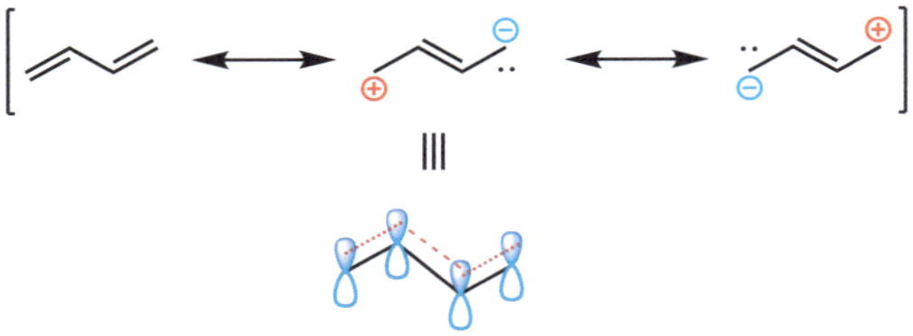

Alkenes, including polyenes, can engage in addition reactions (ORG 4.2.1). The notable exceptions include aromatic compounds (conjugated double bonds in a ring; ORG 5.1) which cannot engage in addition reactions which will be discussed in the next chapter.

Polyenes have multiple double bonds, such as dienes, trienes, tetraenes and many more are possible. In fact, consider the molecular structure of beta-carotene below. Notice that: 1) there are eleven conjugated double bonds highlighted in red; 2) the configuration at those double bonds is all-*trans* (i.e. 0 bonds in the *cis* configuration; ORG 2.2.1); 3) placing the double bond (*pi bond*) above or below the first bond (*sigma bond*) in such an image is irrelevant. It is simply a symbol of the bond between 2 carbons, C=C.

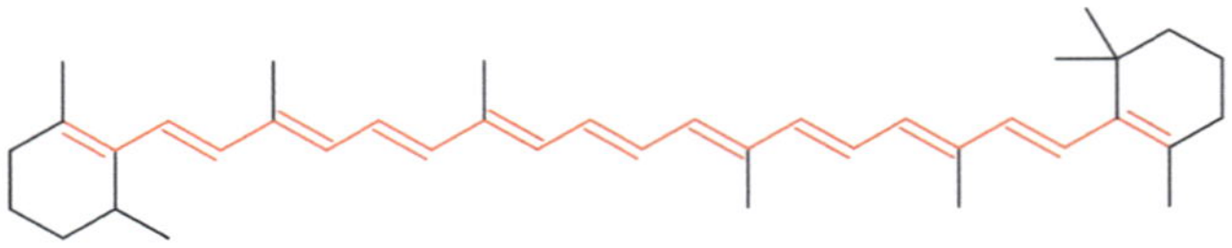

• Synthesis of Alkenes: The two most common alkene-forming reactions involve elimination reactions of either HX from an alkyl halide or H_2O from an alcohol (*see* the following reactions). Dehydrohalogenation occurs by the reaction of an alkyl halide with a strong base. Dehydration (*loss of water*) occurs by reacting an alcohol with a strong acid.

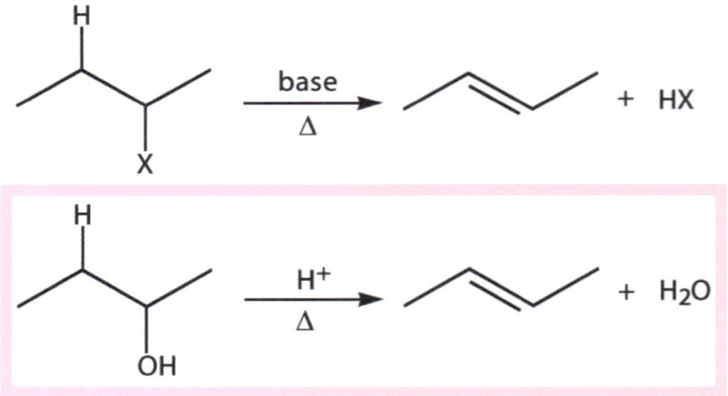

We will discuss elimination reactions (E1 and E2), which can be used to synthesise alkenes, in ORG 6.2.4 (alcohols).

Medium-level Importance

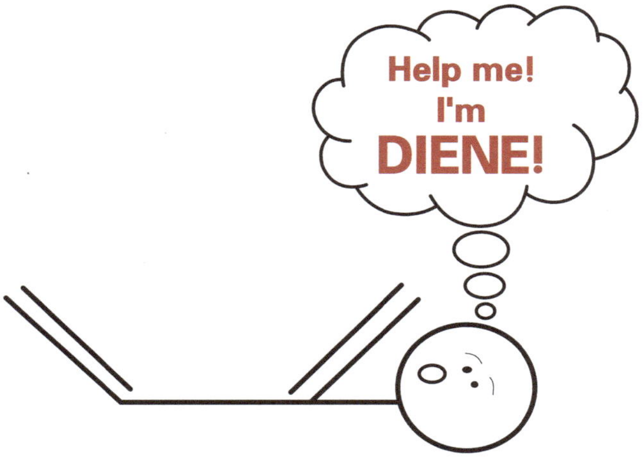

4.1.1 Foundational Nomenclature Exercises: Alkenes and Alkynes

Name the following ten compounds. If it is your first time, feel free to consult the nomenclature rules from ORG 3.1 and 4.1. The answers are at the end of this chapter. Of course, it is more helpful to you in the long run to give a full effort first - rather than looking at the solutions before trying.

Note that alkynes possess a triple bond. The nomenclature for alkynes is the same as that for alkenes, except that the suffix 'yne' replaces 'ene'.

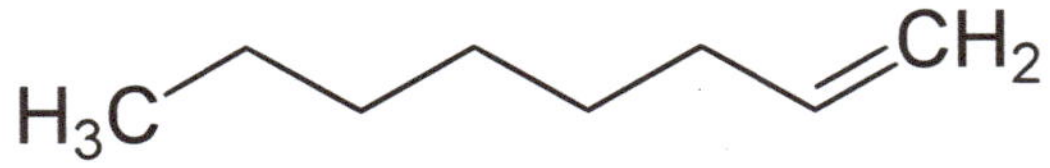

1) ______________________

$H_2C{=}C{=}C{=}CH_2$

2) ______________________

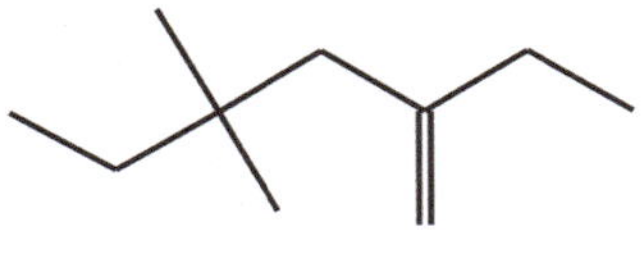

3) ______________________

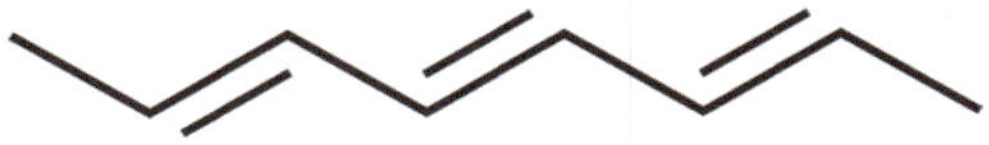

4) ______________________

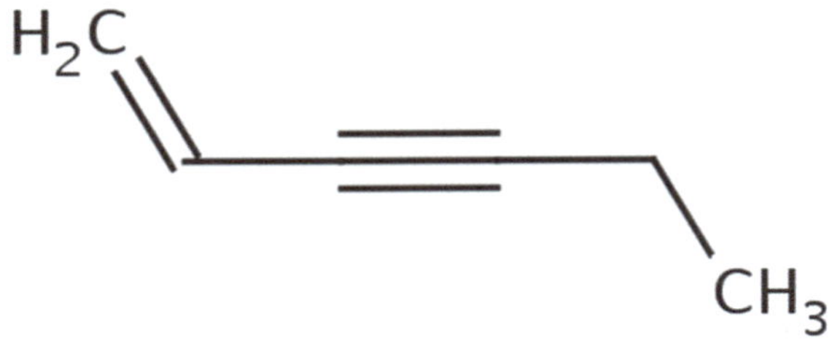

5) ____________________

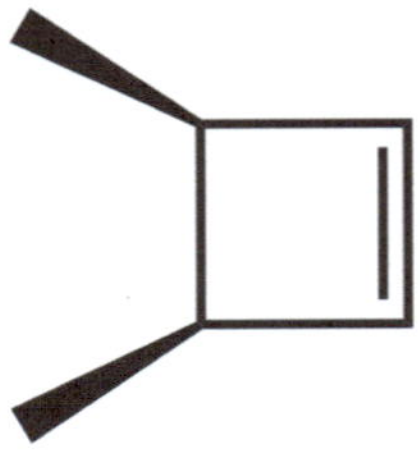

6) ____________________

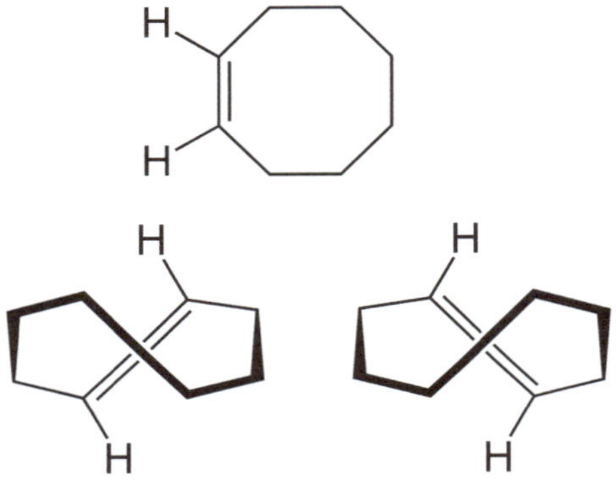

7) ____________________

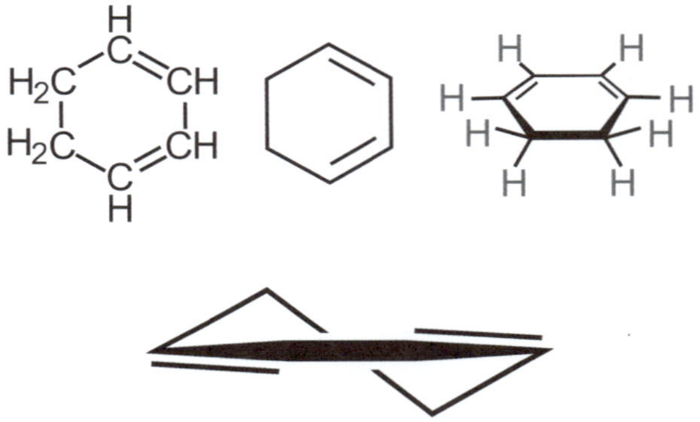

8) ____________________

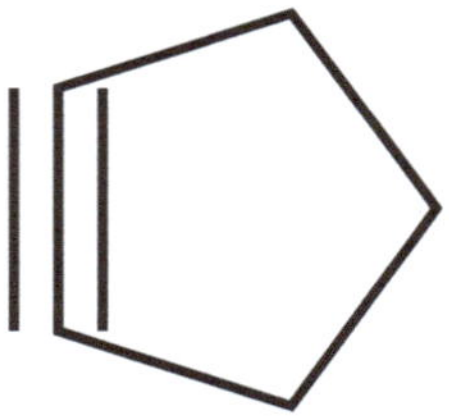

9) ____________________

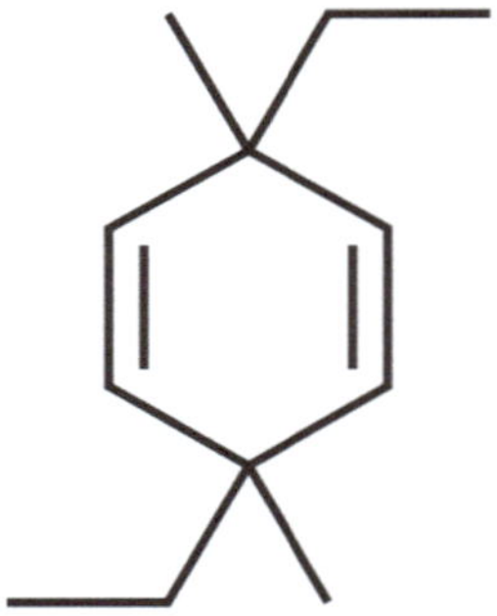

10) ____________________

4.2.1 Electrophilic Addition

The chemistry of alkenes may be understood in terms of their functional group, the double bond. When electrophiles (*substances which seek electrons*) add to alkenes, carbocations (= *carbonium ions*) are formed. An important electrophile is H^+ (i.e. in HBr, H_2O, etc.). A nucleophile (ORG 1.6) is a molecule with a free pair of electrons, and sometimes a negative charge, that seeks out partially or completely positively charged species (i.e. a carbon nucleus). Some important nucleophiles are OH^- and CN^-.

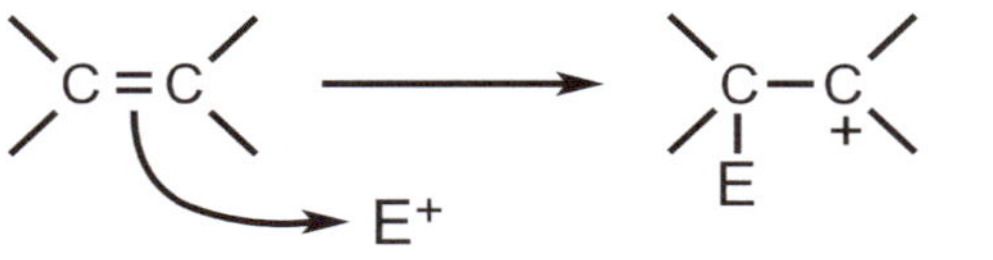

E = electrophile

carbocation (intermediate)

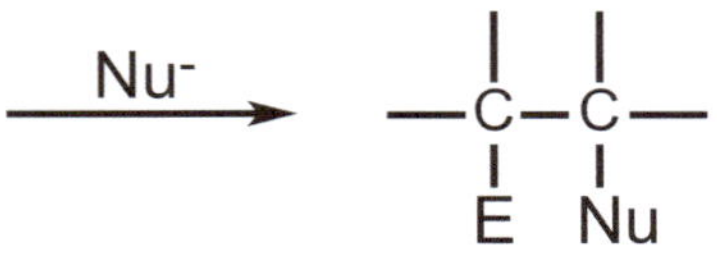

Nu = nucleophile

Note that the carbon-carbon double bond is electron rich (nucleophilic) and can donate a pair of electrons to an electrophile (= "electron loving") during reactions. Electrons from the π bond attack the electrophile. As the π bond is weaker than the σ bond, it can be broken without breaking the σ bond. As a result, the carbon skeleton can remain intact. Electrophilic addition to an unsymmetrically substituted alkene gives the more highly substituted carbocation (i.e. the most stable intermediate). We will soon see that Markovnikov's rule is a guide to determine the outcome of addition reactions.

Another important property of the double bond is its ability to stabilise carbocations, carbanions or radicals attached to adjacent carbons (*allylic carbons*). Note that all the following are resonance stabilised:

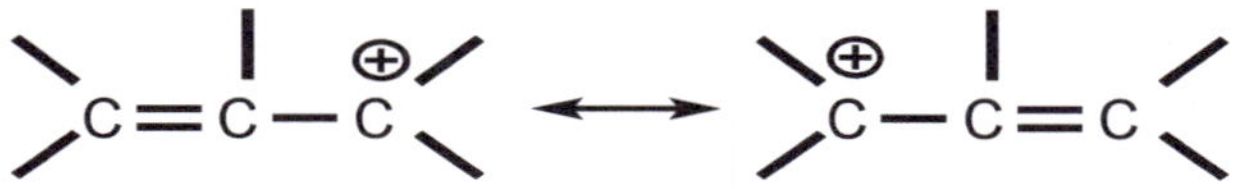

carbocation

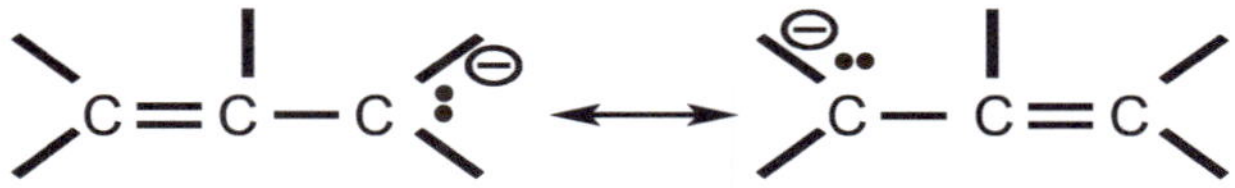

carbanion

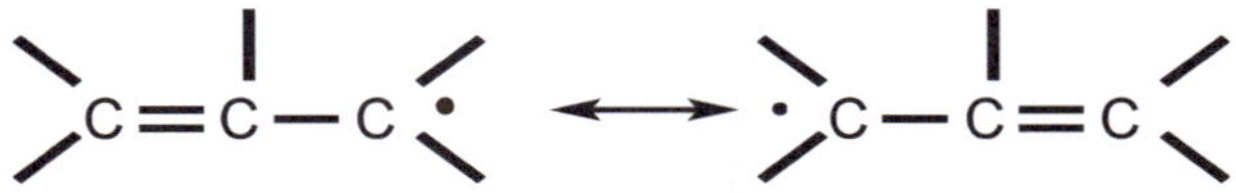

carbon radical

The stability of the intermediate carbocation depends on the groups attached to it, which can either stabilise or destabilise it. As well, groups which place a partial or total positive charge adjacent to the carbocation withdraw electrons inductively, by sigma bonds, to destabilise it. More highly substituted carbocations are more stable than less highly substituted ones.

These points are useful in predicting which carbon will become the carbocation,

Medium-level Importance

Medium-level Importance

and to which carbon the electrophile and nucleophile will bond. The intermediate carbocation formed must be the most stable. **Markovnikov's rule** is a result of this, and it states: *the nucleophile will be bonded to the most substituted carbon* (fewest hydrogens attached) *in the product. Equivalently, the electrophile will be bonded to the least substituted carbon* (most hydrogens attached) *in the product*. An example of this is:

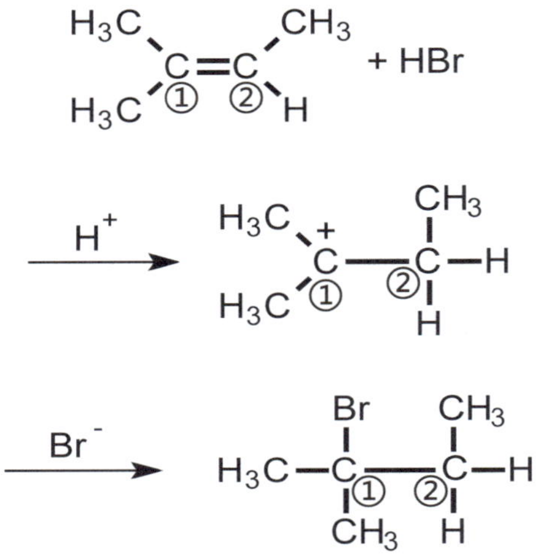

H^+ = electrophile
Br^- = nucleophile
① most substituted carbon
② least substituted carbon
① forms the most stable carbonium ion.

The product, 2-bromo-2-methyl butane, is the more likely or major product (*the Markovnikov product*). Had the H^+ added to the most substituted carbon (which has a much lower probability of occurrence) the less likely or minor product would be formed (*the anti-Markovnikov product*). {Memory guide for Markovnikov's rule: *"Hydrogen prefers to add to the carbon in the double bond where most of its friends are"* (this works because the least substituted carbon has the most bonds to hydrogen atoms)} Example:

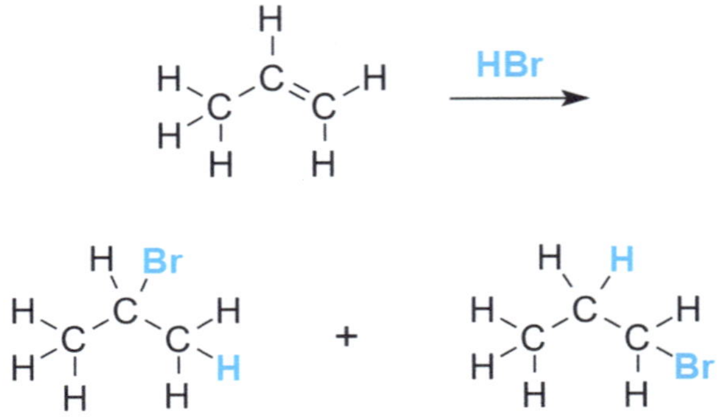

major minor

Carbocation intermediate rearrangement: In both *hydride shift* and *alkyl group shift*, H or CH_3 moves to a positively charged carbon, taking its electron pair with it. As a result, a less stable carbocation rearranges to a more stable one (more substituted).

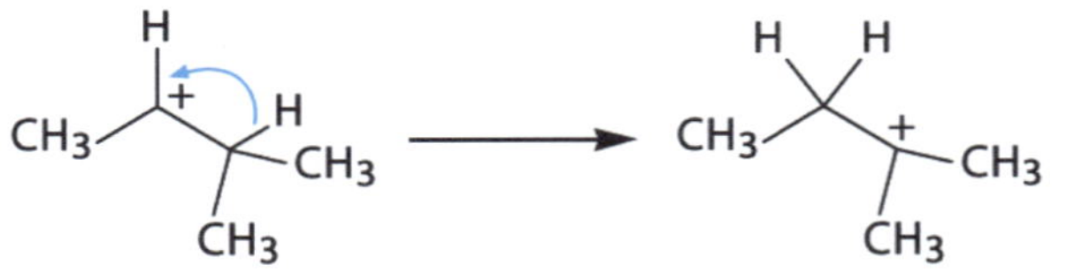

secondary carbocation tertiary carbocation

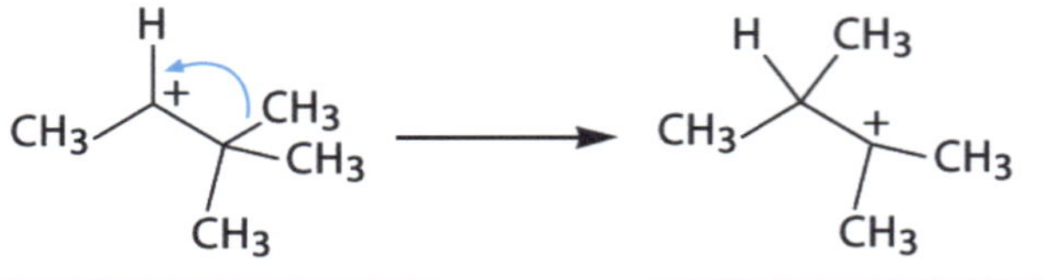

secondary carbocation tertiary carbocation

Markovnikov's rule is true for the ionic conditions presented in the preceding reaction. However, for radical conditions the reverse occurs. Thus *anti-Markovnikov* products are the major products under free radical conditions.

• Addition of halogens: This is a simple and rapid laboratory diagnostic tool to test for the presence of unsaturation (C=C). Immediate disappearance of the reddish Br_2 colour indicates that the sample is an alkene. The general chemical formula of the halogen addition reaction is:

$$C=C + X_2 \longrightarrow X-C-C-X$$

The π electron pair of the double bond attacks the bromine, or X_2 molecule, setting up an induced dipole (*see* CHM 4.2) and then displacing the bromide ion. The intermediate forms a cyclic bromonium ion R_2Br^+, which is then attacked by Br^-, giving the dibromo addition product.

Since the intermediate is a bromonium ion, the bromide anion can only attack from the opposite side, yielding an anti product.

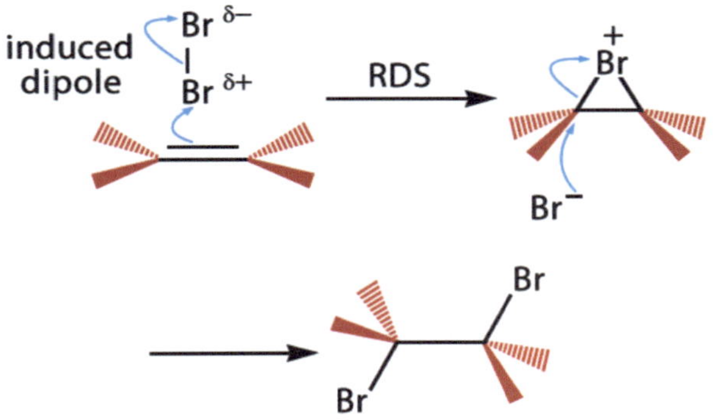

RDS = rate-determining step (CHM 9.4)

Halogen addition does not occur in saturated hydrocarbons (i.e. cyclohexane) which lack the electron rich double bond, nor do the reactions occur within an aromatic ring because of the increased stability afforded by conjugation in a ring system due to resonance.

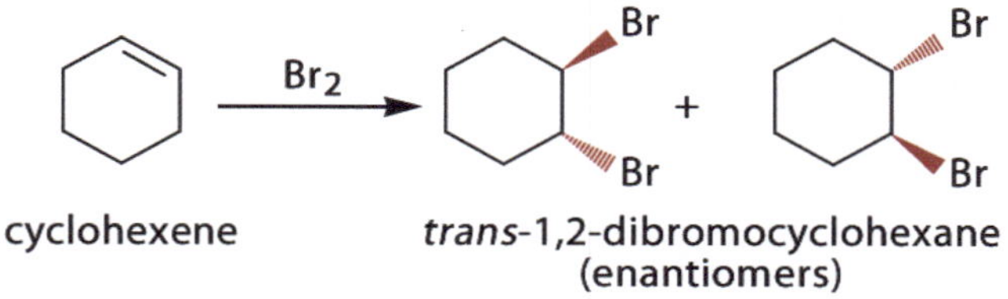

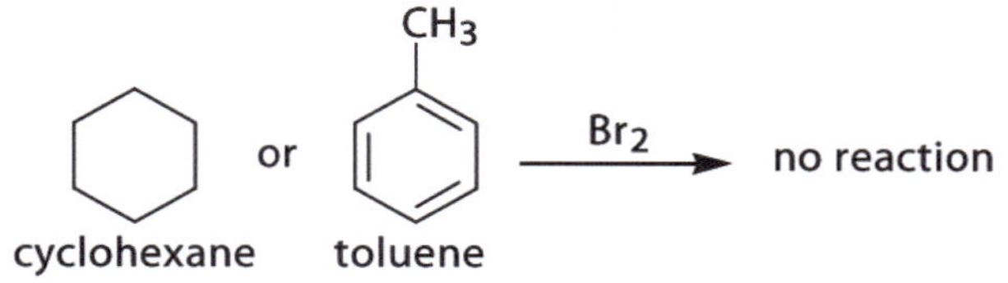

• Halohydrin formation reaction: A halohydrin (or haloalcohol) is a functional group where one carbon atom has a halogen substituent and an adjacent carbon atom has a hydroxyl substituent. This addition, which produces a halohydrin, is done by reacting an alkene with a halogen X_2 in the presence of water. The intermediate forms a cyclic bromonium ion R_2Br^+. The water molecule competes with the bromide ion as a nucleophile and reacts with the bromonium ion to form the halohydrin. The net effect is the addition of HO-X to the alkene.

In practice, the bromohydrin reaction is carried out using a reagent called NBS. Markovnikov regiochemistry and anti addition is observed.

• Addition of HX: As we have seen earlier in this section, this reaction occurs via a carbocation intermediate. The halide ion then combines with the carbocation to give an alkyl halide. The proton will add to the less substituted carbon atom, yielding a more substituted (stabilised) carbocation. Markovnikov regiochemistry is observed. This can be seen in the first two mechanisms shown in this section (ORG 4.2.1).

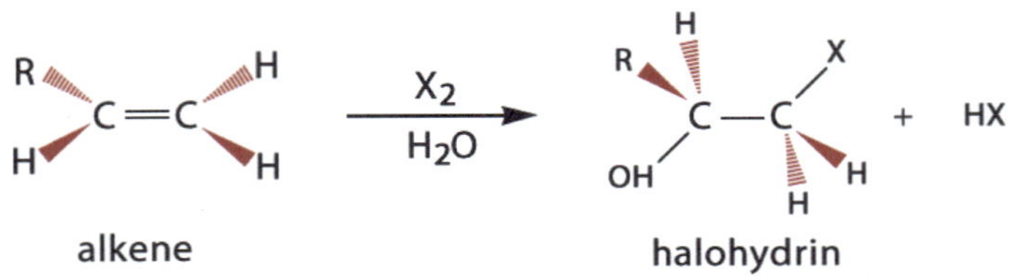

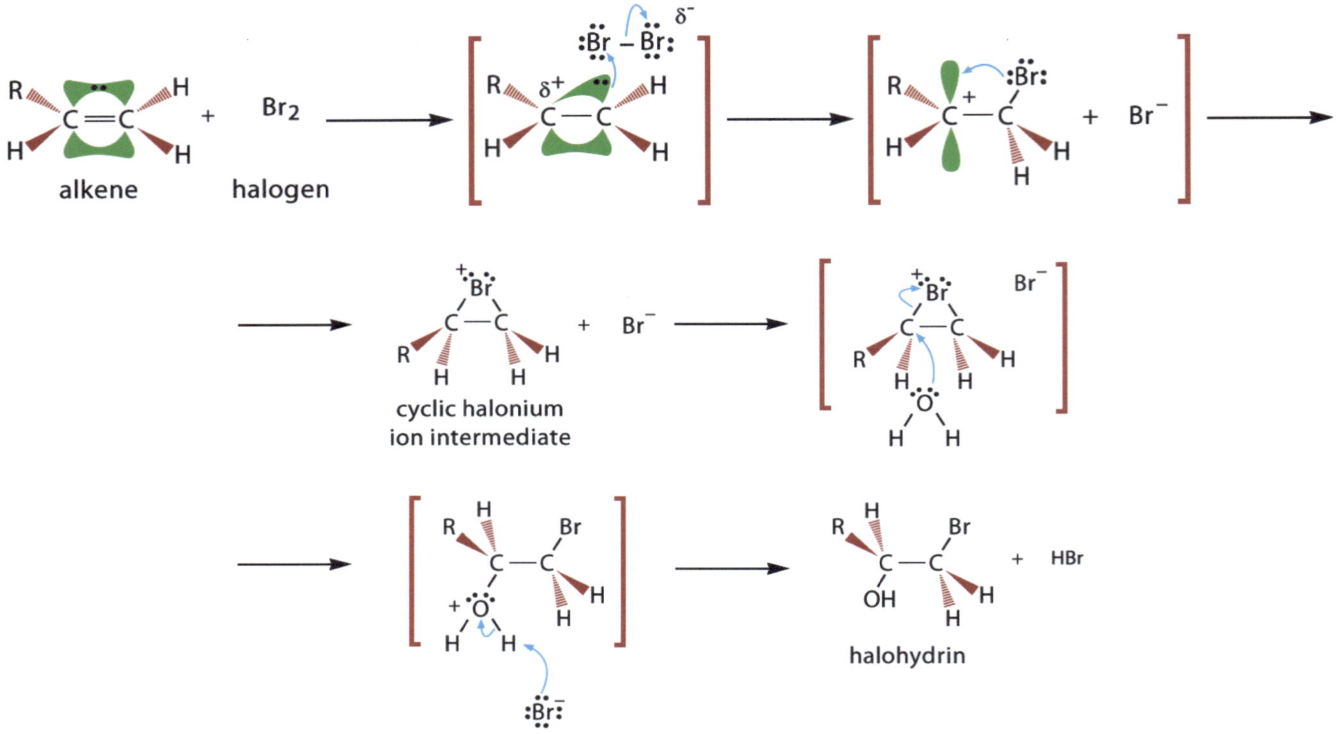

"Should I memorise these reaction mechanisms and the ones on the way?"

That would not be very helpful. If a related question were asked, normally the passage or question stem would begin by spelling out the mechanism and then the questions would lean towards your skills involving nomenclature, geometry, pattern recognition and time efficiency. Mechanisms should be followed like a good story that contains a consistent, reasonable plot. The key is to follow the plot, not to memorise it. If the plot can be reasoned then, if given a blueprint and different characters during an exam (or practice), you should be able to determine the conclusion, and how the examiners arrived at that conclusion (i.e. the intermediates when necessary).

Geometry and pattern recognition allow you to follow if an addition is cis (= syn) or trans (= anti, i.e. halohydrin formation). They also help you: follow where the different R groups end up (i.e. alkene oxidation; ORG 4.2.2); recognise unusual product geometries once you have a blueprint (i.e. Diels-Alder reaction; ORG 4.2.4); etc. As often as possible, get in the habit of drawing molecules shorthand while completing your end-of-chapter practice questions. Drawing and practice questions are important components of GAMSAT Organic Chemistry preparation.

- Free radical addition of HBr to alkenes: Once a bromine free radical has formed in an initiation step (ORG 3.2.2), it adds to the alkene double bond, yielding an alkyl radical. The regiochemistry of this free radical addition is determined in the first propagation step because, instead of H attacking first in electrophilic addition, the bromine radical adds first to the alkene. Thus anti-Markovnikov addition is observed.

The stability order of radicals is identical to the stability order of carbocations, tertiary being the most stable and methyl the least. Notice that the free radical reaction mechanism that follows uses single headed (blue) arrows to follow the movement of single electrons, as opposed to the normal arrows that we have seen which follow the movement of electron pairs.

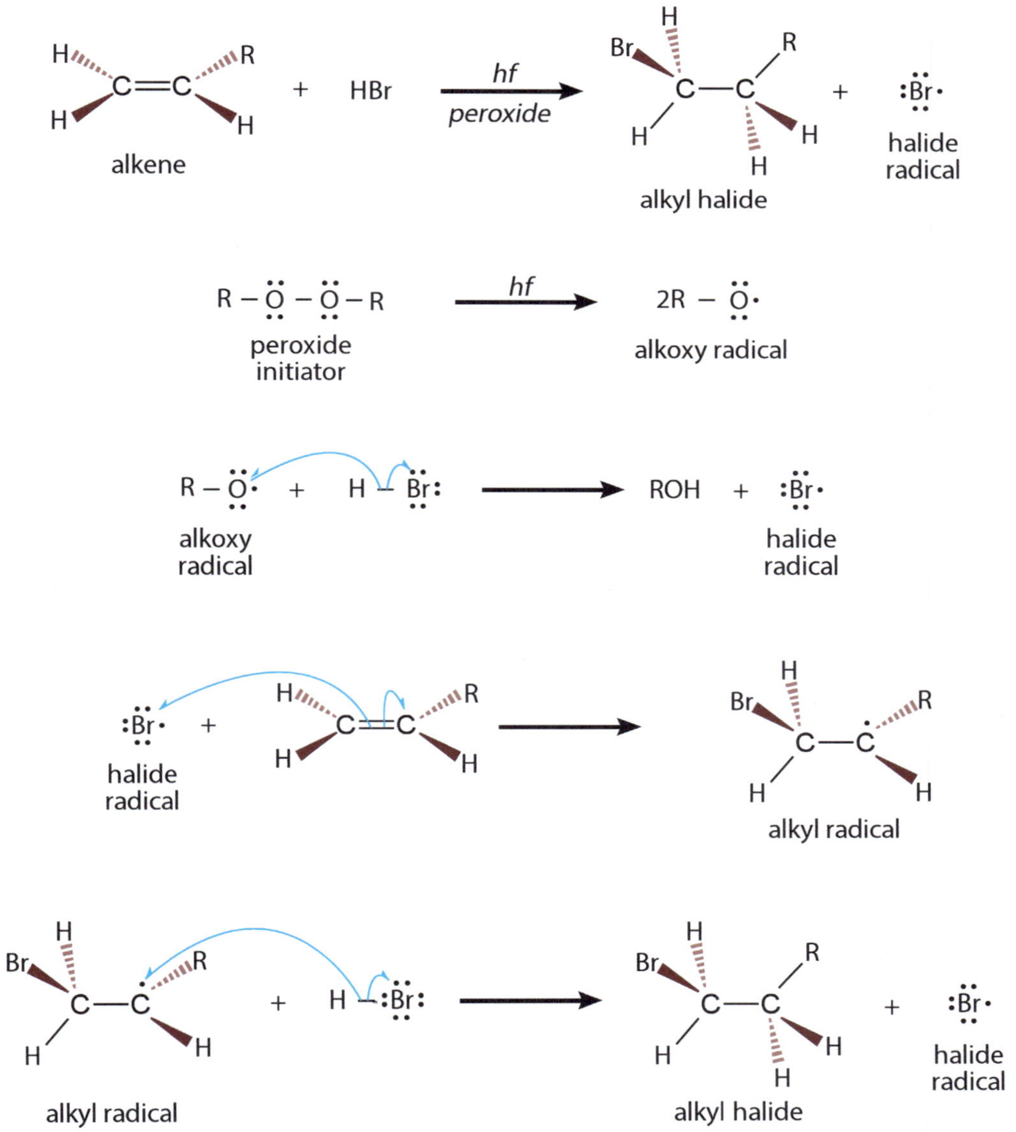

4.2.2 Oxidation

Alkenes can undergo a variety of reactions in which the carbon-carbon double bond is oxidised. Using potassium permanganate ($KMnO_4$) under mild conditions (*no heat*), or osmium tetroxide (OsO_4), a glycol (= *a diol* = *a "dialcohol"*) can be produced.

In the following chapters, you will learn how to derive systematic nomenclature (these are names of compounds based on rules as opposed to "common" names often based on tradition). IUPAC (official) nomenclature is usually systematic (i.e. ethane-1,2-diol) but sometimes it is not (i.e. acetic acid). Knowing both the common and the systematic names is the safest way to approach the GAMSAT.

The first reaction that follows is the oxidation of ethene (= ethylene) under mild conditions and the second is the oxidation of 2-butene under abrasive conditions.

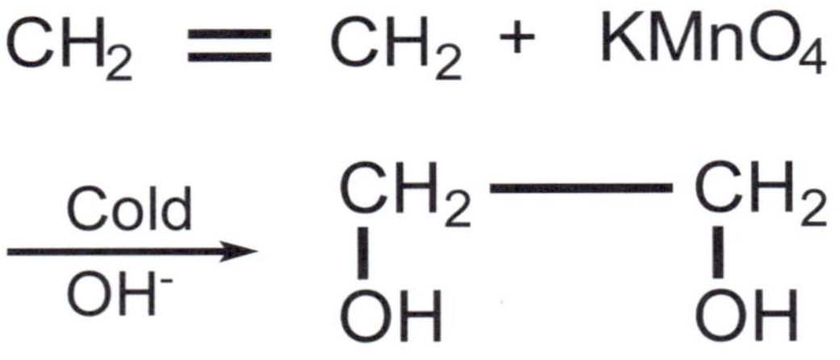

Ethylene glycol
(1,2-ethanediol or
ethane-1,2-diol)

Using $KMnO_4$ under more abrasive conditions leads to an oxidative cleavage of the double bond:

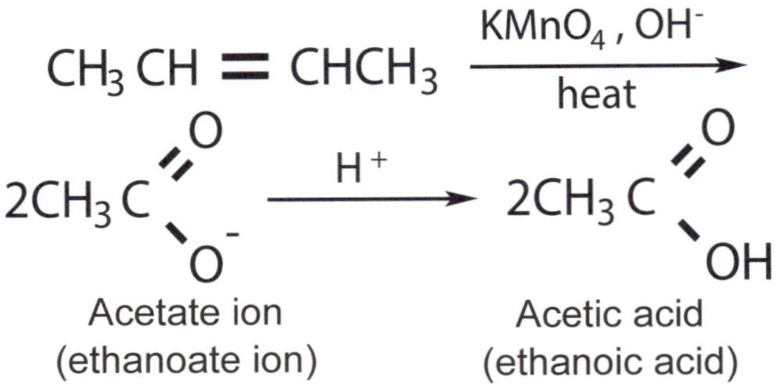

Specifically, cold dilute $KMnO_4$ produces 1,2-diols with the syn orientation. Hot, basic $KMnO_4$ leads to oxidative cleavage of the double bonds with the double bond being replaced with a C=O bond and an O atom added to each H atom that was connected to the central carbon.

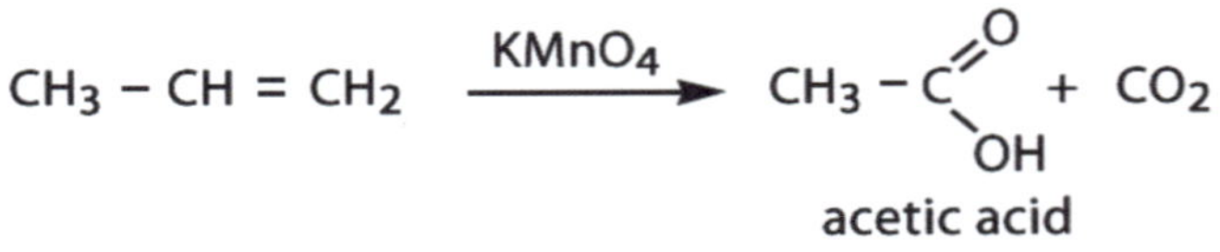

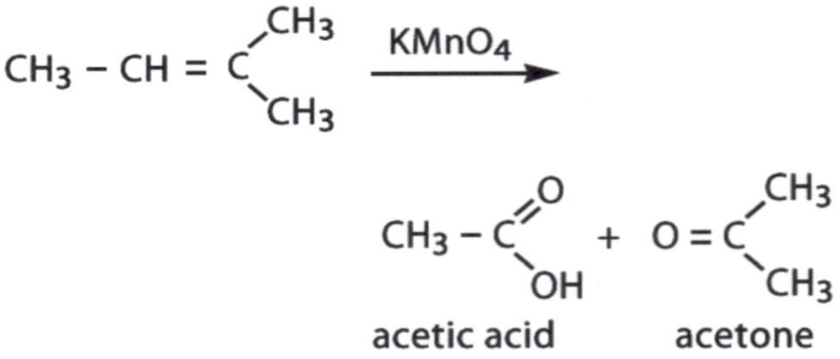

$$CH_2 = CH - CH = CH_2 \xrightarrow{KMnO_4} CO_2 + H_2O$$

Ozone (O_3) reacts vigorously with alkenes. The reaction (= *ozonolysis*) leads to an oxidative cleavage of the double bond which can produce a ketone and an aldehyde:

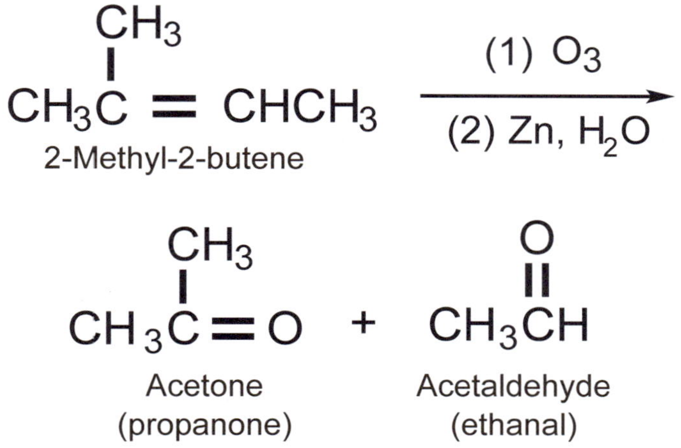

Note that the second step in the reaction uses a reducing agent such as zinc metal.

If the starting alkene has a tetra-substituted double bond (i.e. 4 R groups), two ketones will be formed. If it has a tri-substituted double bond, a ketone and an aldehyde will be formed as in the reaction shown. If it has a di-substituted double bond (e.g. R-CH=CH-R), two aldehydes are possible.

The hydroboration–oxidation reaction is a two-step organic reaction that converts an alkene into an alcohol by the addition of water across the double bond. The hydrogen and hydroxyl group are added in a syn addition leading to *cis* stereochemistry. Hydroboration–oxidation is an anti-Markovnikov reaction since the hydroxyl group (not the hydrogen) attaches to the less substituted carbon.

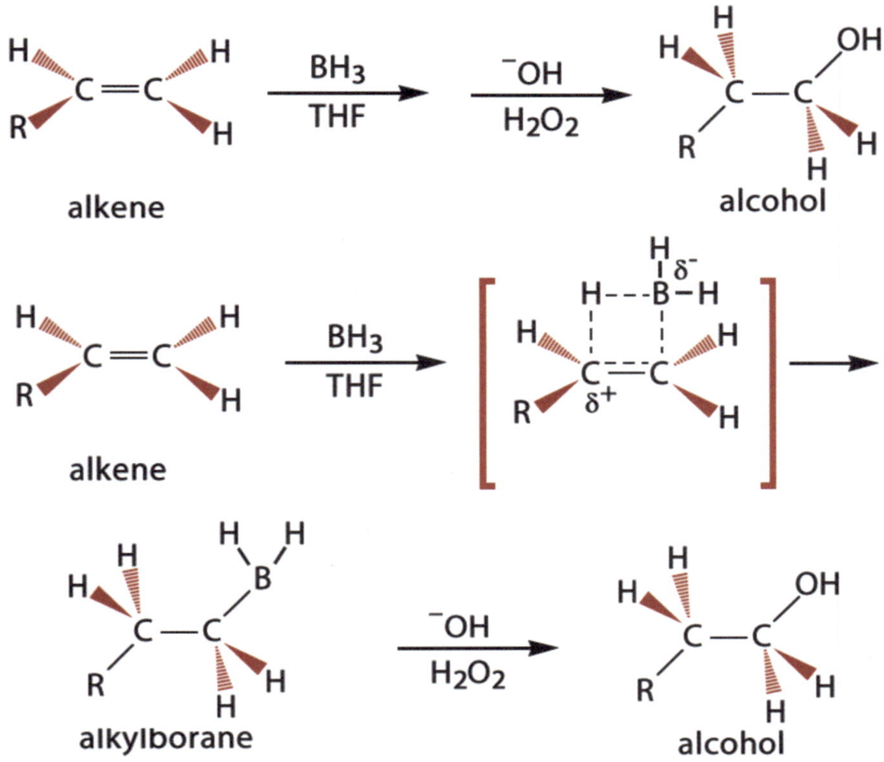

- Epoxide Formation: Alkenes can be oxidised with peroxycarboxylic acids (i.e. CH_3CO_3H or mCPBA). The product is an oxirane (discussed in ORG 10.1.1, ethers).

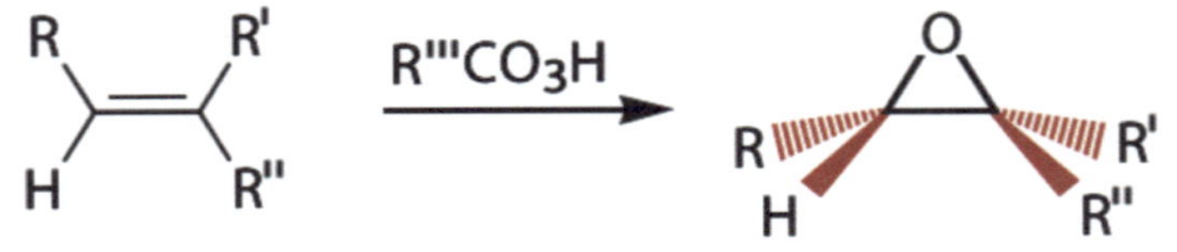

4.2.3 Hydrogenation

Medium-level Importance

Alkenes react with hydrogen in the presence of a variety of metal catalysts (i.e. Ni – nickel, Pd – palladium, Pt – platinum). The reaction that occurs is an *addition* reaction since one atom of hydrogen adds to each carbon of the double bond (= *hydrogenation*). Both hydrogens add to the double bond from the same metal catalyst surface, thus syn addition is observed. Since there are two phases present in the process of hydrogenation (the hydrogen and the metal catalyst), the process is referred to as a heterogenous catalysis.

A carbon with multiple bonds is not bonded to the maximum number of atoms that potentially that carbon could possess. Thus it is *unsaturated*. Alkanes, which can be formed by hydrogenation, are *saturated* since each carbon is bonded to the maximum number of atoms it could possess (= *four*). Thus hydrogenation is sometimes called the process of saturation.

$$CH_3CH = CH_2 + H_2 \longrightarrow CH_3CH_2 - CH_3$$

Alkenes are much more reactive than other functional groups towards hydrogenation. As a result, other functional groups such as ketones, aldehydes, esters and nitriles are usually unchanged during the alkene hydrogenation process.

4.2.4 The Diels–Alder Reaction

The Diels–Alder reaction is a cycloaddition reaction between a conjugated diene and a substituted alkene (= the dienophile) to form a substituted cyclohexene system.

Diene + Dienophile = Cyclohexene

All Diels-Alder reactions have four common features: **(1)** the reaction is initiated by heat; **(2)** the reaction forms new six-membered rings; **(3)** three π bonds break and two new C-C σ bonds and one new C-C π bond are formed; **(4)** all bonds break and form in a single step.

The Diels-Alder diene must have the two double bonds on the same side of the single bond in one of the structures, which is called the s-*cis* conformation (s-*cis*: *cis* with respect to the single bond). If double bonds are on the opposite sides of the single bond in the Lewis structure, this is called the s-*trans* conformation (s-*trans*: *trans* with respect to the single bond).

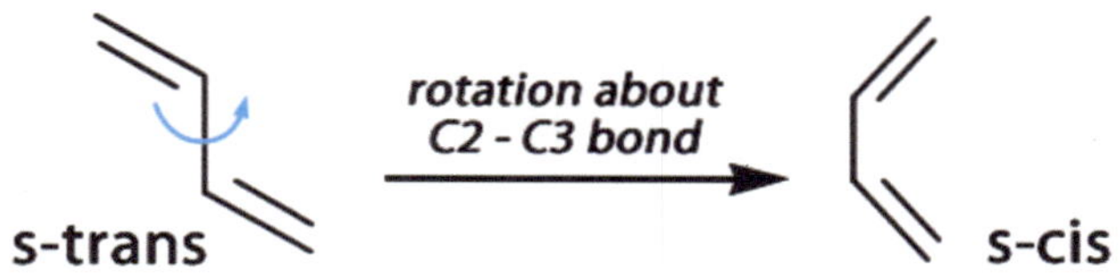

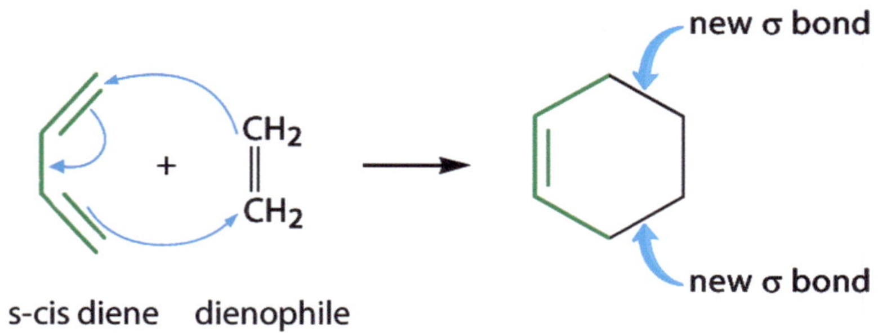

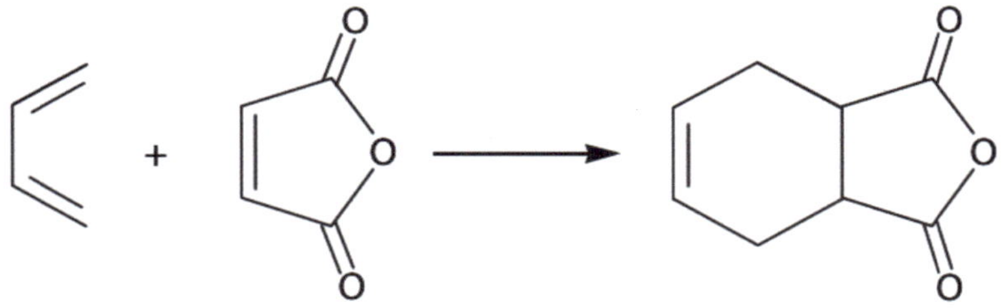

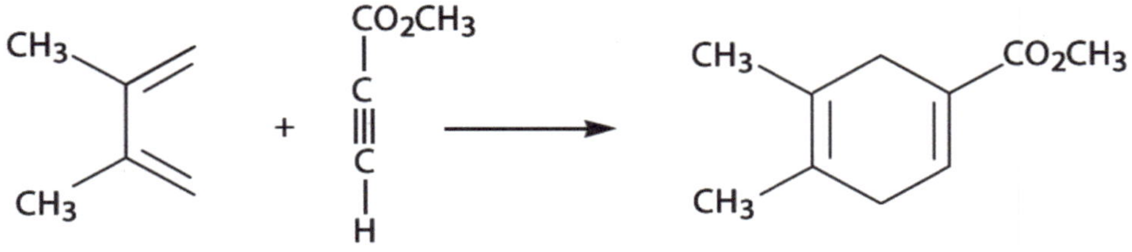

The Diels-Alder reaction is useful because it sometimes creates stereocentres, it always forms a ring, and the reaction is stereospecific (i.e. the reaction mechanism dictates the stereoisomers). For example, a *cis* dienophile generates a ring with *cis* substitution, while a *trans* dienophile generates a ring with *trans* substitution.

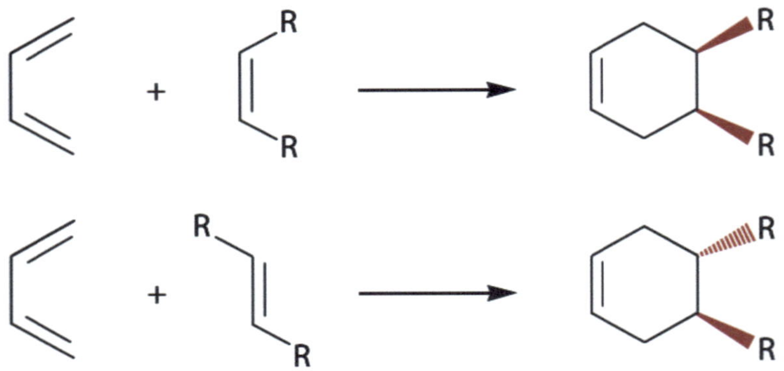

Diels-Alder reactions are reversible (= "Retro-Diels-Alder").

Medium-level Importance

4.2.5 Resonance Revisited

General Chemistry section 3.2 and Organic Chemistry section 1.4 are important to revise before you move on to the next chapter on Aromatics. Many exam questions rely on your understanding of resonance. It is helpful to remember that the only difference between different resonance forms is the placement of π or non-bonding electrons. The atoms themselves do not change positions, create new bonds nor are they "resonating" back and forth. The resonance hybrid with its electrons delocalised is more stable than any single resonance form. The greater the numbers of authentic resonance forms possible, the more stable the molecule.

Consider a typical example of resonance with the allylic carbocation. Here are its two equivalent resonance structures:

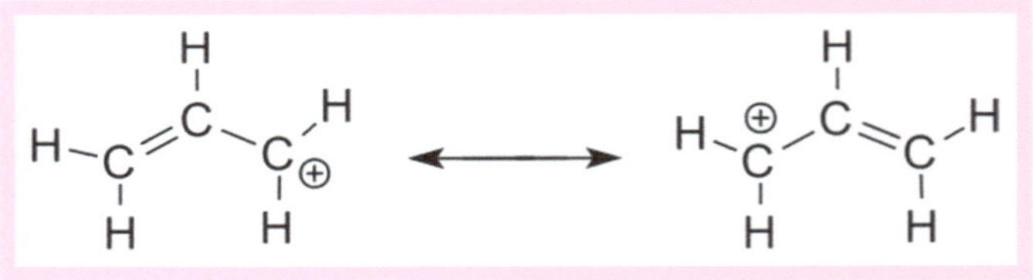

And here are three different ways to represent the identical concept: The true allylic cation does not have a positive charge on one side and a double bond on the other side. Its actual nature is a hybrid structure with the charge delocalised which can be represented in different equivalent ways.

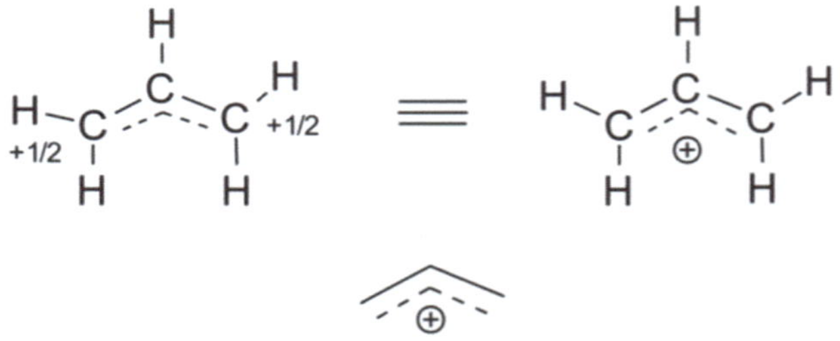

Alkynes are unsaturated hydrocarbon molecules containing carbon-carbon triple bonds (1 sigma + 2 π bonds; ORG 1.3). The nomenclature is the same as that for alkenes, except that the suffix 'yne' replaces 'ene'. Alkynes have a higher boiling point than alkenes or alkanes. Internal alkynes, where the triple bond is in the middle of the compound, boil at higher temperatures than terminal alkynes. Terminal alkynes are relatively acidic.

Basic reactions such as reduction, electrophilic addition, free radical addition and hydroboration proceed in a similar manner to alkenes. Oxidation also follows the same rules and uses the same reactants and catalysts. However, unlike alkenes, alkynes can be partially hydrogenated yielding alkenes with just one equivalent of H_2. The reaction with palladium in Lindlar's catalyst produces the *cis* alkene while sodium or lithium in liquid ammonia will produce the *trans* alkene via a free radical mechanism.

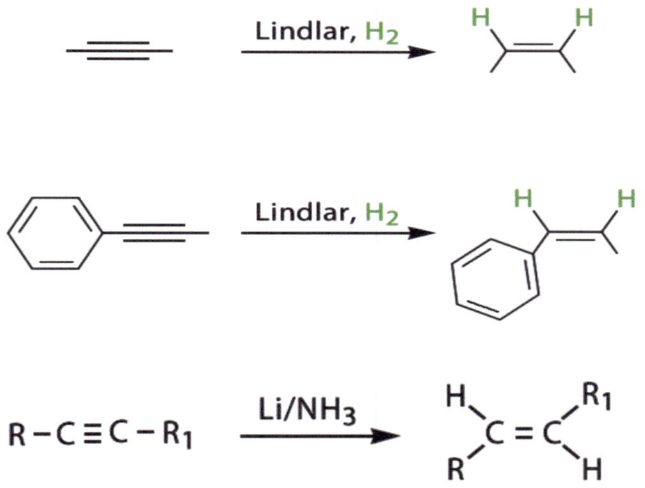

Solutions to Foundational Nomenclature Exercises: Alkenes and Alkynes	
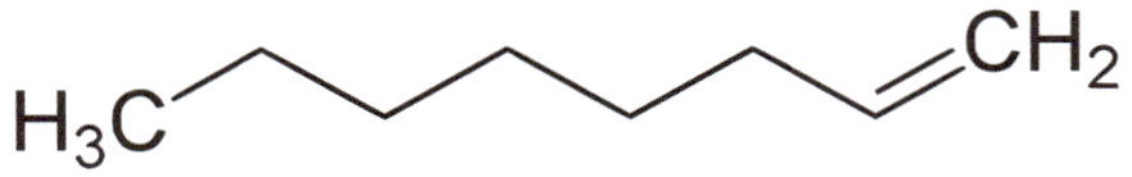 **1)** 1-octene	$H_2C{=}C{=}C{=}CH_2$ **2)** buta-1,2,3-triene (*no* conjugation)
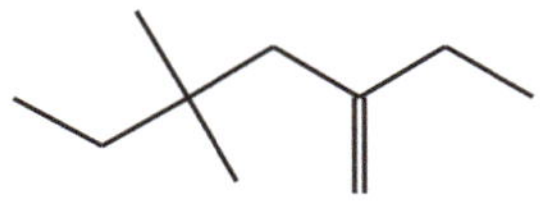 **3)** 4,4-dimethyl-2-ethyl-1-hexene Do not be concerned if you wrote: 2-ethyl-4,4-dimethyl-1-hexene or …hex-1-ene; on an exam, ACER would elucidate the rule. However, if you chose 'heptene' then you counted in a way that did not include the double bond and that is incorrect.	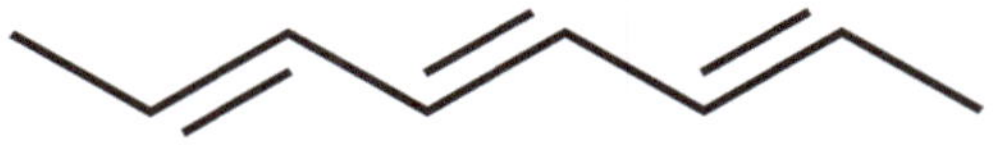 **4)** octa-2,4,6-triene In order to respect the configuration: (*2E,4E,6E*)-octa-2,4,6-triene would be a better name (note that the structure is all *trans* and *fully* conjugated).

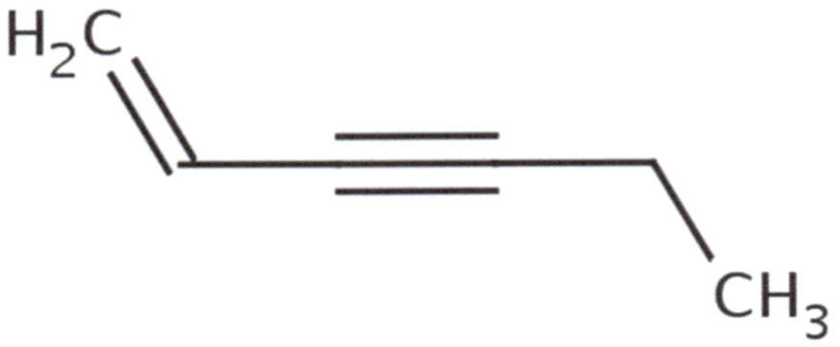

5) hex-1-en-3-yne

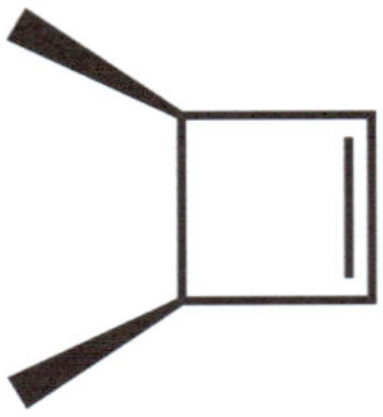

6) *cis*-3,4-dimethylcyclobut-1-ene
(OK: 3,4-dimethylcyclobutene)

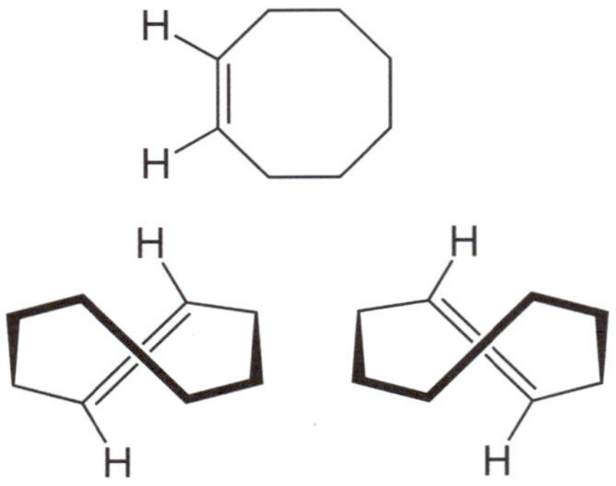

7) *cis* and *trans*-cyclooctene
The first structure is *cis*; the second and third structures are both *trans*. There is only one functional group, so "1-ene" would be redundant.

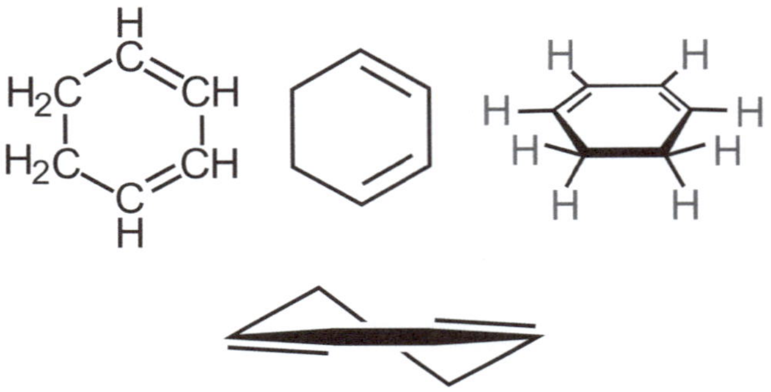

8) cyclohexa-1,3-diene
Yes, all 4 structures are different representations of the identical molecule.

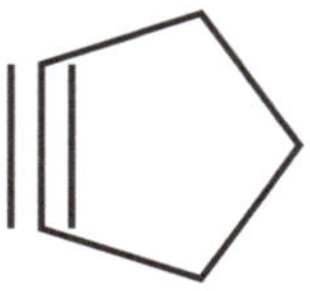

9) cyclopentyne
There is only one functional group, so "1-yne" would be redundant.

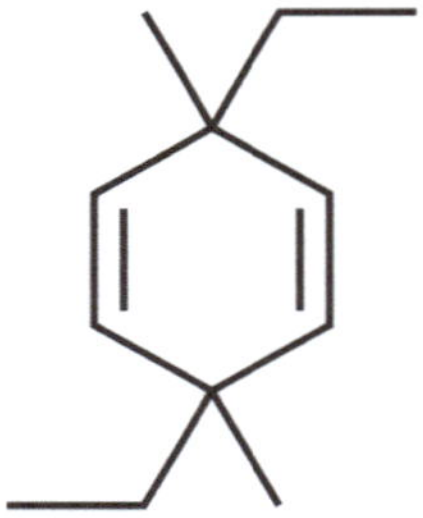

10) 3,6-diethyl-3,6-dimethylcyclohexa-1,4-diene
Do not worry about ending with 1,4-cyclohexadiene, or switching diethyl and dimethyl in the absence of instructions (*although it should be in alphabetical order as above*).

Questions or concerns? gamsat-prep.com/forum

Medium-level Importance

CHAPTER 4: Alkenes

GOLD STANDARD FOUNDATIONAL GAMSAT PRACTICE QUESTIONS

Questions 11–15

You may find some of the information below helpful for the following questions.

A single bond is a *sigma* bond. A double bond has one sigma plus one *pi* bond, and a triple bond has one sigma plus two pi bonds.

Consider Table 1.

When bonded to…	Hybridisation	Shape	Bond angle
2 atoms	sp	linear	180°
3 atoms	sp^2	trigonal (triangular)	120°
4 atoms	sp^3	tetrahedral	109.5°

Table 1: Neutral carbon's bond hybrids

11) How many sigma bonds are there in CH_2=CH-CH_2-CH=CH_2?

A. 6
B. 9
C. 12
D. 14

12) How many sigma bonds are there in the following compound?

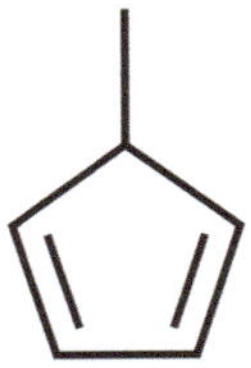

A. 6
B. 8
C. 12
D. 14

13) How many pi-bonds are there in the following compound? (Note: Take the dot on the right as representing a carbon atom.)

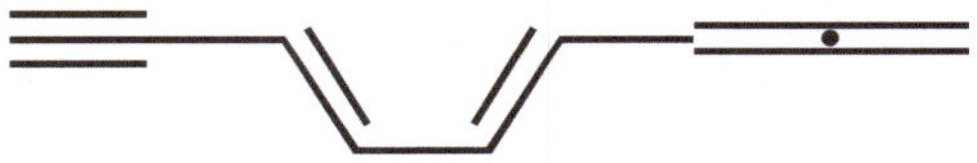

A. 4
B. 5
C. 6
D. 7

14) Identify the orbitals involved with the C-C sigma-bonding framework in ethyne.

A. (2s, 1s)
B. (2sp, 2sp)
C. ($2sp^2$, $2sp^2$)
D. ($2sp^3$, $2sp^3$)

15) Which of the following molecules contains sp-hybridisation?

I

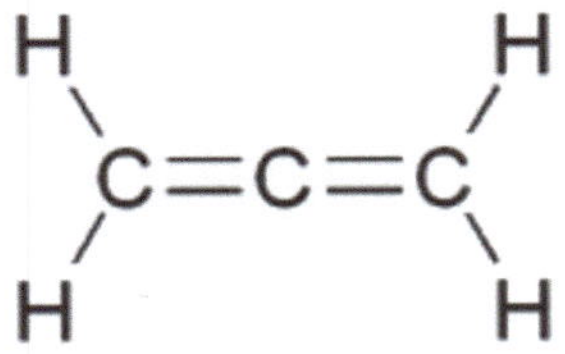

II

A. I only
B. II only
C. Both I and II
D. Neither I nor II

Medium-level Importance

High-level Importance

GOLD STANDARD GAMSAT-LEVEL PRACTICE QUESTIONS

Questions 16–20

There are many conditions that can affect the stability of molecules and related species.

A conjugated system is a system of connected p orbitals with delocalised electrons in a molecule, which in general lowers the overall energy of the molecule and increases stability. It is conventionally represented as having alternating single and multiple bonds. Lone pairs, free radicals or even carbocations may be part of the system, which may be cyclic, acyclic, linear or mixed.

Carbocations and free radicals have the same trend in molecular stability. Their stability increases in the order methyl < primary < secondary < tertiary.

For geometric cis-trans isomers, trans isomers are more stable than cis isomers. This is typically due to the increased unfavorable steric interaction of the substituents in the cis isomer.

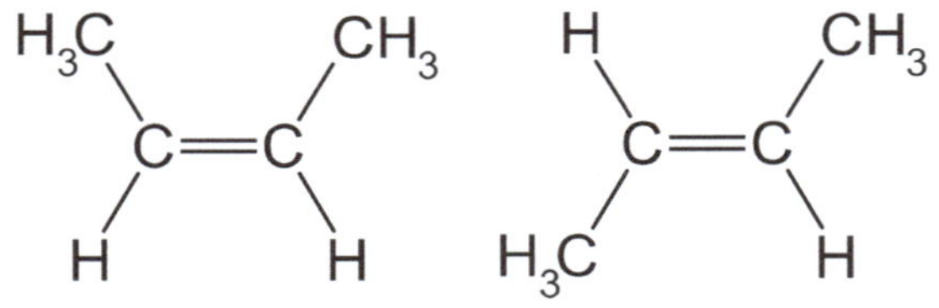

cis-but-2-ene trans-but-2-ene

16) Choose the carbocation which is most stable.

A. 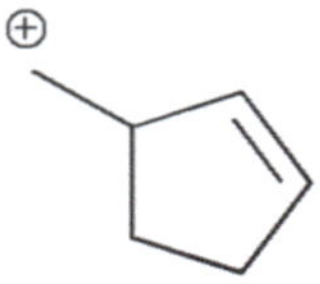

B. 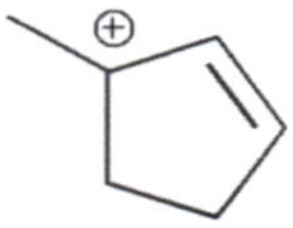

C. 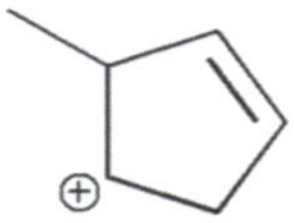

D. 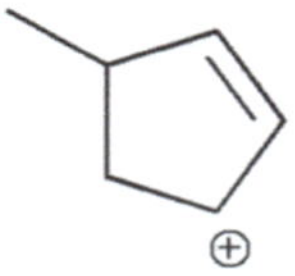

17) Choose the most stable isomer of hexa-2,4-diene?

A. 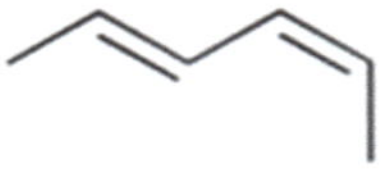

B. 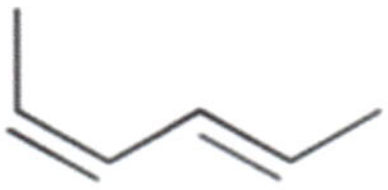

C. 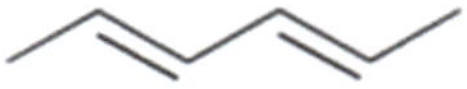

D. 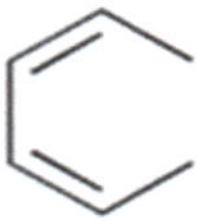

18) Identify the most stable free radical.

A. 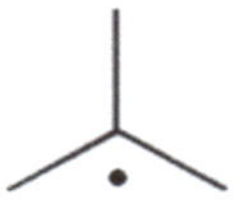

B. 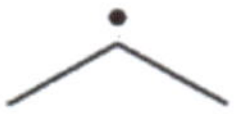

C. 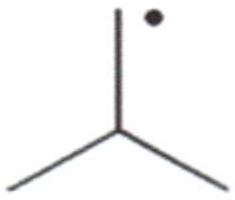

D. 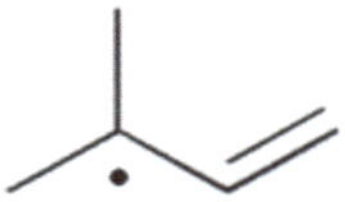

19) Which of the following free radicals is most stable?

A. 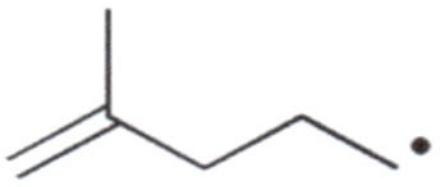

B. 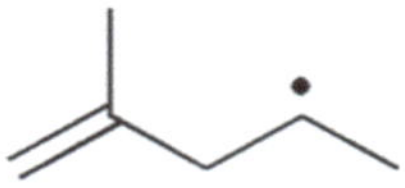

C. 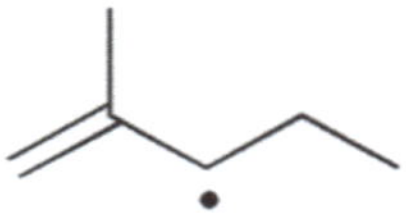

D. 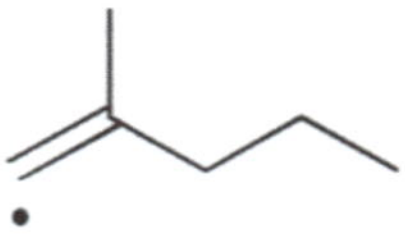

20) Which of these carbocations is most stable?

A. 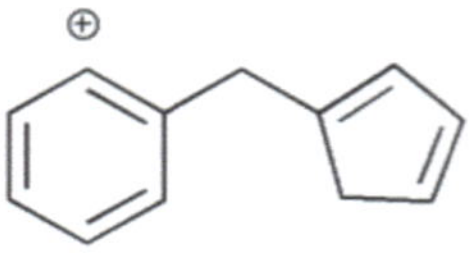

B. 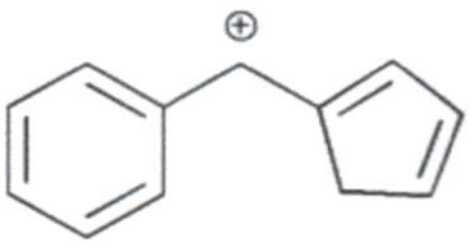

C. 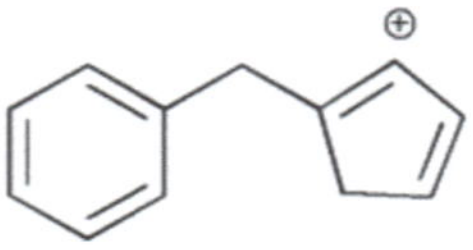

D. 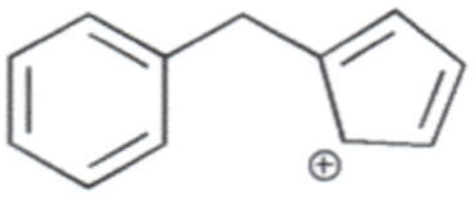

Questions 21–23

A hydrohalogenation reaction is the electrophilic addition of hydrohalic acids like hydrogen chloride or hydrogen bromide to alkenes to yield the corresponding haloalkanes. For example, consider the hydrogen bromide addition to an alkene below.

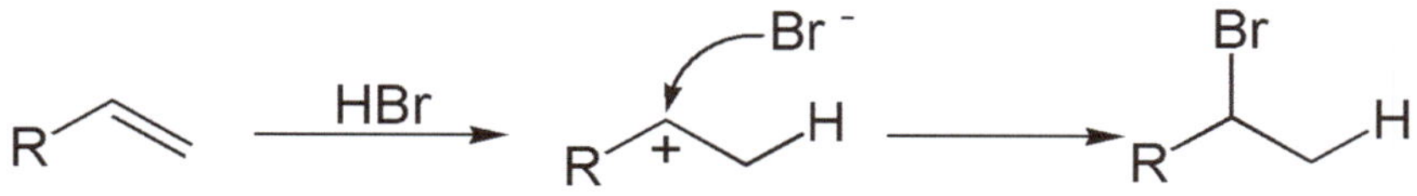

If the two carbon atoms at the alkene's double bond are linked to a different number of hydrogen atoms, the halogen is found preferentially at the carbon with fewer hydrogen substituents, an observation known as *Markovnikov's rule*. This is largely due to the abstraction of a hydrogen atom by the alkene from the acid (HX) to form the most stable carbocation (relative stability: 3°>2°>1°>methyl).

Note that pi bond conjugation can increase the stability of the carbocation intermediate which increases the reactivity of the compound.

21) Identify the product for the following reaction consistent with Markovnikov's rule.

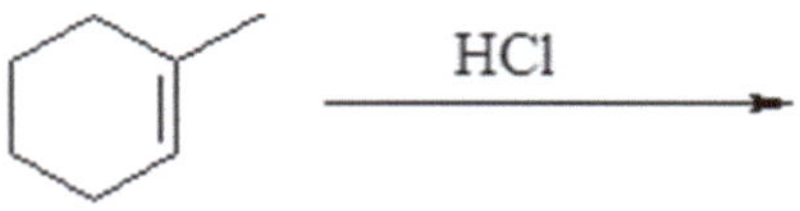

A. 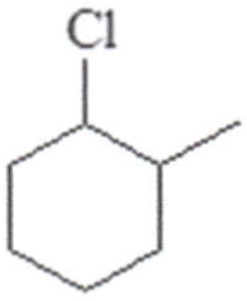

C. 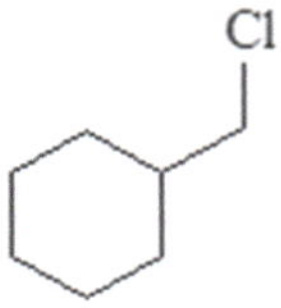

B. 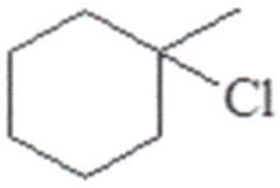

D. 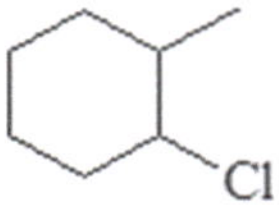

22) Given a reaction with hydrogen bromide obeying Markovnikov's rule, which of the following alkenes would give a product that is different from the products of the other three alkenes?

A. 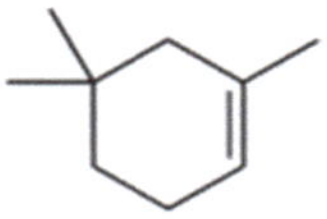

C. 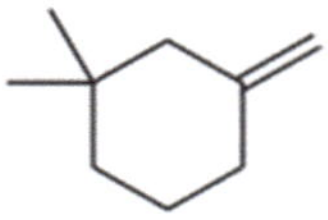

B. 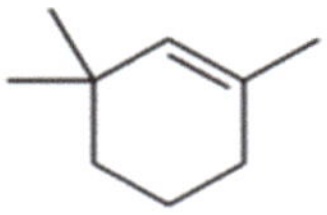

D. 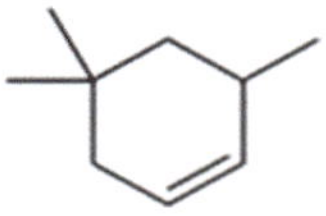

23) Which alkene is **least** reactive with hydrogen chloride?

A. 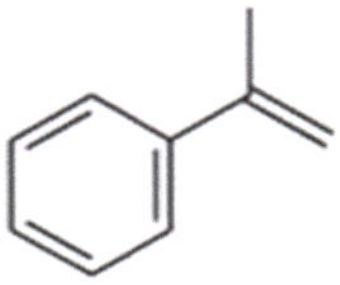

C. 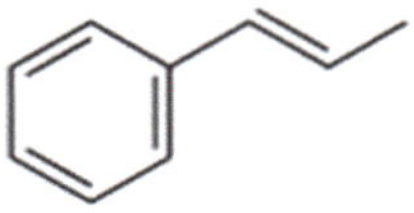

B. 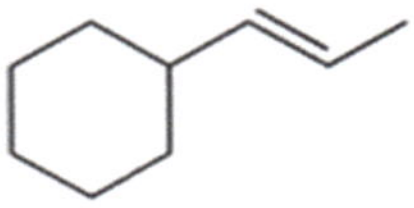

D. 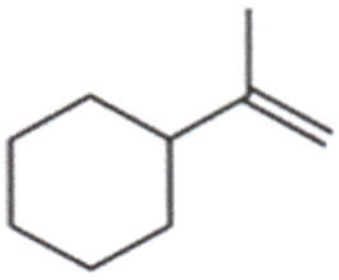

High-level Importance

Questions 24–28

The Diels–Alder reaction is a cycloaddition reaction that can occur between a conjugated diene (= 2 double bonds separated by a single bond) and a substituted alkene (= the dienophile) to form a substituted cyclohexene system.

Diene + dienophile = cyclohexene

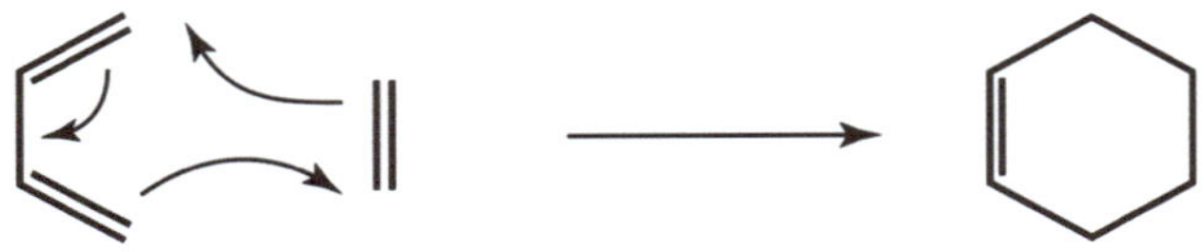

diene + dienophile

All Diels-Alder reactions have four common features: (1) the reaction is initiated by heat; (2) the reaction forms new six-membered rings; (3) three π bonds break and two new C-C σ bonds and one new C-C π bond are formed; (4) all bonds break and form in a single step.

The Diels-Alder diene must have the two double bonds on the same side of the single bond in one of the structures, which is called the *s-cis* conformation (= *cis* with respect to the single bond). If double bonds are on the opposite sides of the single bond in the Lewis structure, this is called the *s-trans* conformation (= *trans* with respect to the single bond).

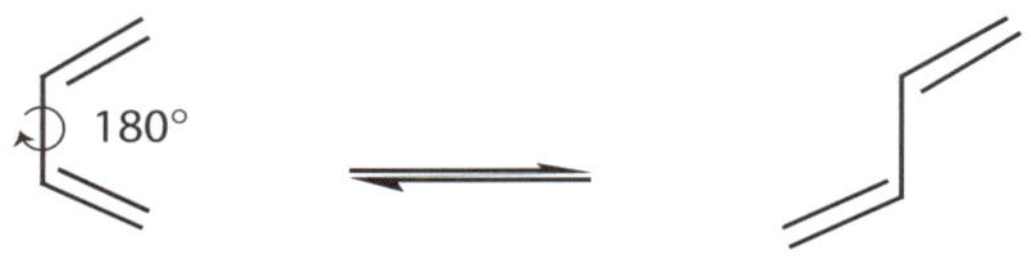

s-cis (reactive conformation) *s-trans* (unreactive conformation)

24) Consider Table 1.

When bonded to...	Hybridisation	Shape	Bond angle
2 atoms	sp	linear	180°
3 atoms	sp^2	trigonal (triangular)	120°
4 atoms	sp^3	tetrahedral	109.5°

Table 1: Neutral carbon's bond hybrids

All of the following are true regarding the neutral, non-cyclic molecule, *allene* (C_3H_4) EXCEPT one. Which one is the EXCEPTION?

A. The C-H bond angles are 120°.
B. The hybridisation of the carbon atoms are sp and sp^2.
C. The bond angle formed by the three carbons is 180°.
D. Allene is a conjugated diene.

25) Which of the following would be the least reactive diene in a Diels-Alder reaction?

A. 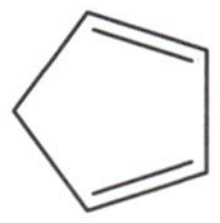

C. 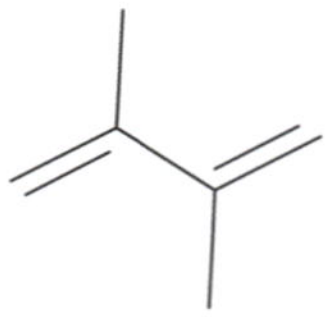

B. 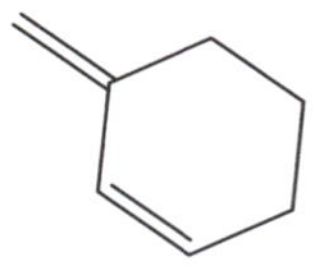

D. 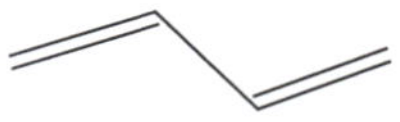

26) The number of conjugated dienes among the 5 structures below is:

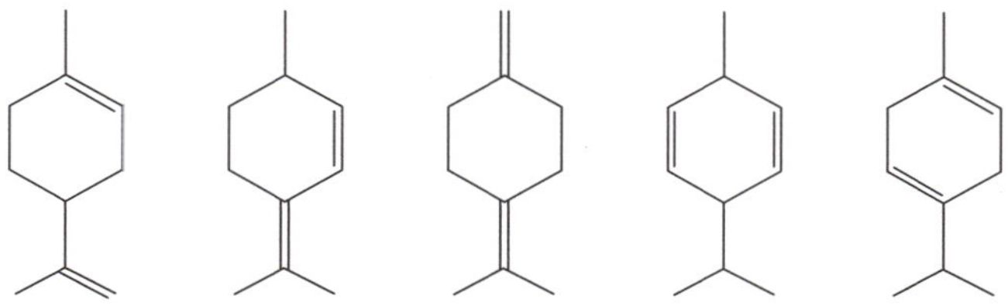

A. 1 only.
B. 2 only.
C. 3 only.
D. more than 3.

27) Choose the diene and dienophile that could be used to produce the Diels-Alder product.

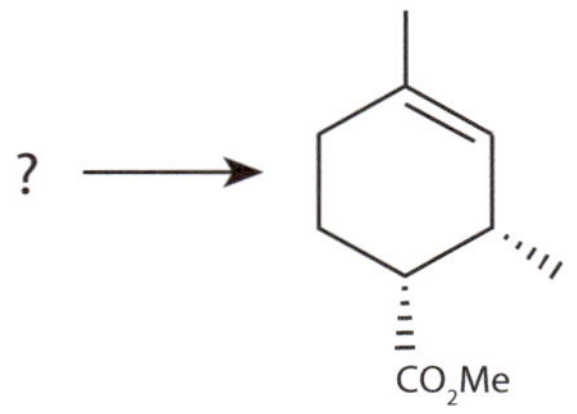

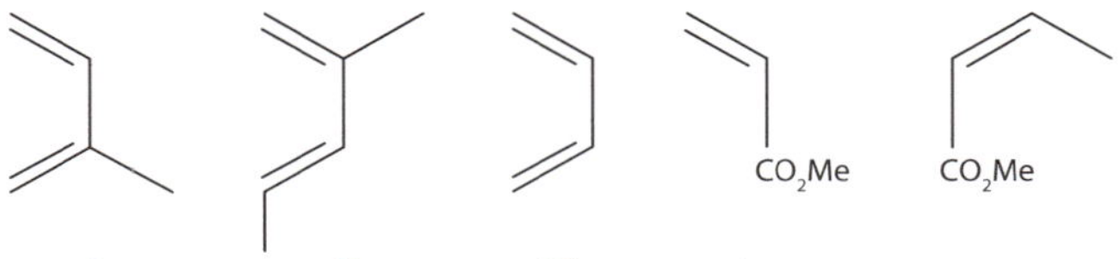

i ii iii iv v

A. **i** and **iv**
B. **ii** and **iv**
C. **iii** and **iv**
D. **iii** and **v**

28) Consider the following dienophile.

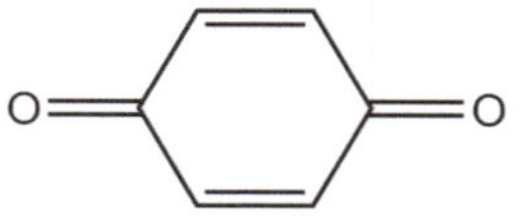

If 1 equivalent of the dienophile would react with 2 equivalents of cyclopenta-1,3-diene, which of the following would be most consistent with the product of a Diels-Alder reaction?

A. 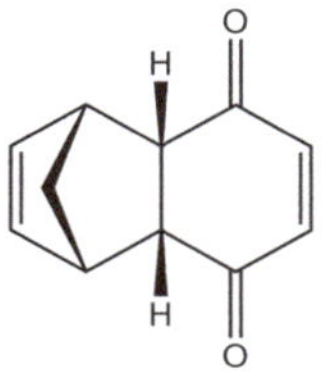

C. 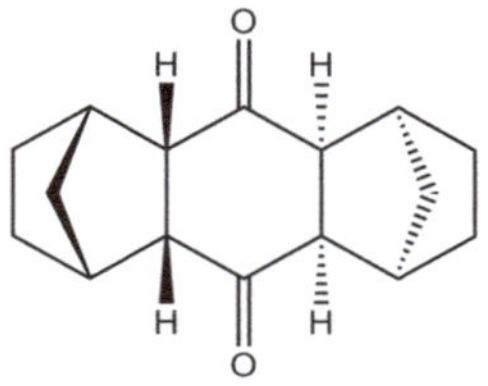

B. 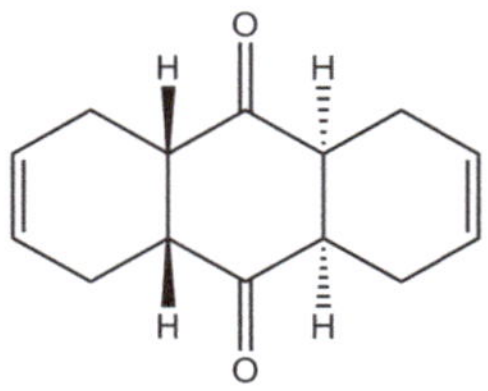

D. 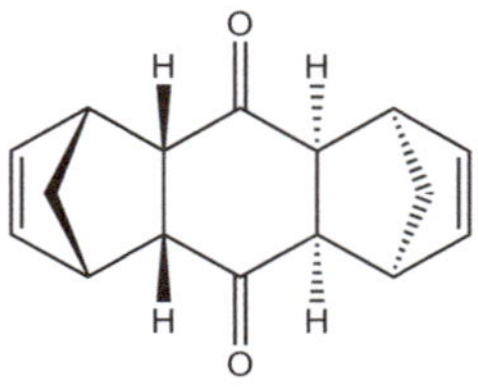

29) Which of the following are **not** resonance forms of one another?

A. 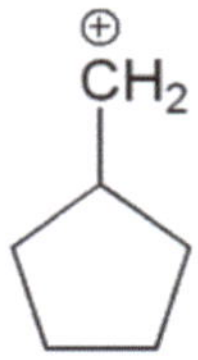 and 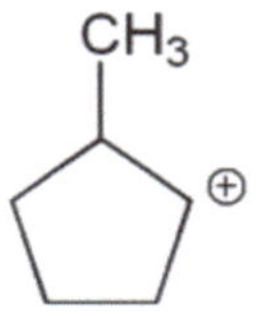

B. 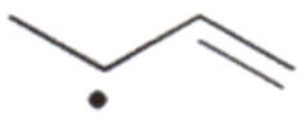 and 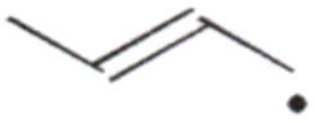

C. 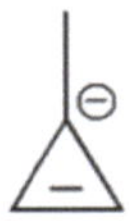 and 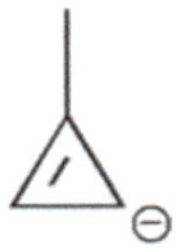

D. 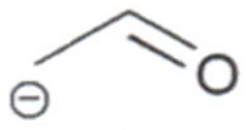 and 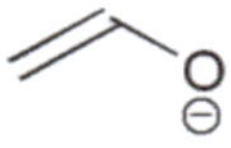

High-level Importance

Note: Being able to name (i.e. *the nomenclature of*) alcohols, aldehydes, ketones and carboxylic acids, represents a GAMSAT-level skill. If you have no experience naming such organic compounds, skip this unit and do not look at the worked solutions; instead, try this unit after you have read sections 6.1, 7.1 and 8.1. Alternatively, you can read those sections now and then attempt the questions in this unit.

Questions 30–37

Ozone (O_3) reacts vigorously with alkenes. The reaction (= *ozonolysis*) breaks carbon-carbon double bonds to generate carbon-oxygen double bonds (= *oxidative cleavage*) which can produce ketones, aldehydes or a combination thereof. The overall reaction is illustrated below.

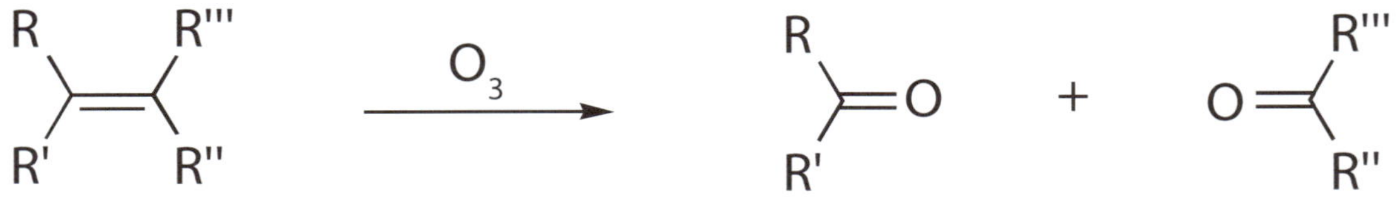

For the reaction above to occur, a reducing agent such as zinc metal or dimethyl sulfide must be used. Alternatively, an oxidative workup would oxidise any aldehydes to carboxylic acids (i.e. *complete oxidation*).

Note that:

- R, R′, R″ and R‴ can each be any of hydrogen, an alkyl or an aryl group.
- if the starting material is an alkyne, the result of ozonolysis with oxidative workup is oxidative cleavage and complete oxidation.

30) Which of the following is consistent with the ozonolysis of a disubstituted alkene?

A. R = R′ = R″ = R‴ = ethyl
B. R = R′ = butyl; R″ = R‴ = methyl
C. R = H; R′ = propyl; R″ = R‴ = H
D. R = methyl; R′ = H; R″ = ethyl; R‴ = H

31) If the starting compound is a disubstituted alkene, which of the following must be true?

A. Formaldehyde must be one of the 2 products
B. At least one aldehyde must be one of the 2 products
C. Two aldehydes must be the 2 products
D. Both **A** and **B** are correct.

32) If ozonolysis with a reductive workup produces acetone and ethanal, which of the following would be consistent with the starting material?

A. 2-methyl-2-butene
B. 2,3-dimethyl-2-butene
C. 1-butene
D. 2-methyl-3-propyl-1-butene

33) Ozonolysis of 5-chlorohex-1-ene under reductive workup would be expected to produce 2 products. Which of the following would be one of those 2 products?

A. Methanal
B. Methanoic acid chloride
C. Acetic acid
D. Acetic acid chloride

34) Ozonolysis of cyclopentene under reductive workup would be expected to produce which of the following products?

A. *cis*-Cyclopentane-1,2-diol
B. *trans*-Cyclopentane-1,2-diol
C. Pentane-2,4-dione
D. Pentanedial

35) Ozonolysis of cyclodecyne under oxidative workup would be expected to produce which of the following products?

A. *trans*-1,2-dihydroxycyclodecanene
B. Decanedioic acid
C. Decanone
D. Decanedial

36) Ozonolysis of compound **Z** gives the following products. Deduce the structure of compound **Z**:

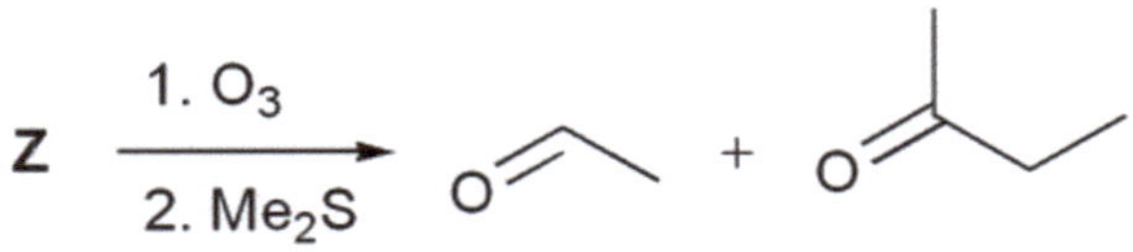

A. 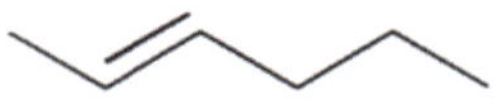

B. 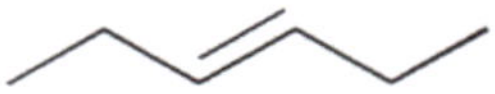

C. 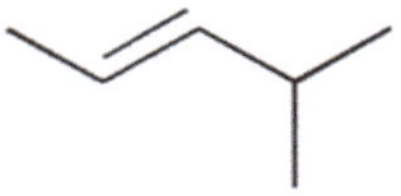

D. 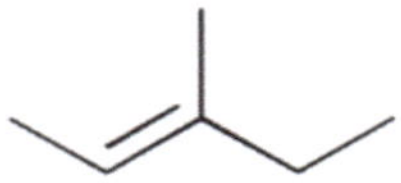

37) Ozonolysis of compound **Z** gives the following products. Identify likely structures that could represent compound **Z**:

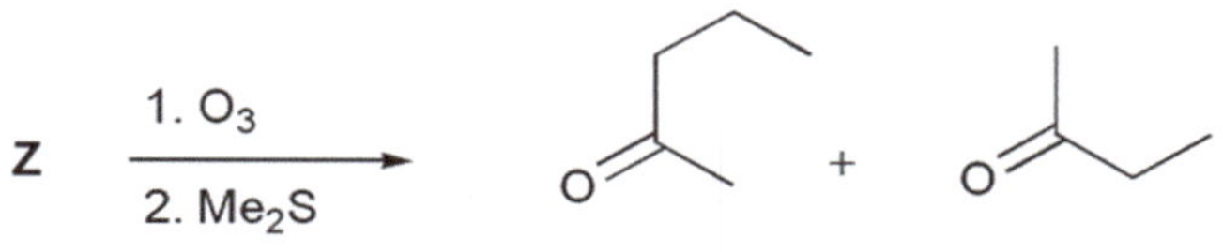

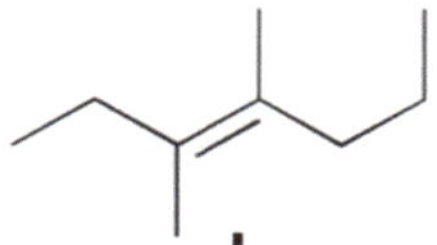
I

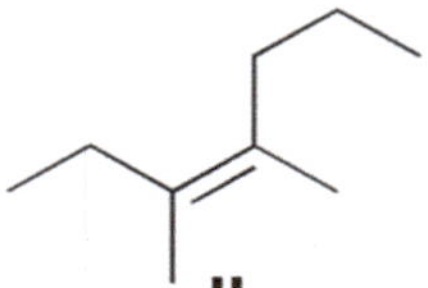
II

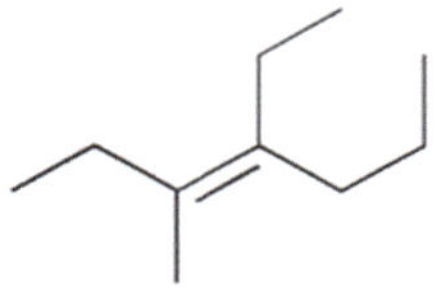
III

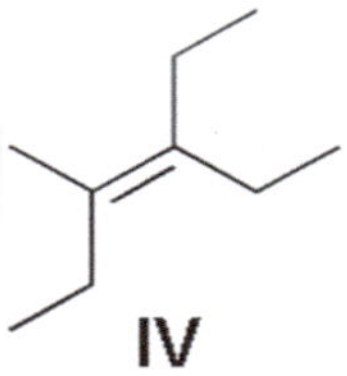
IV

A. **I** and **II**
B. **II** and **III**
C. **III** and **IV**
D. **I** and **IV**

High-level Importance

Questions 38–39

A sigmatropic reaction in organic chemistry is a pericyclic reaction wherein the net result is one sigma (σ) bond is changed to another σ bond in an uncatalysed intramolecular reaction. The sigma (σ) bond is adjacent to one or more pi (π) systems, with the π systems becoming reorganised in the process.

Cope and Claisen rearrangements are the most studied and they both involve a [3,3]-sigmatropic rearrangement of 1,5-hexadiene components of the respective molecules.

The Cope rearrangement:

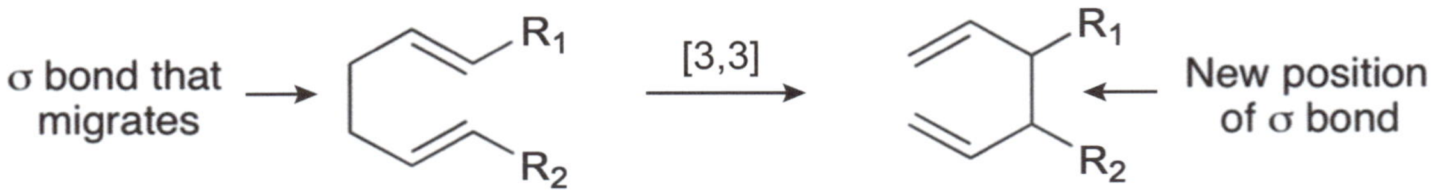

The Claisen rearrangement:

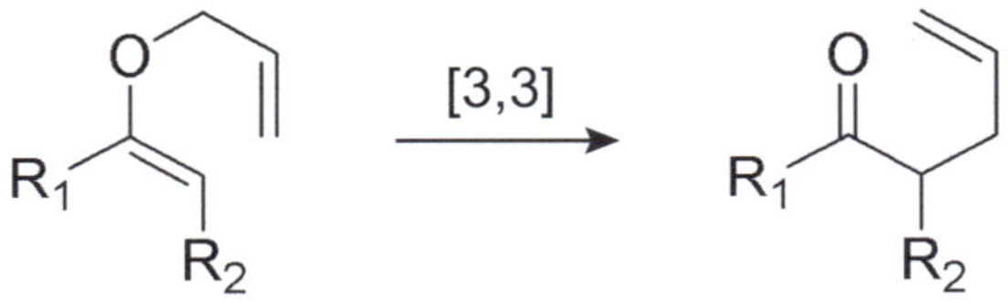

38) Which of the following would be expected to undergo neither a Cope nor a Claisen rearrangement?

A. 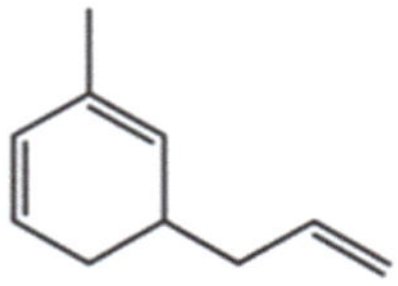

C. 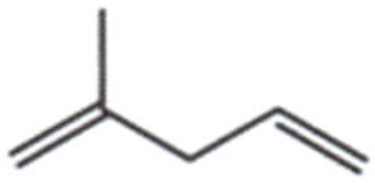

B. 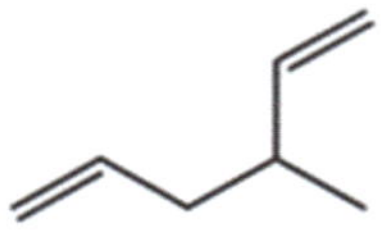

D. 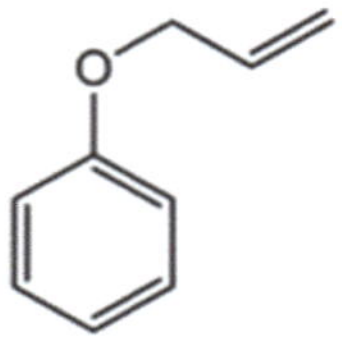

39) Choose the likely result of a sigmatropic reaction.

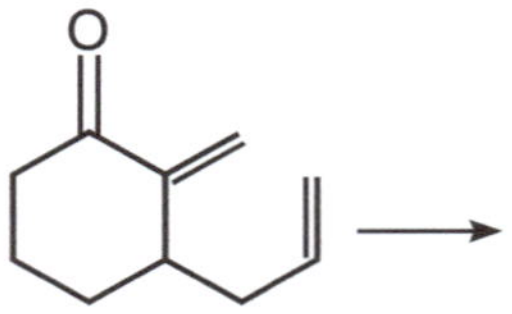

A. 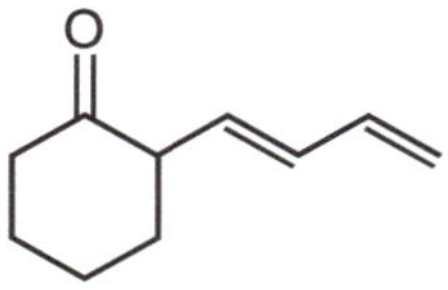

C. 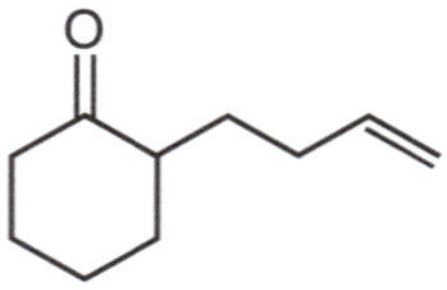

B. 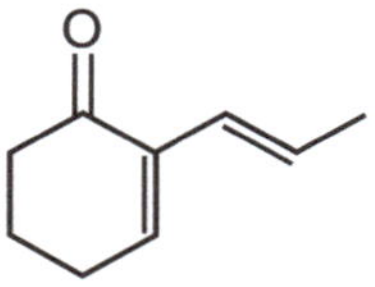

D. 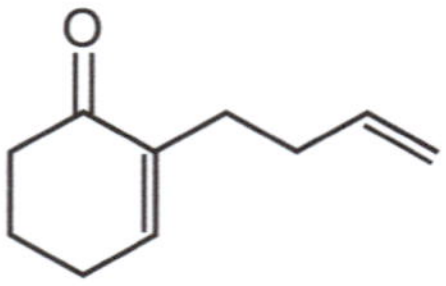

40) Electrocyclic reactions may occur under "thermal" conditions (i.e. heating but no UV light; symbol: Δ), which results in different products than are obtained under "photochemical" conditions (i.e. irradiation with UV light; symbol: hν). The configuration of the reactant is an important factor in determining the outcome based on the conditions. Consider the reactions below.

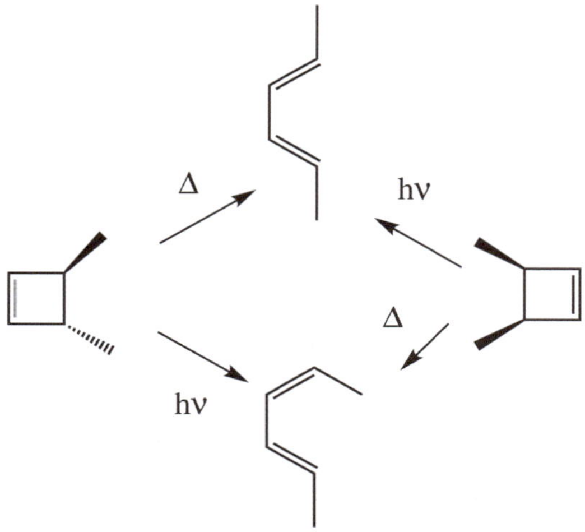

If the following reactant is **not** thermally, but rather photochemically exposed, which of the following would be the expected product?

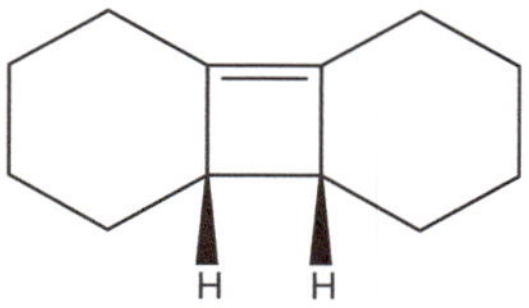

A. 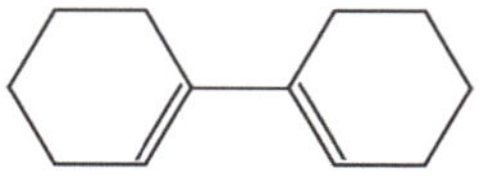

C. 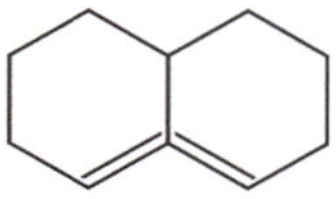

B. 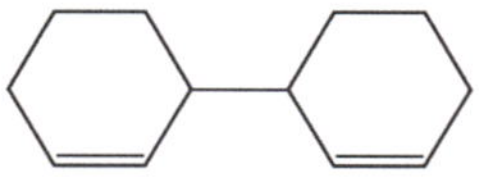

D. 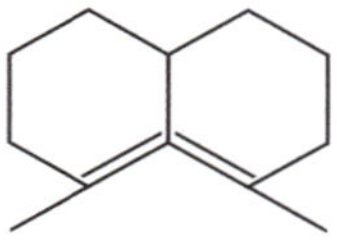

SPOILER ALERT

Gold Standard has cross-referenced the content in this chapter to examples from ACER's official GAMSAT practice materials. It is for you to decide when you want to explore these questions since you may want to preserve some of ACER's materials for timed mock-exam practice.

Examples – Retrocyclisation of cyclobutenes to form butadienes under thermal or photochemical conditions (basically, a ring-opening mechanism similar to the last question in this chapter but with some different twists): Q22-24 of 5; counting the number of conjugated bonds: Q83 of 5. Note that "Q" is followed by the question number, and, for example, "of 1" refers to booklet number 1 which is referenced in the Spoiler Alert table at the end of Chapter 1. The 15 full-length GAMSAT practice tests by Gold Standard, HEAPS-1 through HEAPS-15, contain specific cross-references to this chapter within the worked solutions. Note that the Diels-Alder reaction unit is mostly from HEAPS-6 but 1 question, the last one, is a rare visitor from HEAPS-1; 'ozone (O_3) reacts vigorously' is from HEAPS-6 with 4 new questions added.

High-level Importance

Chapter Checklist

- ☐ Access your online account to view answers, worked solutions and discussion boards.
- ☐ Reassess your 'learning objectives' for this chapter: Go back to the first page of this chapter and re-evaluate the top 3 boxes and the Introduction.
  - ☐ Please be sure that you have completed the *Need for Speed* exercises at the beginning of this chapter.
- ☐ Complete a maximum of 1 page of notes using symbols/abbreviations to represent the entire chapter based on your learning objectives. These are your Gold Notes.
- ☐ Consider your multimedia options based on your optimal way of learning:
  - ☐ Download the free Gold Standard GAMSAT app for your Android device or iPhone.
  - ☐ Create your own, tangible study cards or try the free app: Anki.
  - ☐ Record your voice reading your Gold Notes onto your smartphone (audio files, e.g., *memo* or MP3s) and listen during exercise, transportation, etc.
  - ☐ Try out the Gold Standard GAMSAT online videos at gamsat-prep.com, or you can try other options on YouTube like Khan Academy or Crash Course Organic Chemistry.
- ☐ Reassess your schedule for your full-length GAMSAT practice tests: ACER and/or HEAPS exams. Ensure that you have scheduled one full day to complete a practice test and 1-2 days for a thorough assessment of worked solutions while adding to your abbreviated Gold Notes.
- ☐ Reassess your progress in scheduling and/or evaluating stress reduction techniques such as regular exercise (sports), yoga, meditation and/or mindfulness exercises (*see* YouTube for suggestions).

AROMATICS

Chapter 5

Memorise	Understand	Importance
* Benzene: Structure, resonance, stability	* Electrophilic aromatic substitution * How to apply Hückel's rule	**Low level: 2% of GAMSAT Organic Chemistry** questions released by ACER are related to content in this chapter (in our estimation). * Note that approximately 60% of the questions in GAMSAT Organic Chemistry are related to just 4 chapters: 2, 6, 7 and 12.

GAMSAT-Prep.com

Introduction

Aromatics are cyclic compounds with unusual stability due to cyclic delocalisation and resonance.

Among the chapters of this book, only a few will not benefit from *Need for Speed* nor nomenclature exercises. Chapter 5 is one of those rare chapters. Of course, you need to be able to identify benzene and appreciate its special properties. However, nomenclature and reactions will be clarified, if necessary, during the passage preceding any relevant questions on the real GAMSAT.

As for all chapters, the GAMSAT-level practice questions are "High-level Importance" because they use reasoning relevant to your upcoming exam. Thus, a minimal approach to this chapter would be to glance at the content and attack all of the practice questions.

Multimedia Resources at GAMSAT-Prep.com

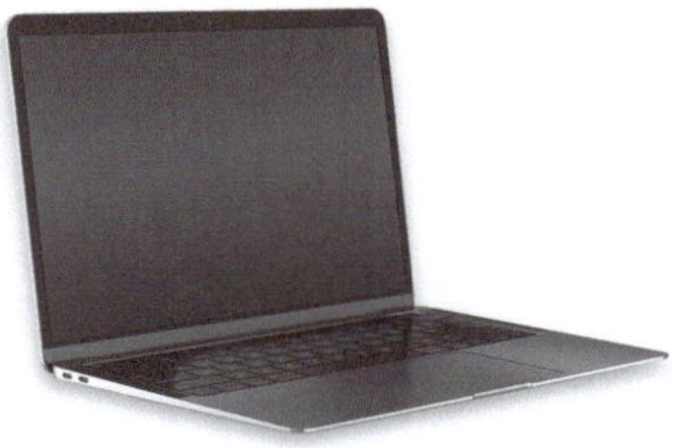

Open Discussion Boards
(*gamsat-prep.com/forum*)

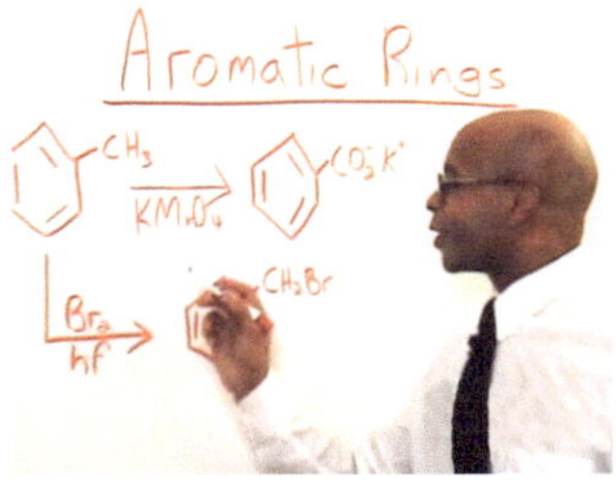

Science Preparation Videos

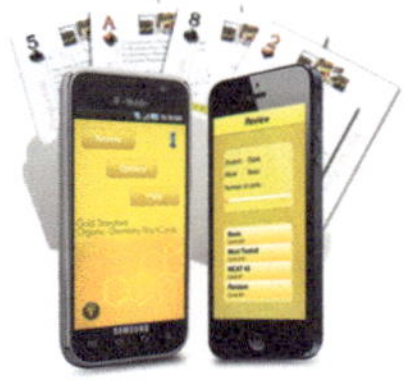

Flashcards

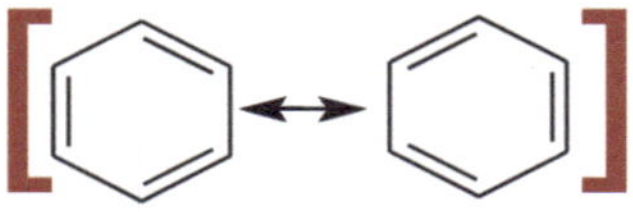

Special Guest

* The real GAMSAT may have advanced-level information presented (i.e. in a passage) but previous knowledge of said information is not required to answer the questions that would follow. Practice questions at the end of this chapter, as well as ACER and GS (HEAPS) practice GAMSATs can help you clarify this point.

5.1 Description and Nomenclature

Low-level Importance

Aromatic compounds are cyclic and have their π electrons delocalised over the entire ring and are thus stabilised by π-electron delocalisation. Benzene is the simplest of all the aromatic hydrocarbons. The term *aromatic* has historical significance in that many well known fragrant compounds were found to be derivatives of benzene. Although at present, it is known that not all benzene derivatives have fragrance, the term remains in use today to describe benzene derivatives and related compounds.

Benzene is known to have only one type of carbon-carbon bond, with a bond length of ≈ 1.4 Å (angstroms, 10^{-10} m), somewhere between that of a single and double bond. Benzene is a hexagonal, flat symmetrical molecule. All C-C-C bond angles are 120° and all C-C bonds are of equal length; all six carbon atoms are sp^2 hybridised; and, all carbons have a p orbital perpendicular to the benzene ring, leading to six π electrons delocalised around the ring.

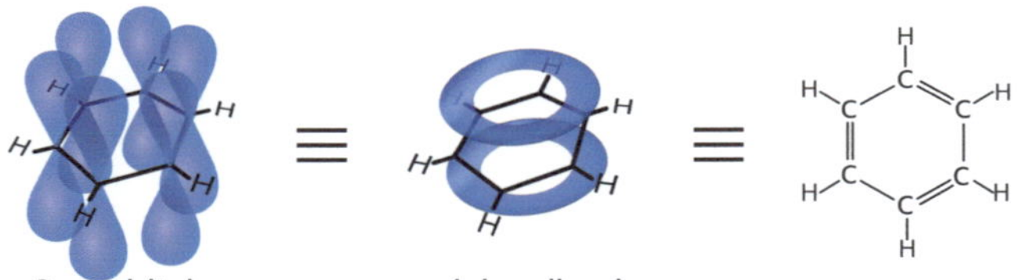

6 p-orbitals ≡ delocalized ≡

Benzene can also be represented by two different resonance structures, showing it to be the average of the two:

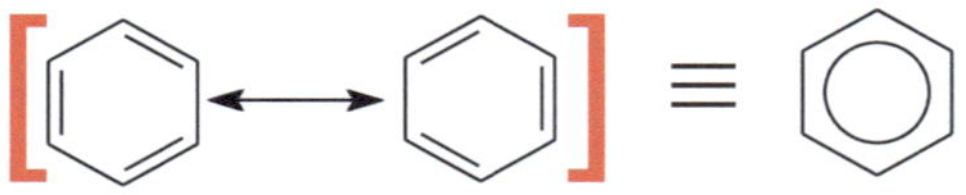

Many monosubstituted benzenes have common names by which they are known. Others are named by substituents attached to the aromatic ring. Some of these are:

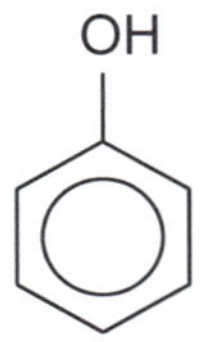

phenol

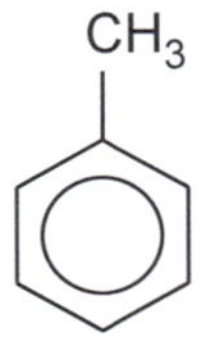

toluene

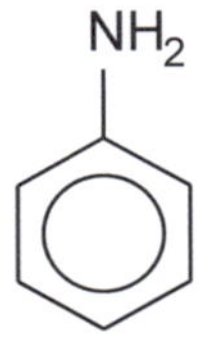

aniline

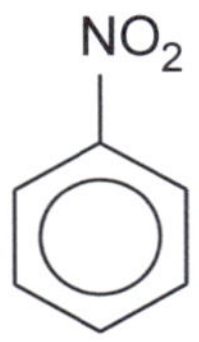

nitrobenzene

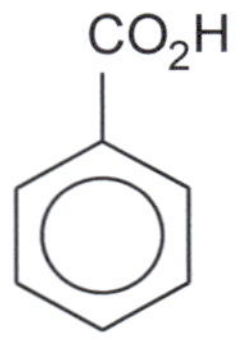

benzoic acid

Disubstituted benzenes are named as derivatives of their primary substituents. In this case, either the usual numbering or the ortho-meta-para system may be used. Ortho (*o*) substituents are at the 2nd position from the primary substituent; meta (*m*) substituents are at the 3rd position; para (*p*) substituents are at the 4th position. If there are more than two substituents on the aromatic ring, the numbering system is used.

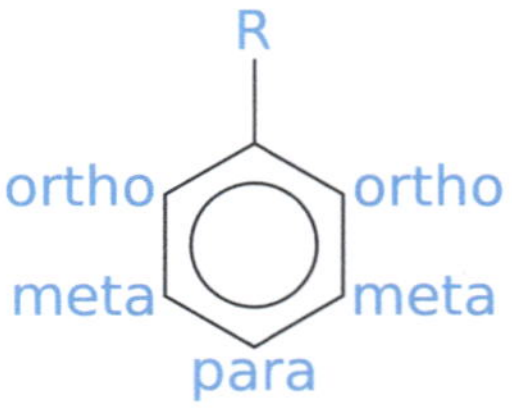

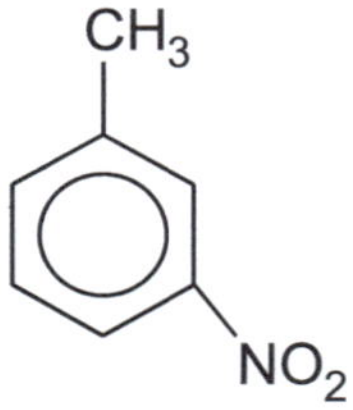

m - Nitrotoluene

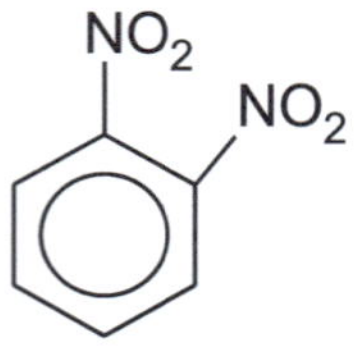

o - Dinitrobenzene

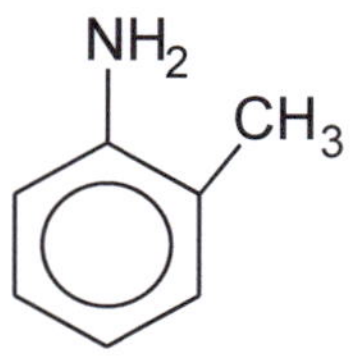

o - Methylaniline
o - Aminotoluene

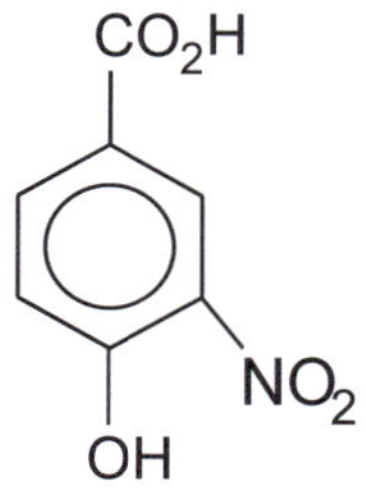

3-nitro-4-hydroxybenzoic acid

When benzene is a substituent, it is called a *phenyl or aryl group*. The shorthand for phenyl is Ph. Toluene without a hydrogen on the methyl substituent is called a *benzyl group.*

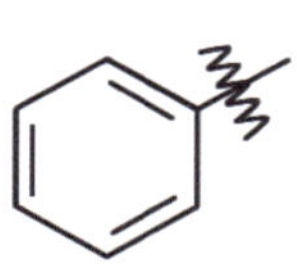

phenyl group

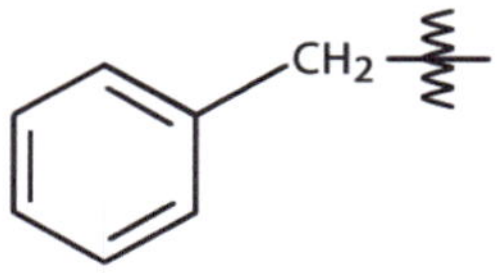

benzyl group

Benzene undergoes substitution reactions that retain the cyclic conjugation as opposed to electrophilic addition reactions.

5.1.1 Hückel's Rule

If a compound does not meet all the following criteria, it is likely not aromatic.

1. The molecule is cyclic.
2. The molecule is planar.
3. The molecule is fully conjugated (i.e. p orbitals at every atom in the ring; ORG 1.4, 4.1, 4.2.5; 5.1).
4. The molecule has $4n + 2$ π electrons.

If rules **1.**, **2.** and/or **3.** are broken, then the molecule is non-aromatic. If rule **4.** is broken then the molecule is antiaromatic.

Notice that the number of π delocalised electrons must be even but NOT a multiple of 4. So $4n + 2$ number of π electrons, where n = 0, 1, 2, 3, and so on, is known as Hückel's Rule. Thus the number of pi electrons can be 2, 6, 10, etc. Of course, benzene is aromatic (6 electrons, from 3 double bonds), but cyclobutadiene is not, since the number of π delocalised electrons is 4. Note that a cyclic molecule with conjugated double bonds in a monocyclic (= 1 ring) hydrocarbon is called an annulene. So cyclobutadiene can be called [4] annulene.

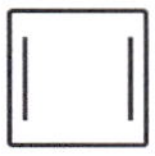

[4]annulene
$4n$ π electrons
n = 1
antiaromatic

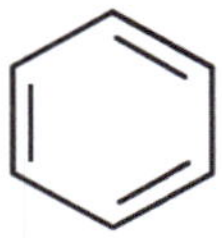

[6]annulene
$4n + 2$ π electrons
n = 1
aromatic

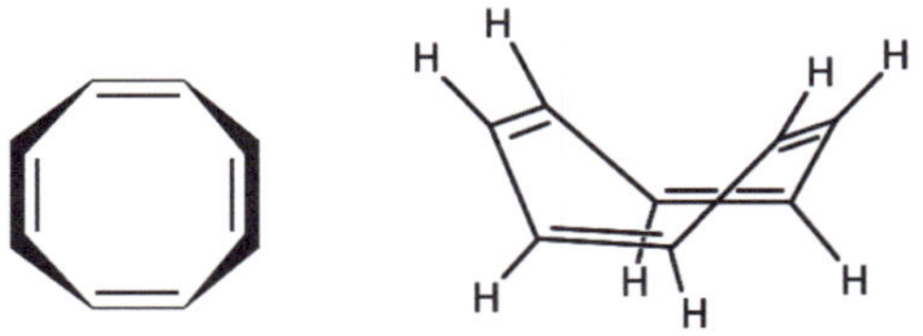

[8]annulene (cyclooctatetraene)
$4n$ π electrons, n = 2
non-planar "tub shape"
non-aromatic

A GAMSAT question on Hückel's rule would normally be preceded by Hückel's rule. The point is to verify that you understand its application. There is no need to memorise Hückel's rule.

Low-level Importance

The number of p orbitals and the number of π electrons can be different, which means, whether a molecule is neutral, a cation or an anion, it can be aromatic. Note that *aliphatic* describes all hydrocarbons that are not aromatic. A cyclic compound containing only 4n electrons is said to be anti-aromatic.

- Cyclopentadienide anion:

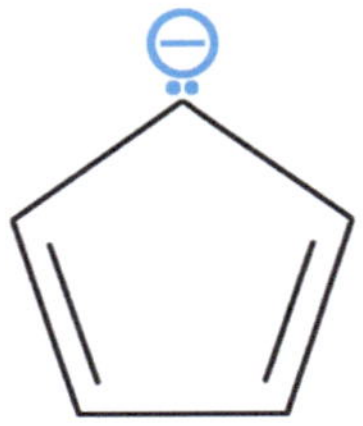

Because of the lone pair, there are 6 π electrons, which meets Hückel's number, so it is aromatic. Thus you can see that if an electron pair is added, or subtracted, a molecule can then become aromatic by fulfilling Hückel's rule. Therefore, if 2 electrons are added to [8]annalene, it will then become a more stable molecule. Specifically, the cyclooctatetraenide dianion ($C_8H_8^{2-}$) is aromatic (thus it has increased stability), and planar, like the cyclopentadienide anion, and both fulfill Hückel's rule.

- Cycloheptatrienyl cation:

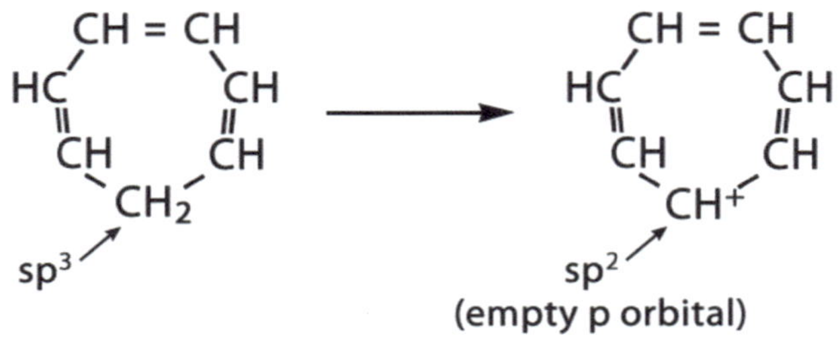

6 π electrons with conjugation through resonance because of the cation, meets Hückel's number, so it is aromatic.

Heterocyclic compounds (usu. = a ring with C + another atom) can also be aromatic.

- Pyridine:

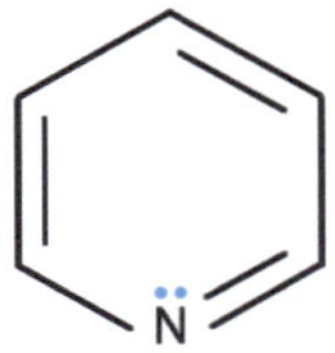

Each sp^2 hybridised carbon atom has a p orbital and contains one π electron. The nitrogen atom is also sp^2 hybridised and has one electron in the p orbital, bringing the total to six π electrons. The nitrogen nonbonding electron pair is in a sp^2 orbital perpendicular to other p orbitals and is not involved with the π system. Thus pyridine is aromatic.

- Pyrrole:

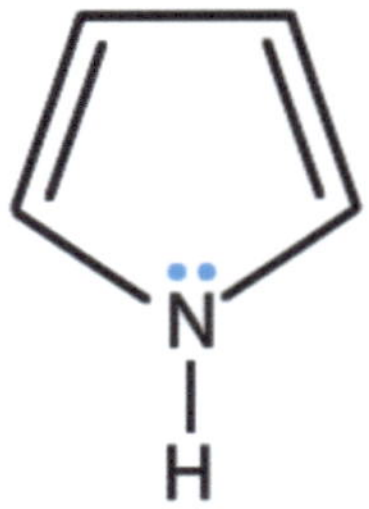

Each sp^2 hybridised carbon atom has a p orbital and contains one π electron. The nitrogen atom is also sp^2 hybridised with its nonbonding electron pair sitting in the p orbital, bringing the total to six π electrons. Thus pyrrole is aromatic.

5.2 Electrophilic Aromatic Substitution

One important reaction of aromatic compounds is known as electrophilic aromatic substitution, which occurs with electrophilic reagents. The reaction is similar to a S_N1 mechanism in that an addition leads to a rearrangement which produces a substitution. However, in this case it is the electrophile (*not a nucleophile*) which substitutes for an atom in the original molecule. An electrophile is quite literally *electron loving*. Thus we cannot be surprised that an electrophile has a positive charge. The reaction may be summarised:

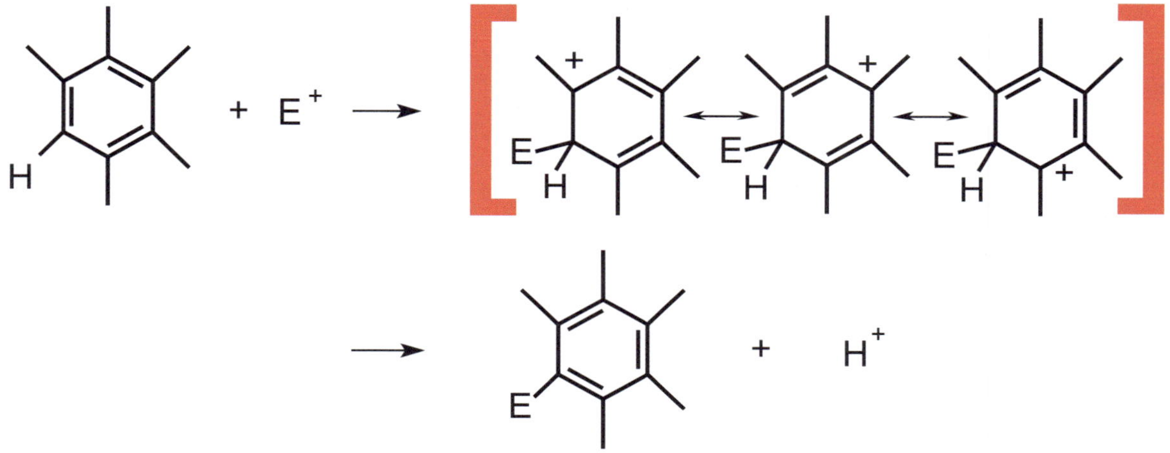

Note that the intermediate positive charge is stabilised by resonance.

It is important to understand that the electrophile used in electrophilic aromatic substitution must always be a powerful electrophile. After all, the resonance stabilised aromatic ring is resistant to many types of routine chemical reactions (i.e. oxidation with $KMnO_4$ – ORG 4.2.2, electrophilic addition with acid - ORG 4.2.1, and hydrogenation - ORG 4.2.3). Remembering that Br, a halide, is already very electronegative (CHM 2.3), Br^+ is an example of a powerful electrophile. In a reaction called bromination, $Br_2/FeBr_3$ is used to generate the Br^+ species which adds to the aromatic ring.

Similar reactions are performed to "juice up" other potential substituents (i.e. alkyl, acyl, iodine, etc.) to become powerful electrophiles to add to the aromatic ring.

- Aromatic halogenation: The benzene ring with its 6 π electrons in a conjugated system acts as an electron nucleophile (electron donor) in most chemical reactions. It reacts with bromine, chlorine or iodine to produce mono-substituted products. Fluorine is too reactive and tends to produce multi-substituted products. Therefore, the electrophilic substitution reaction is characteristic of aromaticity and can be used as a diagnostic tool to test the presence of an aromatic ring.

Low-level Importance

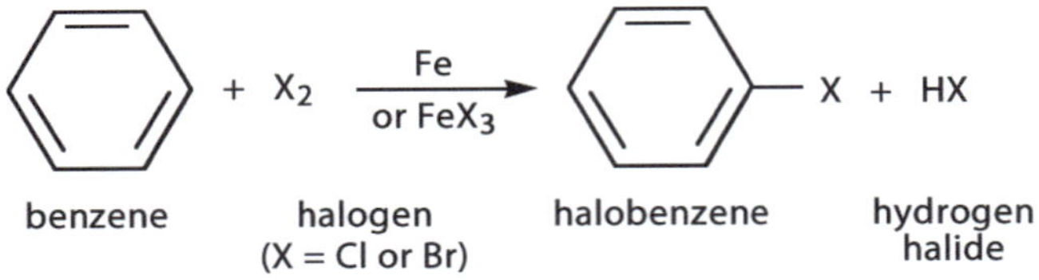

- <u>Aromatic nitration</u>: The aromatic ring can be nitrated when reacted with a mixture of nitric and sulfuric acid. The benzene ring reacts with the electrophile in this reaction, the nitronium ion NO_2^+, yielding a carbocation intermediate in a similar way as the aromatic halogenation reaction.

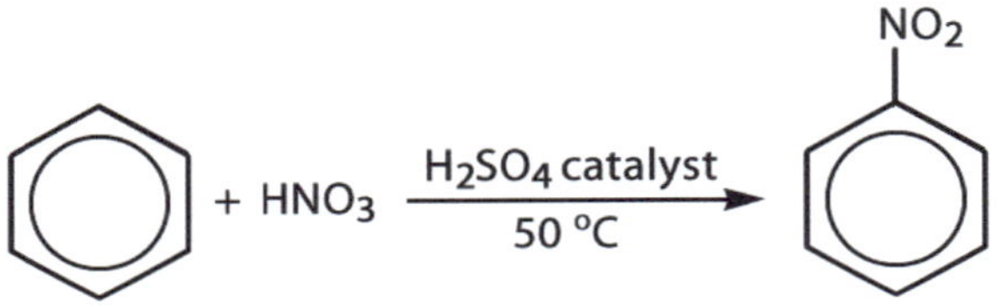

- <u>Aromatic sulfonation</u>: Aromatic rings can react with a mixture of sulfuric acid and sulfur trioxide (H_2SO_4/SO_3) to form sulfonic acid. The electrophile in this reaction is either HSO_3 or SO_3.

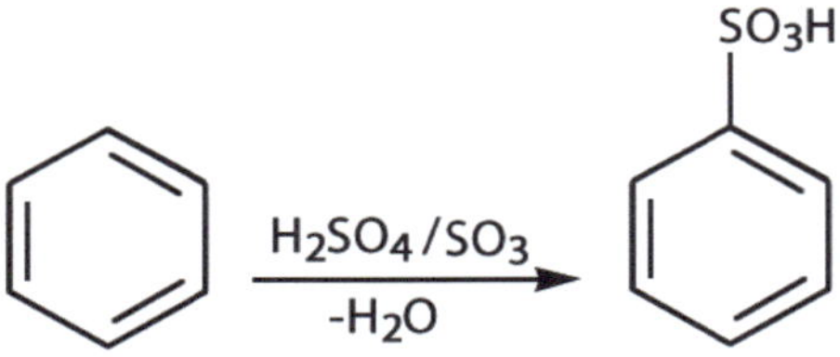

- <u>Friedel-Crafts alkylation</u>: This is an electrophilic aromatic substitution in which the benzene ring is alkylated when it reacts with an alkyl halide. The benzene ring attacks the alkyl cation electrophile, yielding an alkyl-substituted benzene product.

There are several limitations to this reaction:

1. The reaction does not proceed on an aromatic ring that has a strong, deactivating substituent group (ORG 5.2.2).

2. Because the product is attacked even faster by alkyl carbocations than the starting material, polyalkylation is often observed.

3. Skeletal rearrangement of the alkyl group sometimes occurs. A hydride shift or an alkyl shift may produce a more stable carbocation (*see* ORG 4.2.1).

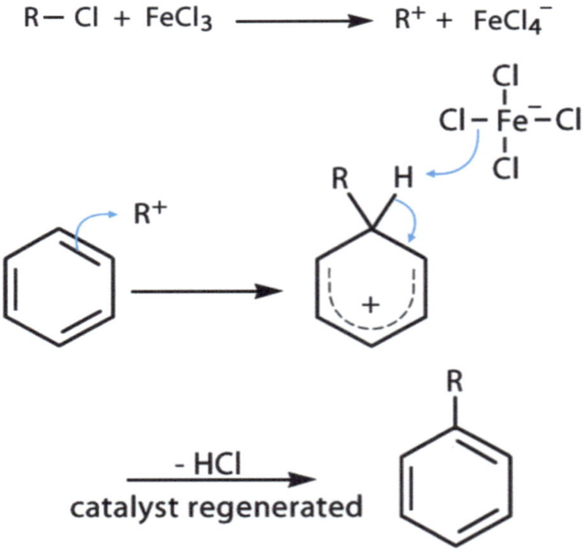

- <u>Friedel-Crafts acylation</u>: An electrophilic aromatic substitution in which the benzene ring is acylated when an acyl group is introduced to the ring. The mechanism is similar to that of Friedel-Crafts alkylation. The electrophile is an acyl cation generated by the reaction between the acyl halide and $AlCl_3$. Because the product is less reactive than the starting material, only mono-substitution is observed.

Low-level Importance

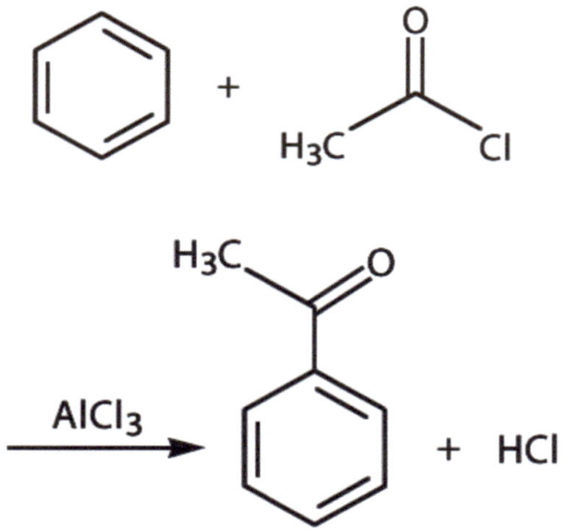

When groups are attached to the aromatic ring, the intermediate charge delocalisation is affected. Thus the nature of the first substituent on the ring determines the position of the second substituent.

Substituents can be classified into three classes: ortho-para (o-p) directing activators, ortho-para directing deactivators, and meta-directing deactivators. As implied, these groups indicate where most of the electrophile will end up in the reaction.

5.2.1 O-P Directors

If a substituted benzene reacts more rapidly than a benzene alone, the substituent group is said to be an <u>activating group</u>. Activating groups can *donate* electrons to the ring. Thus the ring is more attractive to an electrophile. All activating groups are o/p directors. Some examples are –OH,–NH_2, –OR, –NR_2, -OCOR and alkyl groups.

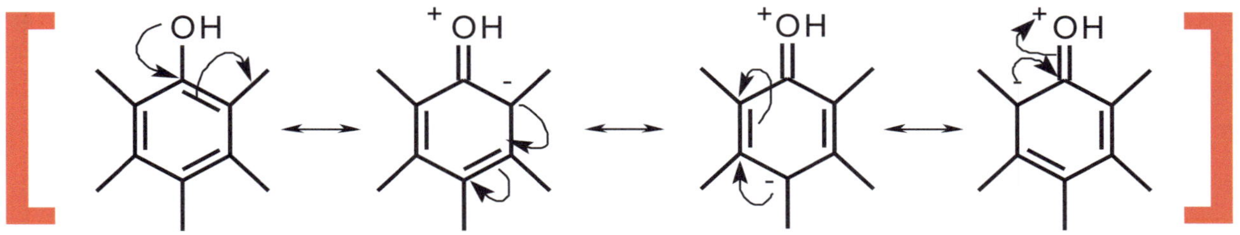

Note that the partial electron density (δ⁻) is at the ortho and para positions, so the electrophile favors attack at these positions. Good stabilisation results with a substituent at the ortho or para positions preferentially.

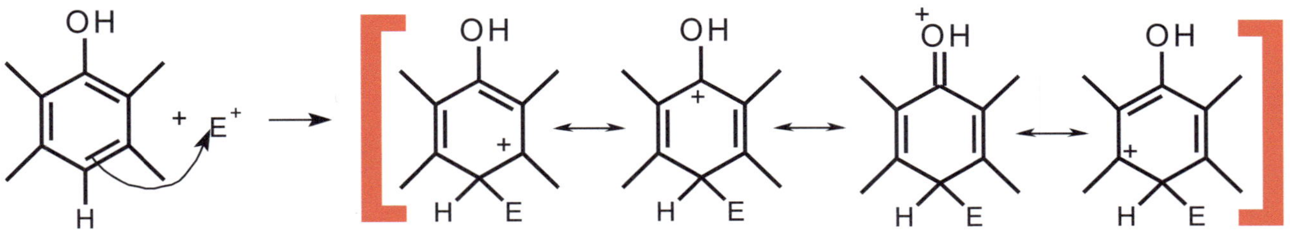

Low-level Importance

When there is a substituent at the meta position, the –OH can no longer help to delocalise the positive charge, so the o-p positions are favored over the meta:

Note that even though the substituents are o-p directors, probability suggests that there will still be a small percentage of the electrophile that will add at the meta position.

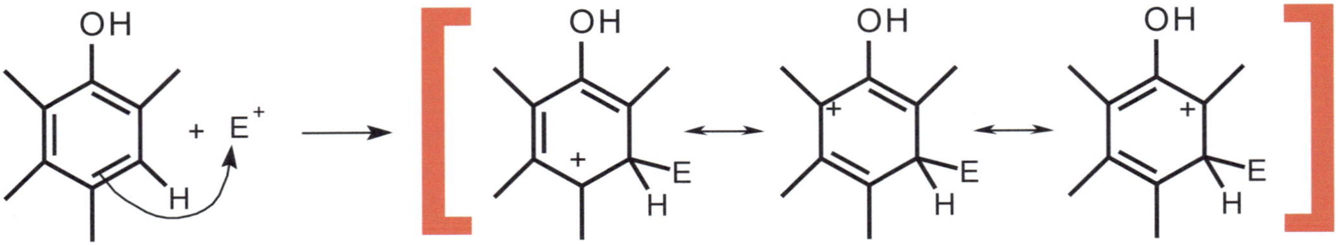

5.2.2 Meta Directors

If a substituted benzene reacts more slowly than the benzene alone, the substituent group is said to be a deactivating group. Deactivating groups can *withdraw* electrons from the ring. Thus the ring is less attractive to an electrophile. All deactivating groups are meta directors, with the exception of the weakly deactivating halides which are o–p directors (-F, -Cl, -Br, -I). Some examples of meta directors are $-NO_2$, $-SO_2$, $-CN$, $-SO_3H$, -COOH, -COOR, -COR, CHO.

Without any substituents, the partial positive charge density (δ^+) will be at the o–p positions. Thus the electrophile avoids the positive charge and favors attack at the meta position:

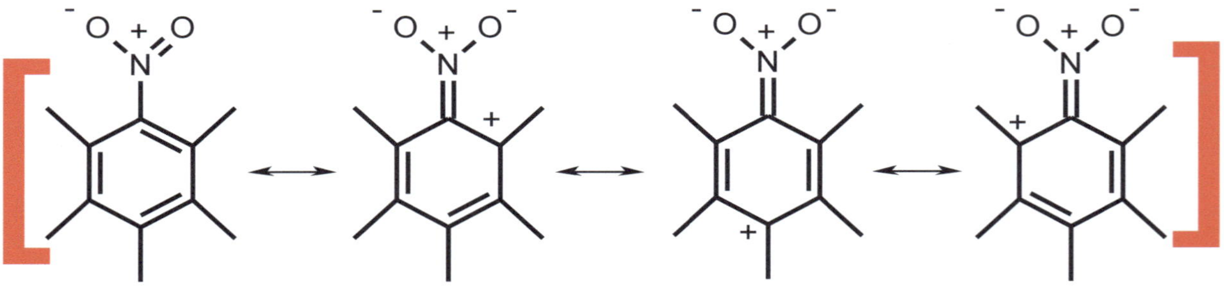

If you are seeking another way to learn, consider logging into your GAMSAT-prep.com account and clicking on Videos to choose the Aromatic Chemistry videos.

With a substituent at the meta position:

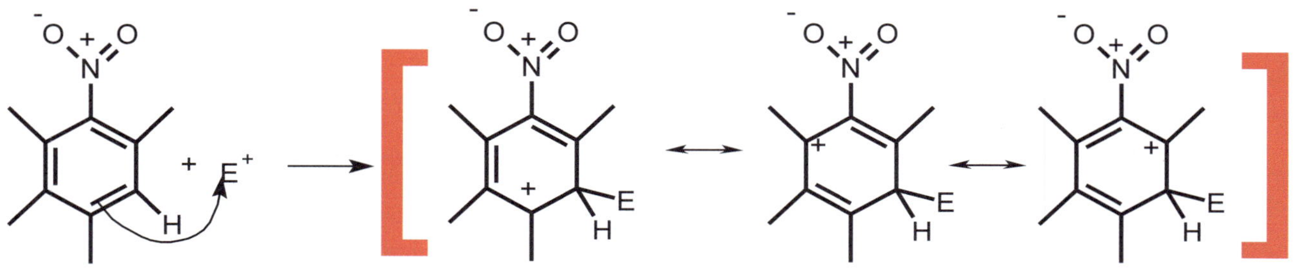

Note that even though the substituents are meta directors, probability suggests that there will still be a smaller percentage of the electrophile that will add at the o–p positions.

5.2.3 Reactions with the Alkylbenzene Side Chain

- Oxidation: Alkyl groups on the benzene ring react rapidly with oxidising agents and are converted into a carboxyl group. The net result is the conversion of an alkylbenzene into benzoic acid.

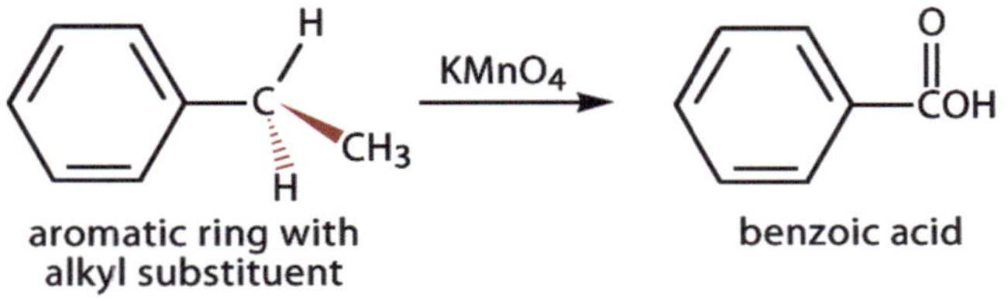

- Bromination: NBS (N-bromosuccinimide) reacts with alkylbenzene through a radical chain mechanism (ORG 3.2.2): the benzyl radical generated from NBS in the presence of benzoyl peroxide reacts with Br_2 to yield the final product and bromine radical, which will cycle back into the reaction to act as a radical initiator. The reaction occurs exclusively at the benzyl position because the benzyl radical is highly stabilised through different forms of resonance.

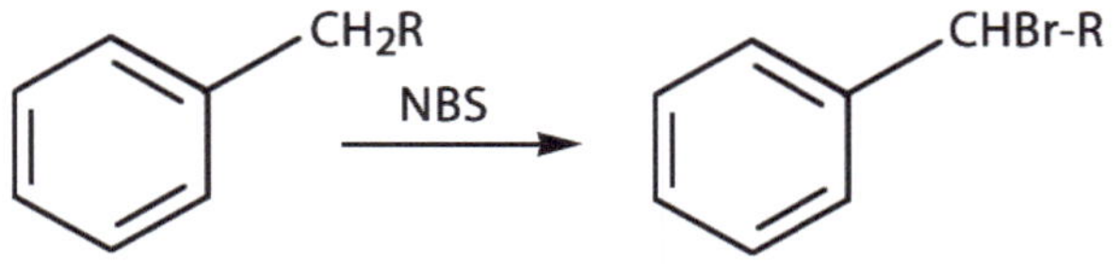

- Reduction: Reductions of aryl alkyl ketones in the presence of H_2 and Pd/C can be used to convert the aryl alkyl ketone generated by the Friedel-Crafts acylation reaction into an alkylbenzene.

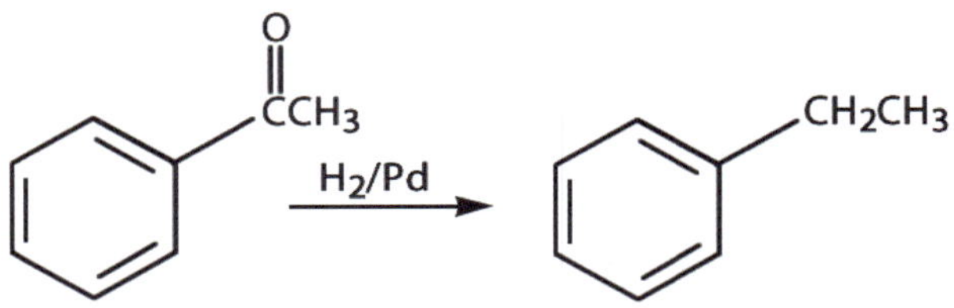

Low-level Importance

CHAPTER 5: Aromatics

GOLD STANDARD FOUNDATIONAL GAMSAT PRACTICE QUESTIONS

1) Which of the following molecules have the same number of pi-electrons?

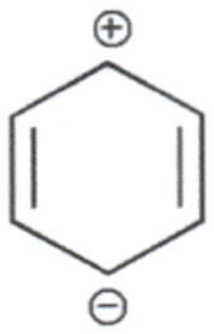
I

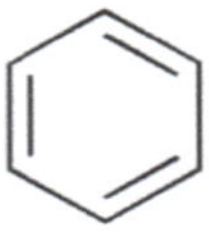
II

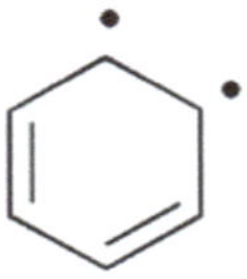
III

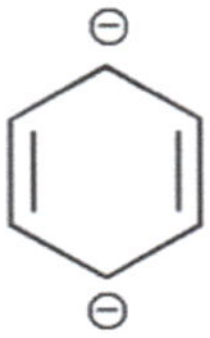
IV

A. **I** and **II** only
B. **III** and **IV** only
C. **I**, **II**, and **III** only
D. **I**, **II**, **III** and **IV**

2) Which of the following molecules have approximately a molecular weight of 156? (hint: no periodic table required!)

Note that:

1) Me = methyl
2) Sulfur's amu is twice that of oxygen.

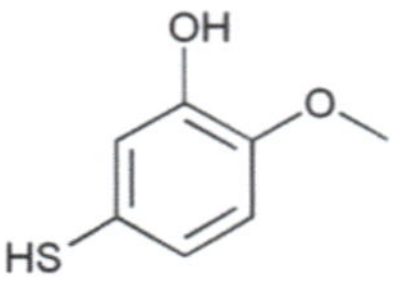

I

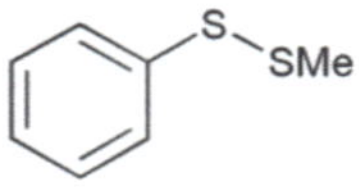

II

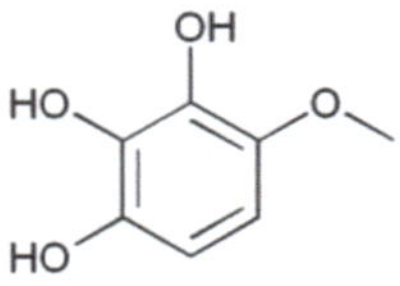

III

A. **I** only
B. **I** and **II** only
C. **I** and **III** only
D. **I**, **II** and **III**

3) Which of the following is correct?

A.
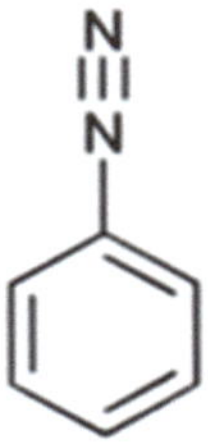

C.
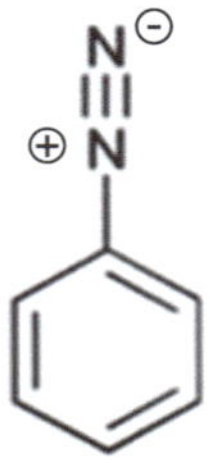

B.
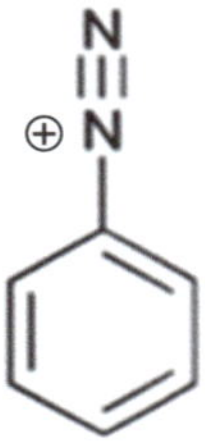

D.
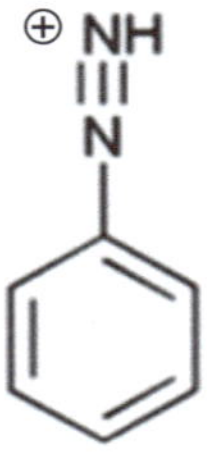

4) What is the relationship between the following three molecules?

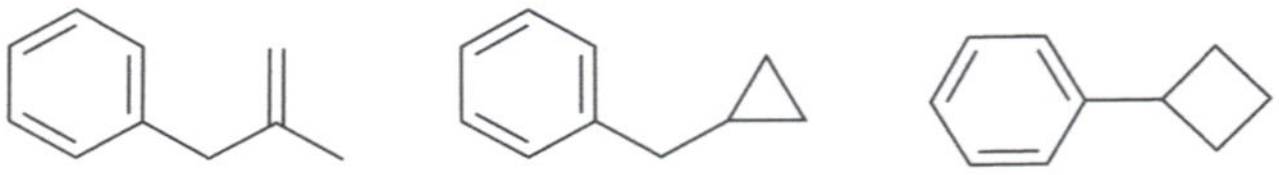

A. Stereoisomers
B. Structural isomers
C. They are not related.
D. They are the same molecule.

5) How many monosubstituted isomers of the benzene ring are possible?

A. 2
B. 3
C. 4
D. None of the above

Low-level Importance

6) How many disubstituted isomers of the benzene ring are possible (i.e. $C_6H_4(X)_2$)?

A. 1
B. 2
C. 3
D. More than 3

7) How many of the following molecules are fully conjugated?

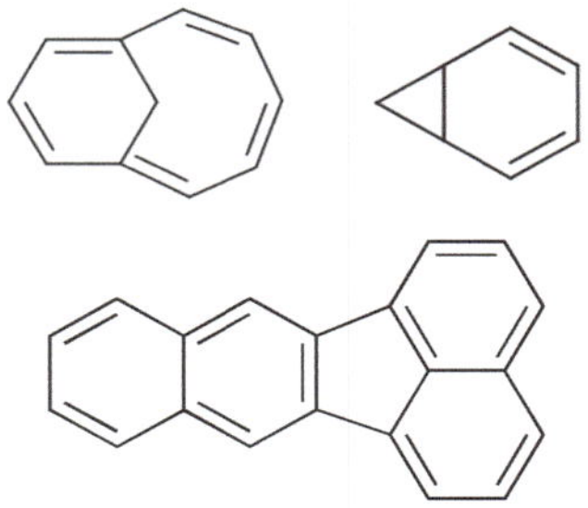

A. None
B. 1
C. 2
D. All 3

GOLD STANDARD GAMSAT-LEVEL PRACTICE QUESTIONS

8) Consider the following disubstituted benzene rings with substituents at the ortho, meta and para positions.

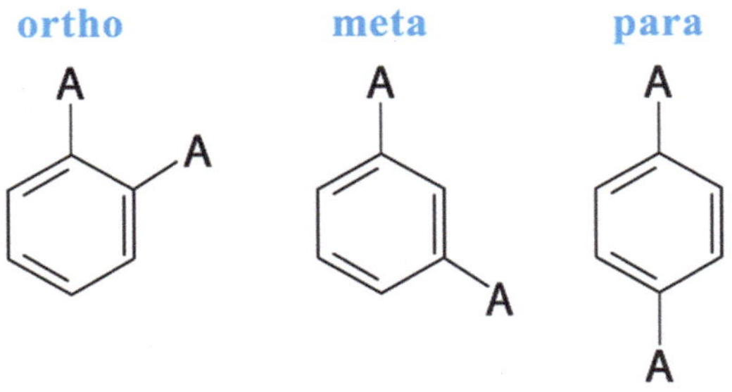

If a third substituent is added to each of the 3 rings, what can be said regarding the number of possible isomers of each of the 3 molecules above?

A. All 3 rings would have 3 possible isomers.
B. 2 rings would have 3 possible isomers, and 1 ring would have 2 possible isomers.
C. 1 ring would have 3 possible isomers, and 2 rings would have 2 possible isomers.
D. 1 ring would have 3 possible isomers, 1 ring would have 2 possible isomers, and 1 ring would have 1 possible isomer.

9) Consider the structure of toluene below.

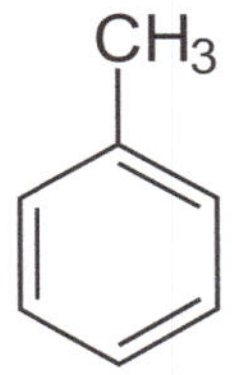

How many different difluorotoluenes are possible?

A. 6
B. 8
C. 9
D. 10

Questions 10–13

Matrices are an array of numbers arranged into n rows and m columns, and are useful for describing the symmetries of molecules. Matrix M is an example of a 3x3 matrix:

$$M = \begin{bmatrix} 2 & 4 & 8 \\ 3 & 5 & 7 \\ 1 & 6 & 9 \end{bmatrix}$$

The number in the ith row and j^{th} column of matrix M is denoted by element mij. In matrix M, m11=2, m12=4, m22=5 and m33=9. Two matrices can be multiplied by element-by-element multiplying a row of the first matrix by a column of the second. For two example matrices A and B where

$$A = \begin{bmatrix} a_{11} & a_{12} & a_{13} \\ a_{21} & a_{22} & a_{23} \end{bmatrix} \quad \text{and} \quad B = \begin{bmatrix} b_{11} & b_{12} \\ b_{21} & b_{22} \\ b_{31} & b_{32} \end{bmatrix}$$

then the product elements of AB are such that AB_{11} is the first row of A multiplied element-by-element the first column of B, AB_{12} is the first row of A multiplied element-by-element the second column of B, and so on.

$$AB = \begin{bmatrix} a_{11}b_{11} + a_{12}b_{21} + a_{13}b_{31} & a_{11}b_{12} + a_{12}b_{22} + a_{13}b_{32} \\ a_{21}b_{11} + a_{22}b_{21} + a_{23}b_{31} & a_{21}b_{12} + a_{22}b_{22} + a_{23}b_{32} \end{bmatrix}$$

Matrices can help classify molecules by identifying their symmetries. Scientists use these symmetries to study molecules since molecules with the same symmetries tend to have similar chemical properties. A molecule has a symmetry when it looks indistinguishable to the original state after a transformation. Two of these transformations include rotation about an axis and reflection about a plane, as shown in Figure 1 for an ammonia molecule NH_3.

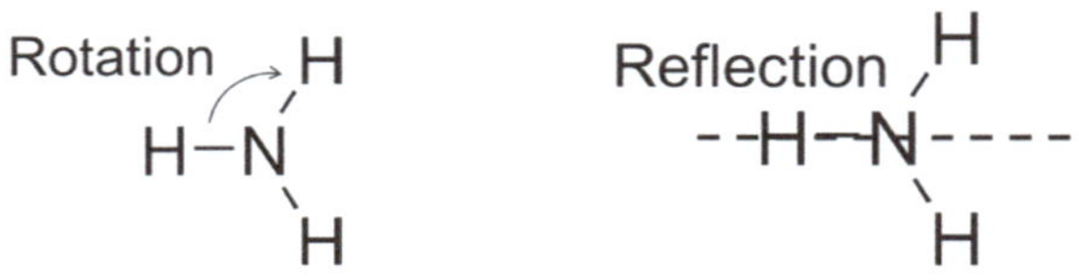

Figure 1: Rotational symmetry about the central nitrogen molecule and reflection about a plane for an ammonia molecule.

To employ matrices for analysing molecular symmetries, consider the hydrogen atoms in the ammonia molecule. Labelling the hydrogen atoms as H_1, H_2 and H_3 to differentiate them, NH_3 can be described as the matrix:

$$\begin{bmatrix} H_1 \\ H_2 \\ H_3 \end{bmatrix}$$

A rotation by 120° about the nitrogen atom as shown in Figure 1 moves H_1 to position 2, H_2 to position 3, and H_3 to position 1. This transformation can be represented using matrices as:

$$M \begin{bmatrix} H_1 \\ H_2 \\ H_3 \end{bmatrix} = \begin{bmatrix} H_3 \\ H_1 \\ H_2 \end{bmatrix}$$

Where it can be shown that:

$$M = \begin{bmatrix} 0 & 0 & 1 \\ 1 & 0 & 0 \\ 0 & 1 & 0 \end{bmatrix}$$

Multiple transformations can be performed by multiplying together each individual transformation and using the rules of matrix multiplication to find the final molecular configuration.

10) What 3x3 matrix represents the transformation in which no atoms change positions?

A. $\begin{bmatrix} 1 & 0 & 0 \\ 0 & 1 & 0 \\ 0 & 0 & 1 \end{bmatrix}$

B. $\begin{bmatrix} 1 & 0 & 0 \\ 1 & 0 & 0 \\ 1 & 0 & 0 \end{bmatrix}$

C. $\begin{bmatrix} 0 & 0 & 1 \\ 0 & 1 & 0 \\ 1 & 0 & 0 \end{bmatrix}$

D. $\begin{bmatrix} 1 & 0 & 0 \\ 0 & 1 & 0 \\ 1 & 0 & 0 \end{bmatrix}$

11) If you rotate the ammonia molecule by 120° and then another 120°, what is the matrix that represents this transformation?

A. $\begin{bmatrix} 0 & 0 & 1 \\ 1 & 0 & 0 \\ 0 & 1 & 0 \end{bmatrix}$

B. $\begin{bmatrix} 0 & 0 & 1 \\ 0 & 1 & 0 \\ 1 & 0 & 0 \end{bmatrix}$

C. $\begin{bmatrix} 0 & 1 & 0 \\ 0 & 0 & 1 \\ 1 & 0 & 0 \end{bmatrix}$

D. $\begin{bmatrix} 0 & 1 & 0 \\ 1 & 0 & 0 \\ 0 & 0 & 1 \end{bmatrix}$

12) Which of the following represents a symmetry of benzene as it is represented below?

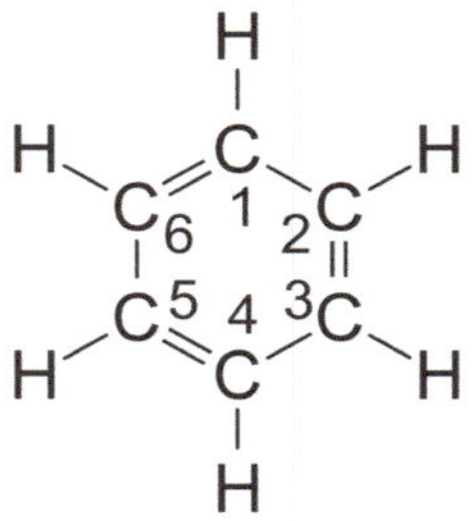

A. Rotation by 60°

B. Rotation by 120°

C. Reflection about the axis passing through carbon 1 and carbon 4

D. Reflection about the axis passing through carbon 2 and carbon 5

13) Consider the following structure of the ammonia molecule with hydrogens labelled 1, 2 and 3.

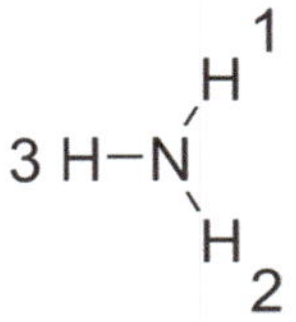

What does the molecule look like under the transformation M?

$$M = \begin{bmatrix} 0 & 1 & 0 \\ 1 & 0 & 0 \\ 0 & 0 & 1 \end{bmatrix}$$

A. 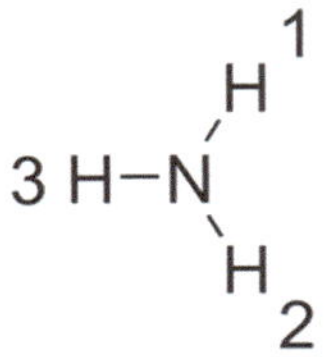

C. 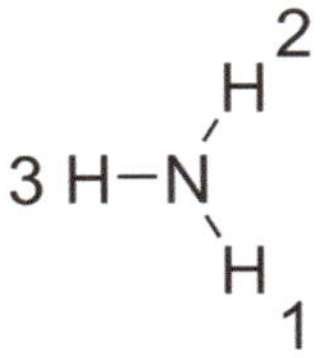

B. 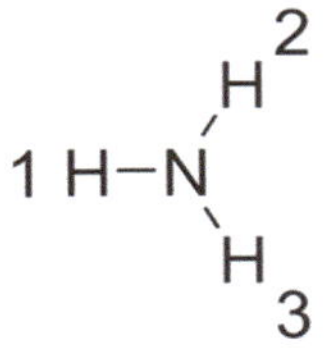

D. 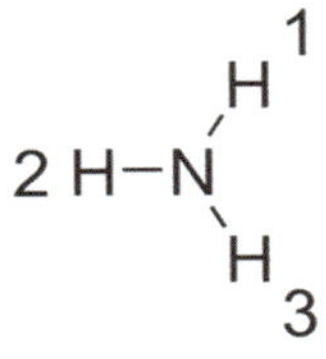

High-level Importance

Questions 14–16

The nature of the first substituent on a benzene ring can:

1) activate or deactivate the ring for further chemical reaction, compared to benzene alone;
2) influence the likely position of any further substituent.

Substituents can be classified into three classes: ortho-para (O-P) directing activators, ortho-para directing deactivators, and meta-directing deactivators. As implied, these groups indicate where most of the new substituent will end up after the chemical reaction.

The following table summarises the effect of substituents attached to the ring where EDG = electron donating group, and EWG = electron withdrawing group.

EDG	EWG	EWG: Halogens
activates the ring	*deactivates the ring*	*weakly deactivating*
O/P Directing	Meta Directing	O/P Directing
e.g., –OH, $-NH_2$, –NHC, NR_2, alkyl groups	e.g., –COOH, –CON, –CHO, nitro ($-NO_2$)	e.g., fluorine, chlorine, bromine, iodine

Table 1

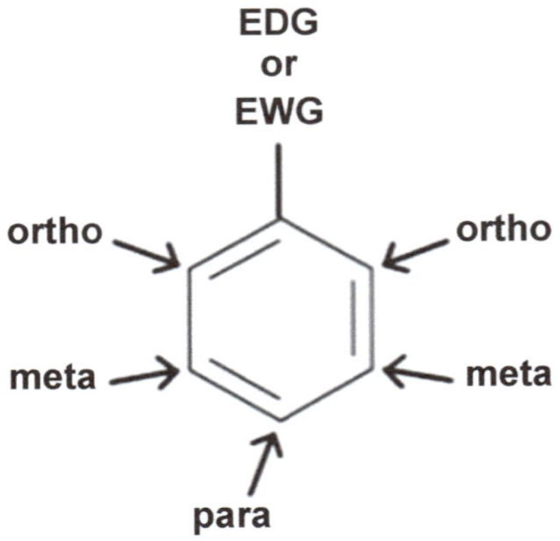

Some common monosubstituted benzene rings:

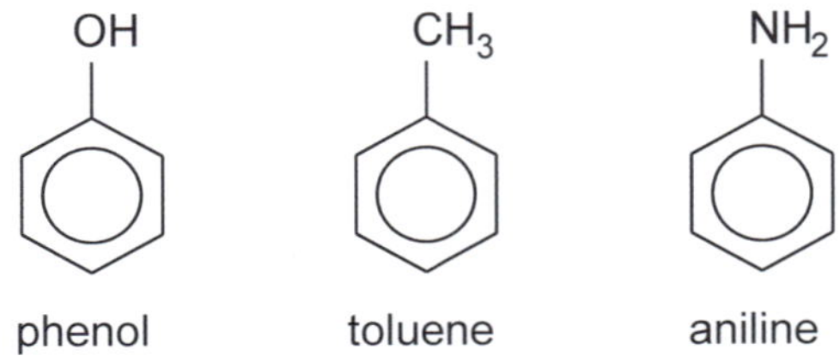

14) When a nitro group is added to the benzene ring, the process is deemed *nitration*. Figure 1 illustrates the energy diagram for the nitration of toluene.

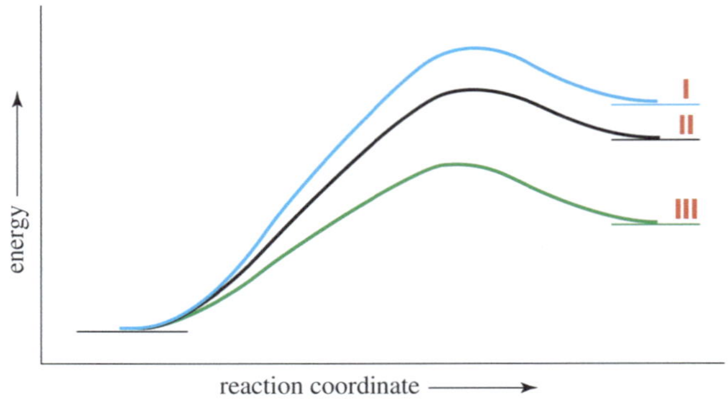

Figure 1

Which of the following is the likely order for the labels in Figure 1 corresponding to ortho-, meta-, and para-nitrotoluene, respectively?

A. **I**, **II** and **III**
B. **III**, **II** and **I**
C. **III**, **I** and **II**
D. **II**, **I** and **III**

15) Bromine (Br) can be added to a benzene ring using $Br_2/FeBr_3$ in a process deemed *bromination*. Based on the information provided, identify the most likely product of the following reaction.

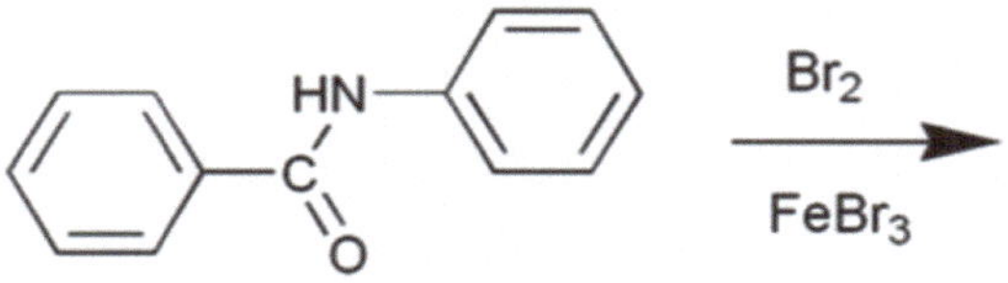

A. 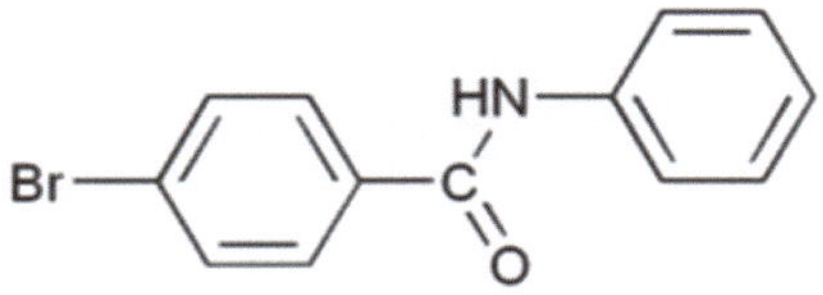

C. 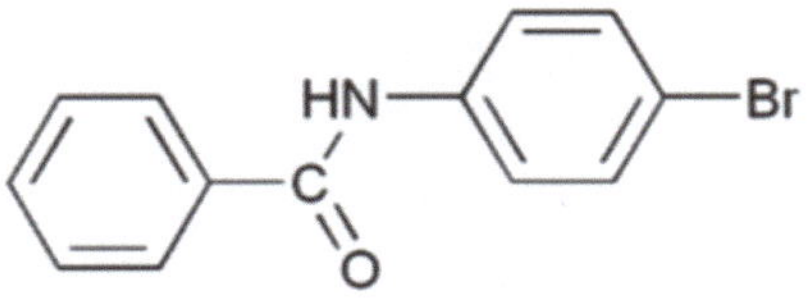

B. 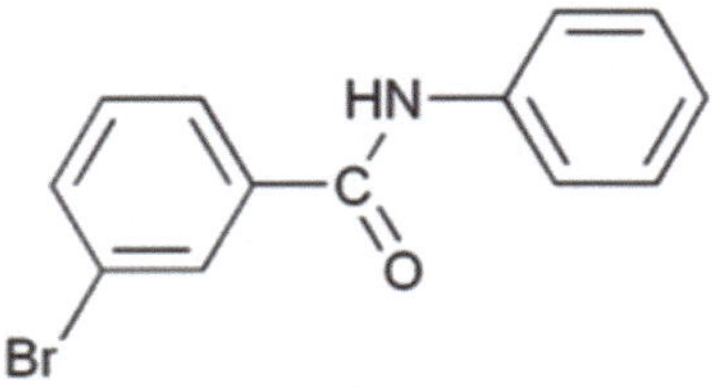

D. 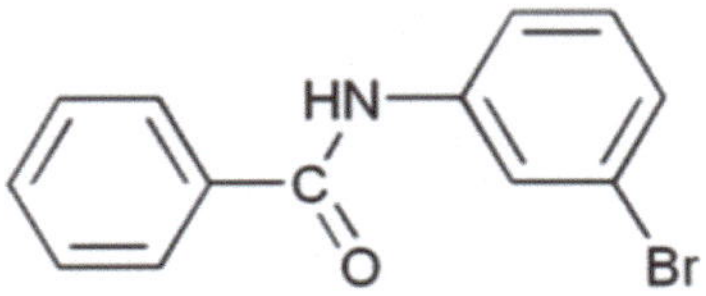

Question 16 also includes the following new information.

Friedel-Crafts alkylation refers to a reaction whereby the benzene ring is alkylated as it reacts with an alkyl halide and, often, $AlCl_3$. The benzene ring attacks the alkyl cation, yielding an alkyl-substituted benzene product.

Note that:

1) poly-alkylation is observed;
2) skeletal rearrangement of the alkyl group sometimes occurs. Specifically, a *hydride shift* could occur to produce a more stable carbocation intermediate (relative stability: 3°>2°>1°>methyl).

16) Based on the information provided, identify the likely product of the following reaction.

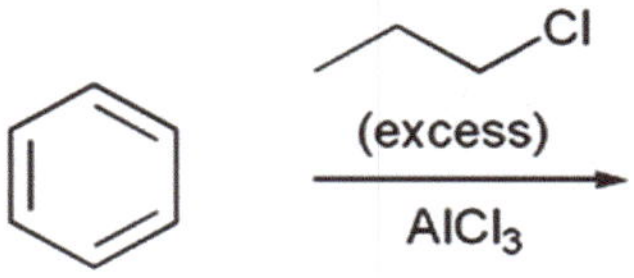

A. 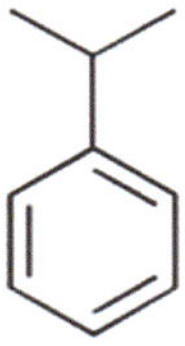

C. 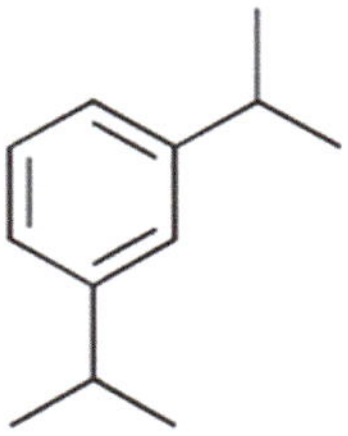

B. 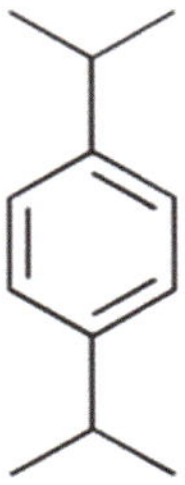

D. 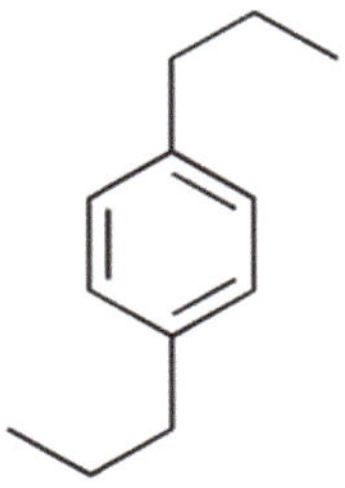

Questions 17–20

Hückel's rule was developed to determine if a planar ring molecule would have aromatic properties.

If a compound does not meet all the following 4 criteria, it is likely not aromatic.

1. The molecule is cyclic (this includes multiple cyclic components).
2. The molecule is planar.
3. The molecule is fully conjugated (i.e. p orbitals at every atom in the ring).
4. The molecule has $4n + 2$ π electrons, where n = 0, 1, 2, 3, and so on.

If rules **1.**, **2.** and/or **3.** are broken, then the molecule is non-aromatic. If only rule **4.** is broken then the molecule is antiaromatic.

Of course, benzene is aromatic (6 π electrons, from 3 double bonds, n = 1), but cyclobutadiene is antiaromatic, since the number of π delocalised electrons is 4. Fused rings can also be regarded as obeying Hückel's rule.

In applying Hückel's rule to any cyclic structure, each doubly-bonded carbon atom contributes one π electron.

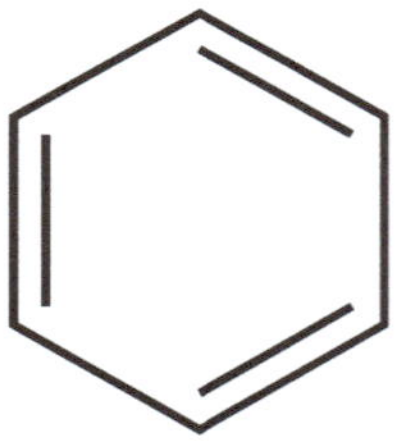

Benzene

Note: All cyclic molecules among the following questions can be assumed to be planar except cyclodecapentaene which has many conformations including a boat-like conformation.

17) Which of the following would you expect to be aromatic?

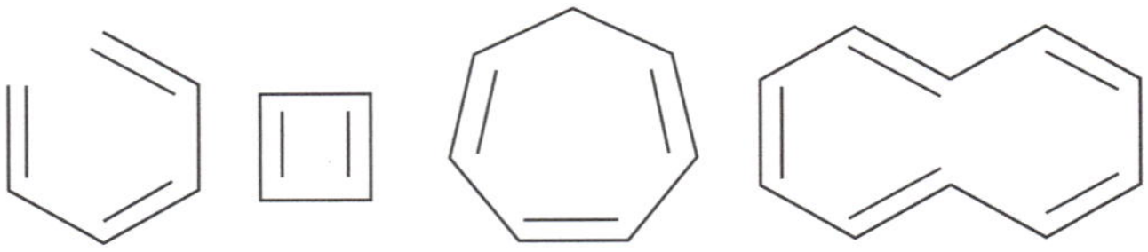

I II III IV

A. None
B. **I** only
C. **II** and **III** only
D. **I**, **II**, **III** and **IV**

Questions 18–20 also depend on the following additional information.

Consider the two planar molecules: hexabenzocoronene (on the left) and pyrene (on the right).

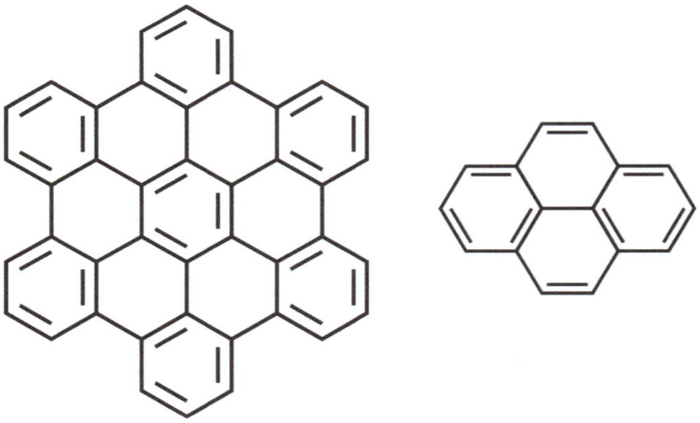

18) Which of the two molecules obeys Hückel's rule?

A. Hexabenzocoronene only
B. Pyrene only
C. Neither
D. Both

19) As compared to pyrene, how many hydrogen atoms does hexabenzocoronene have?

A. The same
B. More but less than twice as many
C. Between twice as many and three times as many
D. More than three times as many

20) What is the best approximation of the simplest structure that can be repeated as needed to recreate hexabenzocoronene?

A. Cyclohexane
B. Benzene
C. Both **A** and **B**
D. Neither **A** nor **B**

SPOILER ALERT

Gold Standard has cross-referenced the content in this chapter to examples from ACER's official GAMSAT practice materials. It is for you to decide when you want to explore these questions since you may want to preserve some of ACER's materials for timed mock-exam practice.

Examples – Delocalisation of electrons over a benzene ring: Q74 of 3; seeking fully-conjugated molecules with benzene-ring substituents: Q82 and Q84 of 5; special mention, but not counted towards the level of importance for this chapter, is assessing an EDG and EWG in the context of carboxylic acids (Chapter 8): Q6 and Q7 of 1; also, special mention, but not counted, is a unit only about structural isomers of benzene (some of the shapes, you have seen in this chapter): Q18-23 of 4 (counted in Chapter 2, Stereochemistry). Note that "Q" is followed by the question number, and, for example, "of 1" refers to booklet number 1 which is referenced in the Spoiler Alert table at the end of Chapter 1. The 15 full-length GAMSAT practice tests by Gold Standard, HEAPS-1 through HEAPS-15, contain specific cross-references to this chapter within the worked solutions. Note that the setup for the EDG and EWG unit is from HEAPS-5 but with different questions; the first question in the unit regarding Hückel's rule is from HEAPS-6; converting structures to a mathematical matrix is a rare visitor from VR-2, Gold Standard's second Virtual Reality practice test.

High-level Importance

Chapter Checklist

- ☐ Access your online account to view answers, worked solutions and discussion boards.
- ☐ Reassess your 'learning objectives' for this chapter: Go back to the first page of this chapter and re-evaluate the top 3 boxes and the Introduction.
- ☐ Complete a maximum of 1 page of notes using symbols/abbreviations to represent the entire chapter based on your learning objectives. These are your Gold Notes.
- ☐ Consider your multimedia options based on your optimal way of learning:
    - ☐ Download the free Gold Standard GAMSAT app for your Android device or iPhone.
    - ☐ Create your own, tangible study cards or try the free app: Anki.
    - ☐ Record your voice reading your Gold Notes onto your smartphone (audio files, e.g., *memo* or MP3s) and listen during exercise, transportation, etc.
    - ☐ Try out the Gold Standard GAMSAT online videos at gamsat-prep.com, or you can try other options on YouTube like Khan Academy or Crash Course Organic Chemistry.
- ☐ Reassess your schedule for your full-length GAMSAT practice tests: ACER and/or HEAPS exams. Ensure that you have scheduled one full day to complete a practice test and 1-2 days for a thorough assessment of worked solutions while adding to your abbreviated Gold Notes.
- ☐ Reassess your progress in scheduling and/or evaluating stress reduction techniques such as regular exercise (sports), yoga, meditation and/or mindfulness exercises (*see* YouTube for suggestions).

ALCOHOLS

Chapter 6

Memorise

* IUPAC nomenclature
* Products of oxidation
* Define: steric hindrance

Understand

* Trends based on length, branching
* Effect of hydrogen bonds
* Dehydration, redox reactions
* Basics: Nucleophilic substitution, elimination

Importance

High level: 10% of GAMSAT Organic Chemistry questions released by ACER are related to content in this chapter (in our estimation).
* Note that approximately 60% of the questions in GAMSAT Organic Chemistry are related to just 4 chapters: 2, 6, 7 and 12.

Introduction

An alcohol is any organic compound in which a hydroxyl group (-OH) is bound to a carbon atom of an alkyl or substituted alkyl group. There is an incredibly wide range of 'alcohols' - although originally, the term only referred to the primary alcohol *ethanol* (ethyl alcohol), the predominant alcohol in alcoholic beverages.

IUPAC nomenclature for alcohols applies the suffix *-ol* to organic molecules where the *hydroxyl* group is the functional group with the highest priority; in substances where a higher priority group is present, the prefix hydroxy- is used. The suffix *-ol* in non-systematic names (such as paracetamol or cholesterol) also usually indicates that the molecule includes a hydroxyl functional group. Some molecules, particularly sugars (e.g. glucose and sucrose, ORG 12.3) contain hydroxyl functional groups without using the suffix *-ol*.

Multimedia Resources at GAMSAT-Prep.com

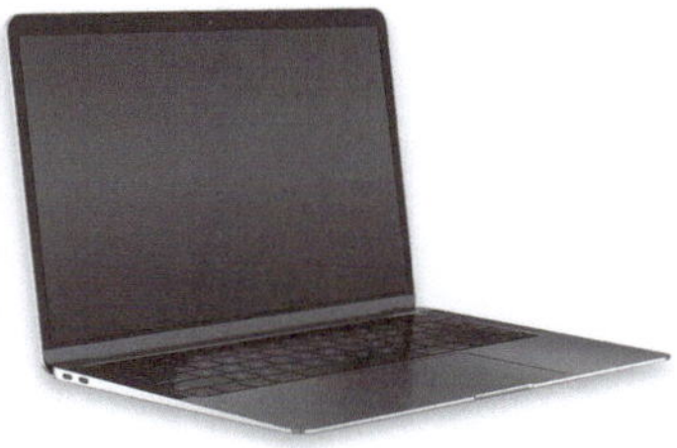

Open Discussion Boards
(*gamsat-prep.com/forum*)

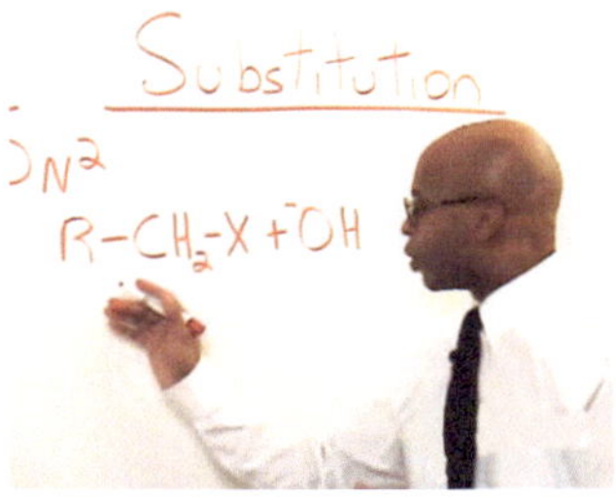

Science Preparation Videos

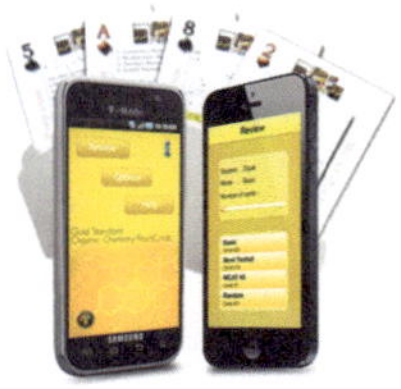

Flashcards

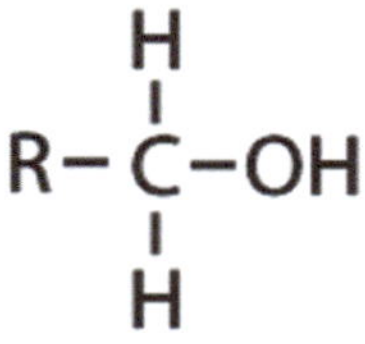

1°

Special Guest

* The real GAMSAT may have advanced-level information presented (i.e. in a passage) but previous knowledge of said information is not required to answer the questions that would follow. Practice questions at the end of this chapter, as well as ACER and GS (HEAPS) practice GAMSATs can help you clarify this point.

6.0 GAMSAT has a *Need for Speed*!

High-level Importance

Section	GAMSAT Organic Chemistry *Need for Speed* Exercises
6.1	Identify each alcohol as either primary (1°), secondary (2°), or tertiary (3°). Note that they are not in the same order as ORG 6.1. 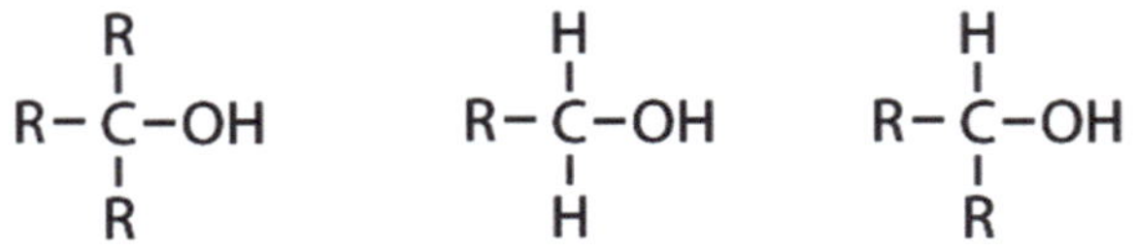
	In order to maintain a balance of charge and atoms, what must be the missing product (*conjugate base*)? $C_2H_5OH + OH^- \rightleftharpoons$ [ ] $+ H_2O$
	Circle one option within each of the square brackets below. Alcohols have [higher / lower] boiling points and a [greater / lower] solubility than comparable alkanes, alkenes, aldehydes, ketones and alkyl halides.
6.1.3	Alcohol synthesis: Is the reaction below oxidation, reduction, or hydration? (later, *see* Spoiler Alert for the rationale for this question) 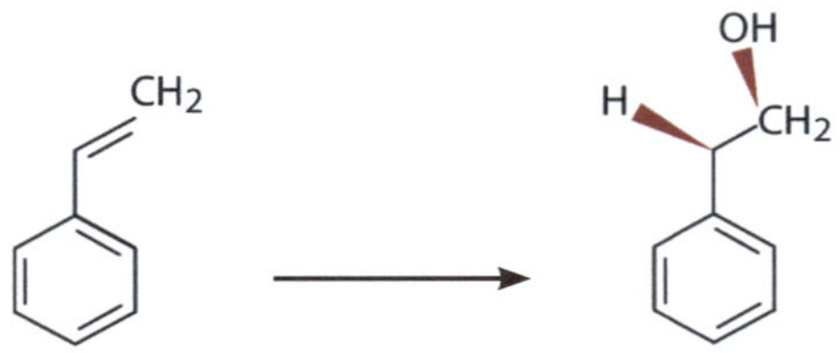
	Grignard reagents (RMgX) react with carbonyl compounds to give alcohols. For the 3 reactions below, draw the missing carbonyl compound (*balance the organic components*). $RMgBr\ +\ \qquad \xrightarrow[2.\ H_3O^+]{1.\ ether} RCH_2OH$ $RMgBr\ +\ \qquad \xrightarrow[2.\ H_3O^+]{1.\ ether}$ 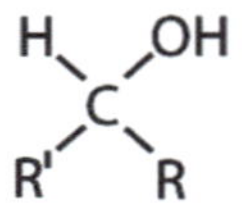 $RMgBr\ +\ \qquad \xrightarrow[2.\ H_3O^+]{1.\ ether}$ 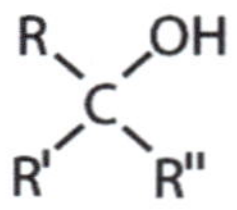

6.2.1	Use a less than < or greater than symbol > to indicate, in each case, which structure is more substituted. 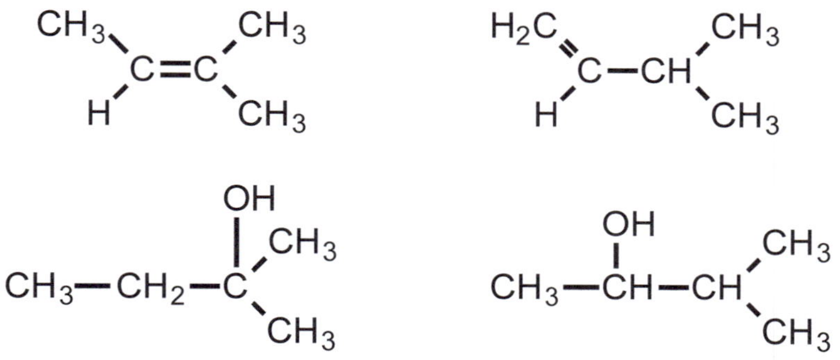
6.2.2	Show the classic results consistent with the oxidation of alcohols. 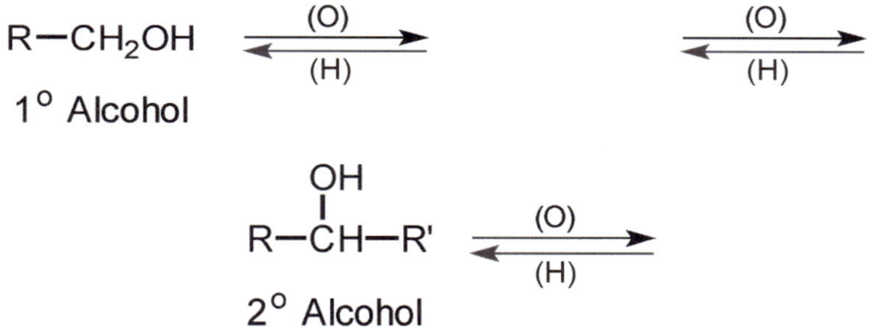
6.2.3	Use a less than < or greater than symbol > below to indicate, in each case, which group is more stable. primary alkyl groups secondary alkyl groups tertiary alkyl groups
6.2.4	Given the reaction below, draw what must be the final product. 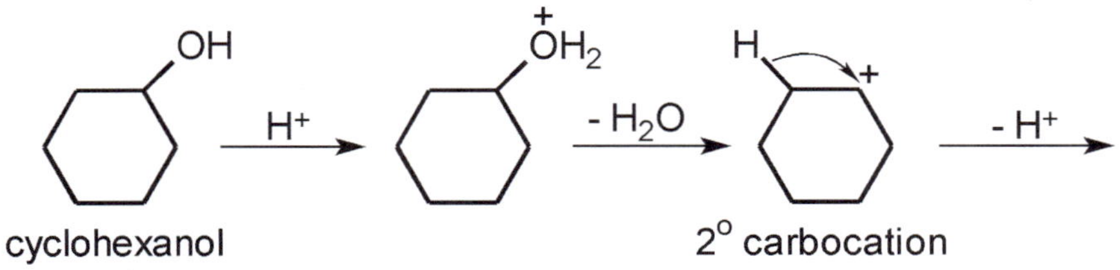

6.1 Description and Nomenclature

The systematic naming of alcohols is accomplished by replacing the *–e* of the corresponding alkane with *–ol*.

Alcohols are compounds that have hydroxyl groups bonded to a saturated carbon atom with the general formula ROH. It can be thought of as a substituted water molecule, with one of the water hydrogens replaced with an alkyl group R. Alcohols are classified as primary (1°), secondary (2°) or tertiary (3°) based on the number of carbon atoms connected to the carbon atom bonded to OH:

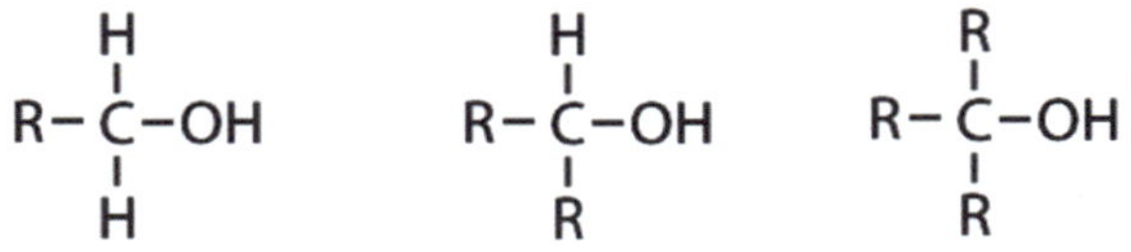

1° 2° 3°

As with alkanes, special names are used for branched groups:

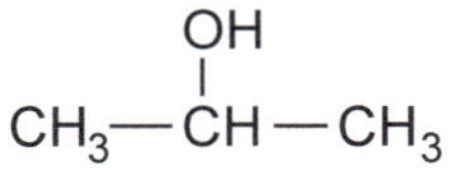

IUPAC: propan-2-ol
- Isopropanol
- Isopropyl alcohol

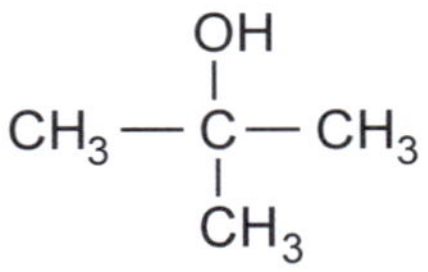

IUPAC: 2-methylpropan-2-ol
- 2-methyl-2-propanol
- tert-butanol

The alcohols are always numbered to give the carbon with the attached hydroxy (–OH) group the lowest number (choose the longest carbon chain that contains the hydroxyl group as the parent):

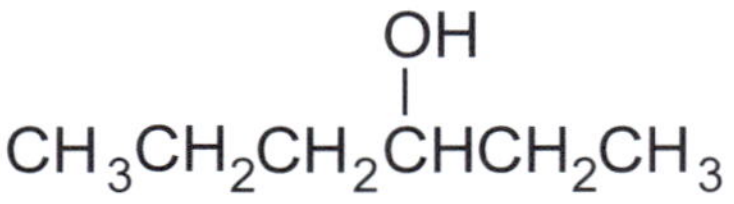

3-hexanol NOT 4-hexanol

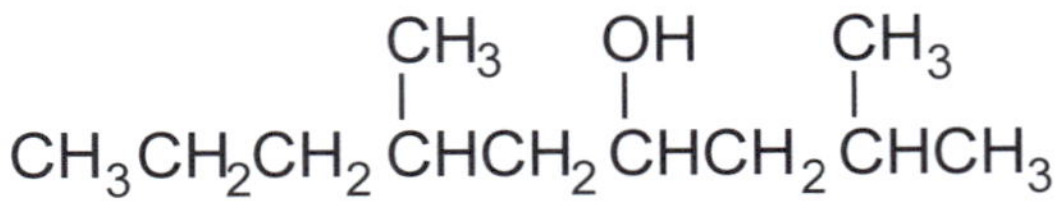

2,6-dimethyl-4-nonanol

The shorthand for methanol is MeOH, and the shorthand for ethanol is EtOH. Alcohols are weak acids ($K_a \approx 10^{-18}$), being weaker acids than water. Their conjugate bases are called alkoxides, very little of which will be present in solution:

$$\underset{\text{ethanol}}{C_2H_5OH} + OH^- \rightleftharpoons \underset{\text{ethoxide}}{C_2H_5O^-} + H_2O$$

The acidity of an alcohol decreases with increasing number of attached carbons. Thus CH_3OH is more acidic than CH_3CH_2OH; and CH_3CH_2OH (a primary alcohol) is more acidic than $(CH_3)_2CHOH$ (a secondary alcohol), which is, in turn, more acidic than $(CH_3)_3COH$ (a tertiary alcohol).

Alcohols have higher boiling points and a greater solubility than comparable alkanes, alkenes, aldehydes, ketones and alkyl halides. The higher boiling point and greater solubility is due to the greater polarity and hydrogen bonding of the alcohol. In alcohols, hydrogen bonding is a weak association of the –OH proton of one molecule, with the oxygen of another. To form the hydrogen bond, both a donor, and an acceptor are required:

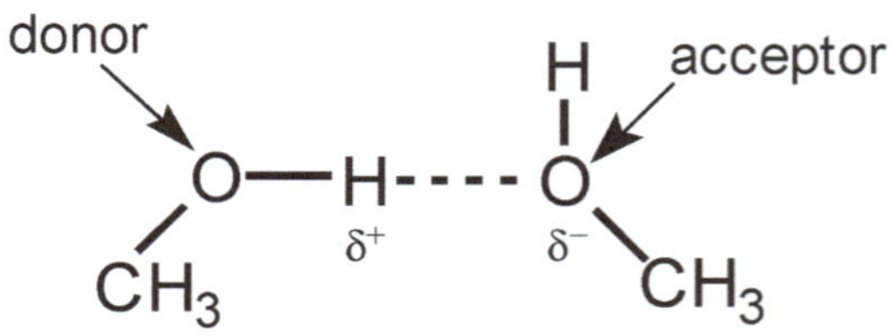

Sometimes an atom may act as both a donor and acceptor of hydrogen bonds. One example of this is the oxygen atom in an alcohol:

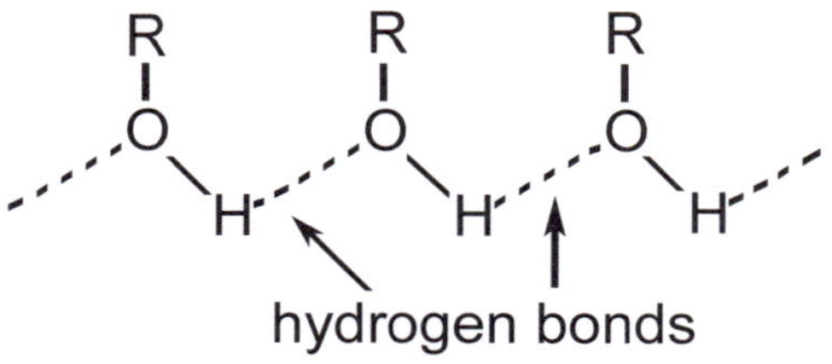

As the length of the carbon chain (= R) of the alcohol molecule increases, the nonpolar chain becomes more meaningful, and the alcohol becomes less water soluble. The hydroxyl group of a primary alcohol is able to form hydrogen bonds with molecules such as water more easily than the hydroxyl group of a tertiary alcohol. The hydroxyl group of a tertiary alcohol is crowded by, for example, the surrounding methyl groups and thus its ability to participate in hydrogen bonds is lessened.

In solution, primary alcohols are more acidic than secondary alcohols, and secondary alcohols are more acidic than tertiary alcohols. In the gas phase, however, the order of acidity is reversed.

6.1.1 Foundational Nomenclature Exercises: Alcohols

Name the following ten compounds. If necessary, feel free to consult the nomenclature rules from ORG 3.1, 4.1 and 6.1. The answers are at the end of this chapter. Of course, it is more helpful to you in the long run to give a full effort first - rather than looking at the solutions before trying. Also, after naming the structure, identify if the molecule is a primary (1°), secondary (2°), or tertiary alcohol (3°).

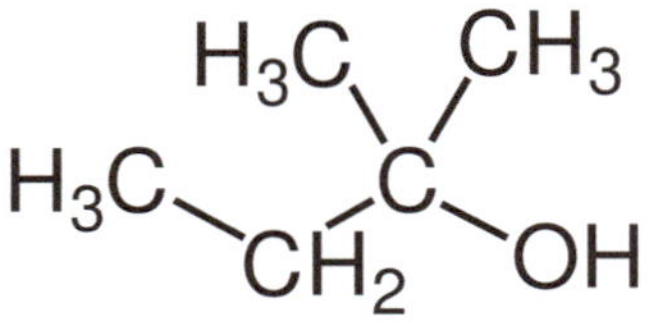

1) ____________________

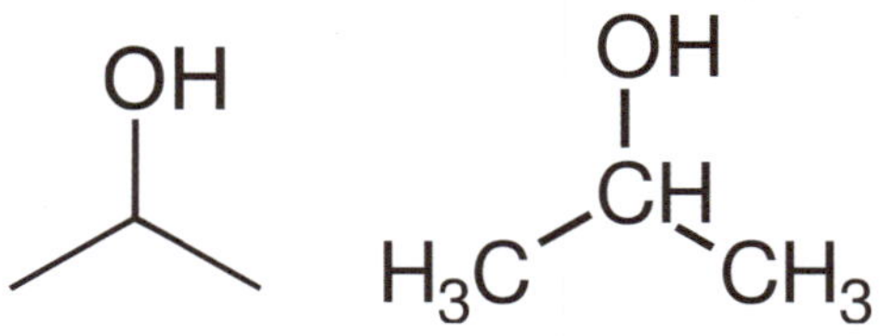

2) ____________________

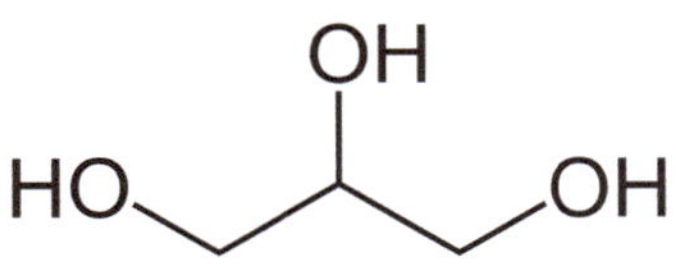

3) ____________________

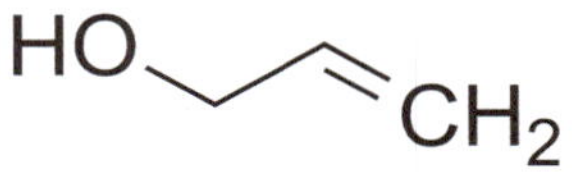

4) ____________________

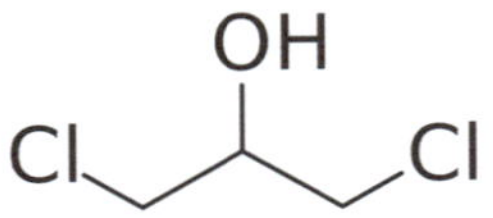

5) ______________________

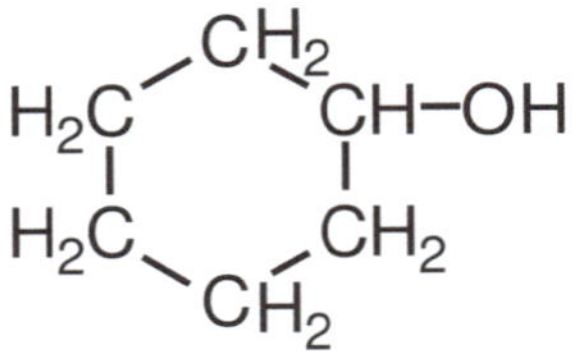

6) ______________________

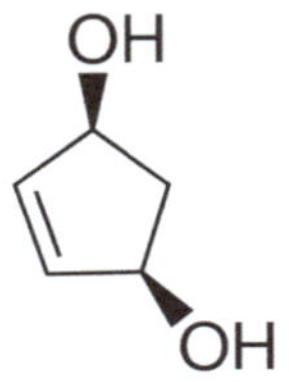

7) ______________________

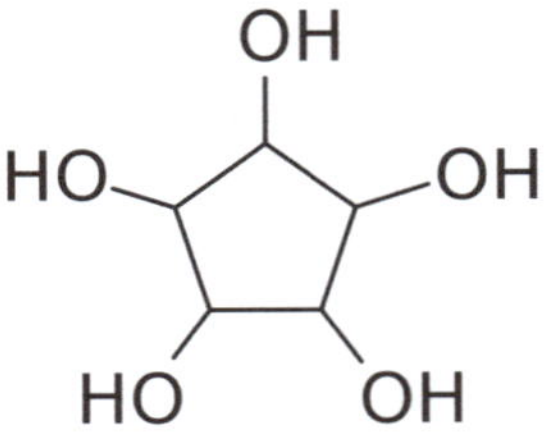

8) ______________________

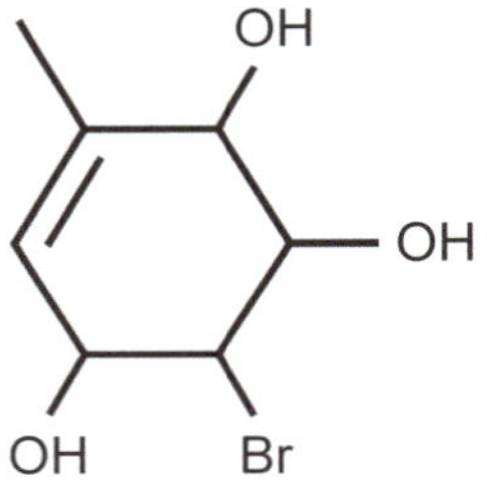

9) ______________________

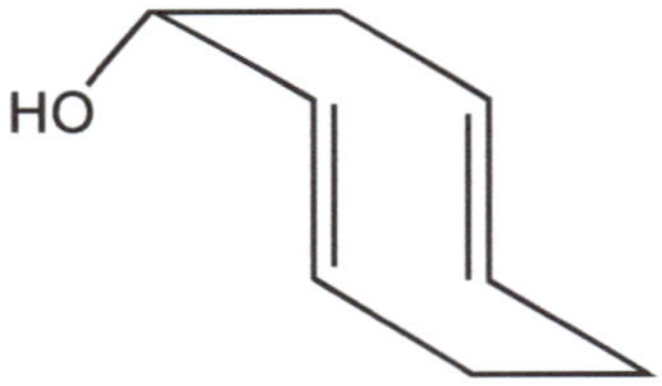

10) ______________________

6.1.2 Acidity and Basicity of Alcohols

Alcohols are both weakly acidic and weakly basic. Alcohols can dissociate into a proton and its conjugate base, the alkoxy ion (alkoxide, RO^-), just as water dissociates into a proton and a hydroxide ion. As weak acids, alcohols act as proton donors, thus $ROH + H_2O \longrightarrow RO^- + H_3O^+$. As weak bases, alcohols act as proton acceptors, thus $ROH + HX \longrightarrow ROH_2^+ + X^-$.

Substituent effects are important in determining alcohol acidity. The more easily the alkoxide ion is accessible to a water molecule, the easier it is stabilised through solvation (CHM 5.3), the more its formation is favored, and the greater the acidity of the alcohol molecule. For example, $(CH_3)_3COH$ is less acidic than CH_3OH.

Inductive effects are also important in determining alcohol acidity. Electron-withdrawing groups stabilise an alkoxide anion by spreading out the charge, thus making the alcohol molecule more acidic. Vice versa, electron-donating groups destabilise an alkoxide anion, thus making the alcohol molecule less acidic. For example, $(CH_3)_3COH$ is less acidic than $(CF_3)_3OH$.

Since alcohols are weak acids, they do not react with weak bases. However, they do react with strong bases such as NaH, $NaNH_2$, or sodium or potassium metal.

$CH_3CH_2OH + NaH \rightarrow CH_3CH_2O^-Na^+ + H_2$

$CH_3CH_2OH + NaNH_2 \rightarrow CH_3CH_2O^-Na^+ + NH_3$

$2CH_3CH_2OH + 2Na \rightarrow 2CH_3CH_2O^-Na^+ + H_2$

High-level Importance

6.1.3 Synthesis of Alcohols: How to Make Alcohols

1. Hydration of alkenes: Alcohols can be prepared through the hydration (= *to combine with water*) of alkenes:

(1) Halohydrin (*one carbon with a halogen and an adjacent carbon with a hydroxyl substituent;* ORG 4.2.1) formation yields a Markovnikov hydration product with anti stereospecificity (i.e. the OH nucleophile adds to the most substituted carbon but *opposite* to the halide);

(2) Hydroboration-oxidation yields a syn stereospecific anti-Markovnikov hydration product (the OH adds to the least substituted carbon);

(3) Oxymercuration-reduction yields a Markovnikov hydration product.

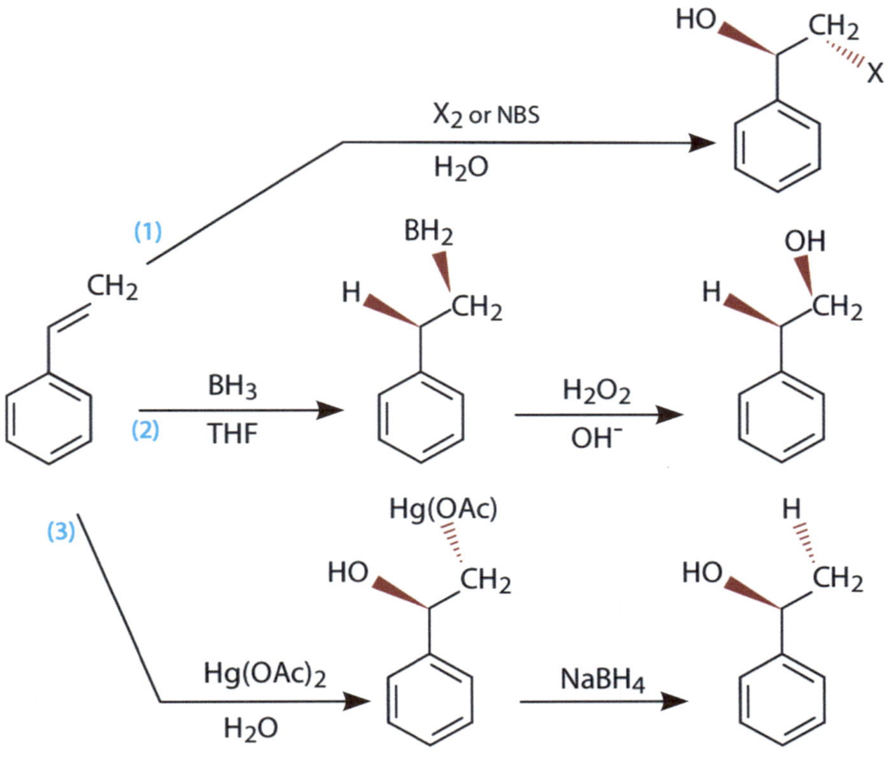

High-level Importance

2. Reduction of carbonyl compounds: An alcohol can be prepared through the reduction of an aldehyde, ketone, carboxylic acid or ester. Aldehydes are converted into primary alcohols and ketones are converted into secondary alcohols in the presence of reducing agents $NaBH_4$ or $LiAlH_4$ (also symbolised as LAH or LithAl). Since $LiAlH_4$ is more powerful and more reactive than $NaBH_4$, it can be used as a reducing agent for the reduction of carboxylic acids and esters to give primary alcohols (*see* ORG 6.2.2).

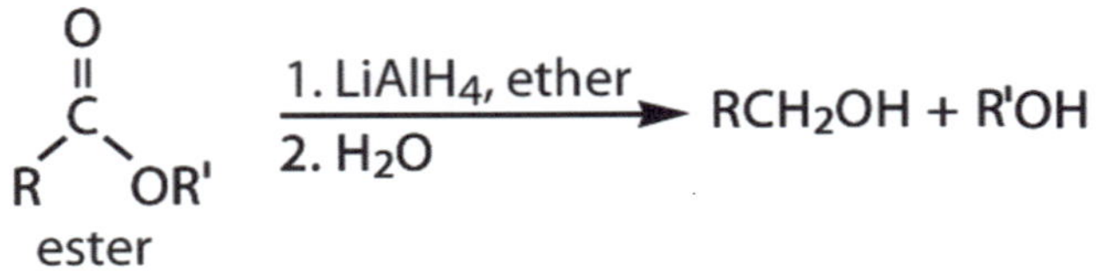

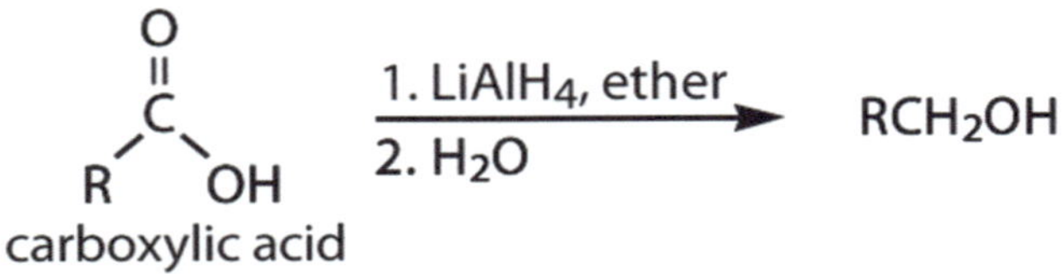

3. Addition reaction with Grignard reagents: Grignard reagents (RMgX) react with carbonyl compounds to give alcohols. Grignard reagents are created by reacting Mg metal with an alkyl (aryl or vinyl) halide.

$$R\text{-}X + Mg \longrightarrow RMgX$$

A number of different alcohol products can be obtained from Grignard reactions with formaldehyde, other aldehydes, ketones or esters. A carboxylic acid does not give an alcohol product because, instead of an addition reaction, the carboxylic acid reacts with the Grignard reagent giving a hydrocarbon and magnesium salt of the acid.

- Formaldehyde: Primary alcohol

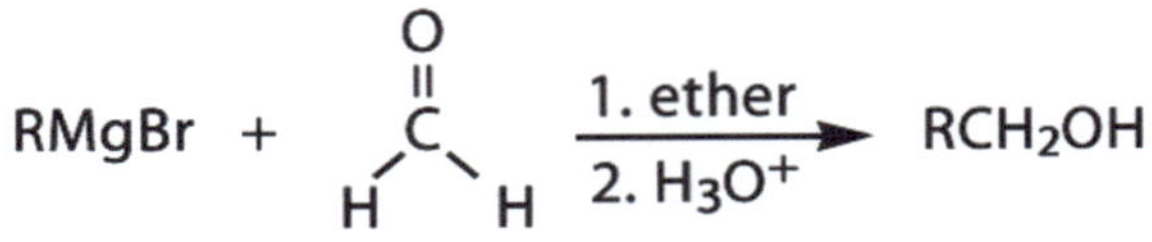

- Aldehyde: Secondary alcohol

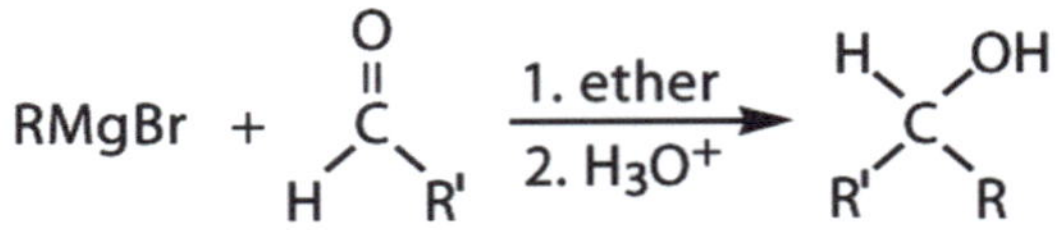

- Ketone: Tertiary alcohol

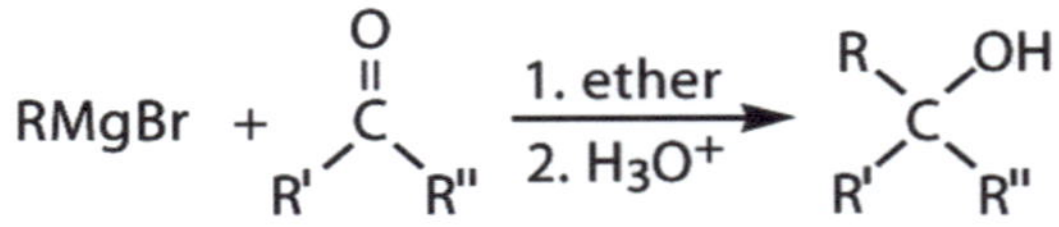

- Ester: Tertiary alcohol

Two substituents from the Grignard reagent are added to the carbonyl-bearing carbon, giving a tertiary alcohol.

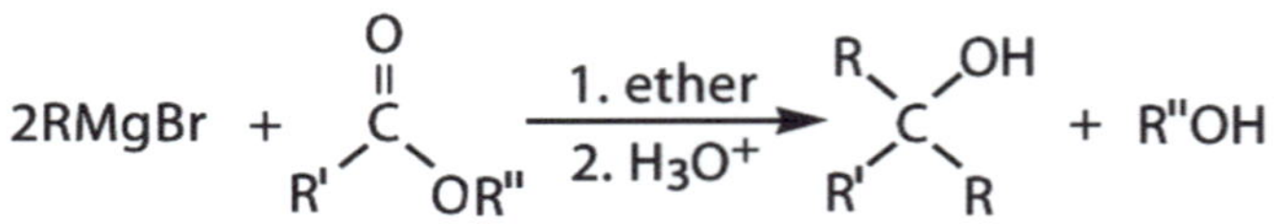

For alkene hydration, reduction of carbonyl, addition with Grignards, and the other reactions, follow the story, follow the geometry, follow the substituents (R, R', R'', etc.) as you have been doing with the other chapters. It is extremely unlikely to be asked a GAMSAT question that requires the memorisation of a reagent (= the chemical added to bring about the reaction, i.e. Grignard, ether, catalysts, etc.). Pattern recognition and geometric reasoning with the reactions above await you at the end of this chapter.

6.2.1 Dehydration

Dehydration (= *loss of water*) reactions of alcohols produce alkenes. The general dehydration reaction is shown in Figure IV.B.6.1.

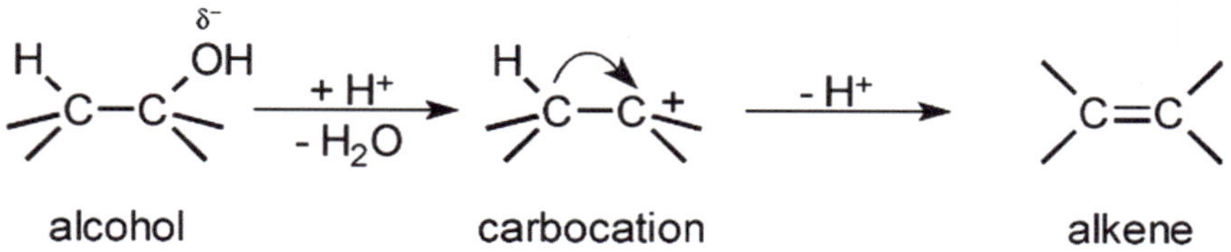

Figure IV.B.6.1: Dehydration of an alcohol. The proton (H^+) is attracted to the partial negative charge of –OH thus water is formed which is a good leaving group. Then electrons are attracted to the positively charged carbon causing a proton to leave. Thus the acid (i.e. proton) increases the reaction rate and is regenerated (= *catalyst;* CHM 9.7).

For the preceding reaction to occur, the temperature must be between 300 and 400 degrees Celsius, and the vapors must be passed over a metal oxide catalyst. Alternatively, strong, hot acids, such as H_2SO_4 or H_3PO_4 at 100 to 200 degrees Celsius may be used.

The reactivity depends upon the type of alcohol. A tertiary alcohol is more reactive than a secondary alcohol which is, in turn, more reactive than a primary alcohol. The faster reactions have the most stable carbocation intermediates. The alkene that is formed is the most stable one. A phenyl group will take preference over one or two alkyl groups, otherwise the most substituted double bond is the most stable (= *major product*) and the least substituted is less stable (= *minor product*).

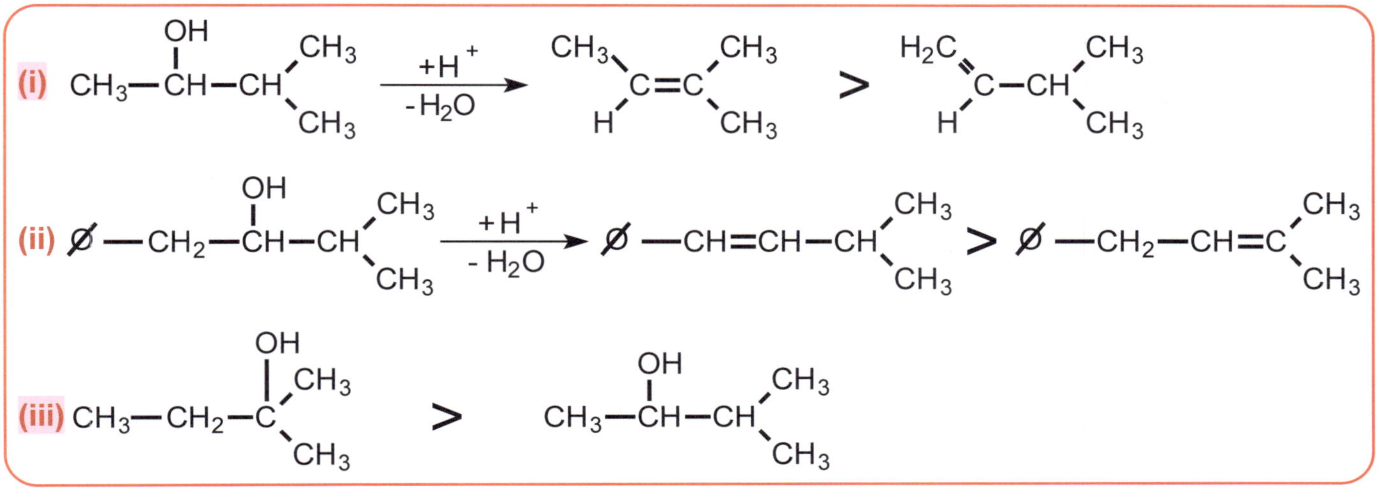

Figure IV.B.6.2: Dehydration of substituted alcohols. Major and minor products, respectively, are represented in reactions (i) and (ii). An example of a reactant with a greater reaction rate due to more substituents as an intermediate is represented by (iii). ϕ = a phenyl group.

High-level Importance

6.2.2 Oxidation-Reduction

In organic chemistry, oxidation (O) is the increasing of oxygen or decreasing of hydrogen content, and reduction (H) is the opposite. Primary alcohols are converted to aldehydes using PCC or $KMnO_4$, under mild conditions (i.e. room temperature, neutral pH). Primary alcohols are converted to carboxylic acids using CrO_3 (the mixture is called a Jones reagent), $K_2Cr_2O_7$, or $KMnO_4$ under abrasive conditions (i.e. increased temperature, presence of OH^-). Secondary alcohols are converted to ketones by any of the preceding oxidising agents. It is *very* difficult to oxidise a tertiary alcohol. Under acidic conditions, tertiary alcohols are unaffected; they may be oxidised under acidic conditions by dehydration and *then* oxidising the double bond of the resultant alkene. The resistance of tertiary alcohols to oxidation is a testable item. Classic reducing agents (H) include $LiAlH_4$ (strong), H_2/metals (strong) and $NaBH_4$ (mild).

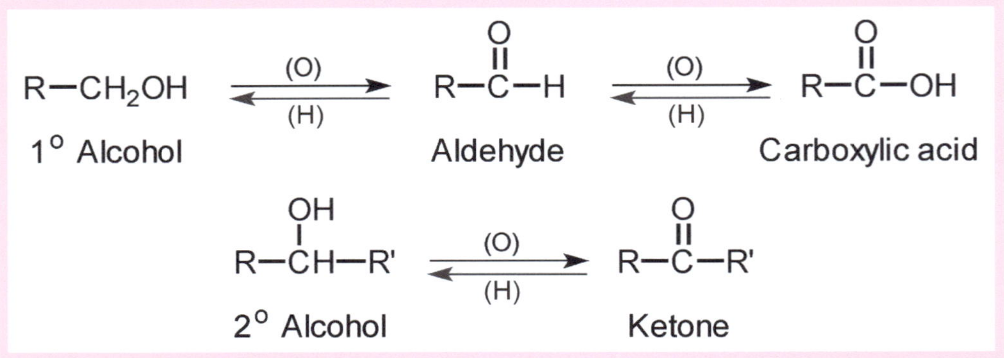

Figure IV.B.6.3: Oxidation-Reduction. In organic chemistry, traditionally the symbols R and R' denote an attached hydrogen, or a hydrocarbon side chain of any length (which is consistent with the reactions above), but sometimes these symbols refer to any group of atoms. For the GAMSAT, when R is used, it is normally defined in the passage preceding the questions.

6.2.3 Substitution

In a substitution reaction, one atom or group is *substituted* or replaced by another atom or group. For an alcohol, the –OH group is replaced (*substituted*) by a halide (usually chlorine or bromine), or vice-versa. For halogenation, a variety of reagents may be used, such as HCl, HBr or PCl_3. There are two different types of substitution reactions, S_N1 and S_N2.

In the $\mathbf{S_N1}$ (***S**ubstitution, **N**ucleophilic **1**st order, or unimolecular*) reaction, the transition state involves a carbocation, the formation of which is the rate-determining step (i.e. *the slowest step in a sequence, determines the overall rate*; CHM 9.4). Alcohol substitutions that proceed by this mechanism are those involving benzyl groups, allyl groups, tertiary and secondary alcohols. The mechanism of this reaction is:

(i) R–L → R^+ + L^-
(ii) Nu^- + R^+ → Nu–R

The important features of this reaction are:

- The reaction is first order (i.e. *the rate of the reaction depends only on the concentration of one compound;* CHM 9.2); thus rate = k[R–L], where R may be an alkyl group, L represents a substituent or ligand, and k is the rate constant.
- There is racemisation (ORG 2.3.2) when a chiral molecule is involved.
- A stable carbonium ion should be formed; thus in terms of reaction rate, benzyl groups = allyl groups > tertiary alcohols > secondary alcohols >> primary alcohols.
- The stability of alkyl groups is as follows: primary alkyl groups < secondary alkyl groups < tertiary alkyl groups.

The mechanism of the **S_N2** (***S**ubstitution, **N**ucleophilic **2**nd order, or bimolecular*) reaction is:

$$Nu^- + R—L \rightarrow [Nu\text{----}R\text{----}L]^- \rightarrow Nu—R + L^-$$

There are several important points to know about this reaction:

- The reaction rate is second order overall (the rate depends on the concentration of two compounds); first order with respect to [R-L] and first order with respect to the concentration of the nucleophile [Nu^-]; thus rate = k [R–L][Nu^-].
- Note that the nucleophile adds to the alkyl group by *backside displacement* (i.e. Nu must add to the *opposite* site to the ligand; *see* Figure IV.B.6.5). Thus optically active alcohols react to give an inversion of configuration, forming the opposite enantiomer (ORG 2.2.2, 2.3.2).
- Large or bulky groups near or at the reacting site may hinder or retard a reaction. This is called *steric hindrance*. Size

Figure IV.B.6.4: S_N1 mechanism in which OH substitutes for Cl producing racemisation via a tertiary carbocation.

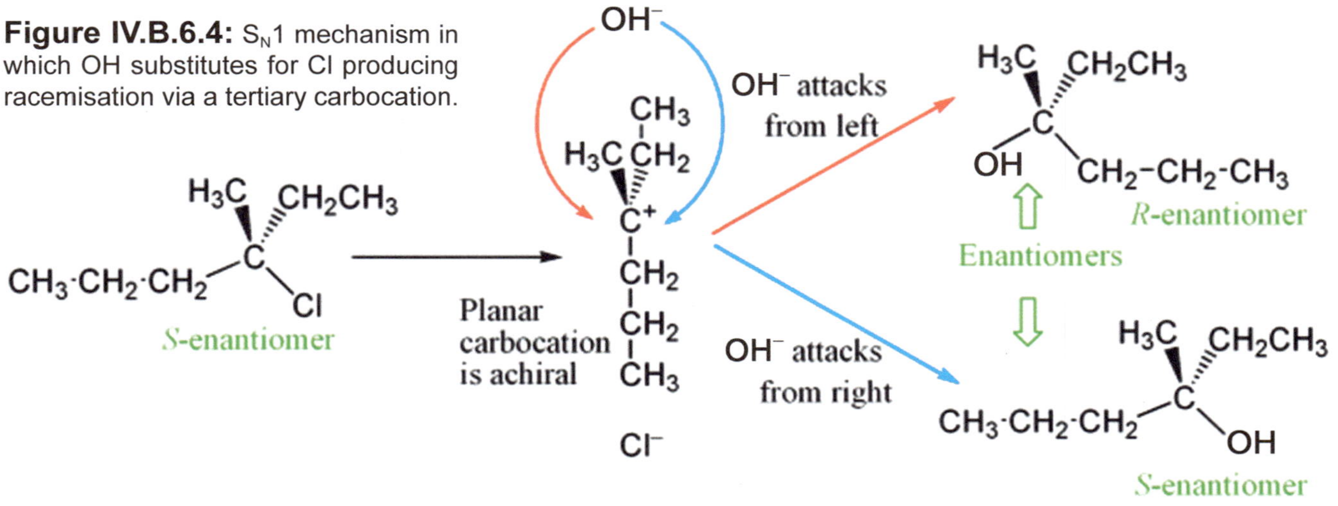

High-level Importance

or steric factors are important since they affect S_N2 reaction rates; in terms of reaction rates, CH_3^- > primary alcohols > secondary alcohols >> tertiary alcohols.

The substitution reactions for methanol (CH_3OH) and other primary alcohols are by the S_N2 reaction mechanism.

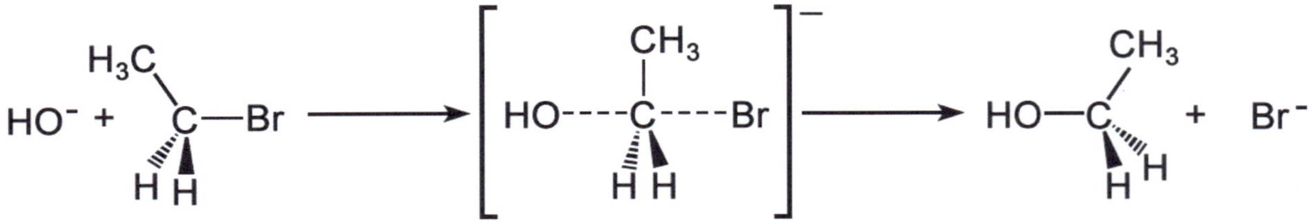

Figure IV.B.6.5: S_N2 mechanism in which OH substitutes for Br producing an alcohol with inversion due to backside displacement.

6.2.4 Elimination

Elimination reactions occur when an atom or a group of atoms is removed (*eliminated*) from adjacent carbons leaving a multiple bond:

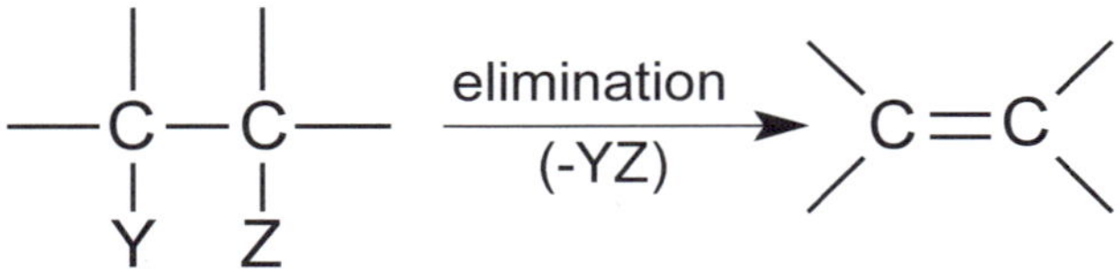

There are two different types of elimination reactions, E1 and E2. In the **E1** (**E**limination, **1**st order) reaction, the rate of reaction depends on the concentration of one compound. E1 often occurs as minor products alongside S_N2 reactions. E1 can occur as major products starting with a *substrate* (reactant) like an alkyl halide, or an alcohol:

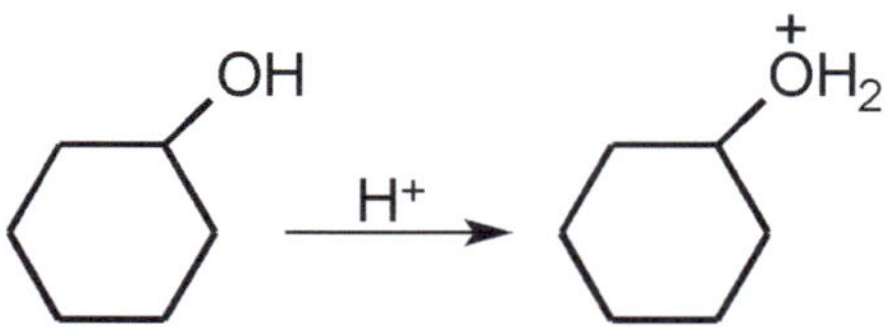

cyclohexanol

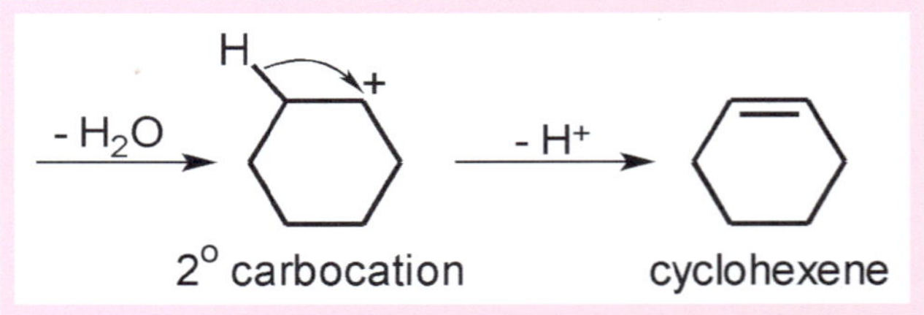

The acid-catalysed dehydration of alcohols is thus an E1 reaction which yields the more highly substituted alkene as the major product. There is a carbocation intermediate formed during the preceding reaction, thus a tertiary alcohol will react faster and yield an alkene in a more stable way than a secondary or primary alcohol.

Secondary and primary alcohols will only react with acids in very harsh conditions (75%-95% H_2SO_4, 100 °C). However, they will react with $POCl_3$ converting the –OH into a good leaving group to yield an alkene. This reaction takes place with an E2 mechanism.

In the **E2** (**E**limination, **2**nd order) reaction, the rate of reaction depends on the concentration of two compounds (CHM 9.2). E2 reactions require strong bases like KOH or the salt of an alcohol (e.g. ORG 6.1.1, *sodium alkoxide*). An alkoxide (RO^-) can be synthesised from an alcohol using either Na(*s*) or NaH (*sodium hydride*) as reducing agents. The hydride ion H^- is a powerful base:

$$\text{R-OH} + \text{NaH} \longrightarrow \underset{\text{sodium alkoxide}}{\text{R-O}^-\text{Na}^+} + H_2$$

Now the alkoxide can be used as a proton acceptor in an E2 reaction involving an alkyl halide:

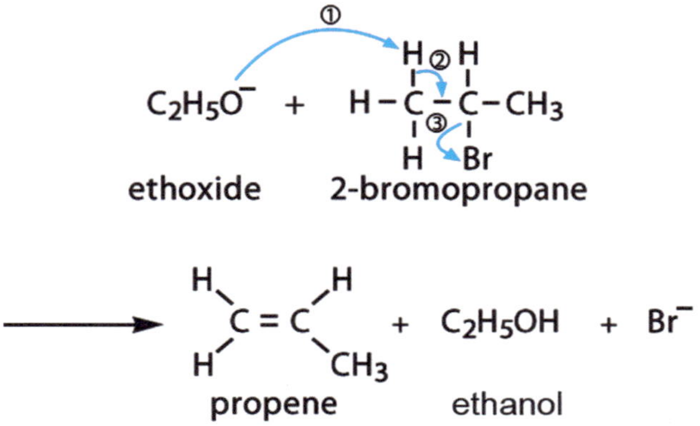

In the preceding reaction, the first step (1) involves the base (ethoxide) removing (*elimination*) a proton, thus carbon has a negative charge (*primary* carbanion, <u>very</u> *unstable*). The electron pair is quickly attracted to the δ^+ neighboring carbon (2) forming a double bond (note that the carbon was δ^+ because it was attached to the electronegative atom Br, *see* ORG 1.5). Simultaneously, Br (*a halide; halides are good leaving groups*) is bumped (3) from the carbon as carbon can have only four bonds. {*Notice that in organic chemistry the curved arrows always follow the movement of electrons.*}

The determination of the quality of a leaving group is quite simple: <u>good leaving groups</u> have *strong* conjugate acids (CHM 6.3). As examples, H_2O is a good leaving group because H_3O^+ is a strong acid, likewise for Br^-/HBr, Cl^-/HCl, HSO_4^-/H_2SO_4, etc.

Substitution and elimination reactions are the most important mechanisms to understand in GAMSAT Organic Chemistry.

High-level Importance

6.2.5 Conversion of Alcohols to Alkyl Halides

Alcohols can participate in substitution reactions only if the hydroxyl group is converted into a better leaving group by either protonation or the formation of an inorganic ester. Tertiary alcohols can be converted into alkyl halides by a reaction with HCl or HBr. This reaction occurs in an S_N1 mechanism. Primary and secondary alcohols do not react with HCl or HBr readily and are converted into halides by $SOCl_2$ or PBr_3. This reaction occurs in an S_N2 mechanism.

$$RCH_2OH + SOCl_2 \longrightarrow RCH_2Cl + SO_2 + HCl$$

$$RCH_2OH + PBr_3 \longrightarrow RCH_2Br + HOPBr_2$$

High-level Importance

Solutions to Foundational Nomenclature Exercises: Alcohols

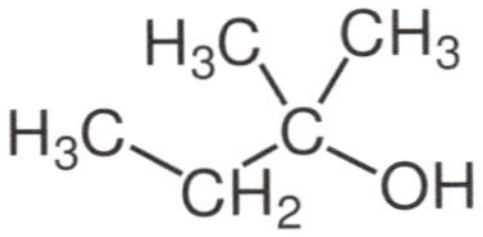

1) 2-methylbutan-2-ol (2-methyl-2-butanol; tertiary alcohol)

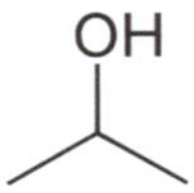

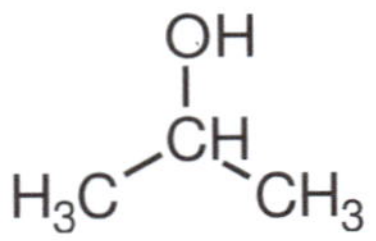

2) 2-propanol (isopropanol, propan-2-ol; secondary alcohol)

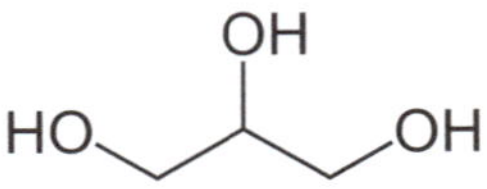

3) propane-1,2,3-triol (do not memorise: *glycerol*; primary – left and right - and secondary – up - alcohol features)

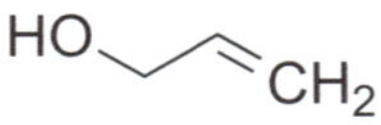

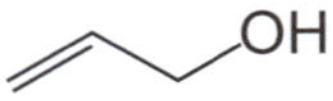

4) prop-2-en-1-ol (identical structures above; do not memorise: *allyl alcohol*; primary alcohol)

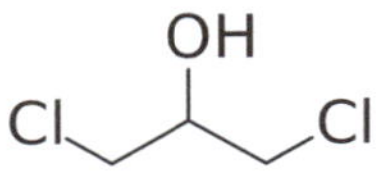

5) 1,3-dichloropropan-2-ol (1,3-dichloro-2-propanol; secondary alcohol)

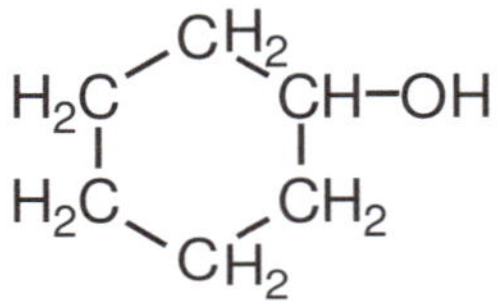

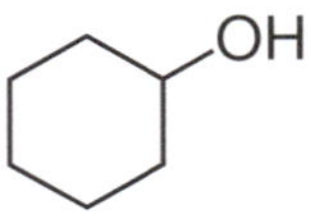

6) Cyclohexanol (secondary alcohol)

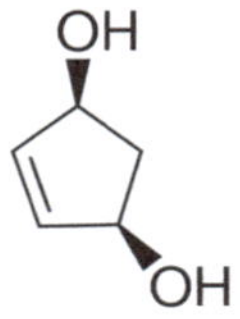

7) *cis*-4-cyclopentene-1,3-diol [(1R,3S)-cyclopent-4-ene-1,3-diol; secondary alcohol]

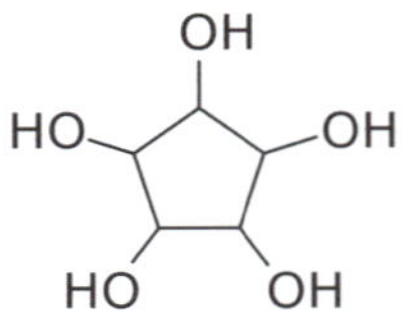

8) cyclopentane-1,2,3,4,5-pentol (1,2,3,4,5-cyclopentanepentol; secondary alcohol)

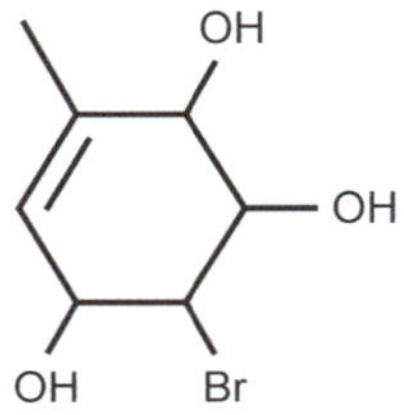

9) 3-bromo-6-methylcyclohex-5-ene-1,2,4-triol (3-bromo-6-methyl-5-cyclohex-ene-1,2,4-triol; secondary alcohol)

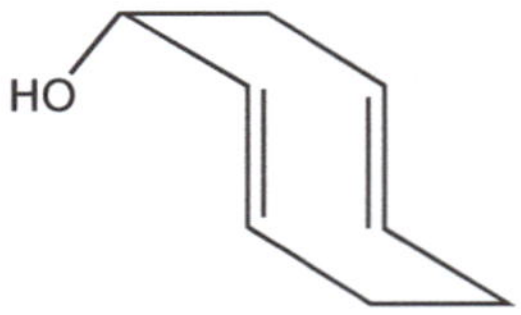

10) (*2E,6E*)-cycloocta-2,6-dien-1-ol (trans,trans-2,6-cyclooctadien-1-ol; secondary alcohol)

Questions or concerns? gamsat-prep.com/forum

CHAPTER 6: Alcohols

GOLD STANDARD FOUNDATIONAL GAMSAT PRACTICE QUESTIONS

11) Which of the consecutive statements below are true for butan-2-ol as compared to butane?

Note: The issue of solubility is with respect to water as the solvent.

A.	More volatile	Less soluble	Is a primary alcohol
B.	More volatile	More soluble	Is a secondary alcohol
C.	Less volatile	Less soluble	Is a tertiary alcohol
D.	Less volatile	More soluble	Is a secondary alcohol

12) A hydrogen bond is represented below as 3 dots. Which of the following correctly represents a hydrogen bond?

A. -O-H···O-X
B. -O-H···H-O-X
C. -O-H···C-O-X
D. -O-H-O-H-X

13) Which of the following substituents would **not** form a hydrogen bond in water?

A. -O-H
B. -C-H
C. -N-H
D. -S-H

14) Which of the following compounds would be expected to have the lowest boiling point?

A. 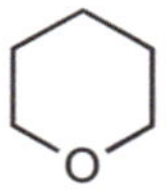

B. 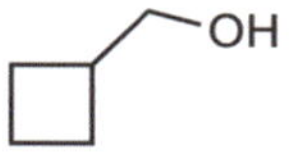

C. 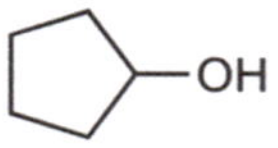

D. 

15) How many of the following structures represent a secondary alcohol?

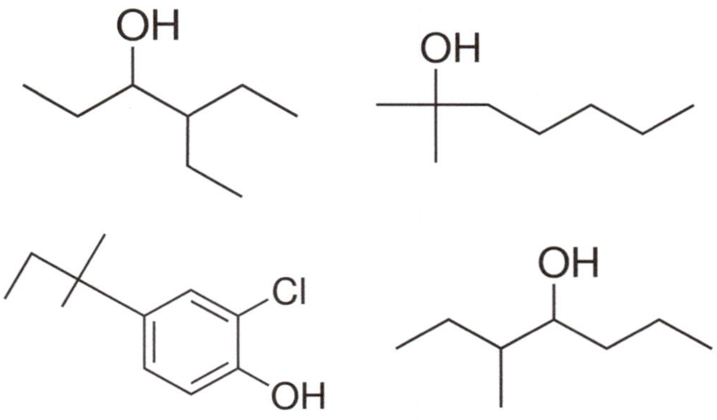

A. 1
B. 2
C. 3
D. 4

High-level Importance

16) Which compound is a tertiary alcohol?

A. 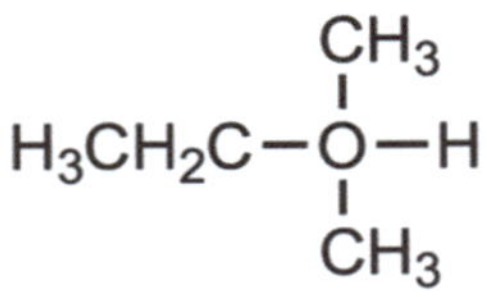

B. 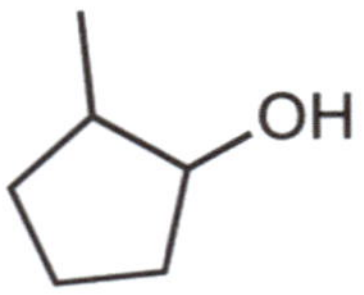

C. 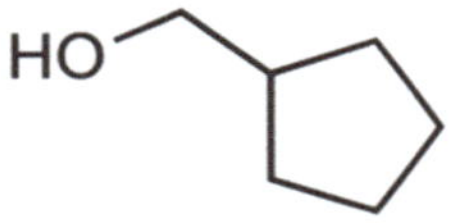

D. 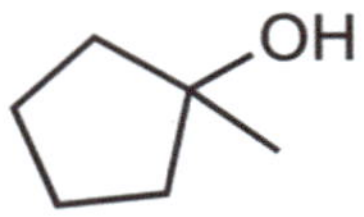

17) Prostaglandin E1, illustrated below, is a naturally occurring prostaglandin which is also used as a medication. Which functional group is not contained in prostaglandin E1?

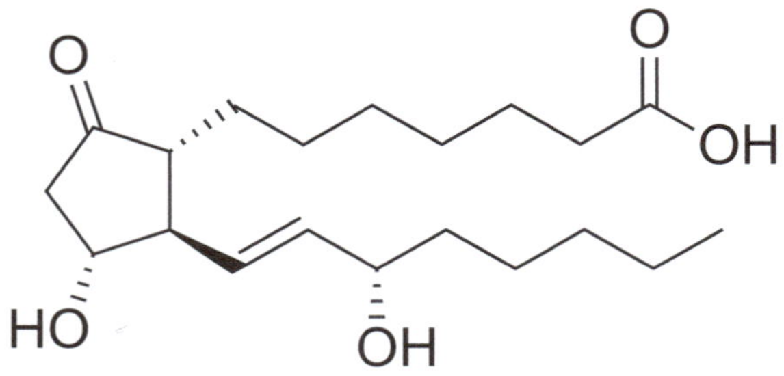

A. Alkene
B. 2° alcohol
C. 3° alcohol
D. Carboxylic acid

18) The compound below is an adrenocortical hormone called *cortisone*. Which functional group is **not** present in cortisone?

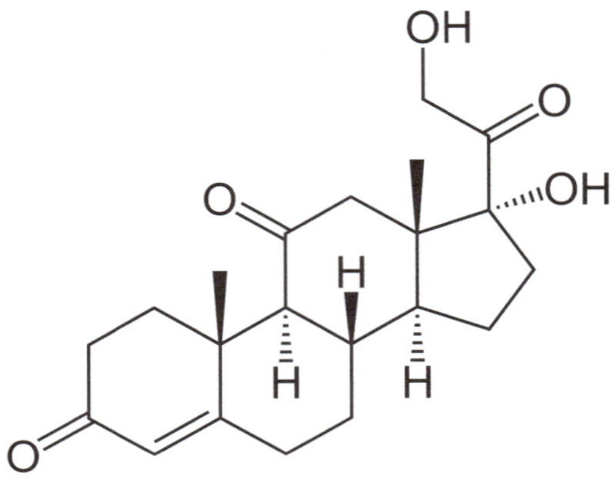

A. Alkene
B. 1° alcohol
C. 2° alcohol
D. 3° alcohol

Being able to name (i.e. *the nomenclature of*) alcohols, ketones and esters, represents a GAMSAT-level skill. If you have no experience naming ketones and esters, skip Questions 19-21 and do not look at the worked solutions; instead, try this unit after you have read sections 7.1, 8.1 and 9.1. Alternatively, you can read those sections now, and then attempt Questions 19-21.

High-level Importance

GOLD STANDARD GAMSAT-LEVEL PRACTICE QUESTIONS

Questions 19–21

The following represents a summary of nucleophilic acyl substitution followed by nucleophilic addition:

- Carboxylic esters, $R'CO_2R''$, react with 2 equivalents of organolithium or Grignard reagents to give tertiary alcohols.
- The tertiary alcohol that results contains 2 identical alkyl groups (R in the mechanism shown).
- The reaction proceeds via a ketone intermediate [Step (1)] which then reacts with the second equivalent of the organometallic reagent or Grignard reagent [Step (2)].
- Et = ethyl

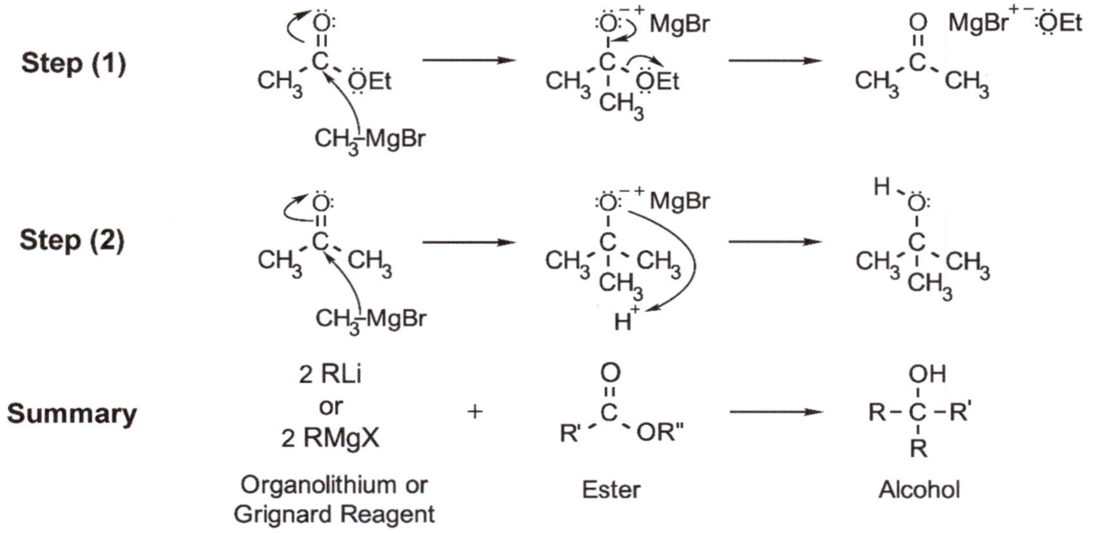

19) Which of the following represents the product of the reaction between propyl ethanoate and 1 equivalent of 2-butyl lithium (*sec*-butyllithium)?

A. 2-hexanone
B. 3-methyl-2-pentanone
C. 4-methyl-3-hexanone
D. 3-heptanone

20) Given the mechanism provided, in order to produce a secondary alcohol, which of the following must be true?

A. R' must be a hydrogen
B. One R must be a hydrogen
C. R' and R" must be hydrogens
D. Either one R or R' must be hydrogen

21) Using 2 equivalents of the first and 1 equivalent of the second, respectively, which of the following pairs of compounds can be used to form the following tertiary alcohol?

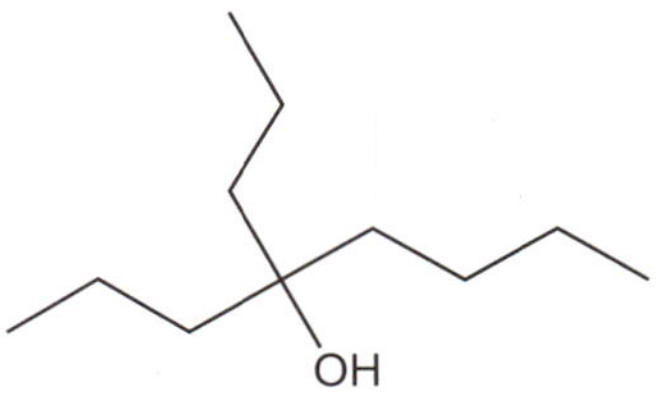

A. Propyl lithium and methyl butanoate
B. Butyl magnesium bromide and propyl butanoate
C. Butyl lithium and pentyl pentanoate
D. Propyl magnesium bromide and hexyl pentanoate

Questions 22–29

The two most important mechanisms of reaction between compounds in Organic Chemistry are *substitution* and *elimination* reactions. The example below shows the result of the 2 mechanisms.

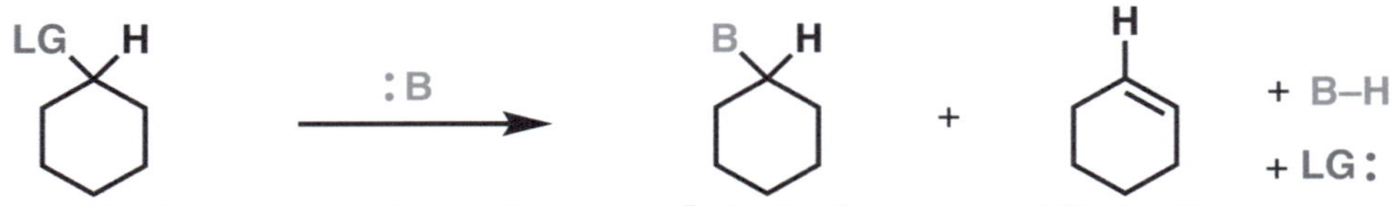

B = **base or nucleophile**
LG = **leaving group**

Substitution product

Elimination product

Substitution reactions often occur when two reactants exchange parts of each molecule to form two new products. If the substitution occurs at a saturated carbon of a single molecule "A" due to a nucleophilic attack "N^-", then the reaction is classified at S_N1 if the rate of the reaction is first order, which means that rate = k[A]. S_N2 signifies that the reaction is second order, thus rate = k[A][N^-].

		S_N1	S_N2
SUBSTITUTION	Mechanism	Two steps (carbocation rearrangements possible)	One step (= *concerted*)
	Rate law	Rate = k[R–X] (unimolecular, 1st order)	Rate = k[R–X][Nuke] (bimolecular, 2nd order)
	Stereochemistry	Loss of stereochemistry (racemization possible)	Stereospecific (inversion due to backside displacement)
	Substrate	Cation stability (benzylic > allylic > 3° > 2°) No 1° or methyl R^+ without extra stabilization.	Sterics (methyl > 1° > 2°) No S_N2 with 3°
	Nucleophile	Not Important	Strong/Moderate required •strong: RS^-, I^-, R_2N^-, R_2NH, RO^-, CN^- •moderate: RSH, Br^-, RCO_2^-
	Leaving group	Very important (–OSO_2CF_3 > –OSO_2F >> derivatives of 4-toluenesulfonyl chloride >> –I > –Br > –Cl)	Moderately important (same trend as S_N1)
	Solvent	Polar protic (water, most alcohols, formic acid, HF, ammonia)	Polar aprotic (acetonitrile, DMF, HMPA, DMSO - dimethyl sulfoxide)

Elimination reactions occur when a single reactant loses parts of the molecule from adjacent carbons. The organic product ends up with a double bond between the two carbons that each lost an attachment. If the elimination occurs in 2 steps at a saturated carbon of molecule "A" due to an attack from base "B^-", then the reaction is classified at E1 as the reaction rate is first order, thus rate = k[A]. E2 signifies that the reaction is second order, thus rate = k[A][B^-].

ELIMINATION		E1	E2
	Mechanism	Two steps (carbocation rearrangements possible)	One step (= *concerted*)
	Rate law	Rate = k[R–X] (unimolecular, 1st order)	Rate = k[R–X][Base] (bimolecular, 2nd order)
	Stereochemistry	Not stereospecific	Stereospecific (antiperiplanar transition state)
	Substrate	Cation stability (benzylic > allylic > 3° > 2°)	Alkene stability (3° > 2° > 1°)
	Base	Not important: usually weak (ROH, R_2NH)	Strong base required (RO^-, R_2N^-)
	Leaving group	Very important (same trend as S_N1)	Moderately important (same trend as S_N1)
	Solvent	Polar protic (water, most alcohols, formic acid, HF, ammonia)	Wide range of solvents
	Product ratio	Zaitsev's Rule (or Saytzeff's Rule): The most highly substituted alkene usually predominates. Hofmann Product: Using a sterically hindered base (i.e. t-BuO⁻ or LDA), results in formation of the least substituted alkene (Hofmann product). High temperature favors elimination.	

22) Consider the following S_N2 reaction: The reactants are on the left, in the middle is the transition state (a momentary intermediate *en route* to the products on the right), and the dashed horizontal lines ---- indicate bonds being created and formed at the same time.

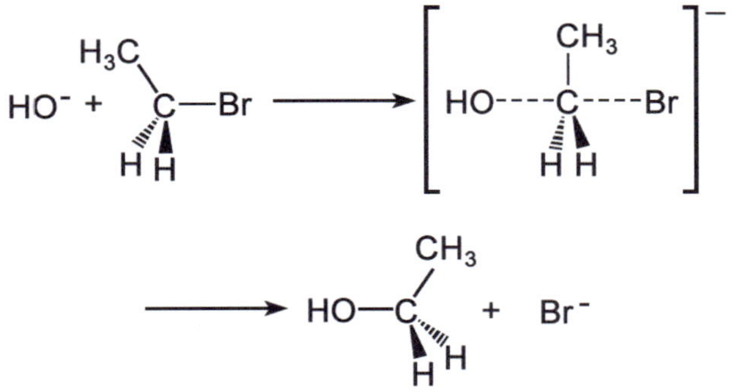

What would be the effect on the reaction rate if the concentrations of the alkyl bromide and hydroxide ions were doubled?

A. Increase the rate exponentially
B. Increase the rate by four times
C. Increase the rate by two times
D. No net effect on the rate

23) The following reaction occurs by substitution. Choose the major organic product from the reaction.

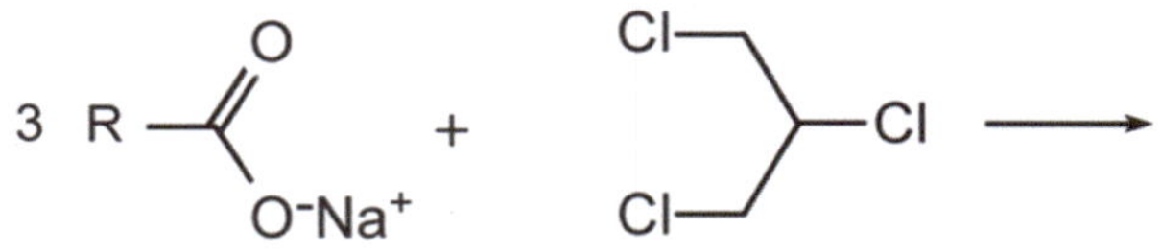

A.

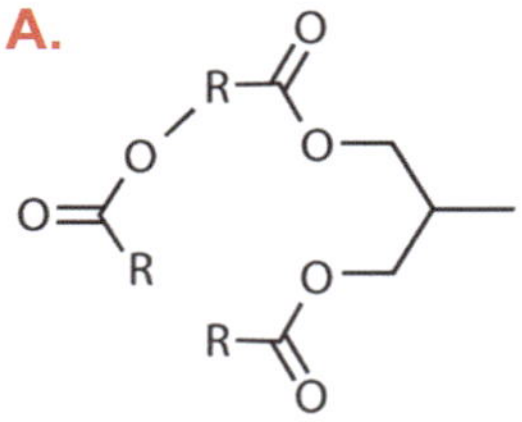

C.

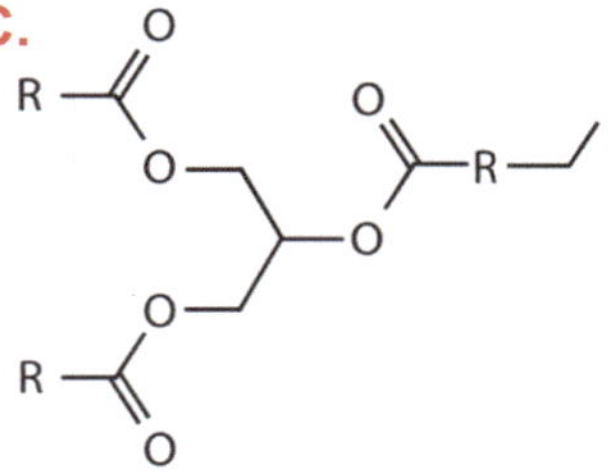

B.

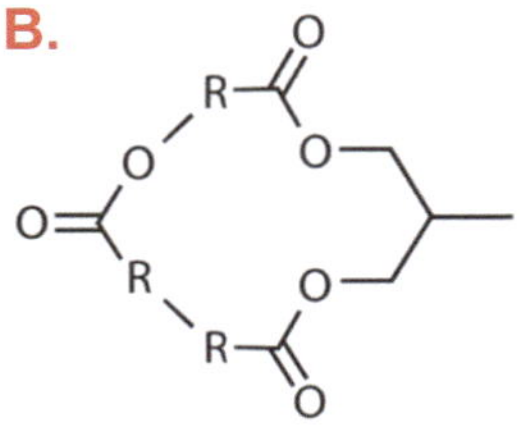

D.

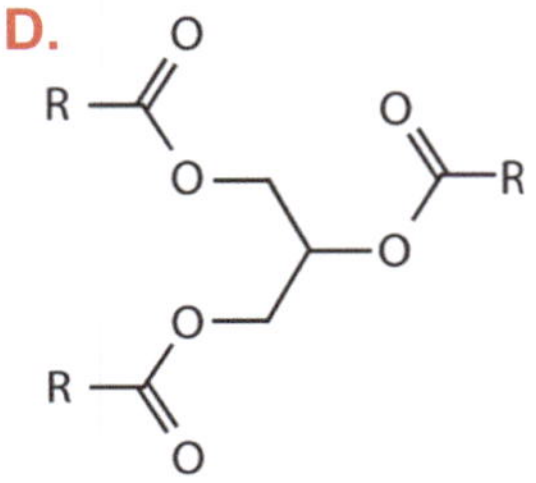

24) What product(s) would you expect from the following S_N2 reaction?

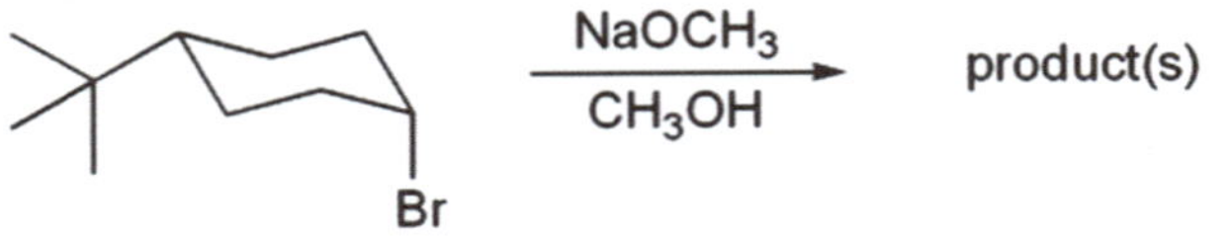

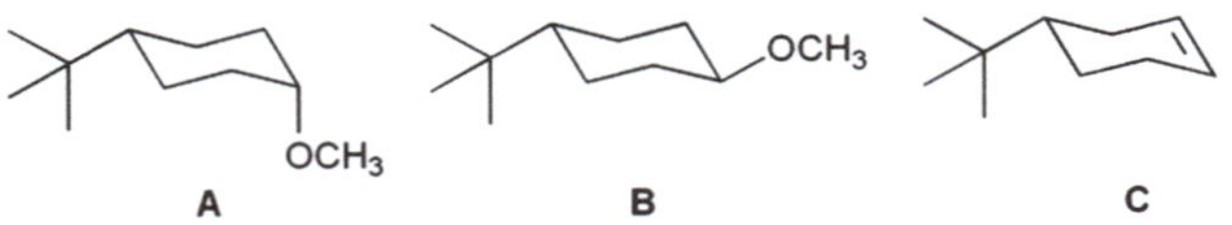

A. A
B. B
C. C
D. An equimolar mixture of **A** and **B**

25) Consider the 5 following bromoalkanes.

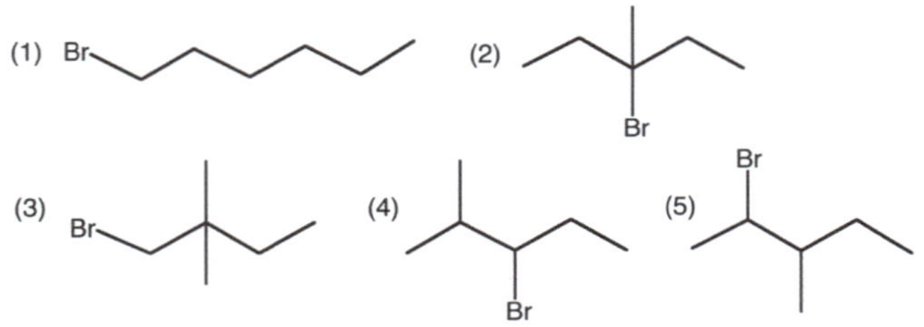

Ignoring any possible rearrangements, how many of the five bromoalkanes would produce exactly one elimination product after the removal of HBr?

A. 1
B. 2
C. 3
D. More than 3

26) Sometimes an intermediate to a chemical reaction undergoes an internal rearrangement of atoms which may increase stability. Examples include rearrangements such as hydride and alkyl shifts, and sigmatropic rearrangements such as Claisen and Cope. In a hydride shift, H moves to a positively-charged adjacent carbon, taking its electron pair with it. As a result, a less stable carbocation rearranges to a more stable one (more substituted). Consider the following example.

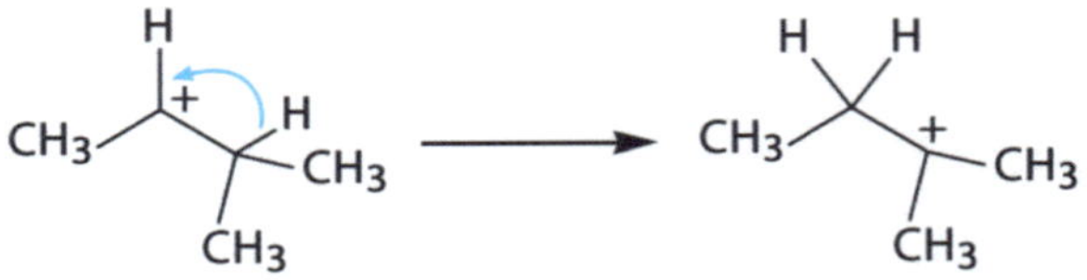

secondary carbocation

tertiary carbocation

Based on the information provided, how many of the five bromoalkanes from the previous question could produce a hydride shift after the removal of the Br⁻ anion?

A. 1
B. 2
C. 3
D. More than 3

27) Consider the following products from 2 different elimination reactions.

Reaction I

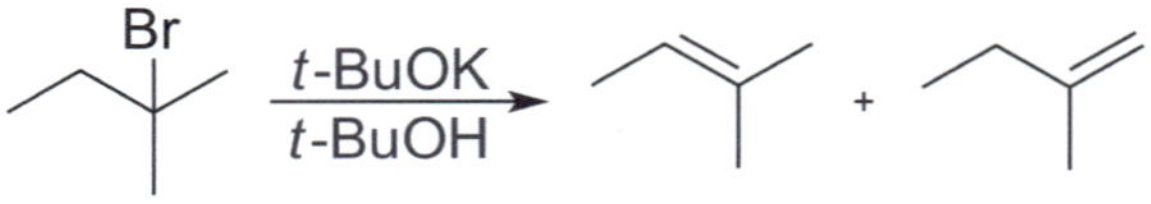

Reaction II

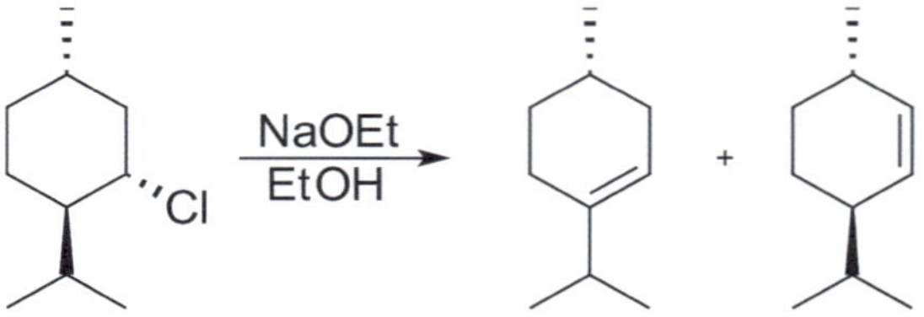

Based on the information provided, in which instance(s) is the Hofmann product on the left with the Zaitsev product on the right?

A. In neither case
B. Reaction I only
C. Reaction II only
D. In both cases

28) Consider the following chart in context with the previous information regarding substitution and elimination reactions (t–Bu = tertiary butyl).

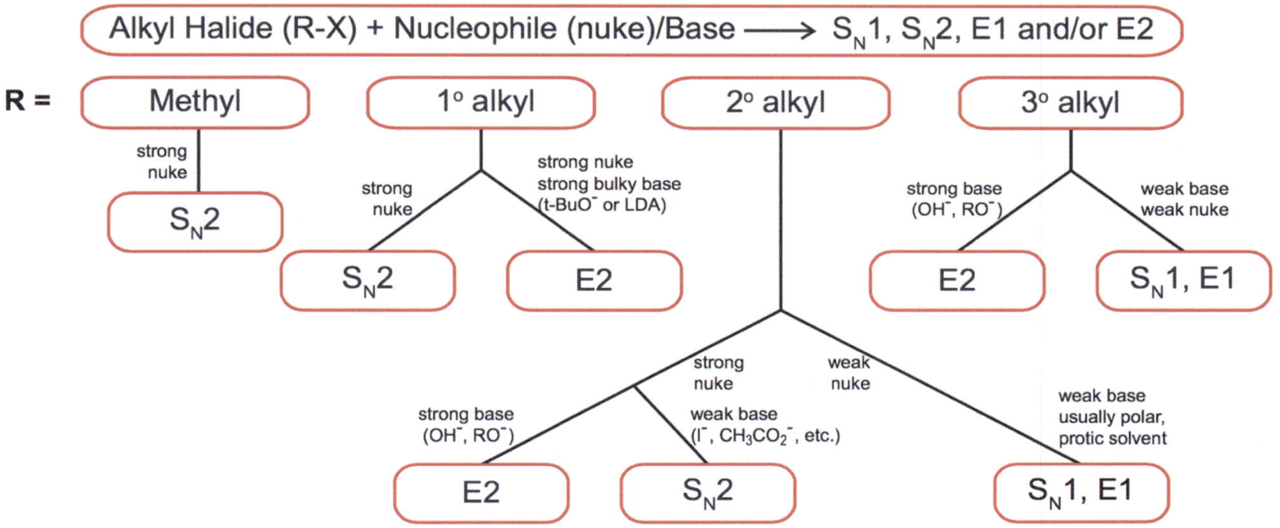

In all likelihood, which of the following represents the mechanisms responsible for the two organic products below, respectively?

$$CH_3CH_2CH_2CH_2Cl + CH_3CH_2O^-Na^+ \longrightarrow CH_2{=}CHCH_2CH_3 + CH_3(CH_2)_3OCH_2CH_3 + NaCl$$

A. E1, S_N1
B. E1, S_N2
C. E2, S_N1
D. E2, S_N2

29) Based on the information provided in this unit, identify the main product of the following reaction. (note: Me = methyl)

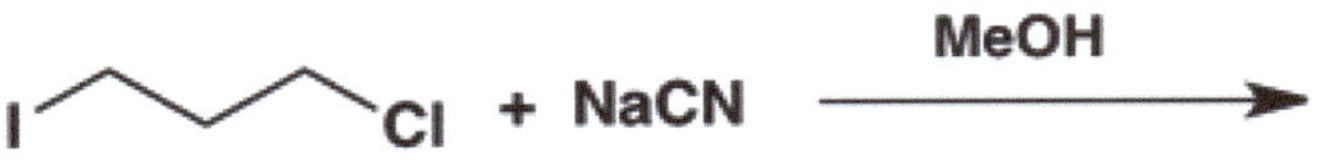

A. 

B. 

C. 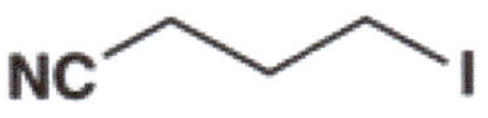

D. 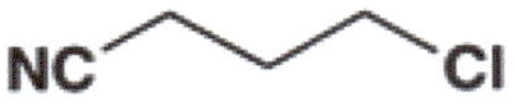

Questions 30–33

Alcohols can be prepared through the hydration (= *to combine with water*) of alkenes. There are 3 common methods:

(1) Halohydrin (one carbon with X, a halogen, and an adjacent carbon with a hydroxyl substituent); the formation yields a Markovnikov hydration product with anti stereospecificity (i.e. the OH group adds to the most substituted carbon but *opposite* to the halide);

(2) Hydroboration-oxidation yields a syn stereospecific anti-Markovnikov hydration product (the OH adds to the least substituted carbon); this *syn* addition means that both the hydrogen and the hydroxyl add to the same side of the molecule.

(3) Oxymercuration-reduction yields a Markovnikov hydration product.

Consider the summary in Figure 1 of the 3 methods of hydration labelled (1), (2) and (3).

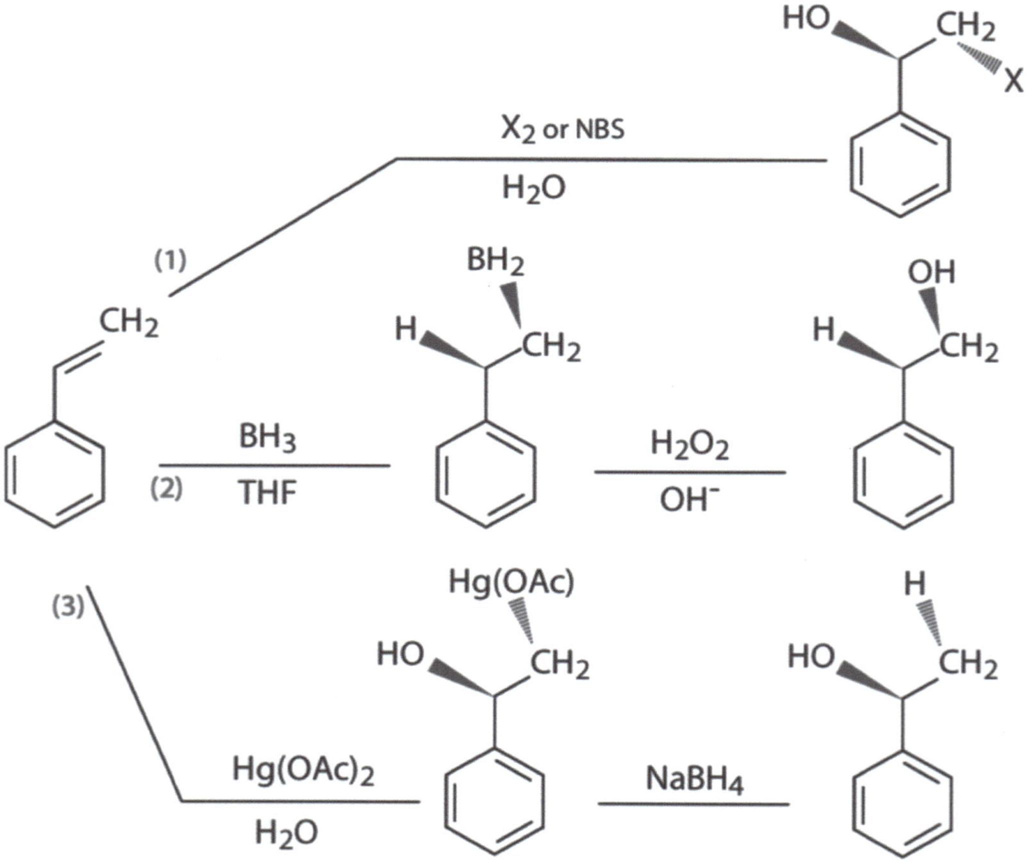

Figure 1

30) Based on Figure 1, what would be the expected product of the hydroboration–oxidation of 1-pentene?

- A. 1-pentanol
- B. 2-pentanol
- C. 3-pentanol
- D. 4-pentanol

31) What would be the likely product obtained from the following reaction?

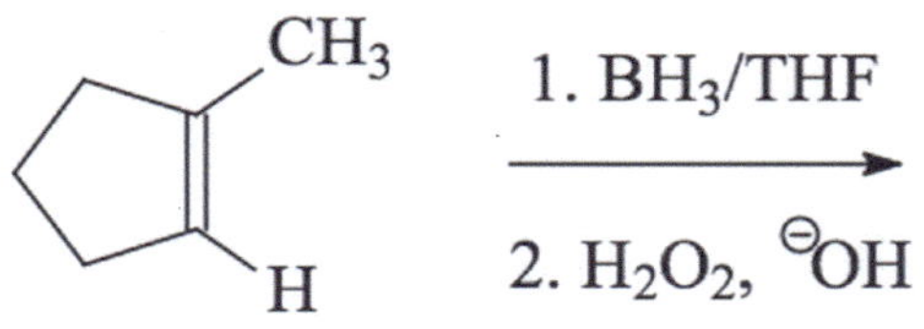

A.
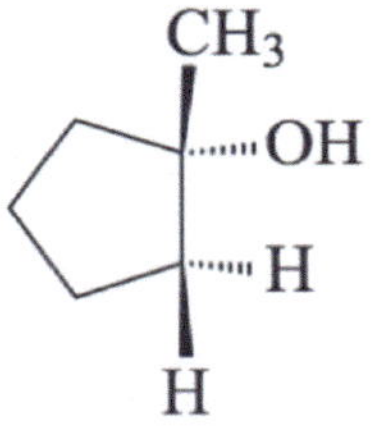

C.
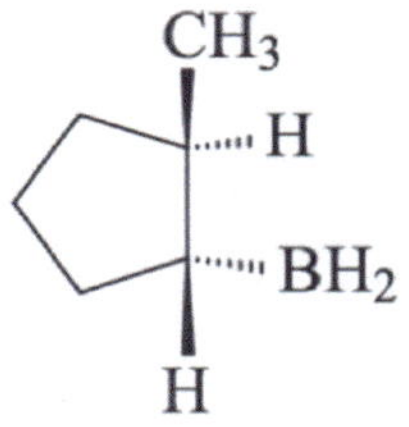

B.
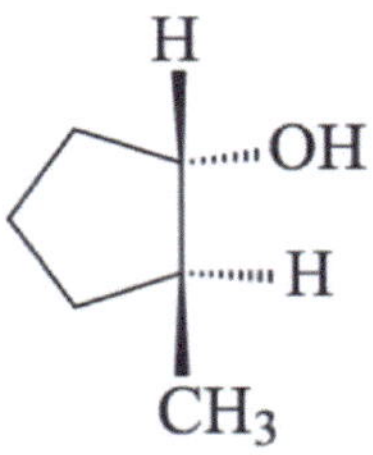

D.
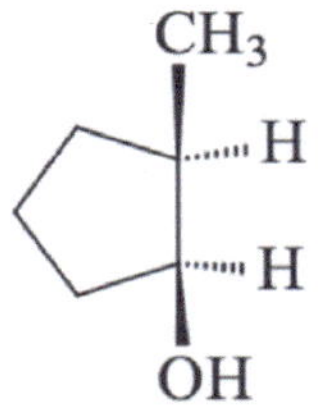

32) For the following reaction, identify the product **Z**.

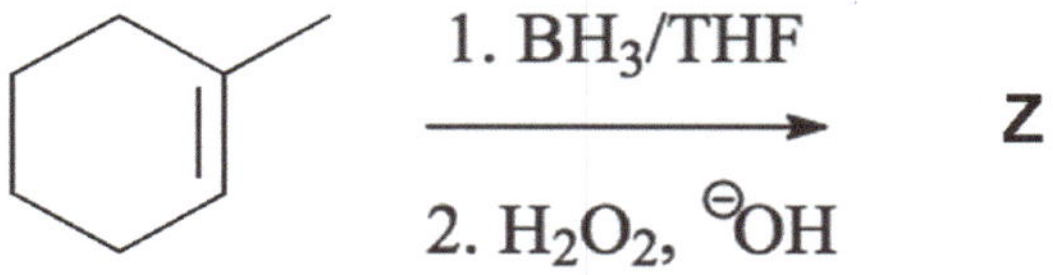

A.
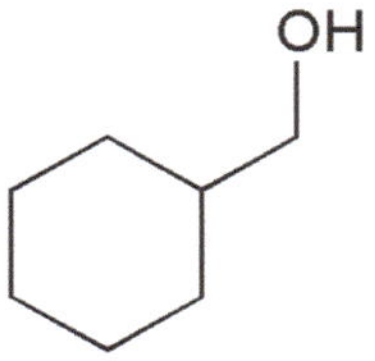

C.
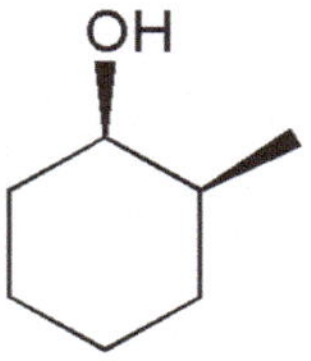

B.
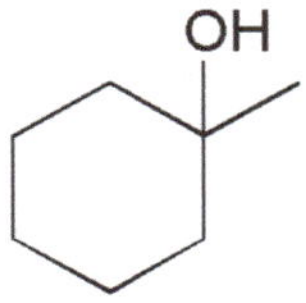

D.
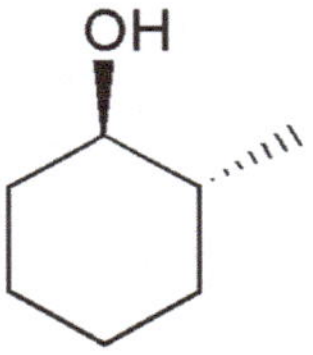

33) Which of the 3 numbered reactions from Figure 1 would be expected to produce the following product?

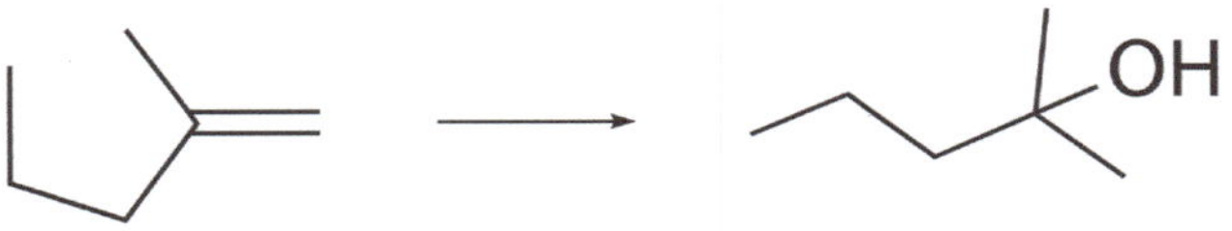

- A. (1)
- B. (2)
- C. (3)
- D. None of the above

High-level Importance

Being able to name (i.e. *the nomenclature of*) alcohols, aldehydes, ketones and carboxylic acids, represents a GAMSAT-level skill. If you have no experience naming aldehydes and ketones, skip this unit and do not look at the worked solutions; instead, try this unit after you have read section 7.1. Alternatively, you can read that section now, and then attempt the questions in this unit.

Questions 34–35

Ethanol metabolism in yeast and in the human liver begins with oxidation by alcohol dehydrogenase (ADH) and NAD^+ to give acetaldehyde and NADH. The reaction can be summarised as follows:

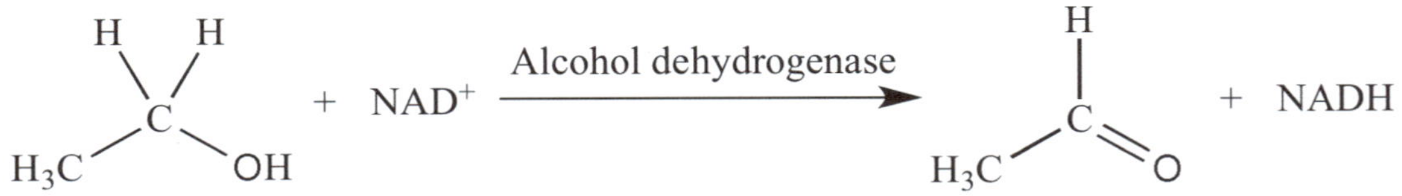

Aside from ethanol, ADH is able to oxidise many other types of alcohols with the same mechanism: Only if the OH group is attached to a carbon that has at least one C-H bond, ADH can remove the H from that carbon and remove the H from the OH resulting in a C=O bond. The reaction serves to break down alcohols that otherwise are toxic, and the reaction may produce useful aldehydes or even ketones, depending on the structure of the alcohol.

In the reverse reaction, ADH uses NADH to alter the aldehyde or ketone to produce an alcohol.

34) The reaction with ADH, NADH and a ketone is an example of which of the following?

- **A.** Dehydration
- **B.** Dehydrogenation
- **C.** Oxidation
- **D.** Reduction

35) Consider the structure of the following molecule.

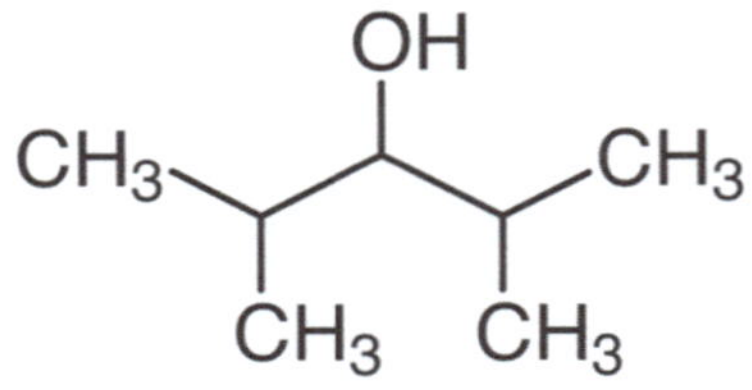

What would be the expected product if the molecule above is placed in a reaction vessel with ADH and NAD^+?

- **A.** 2,4-dimethyl-3-pentanone
- **B.** 2,4-dimethyl-3-pentanal
- **C.** 2,4-dimethyl-3-pentanol
- **D.** The reaction cannot occur with a tertiary alcohol.

SPOILER ALERT

Gold Standard has cross-referenced the content in this chapter to examples from ACER's official GAMSAT practice materials. It is for you to decide when you want to explore these questions since you may want to preserve some of ACER's materials for timed mock-exam practice.

Examples – Creating an alcohol functional group by adding water across a double bond: is that oxidation or hydration? (*see Need for Speed*): Q38 of 1; alcohol oxidation and reduction with the enzyme alcohol dehydrogenase (ADH): Q53-55 of 2; alcohols, Grignard reagents, aldehydes and ketones: Q95-99 of 4 (this unit will get a special mention in chapter 7!); alcohol, oxidation and a device to prevent a drunk person from driving (BAIID): Q40-42 of 5; alcohol oxidation with ADH and NAD^+, again: Q69-72 of 5. Special mention, but not counted towards the importance of this chapter, a biological molecule and its solubility related to H-bonds: Q66 of 5. Note that "Q" is followed by the question number, and, for example, "of 1" refers to booklet number 1 which is referenced in the Spoiler Alert table at the end of Chapter 1. The 15 full-length GAMSAT practice tests by Gold Standard, HEAPS-1 through HEAPS-15, contain specific cross-references to this chapter within the worked solutions. Note that the epic unit discussing S_N1, S_N2, E1, E2 and hydride/methyl shifts, is from HEAPS-3; the challenging unit making alcohols with the help of Grignard reagents, alkyl lithiums, aldehydes and ketones is from HEAPS-6; the BH_3-hydroboration oxidation is a rare visitor from VR-2, the second virtual reality mock exam.

High-level Importance

Chapter Checklist

- ☐ Access your online account to view answers, worked solutions and discussion boards.
- ☐ Reassess your 'learning objectives' for this chapter: Go back to the first page of this chapter and re-evaluate the top 3 boxes and the Introduction.
    - ☐ Please be sure that you have completed the *Need for Speed* exercises at the beginning of this chapter.
- ☐ Complete a maximum of 1 page of notes using symbols/abbreviations to represent the entire chapter based on your learning objectives. These are your Gold Notes.
- ☐ Consider your multimedia options based on your optimal way of learning:
    - ☐ Download the free Gold Standard GAMSAT app for your Android device or iPhone.
    - ☐ Create your own, tangible study cards or try the free app: Anki.
    - ☐ Record your voice reading your Gold Notes onto your smartphone (audio files, e.g., *memo* or MP3s) and listen during exercise, transportation, etc.
    - ☐ Try out the Gold Standard GAMSAT online videos at gamsat-prep.com, or you can try other options on YouTube like Khan Academy or Crash Course Organic Chemistry.
- ☐ Reassess your schedule for your full-length GAMSAT practice tests: ACER and/or HEAPS exams. Ensure that you have scheduled one full day to complete a practice test and 1-2 days for a thorough assessment of worked solutions while adding to your abbreviated Gold Notes.
- ☐ Reassess your progress in scheduling and/or evaluating stress reduction techniques such as regular exercise (sports), yoga, meditation and/or mindfulness exercises (*see* YouTube for suggestions).

ALDEHYDES AND KETONES

Chapter 7

Memorise

* IUPAC nomenclature

Understand

* Effect of hydrogen bonds
* Mechanisms of reactions
* Acidity of the alpha H
* Resonance, polarity
* Grignards, organometallic reagents
* Redox reactions

Importance

High level: 15% of GAMSAT Organic Chemistry

questions released by ACER are related to content in this chapter (in our estimation).
* Note that approximately 60% of the questions in GAMSAT Organic Chemistry are related to just 4 chapters: 2, 6, 7 and 12.

GAMSAT-Prep.com

Introduction

An aldehyde contains a terminal carbonyl group. The functional group is a carbon atom bonded to a hydrogen atom and double-bonded to an oxygen atom (O=CH-) and is called the aldehyde group. A ketone contains a carbonyl group (C=O) bonded to two other carbon atoms: R(CO)R'. Consider revising the functional groups presented in ORG 1.6.

Nomenclature for alkanes, alkenes, alcohols, aldehydes, carboxylic acids and their derivatives, is a fundamental aspect to proper GAMSAT preparation. This chapter includes nomenclature exercises and many practice questions designed to ensure that you can recognise key functional groups (*exercising your pattern recognition and geometric reasoning skills*). *Need for Speed* will retire until you have more content to memorise within a chapter.

Multimedia Resources at GAMSAT-Prep.com

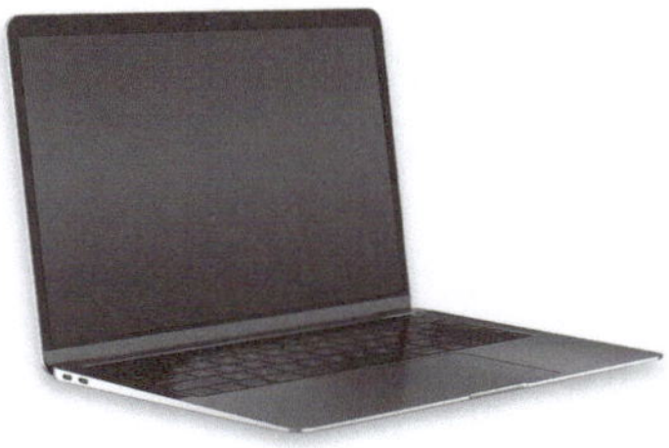

Open Discussion Boards
(*gamsat-prep.com/forum*)

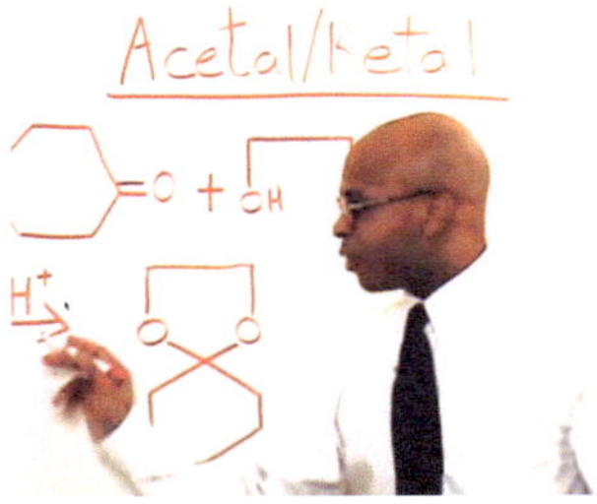

Science Preparation Videos

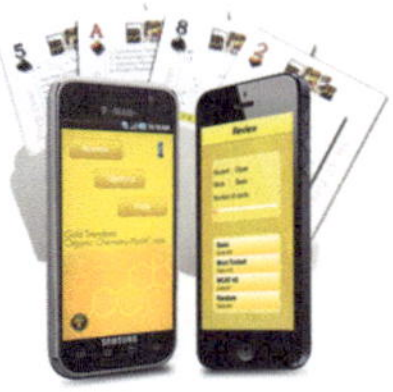

Flashcards

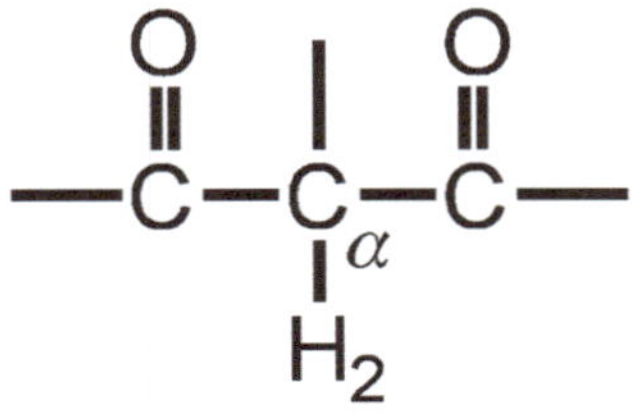

Special Guest

* The real GAMSAT may have advanced-level information presented (i.e. in a passage) but previous knowledge of said information is not required to answer the questions that would follow. Practice questions at the end of this chapter, as well as ACER and GS (HEAPS) practice GAMSATs can help you clarify this point.

7.1 Description and Nomenclature

Aldehydes and ketones are two types of molecules, both containing the carbonyl group, C=O, which is the basis for their chemistry.

The carbonyl functional group is planar (*flat*) with bond angles of approximately 120°. The carbonyl carbon atom is sp^2 hybridised and forms three σ bonds. The C=O double bond is both stronger and shorter than the C-O single bond.

The general structure of aldehydes and ketones is:

Aldehydes have at least one hydrogen bonded to the carbonyl carbon, as well as a second hydrogen (= *formaldehyde*) or either an alkyl or an aryl group (= *aromatic ring like benzene but minus one hydrogen*). Ketones have two alkyl or aryl groups bound to the carbonyl carbon (i.e. the carbon forming the double bond with oxygen).

Systematic naming of these compounds is done by replacing the '–e' of the corresponding alkane with '–al' for aldehydes, and '–one' for ketones. For aldehydes, the longest chain chosen as the parent name must contain the -CHO group and the -CHO group must occupy the terminal (1st Carbon, or C1) position. For ketones, the longest chain chosen as the parent name must contain the ketone group and give the lowest possible number to the carbonyl carbon. Non-systematic names are given in brackets:

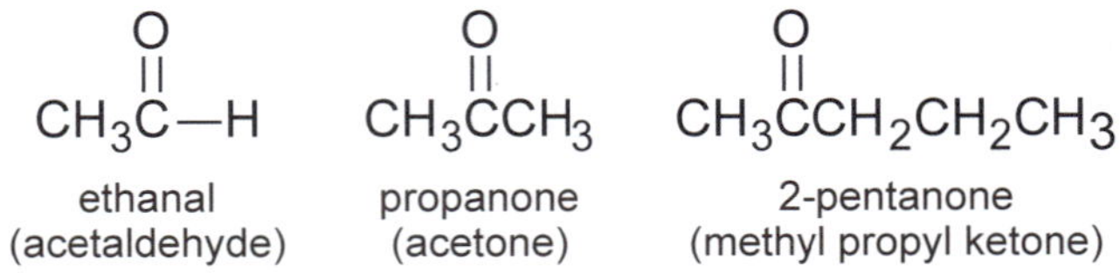

The important features of the carbonyl group are:

- Resonance: There are two resonance forms of the carbonyl group:

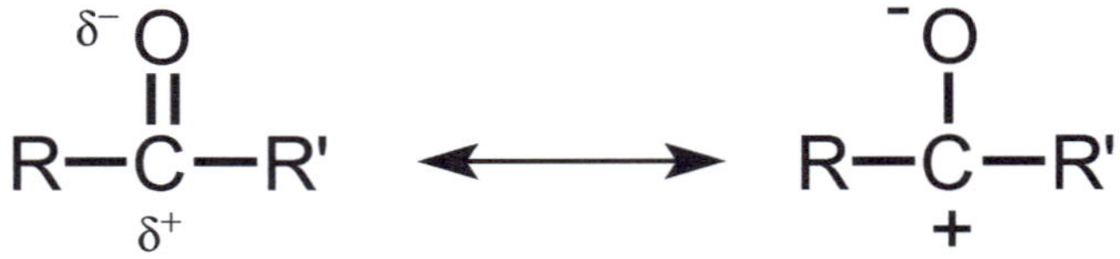

- Polarity: Reactions about this group may be either nucleophilic, or electrophilic. Since opposite charges attract, nucleophiles (Nu^-) attack the δ^+ carbon, and electrophiles (E^+) attack the δ^- oxygen. In both of these types of reactions, the character of the double bond is altered:

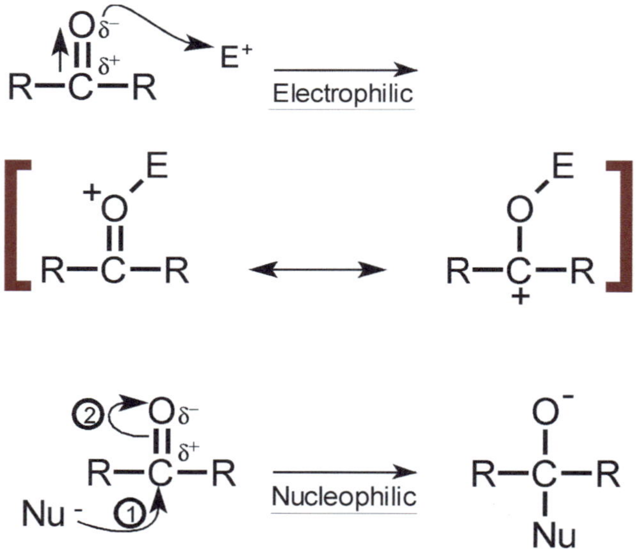

- Acidity of the α-hydrogen: The α-hydrogen is the hydrogen attached to the carbon next to the carbonyl group (the α-carbon). The β-carbon is the carbon adjacent to the α-carbon. The α-hydrogen may be removed by a base. The acidity of this hydrogen is increased if it is between 2 carbonyl groups:

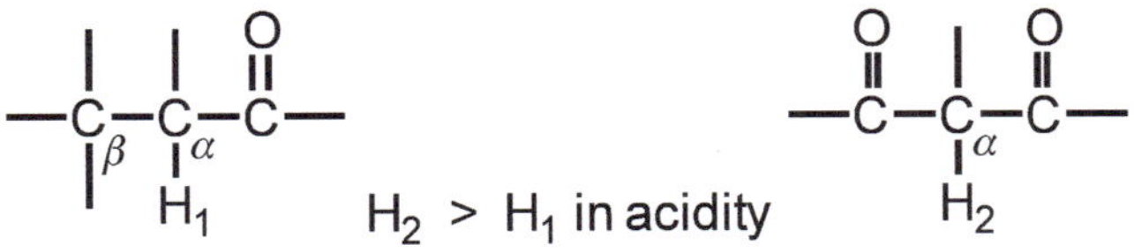

This acidity is a result of the resonance stabilisation of the α-carbanion formed. This stabilisation will also permit addition at the β-carbon in α-β unsaturated carbonyls (*those with double or triple bonds*):

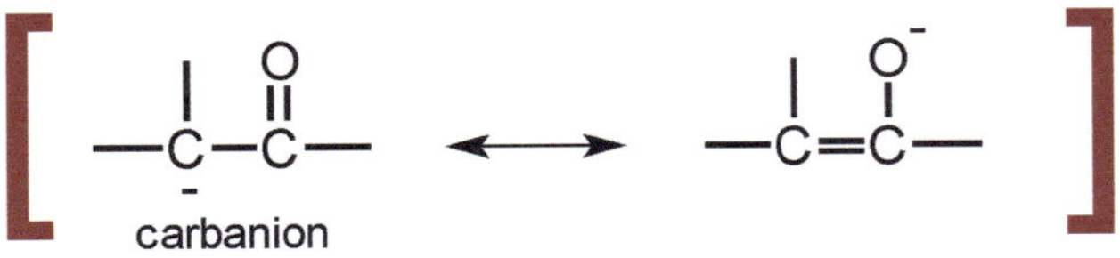

resonance stabilization

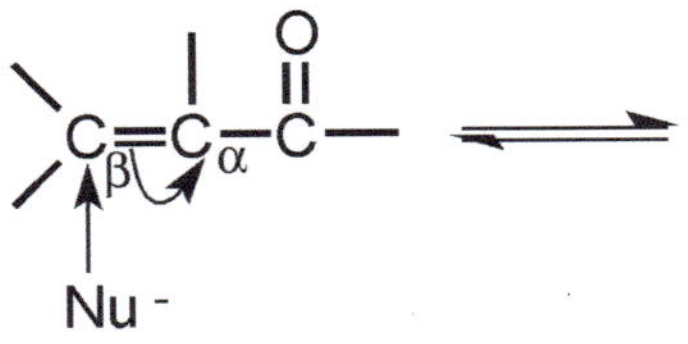

α, β unsaturated carbonyl

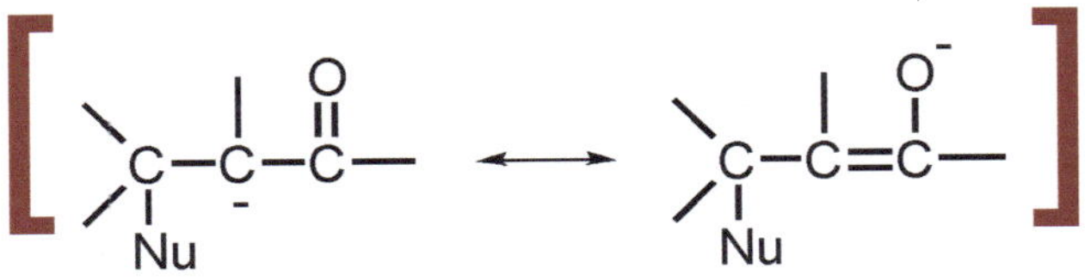

Note that only protons at the α position of carbonyl compounds are acidic. Protons further from the carbonyl carbon (β, gamma - γ, and so on, positions) are not acidic.

- Keto-enol tautomerisation: Tautomers are constitutional isomers (ORG 2.1-2.3) that readily interconvert (= *tautomerisation*). Because the interconversion is so fast, they are usually considered to be the same chemical compound. The carbonyl exists in equilibrium with the enol form of the molecule (enol = alk***ene*** + alcoh***ol***).

Although the carbonyl is usually the predominant one, if the enol double bond can be conjugated with other double bonds, it becomes stable (conjugated double bonds are those which are separated by a single bond; ORG 1.4, 4.1):

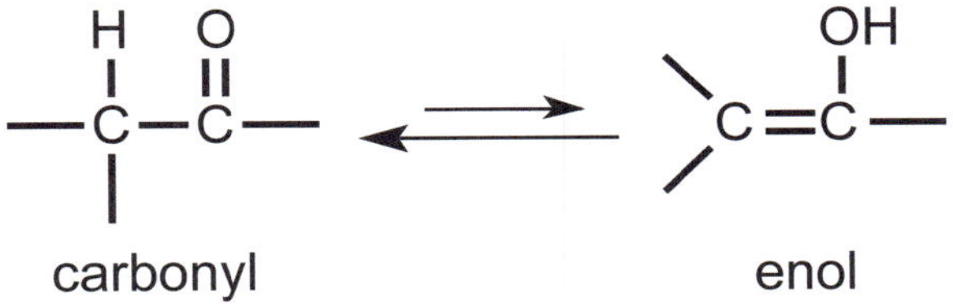

- Hydrogen bonds: The O of the carbonyl forms hydrogen bonds with the hydrogens attached to other electronegative atoms, such as O's or N's:

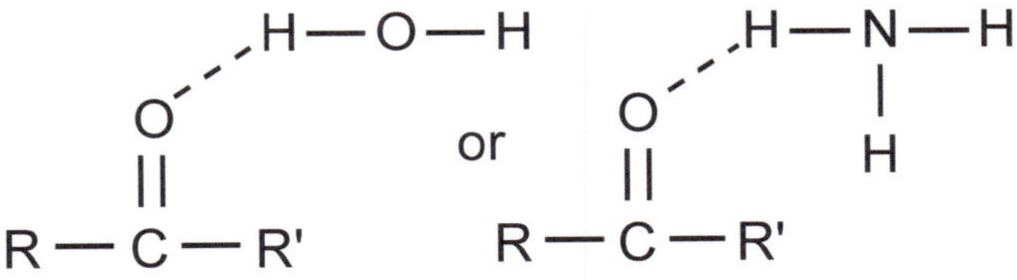

Since there is no hydrogen on the carbonyl oxygen, aldehydes and ketones do not form hydrogen bonds with themselves.

7.1.1 Foundational Nomenclature Exercises: Aldehydes and Ketones

High-level Importance

Name the following ten compounds. If necessary, feel free to consult the nomenclature rules from ORG 3.1, 4.1 and 7.1. The answers are at the end of this chapter. Of course, it is more helpful to you in the long run to give a full effort first - rather than looking at the solutions before trying.

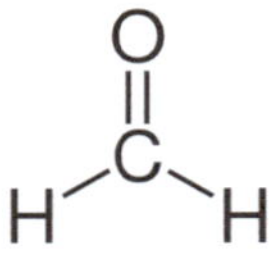

1) ______________________

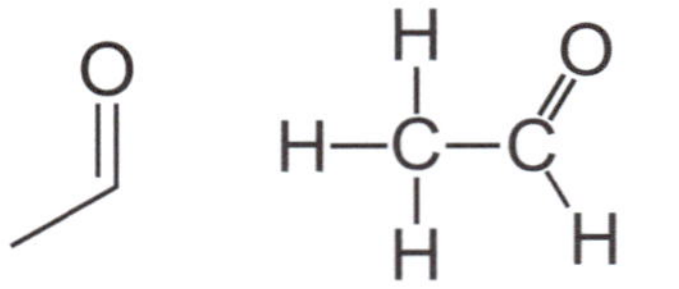

2) ______________________

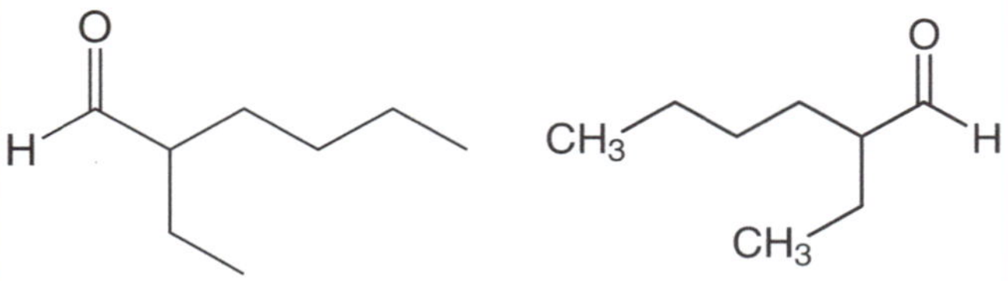

3) ______________________

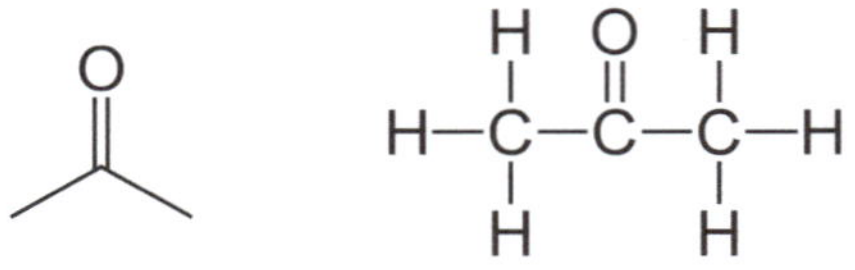

4) ______________________

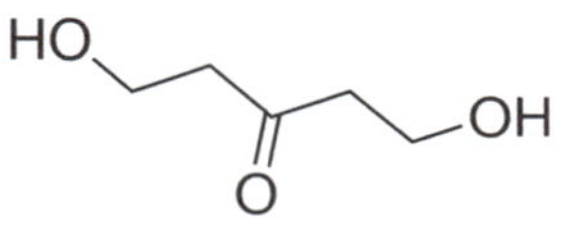

5) ______________________

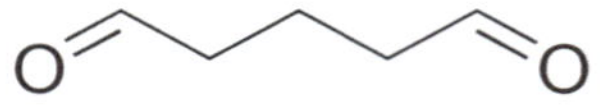

6) ______________________

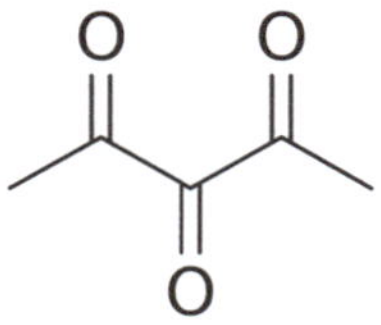

7) ______________________

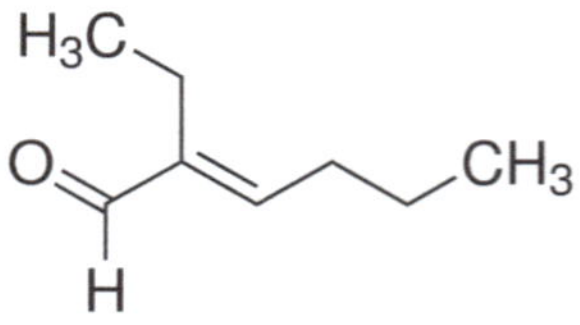

8) ______________________

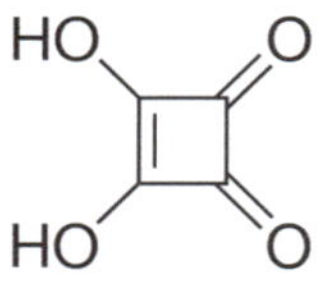

9) ______________________

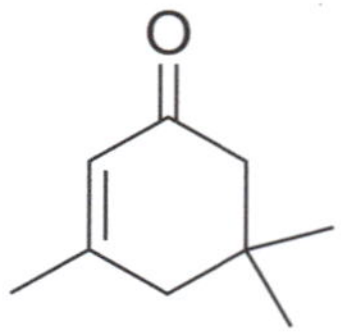

10) ______________________

7.2 Important Reactions of Aldehydes & Ketones

7.2.1 Overview

Since the carbonyl group is the functional group of aldehydes and ketones, groups adjacent to the carbonyl group affect the rate of reaction for the molecule. For example, an electron withdrawing ligand adjacent to the carbonyl group will increase the partial positive charge on the carbon making the carbonyl group more attractive to a nucleophile. Conversely, an electron donating ligand would decrease the reactivity of the carbonyl group.

Generally, aldehydes oxidise easier, and undergo nucleophilic additions easier than ketones. This is a consequence of steric hindrance (ORG 6.2.3).

Aldehydes will be oxidised to carboxylic acids with the standard oxidising agents such as $KMnO_4$, CrO_3 (Jones reagent), HNO_3, Ag_2O (Tollens' reagent). Ketones rarely oxidise. When the Tollens' reagent is used, metallic silver Ag is produced if the aldehyde functional group is present in a molecule of unknown structure, thus making it useful as a diagnostic tool. Therefore, the aldehyde will form a silver precipitate while a ketone will not because ketones cannot be oxidised to carboxylic acid.

There are several methods for preparing aldehydes and ketones. We have already seen ozonolysis (ORG 4.2.2) and the classic redox series of reactions (*see* ORG 6.2.2). To add to the preceding is a reaction called "hydroformylation" shown for the generation of butyraldehyde (butanal) by the hydroformylation of propene:

$$H_2 + CO + CH_3CH{=}CH_2 \longrightarrow CH_3CH_2CH_2CHO$$

Primary alcohols can be oxidised to yield aldehydes. The reaction is performed with the mild oxidation reagent PCC.

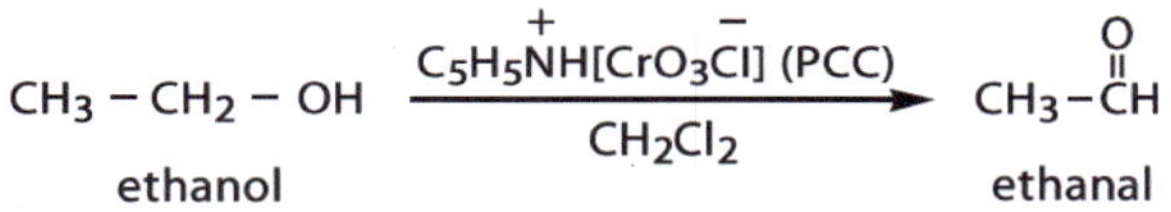

Secondary alcohols can be oxidised to yield ketones. These reactions are usually performed with PCC, Jones reagent (CrO_3), or sodium dichromate, which all form H_2CrO_4:

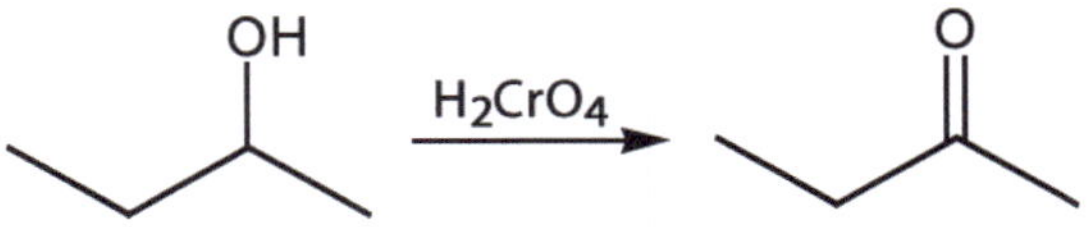

Other reagents include: $K_2Cr_2O_7/H_2SO_4$ or CrO_3/H_2SO_4 or $KMnO_4/OH^-$ or $KMnO_4/H_3O^+$.

Alkenes can be oxidatively cleaved to yield aldehydes when treated with ozone (ORG 4.2.2).

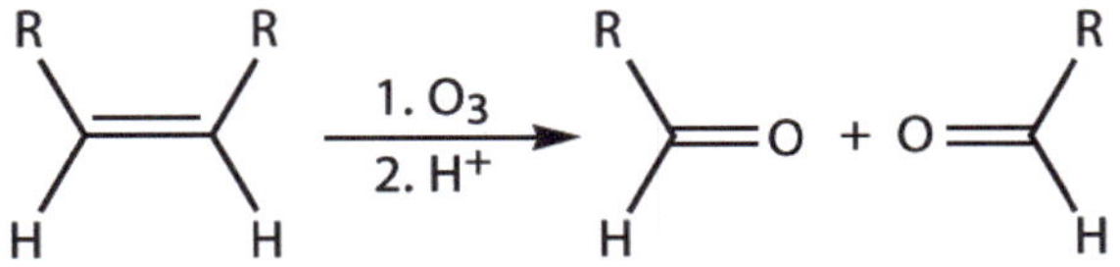

Alkenes can be oxidatively cleaved to yield ketones when treated with ozone if one or both of the double-bonded carbons is (are) disubstituted (i.e. 2 R groups attached).

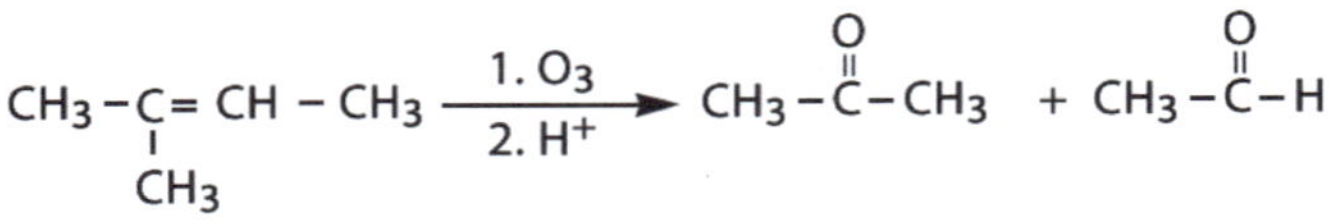

Ketones can also be prepared by Friedel-Crafts acylation of a benzene ring with acyl halide in the presence of an $AlCl_3$ catalyst (ORG 5.2).

Hydration of terminal alkynes will yield methyl ketones in the presence of mercuric ion as catalyst and strong acids. The formation of an unstable vinyl alcohol undergoes keto-enol tautomerisation (ORG 7.1) to form ketones.

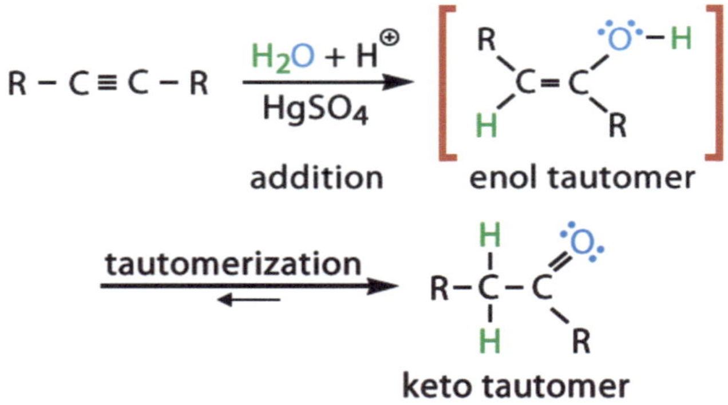

There are two classes of reactions that will be investigated: nucleophilic addition reactions at C=O bond, and reactions at adjacent positions.

The most important reaction of aldehydes and ketones is the nucleophilic addition reaction. A nucleophile attacks the electrophilic carbonyl carbon atom and a tetrahedral alkoxide ion intermediate is formed. The intermediate can lead to the protonation of the carbonyl oxygen atom to form an alcohol or expel the carbonyl oxygen atom as H_2O or OH^- to form a carbon-nucleophile double bond.

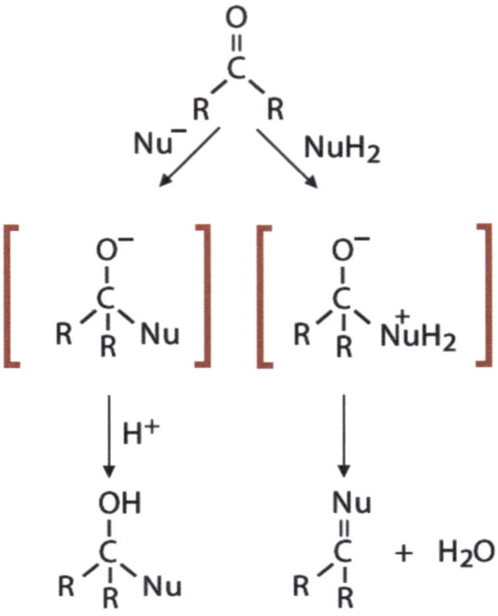

Aldehydes and ketones react with water in the presence of acid or base catalyst to form 1,1-diols, or geminal diols (*gem-diols*). Thus gem-diols are ketone (or aldehyde) *hydrates* and they are unstable (i.e. *they easily convert back to C=O with the loss of water*).

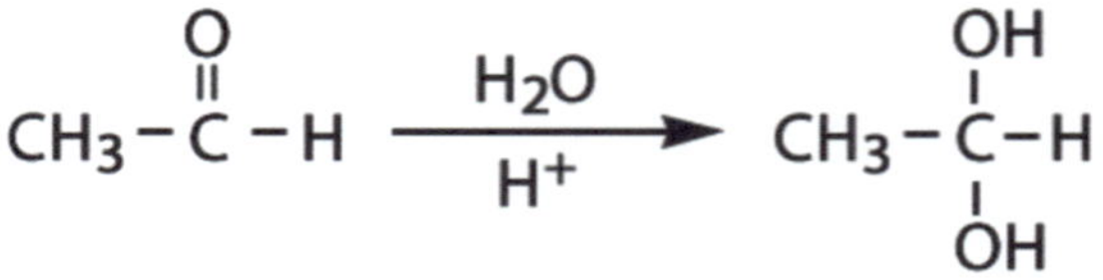

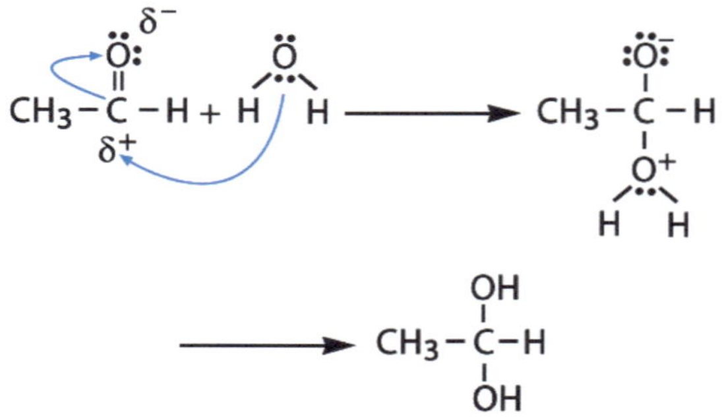

Aldehydes and ketones react with HCN to form cyanohydrin. CN^- attacks the carbonyl carbon atom and protonation of O^- forms a tetrahedral cyanohydrin product.

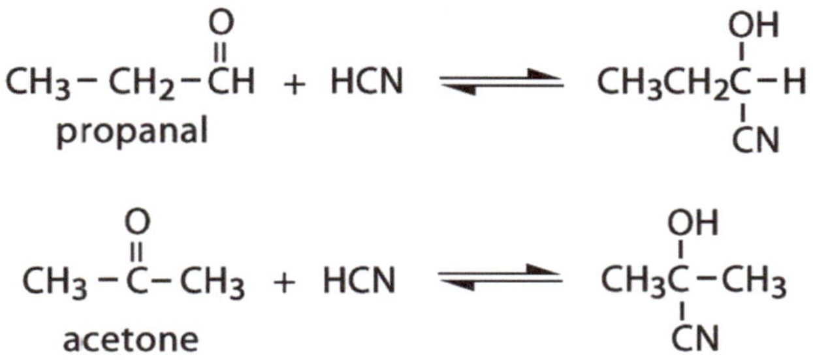

Reduction of aldehydes and ketones with Grignard reagents yields alcohols. Grignard reagents react with formaldehyde to produce primary alcohols, all other aldehydes to produce secondary alcohols, and ketones to produce tertiary alcohols.

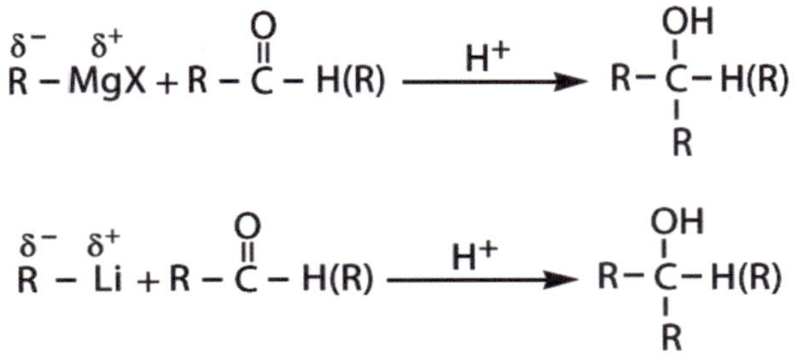

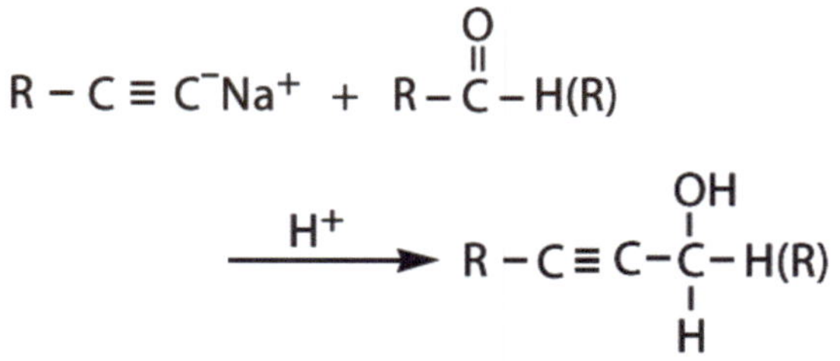

Reducing agents such as $NaBH_4$ and $LiAlH_4$ react with aldehydes and ketones to form alcohols (ORG 6.2.2). The reducing agent functions as if they are hydride ion equivalents and the $H:^-$ attacks the carbonyl carbon atom to form the product.

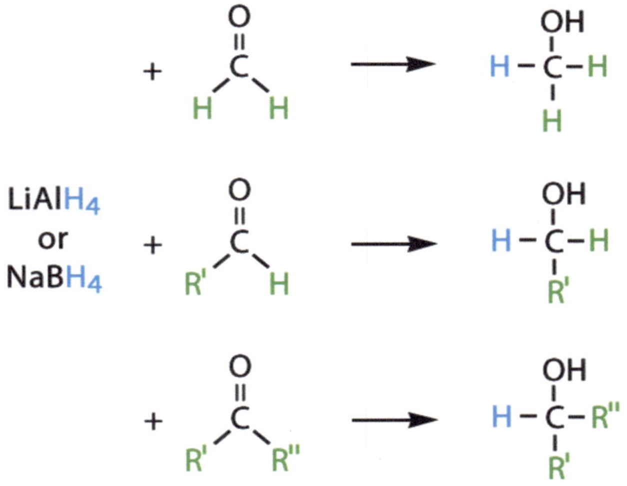

7.2.2 Acetal (ketal) and Hemiacetal (hemiketal) Formation

Aldehydes and ketones will form **hemiacetals** and **hemiketals**, respectively, when dissolved in an excess of a primary alcohol. In addition, if this mixture contains a trace of an acid catalyst, the hemiacetal (hemiketal) will react further to form *acetals* and *ketals*.

An **acetal** is a composite functional group in which two ether functions are joined to a carbon bearing a hydrogen and an alkyl group (important exception: *an acetal formed from formaldehyde has two hydrogens attached to the central carbon*). A **ketal** is a composite functional group in which two ether functions are joined to a carbon bearing two alkyl groups.

This reaction may be summarised:

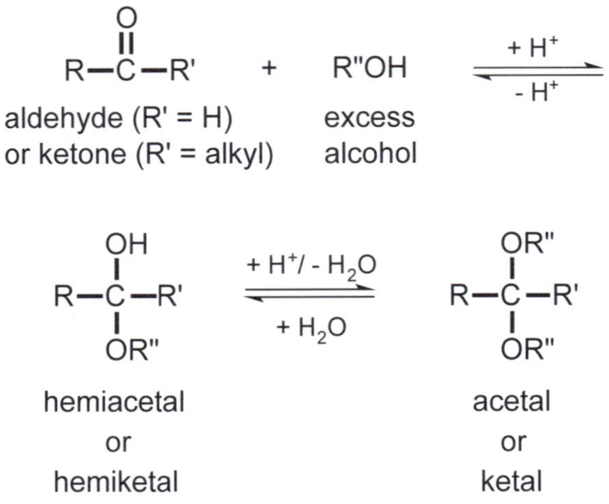

The first step in the above reaction is that the most charged species (+, the hydrogen) attracts electrons from the δ^- oxygen, leaving a carbocation intermediate. The second step involves the δ^- oxygen from the alcohol *quickly* attracted to the current most charged species (+, carbon). A proton is lost which regenerates the catalyst, and produces the hemiacetal or hemiketal. Now the proton may attract electrons from -OH forming H_2O, a good leaving group. Again the δ^- oxygen on the alcohol is attracted to the positive carbocation. And again the alcohol releases its proton, regenerating the catalyst, producing an acetal or ketal. Spoiler Alert contains multiple units with aldehydes/ketones (acetals/ketals), and so you can expect relevant practice among the GAMSAT-level practice questions for this chapter.

Aldehydes and ketones can also react with HCN (hydrogen cyanide) to produce stable compounds called cyanohydrins which owe their stability to the newly formed C-C bond.

7.2.3 Imine and Enamine Formation

Imines and enamines are formed when aldehydes and ketones are allowed to react with amines.

When an aldehyde or ketone reacts with a primary amine, an imine (or Schiff base) is formed. A primary amine is a nitrogen compound with the general formula R-NH_2, where R represents an alkyl or aryl group. In an imine, the carbonyl group of the aldehyde or ketone is replaced with a C=N-R group.

The reaction may be summarised:

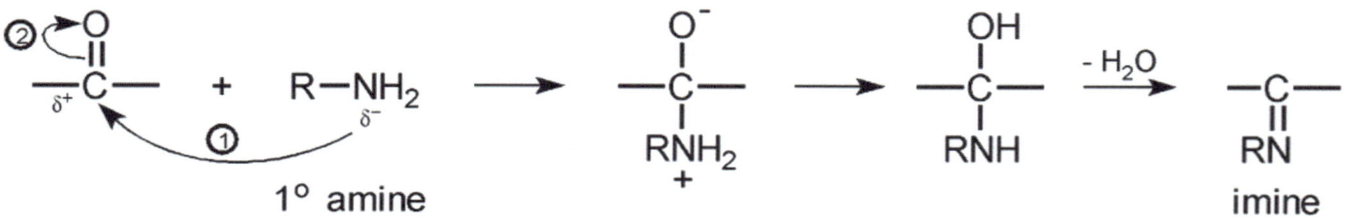

When an aldehyde or ketone reacts with a secondary amine, an enamine is formed. A secondary amine is a nitrogen with the general formula R_2N-H (*see* ORG 1.6 for functional groups), where R represents aryl or alkyl groups (these groups need not be identical).

Tertiary amines (of the general form R_3N) do not react with aldehydes or ketones (*see* Chapter 11 for more details about amines).

7.2.4 Aldol Condensation

Aldol condensation is a base-catalysed reaction of aldehydes and ketones that have α-hydrogens. The intermediate, an aldol, is both an ald*ehyde* and a *alcoh*ol. The aldol undergoes a dehydration reaction producing a carbon-carbon bond in the condensation product, an *enal* (= *alkene* + *aldehyde*).

The reaction may be summarised:

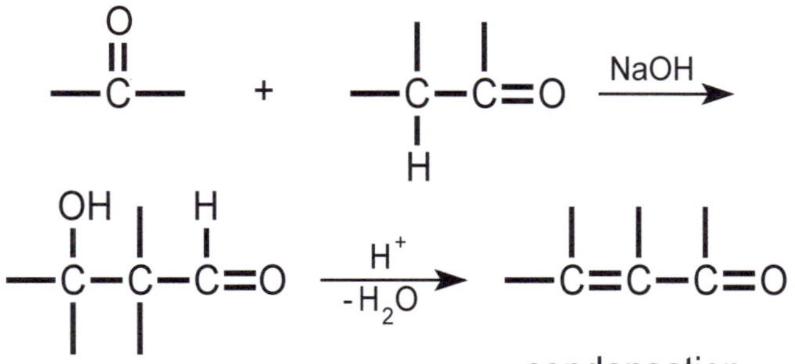

Aldol

condensation product

The reaction mechanism:

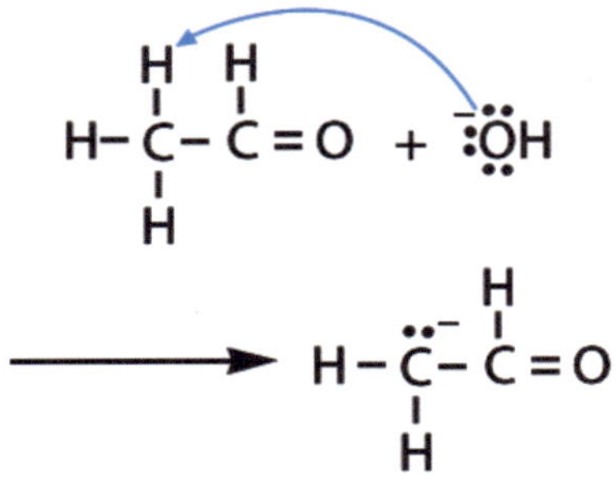

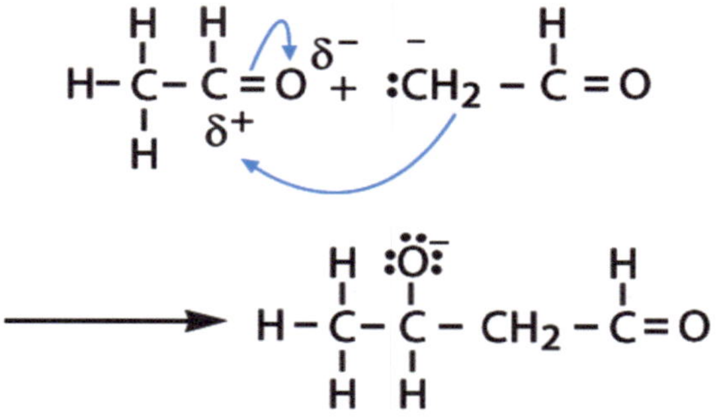

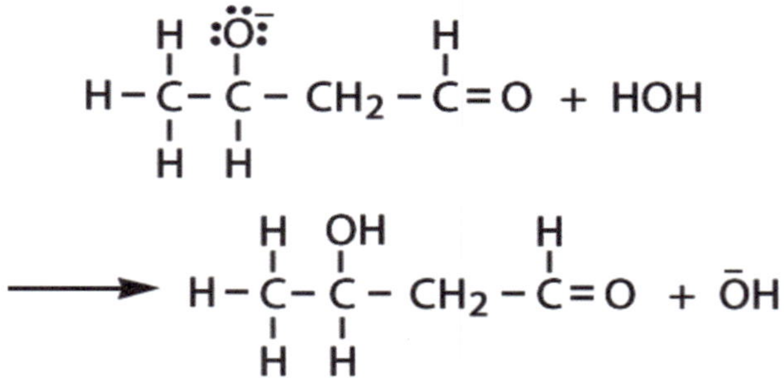

An aldol can now lose H_2O to form a β-unsaturated aldehyde via an E1 mechanism.

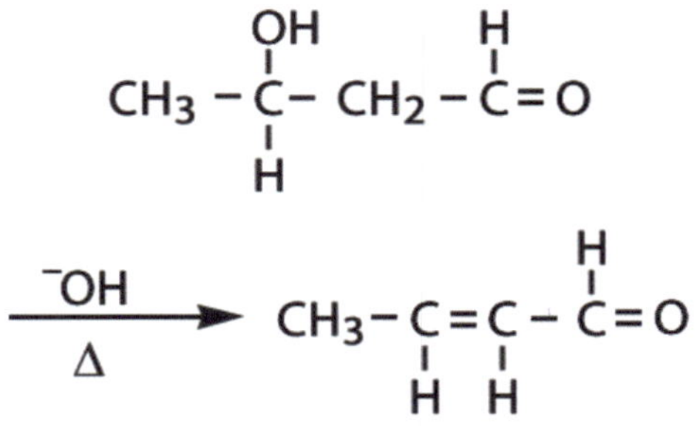

7.2.5 Conjugate Addition to α-β Unsaturated Carbonyls

High-level Importance

α-β unsaturated carbonyls are unusually reactive with nucleophiles. This is best illustrated by example:

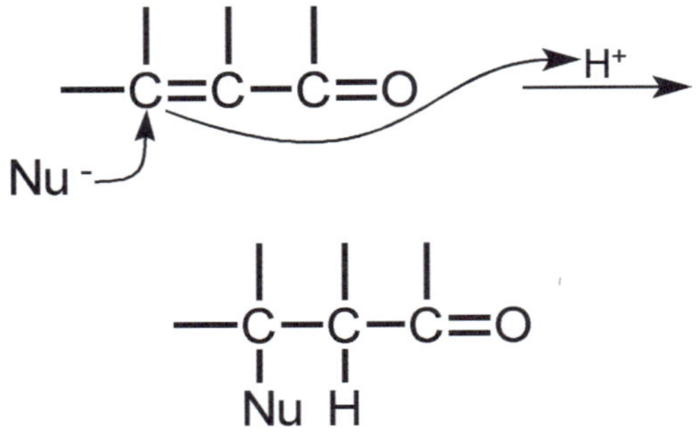

Examples of relevant nucleophiles includes CN^- from HCN, and R^- which can be generated by a Grignard Reagent (= RMgX) or as an alkyl lithium (= RLi).

For example:

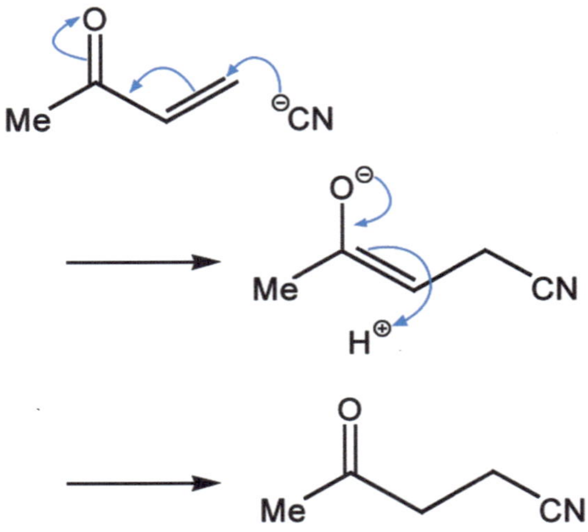

Solutions to Foundational Nomenclature Exercises: Aldehydes and Ketones

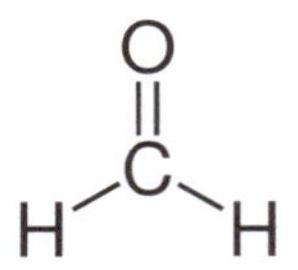

1) Preferred IUPAC name: formaldehyde; systematic IUPAC name: methanal (ACER may use either name or both)

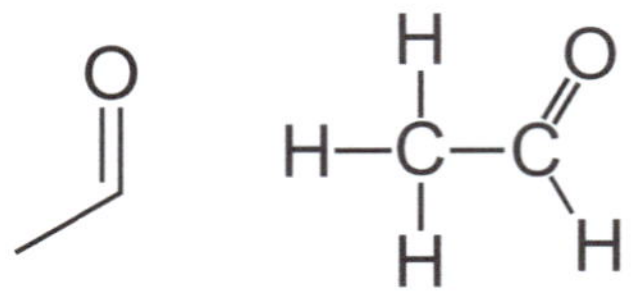

2) Preferred IUPAC name: acetaldehyde; systematic IUPAC name: ethanal (ACER may use either name or both; the two structures are identical)

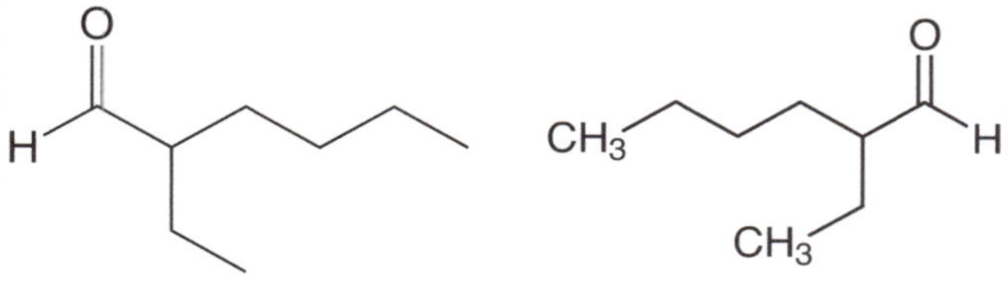

3) 2-ethylhexanal (the two structures are identical)

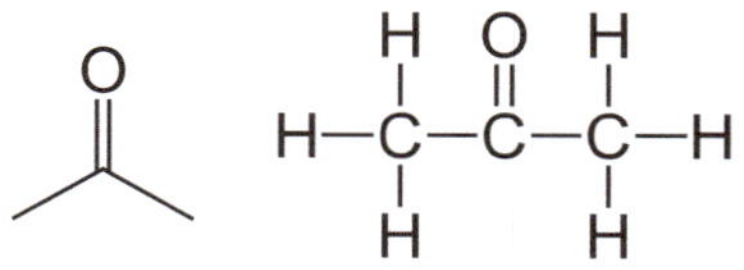

4) IUPAC name: acetone; preferred IUPAC name: propan-2-one (ACER may use either name or both; AKA: dimethyl ketone, $(CH_3)_2CO$; the two structures are identical)

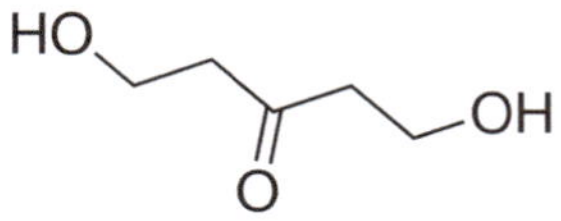

5) 1,5-dihydroxy-pentan-3-one (1,5-dihydroxy-3-pentanone; ketones and aldehydes supersede alcohol functional groups, which supersede alkenes, which supersede alkanes)

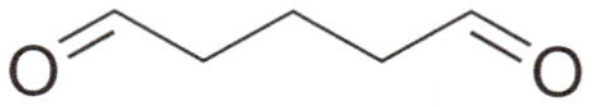

6) IUPAC name: pentanedial (no need: 1,5-pentanedial since aldehydes are always terminal functional groups - always at the end of the line)

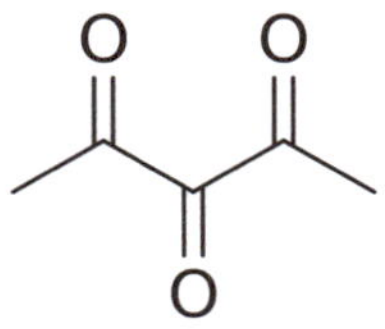

7) pentane-2,3,4-trione [2,3,4-pentanetrione; $CH_3COCOCOCH_3$; $CH_3(C{=}O)(C{=}O)(C{=}O)CH_3$]

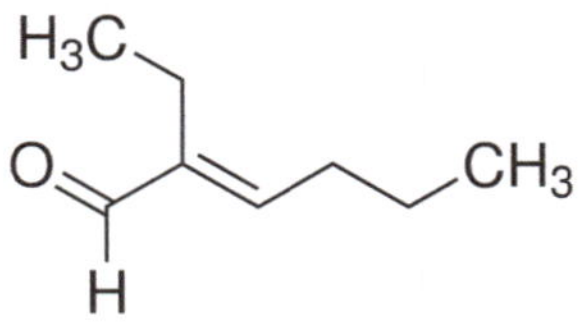

8) 2-ethyl-2-hexenal (2-ethylhex-2-enal; note that you do not need to number the position of the aldehyde group since it must be carbon-1)

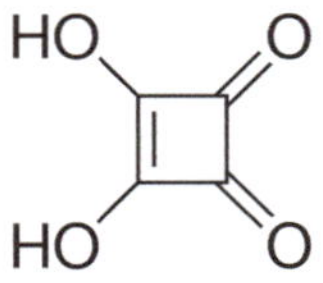

9) 3,4-dihydroxy-3-cyclobutene-1,2-dione (3,4-dihydroxycyclobut-3-ene-1,2-dione; *the most important functional group, the ketone, gets the lowest numbers*)

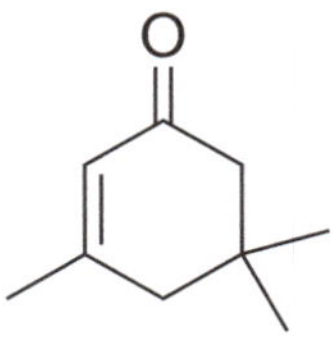

10) 3,5,5-trimethylcyclohex-2-en-1-one (3,5,5-trimethyl-2-cyclohexen-1-one)

Questions or concerns? gamsat-prep.com/forum

High-level Importance

CHAPTER 7: Aldehydes and Ketones

GOLD STANDARD FOUNDATIONAL GAMSAT PRACTICE QUESTIONS

11) Which compound is an aldehyde?

A. 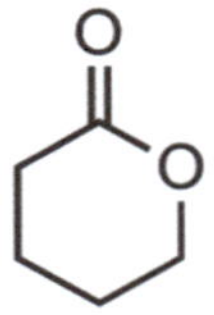

B. 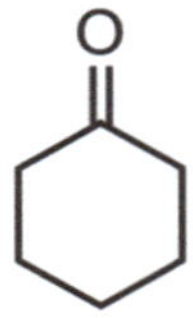

C. 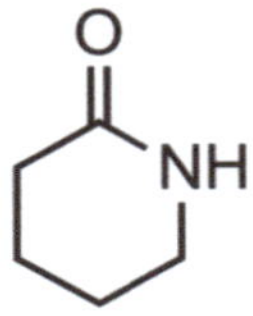

D. 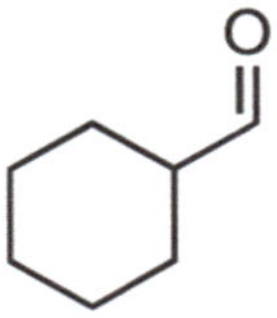

12) Which compound is a ketone?

A. 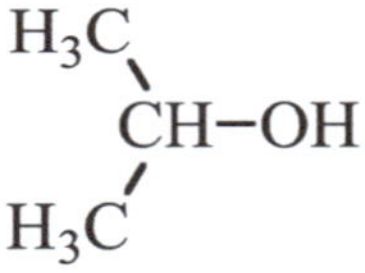

B. 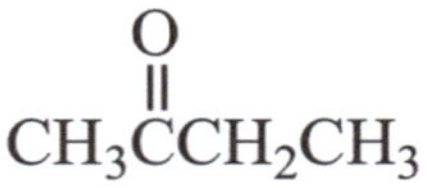

C. 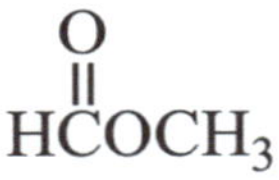

D. 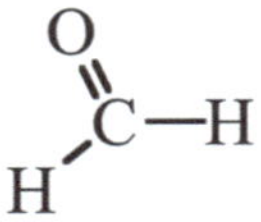

13) Propan-2-one is also known as which of the following?

A. Acetone
B. Dimethyl ketone
C. Propanone
D. All of the above

14) Which compound is a ketone?

- Me = methyl
- Et = ethyl

A. HCOOH
B. MeCOEt
C. HCOOMe
D. HCHO

15) Which of the following molecules is an aldehyde?

A. 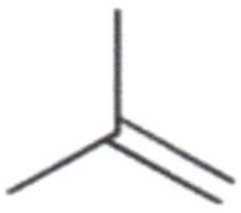

B. 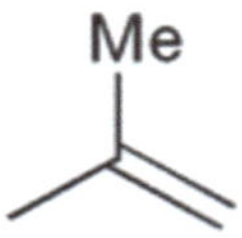

C. 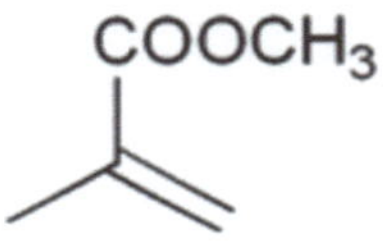

D. 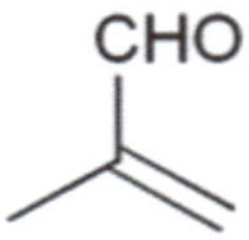

16) Which compound is a hemiacetal?

A. 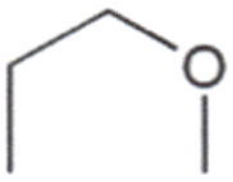

B. 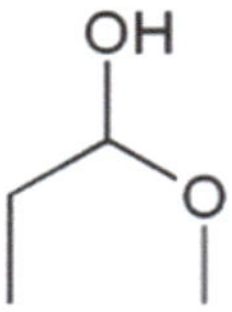

C. 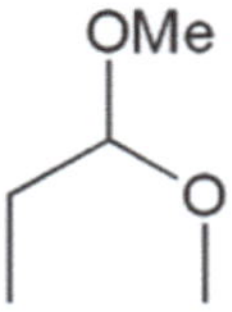

D. 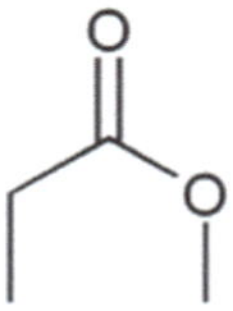

17) Which compound is a ketal?

A. 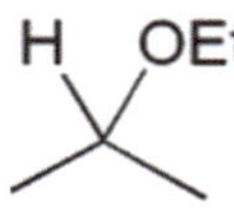

B. 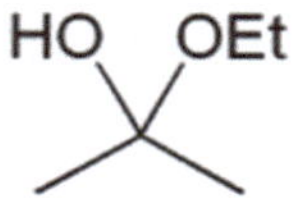

C. 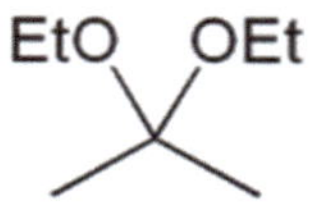

D. 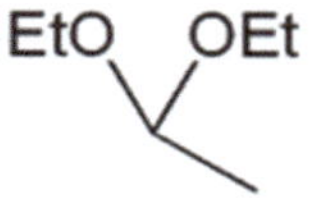

18) Which compound is an acetal?

A. 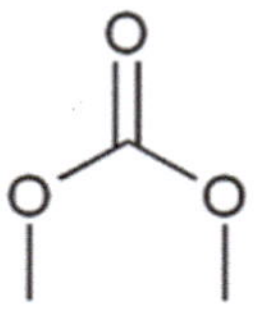

B. 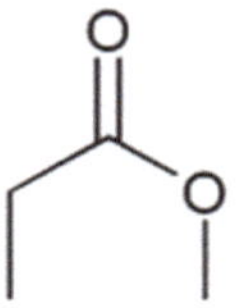

C. 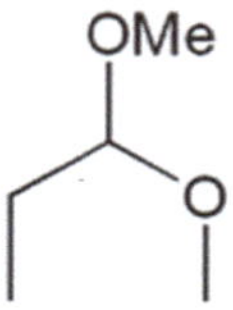

D. 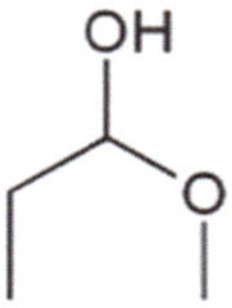

19) Provide the correct IUPAC name for the following molecule.

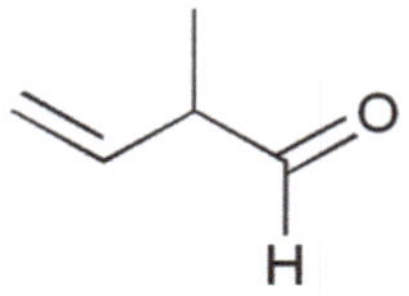

A. 3-formyl-but-1-ene
B. 3-methylbut-2-enal
C. 2-methylbut-3-enal
D. 2-vinylpropanal

High-level Importance

GOLD STANDARD GAMSAT-LEVEL PRACTICE QUESTIONS

Reminder: We started our adventure with GAMSAT-level practice questions in Chapter 1. In section 1.8, unit 3, Questions 19-22, the passage focused on pattern recognition and geometric reasoning as it relates to aldol condensation (ORG 7.2.4). If you did not attempt those questions before, now might be a good time! Those skills will be very useful to help solve the questions in this section.

Questions 20–31

Aldehydes and ketones will form the less stable hemiacetals and hemiketals, respectively, when dissolved in an excess of a primary alcohol. In addition, if this mixture contains a trace of an acid catalyst, the hemiacetal (hemiketal) will react further to form acetals and ketals. The addition of water – with or without an acid catalyst – can reverse the forward reaction.

The reaction can be summarised:

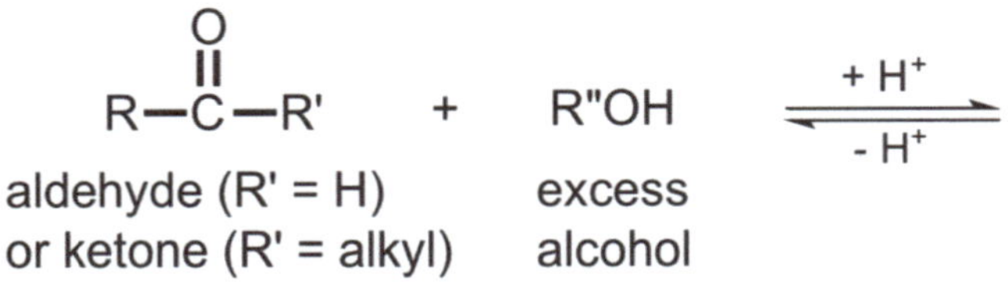

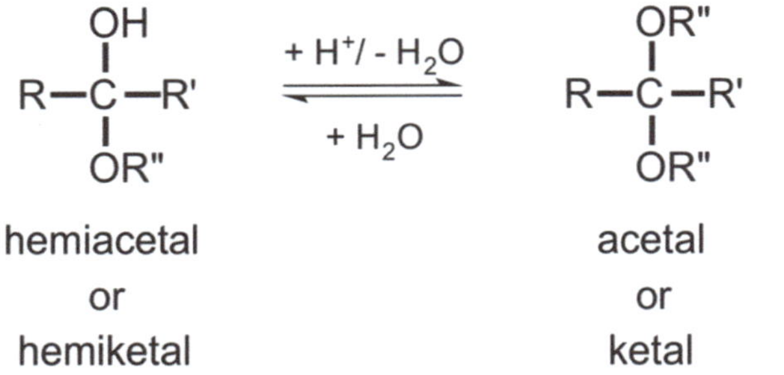

When the key functional groups to make an acetal or ketal are contained in the same molecule then an internal addition can take place forming a cyclic hemiacetal or hemiketal. For example, the C5 hydroxyl group of galactose (*see* below) can add to the aldehyde group (-CHO) which results in a six-membered cyclic hemiacetal, in this case, alpha-D-galactose.

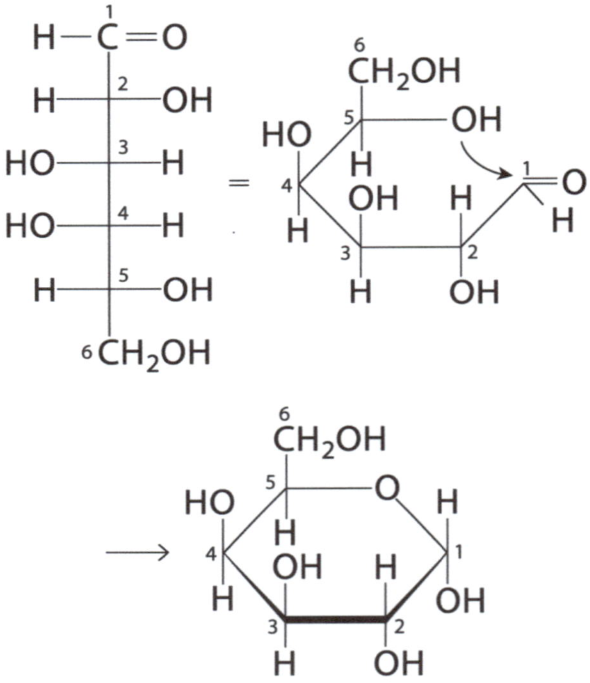

Cyclic products are also possible when diols are used as the primary alcohol.

20) Hydrolysis of an acetal could yield:

A. an aldehyde, a ketone and one alcohol.
B. an aldehyde, a ketone and two alcohols.
C. an aldehyde and one alcohol.
D. an aldehyde and two alcohols.

21) Which pair of compounds can react to form a hemiketal?

A. CH_3CH_2CHO and CH_3COOH
B. CH_3COCH_3 and CH_3CH_2CHO
C. CH_3CH_2CHO and CH_3CH_2OH
D. CH_3COCH_3 and CH_3CH_2OH

22) Glucose, in the cyclic form, is represented below.

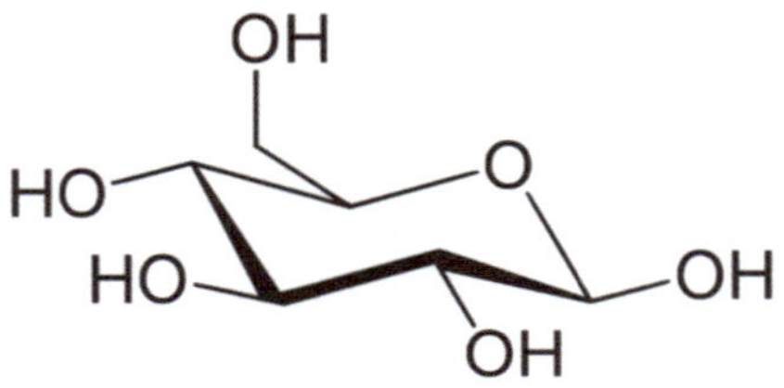

The cyclic form of glucose is a (an):

A. hemiacetal.
B. acetal.
C. ketal.
D. hemiketal.

23) Fructose in cyclic form, is represented below.

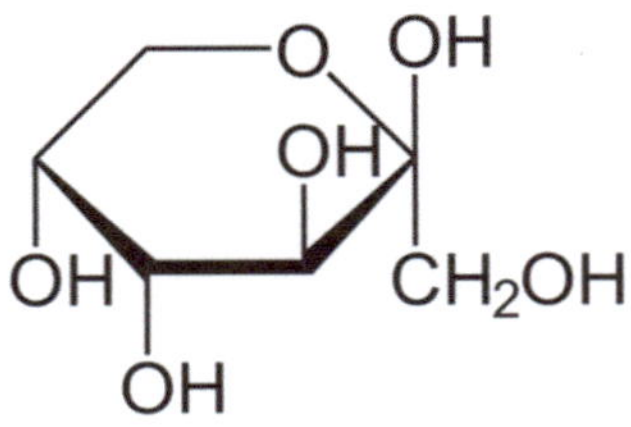

The cyclic form of fructose is a (an):

A. hemiacetal.
B. acetal.
C. ketal.
D. hemiketal.

24) Maltose is a disaccharide made from starch. The structure of maltose is below.

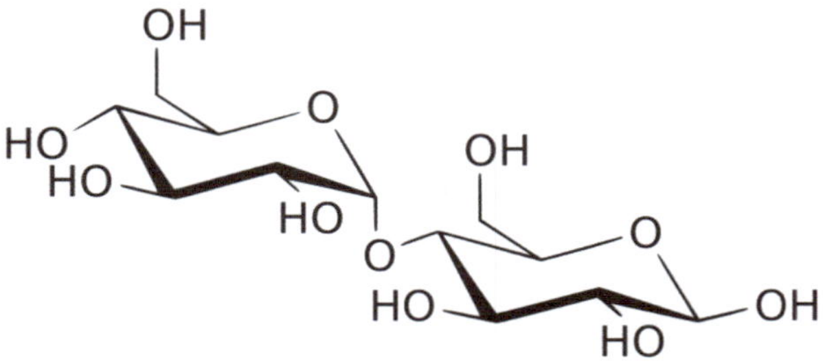

In terms of functional groups, when comparing the number of acetal structures to hemiacetal structures, maltose has:

A. an equal number.
B. one more acetal structure.
C. one more hemiacetal structure.
D. more than one more hemiacetal structure.

25) Given the information provided, predict the most likely end product of hydrolysis for the following reaction.

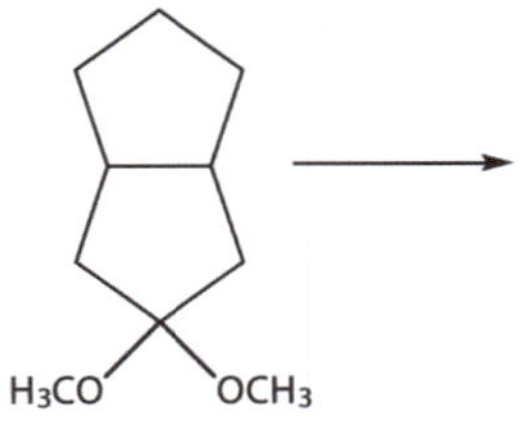

A.

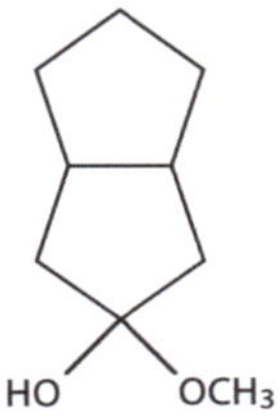

B.

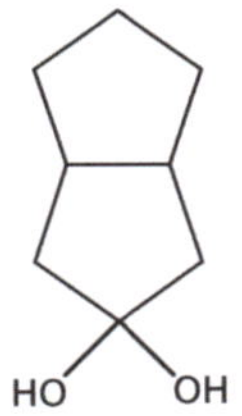

C.

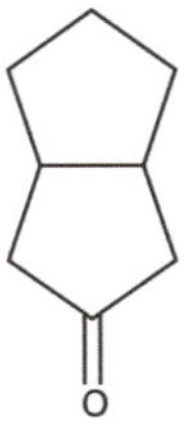

D.

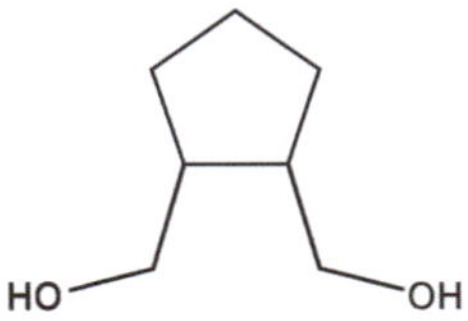

High-level Importance

26) With reference to the reaction summarised in the passage, which of the following is **not** consistent with the production of a ketal?

A. R cannot be H
B. R' cannot be $-CH(CH_3)_2$
C. R'' cannot be $-CH(CH_3)_2$
D. R'' cannot be H

27) The following compound is 1,4-dioxaspiro[4,5] decane.

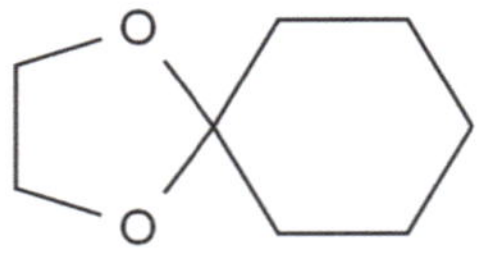

In order to produce 1,4-dioxaspiro[4,5]decane, ethane-1,2-diol ($HOCH_2CH_2OH$) is likely to have reacted with which of the following compounds?

A. 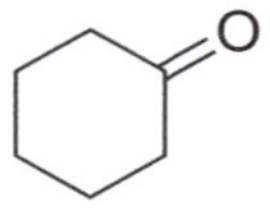

C. 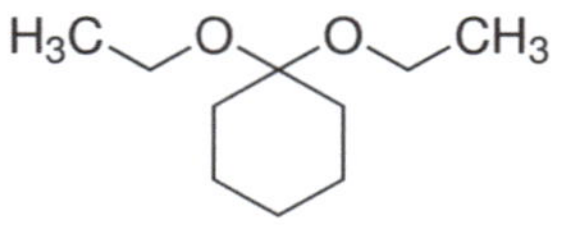

B. 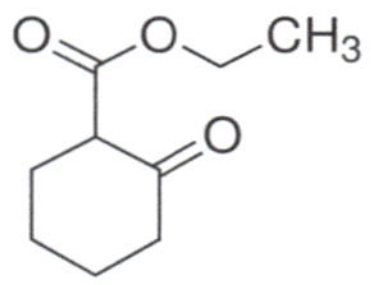

D. 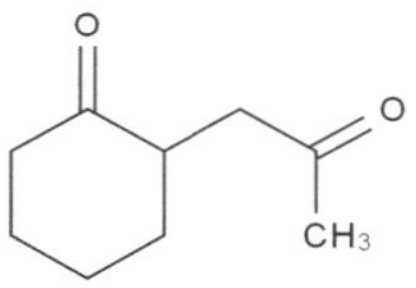

28) How many of the following six compounds are acetals?

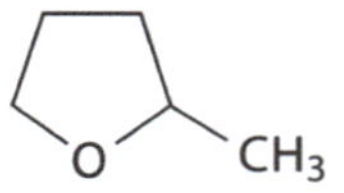

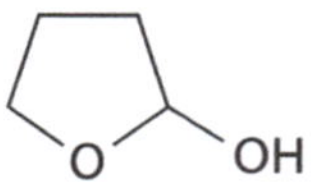

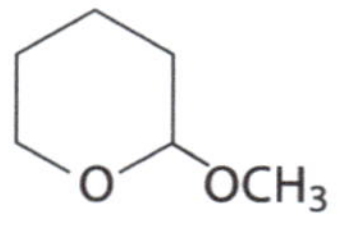

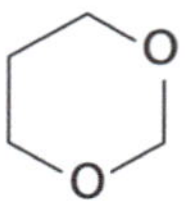

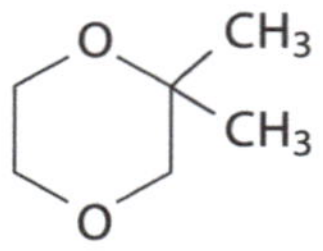

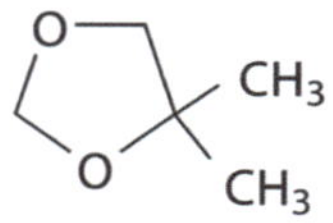

A. 1
B. 2
C. 3
D. More than 3

29) Consider the following reaction.

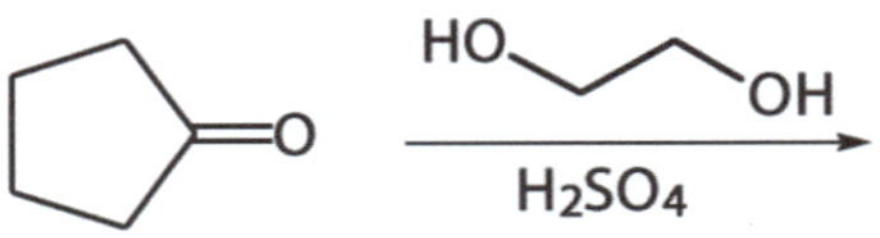

Which of the following would be expected as a major product?

A. 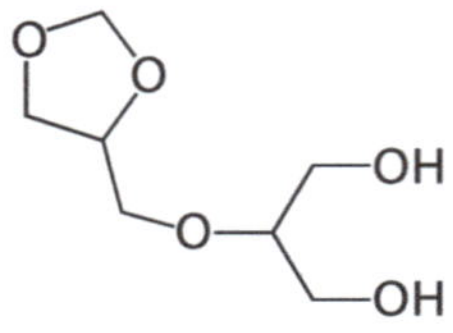

C. 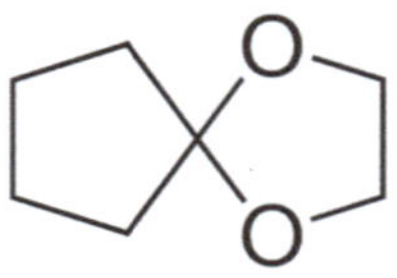

B. 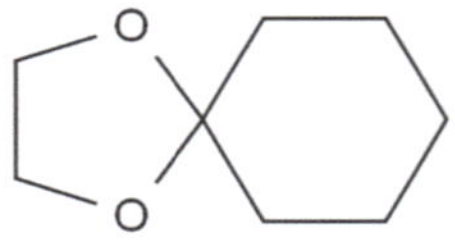

D. 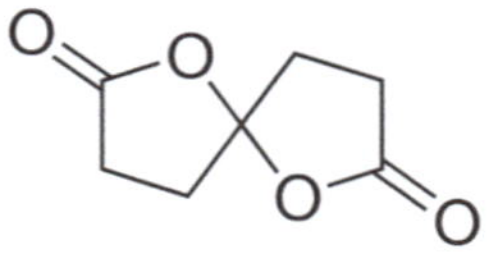

30) Consider the molecular structure of Compound P-54-875.

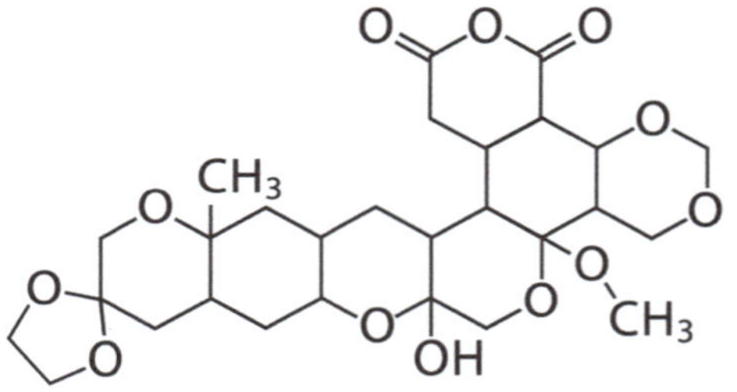

In terms of functional groups, when comparing the number of ketal structures to hemiketal structures, Compound P-54-875 has:

A. an equal number.
B. one more ketal structure.
C. one more hemiketal structure.
D. more than one more ketal structure.

31) How many stereocentres does Compound P-54-875 possess?

A. Less than 11
B. 11
C. 12
D. More than 12

Questions 32–36

Acetaldehyde and methyl ketones react with iodine in the presence of sodium hydroxide to give iodoform and sodium salt of the acid. This reaction is known as the iodoform test. Iodoform is a yellow solid which is insoluble in water. The iodoform test is used for distinguishing methyl ketones from other ketones. It is also used to distinguish ethanol from methanol and other primary alcohols. It can be used to distinguish acetaldehyde from other aldehydes.

Secondary alcohols containing the hydroxyl group on the second carbon atom also undergo this reaction. Ethanol is the only primary alcohol that gives this reaction.

The mechanism of the iodoform reaction is as follows:

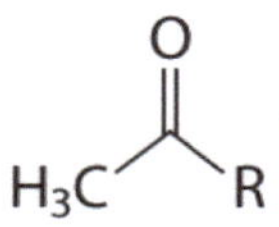

$$+ 3\,I_2 + 4\,NaOH \longrightarrow CHI_3 + RCOONa + 3\,NaI + 3\,H_2O$$

32) Which of the following compounds gives a positive iodoform test?

- **A.** $CH_3CH_2COCH_3$
- **B.** $CH_3CH_2COCH_2CH_3$
- **C.** $CH_3(CH_2)_2COCH_2CH_3$
- **D.** CH_3CH_2COH

33) Which of the following pair of compounds can be most reliably distinguished from each other using the iodoform test?

- **A.** Aldehyde from ketone
- **B.** Acetone from ethyl methyl ketone
- **C.** Propanol from ethanol
- **D.** Acetone from diethyl ketone

34) When ethyl methyl ketone (butanone) reacts with iodine and aqueous sodium hydroxide, which of the following carboxylate compounds is formed?

- **A.** CH_3COONa
- **B.** $HCOONa$
- **C.** C_3H_7COONa
- **D.** CH_3CH_2COONa

35) The iodoform test can be used to convert:

- **A.** ketones into alcohols.
- **B.** aldehydes into ketones.
- **C.** ketones into carboxylic acids.
- **D.** acetaldehydes into propionaldehydes.

36) The number of carbon atoms in the carboxylate formed as a result of the iodoform reaction is:

- **A.** equal to number of carbon atoms in the reactants.
- **B.** one more than the number of carbon atoms in the reactants.
- **C.** is independent of carbon atoms in the reactants.
- **D.** one less than the number of carbon atoms in the reactants.

Questions 37–39

The alpha carbon (Cα) in organic molecules refers to the first carbon atom that attaches to a functional group, such as a carbonyl. The second carbon atom is called the beta carbon (Cβ), and the system continues naming in alphabetical order with Greek letters.

Acidity of the α-hydrogen: The α-hydrogen may be removed by a base. The acidity of this hydrogen is increased if conjugation is possible.

This acidity is a result of the resonance stabilisation of the α-carbanion formed. Note that only protons at the α position of carbonyl compounds are acidic. Protons further from the carbonyl carbon (β, gamma - γ, and so on, positions) are not acidic.

37) Consider the structure of benzylacetone.

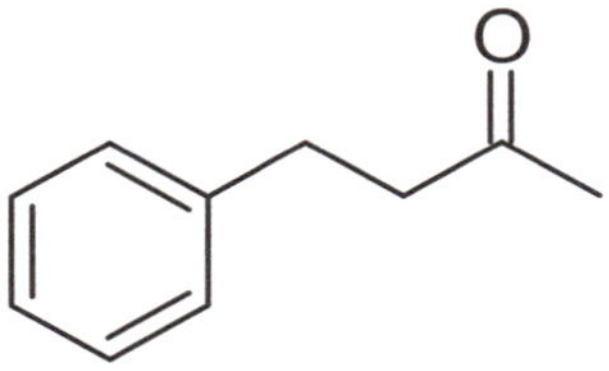

The number of alpha hydrogens minus the number of beta hydrogens = *N*. What is *N* for benzylacetone?

A. 0
B. 1
C. 2
D. More than 2

38) Which is more acidic, **A** or **B**?

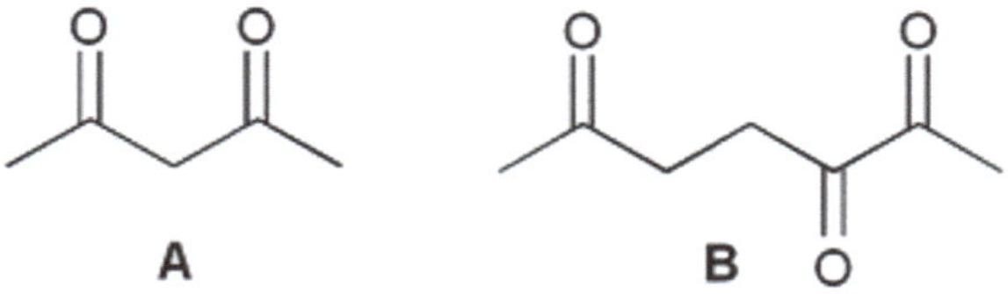

A **B**

A. **A**
B. **B**
C. They are equally acidic.
D. Neither can donate a proton.

39) Which hydrogen is most acidic?

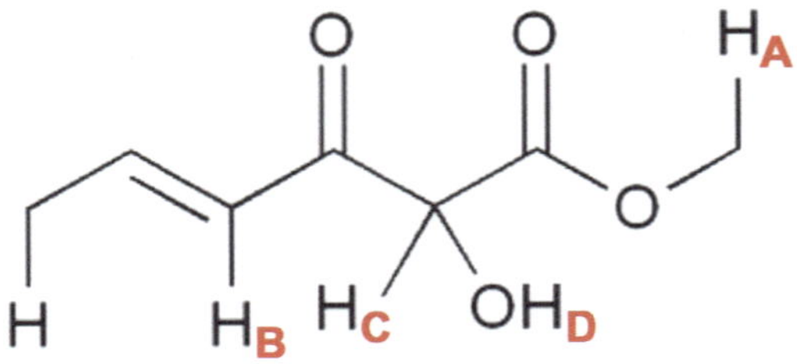

40) The Claisen rearrangement is the first recorded example of a [3,3]-sigmatropic rearrangement. The heating of an allyl vinyl ether will lead to a [3,3]-sigmatropic rearrangement which results in a gamma, delta-unsaturated carbonyl.

Consider the following example.

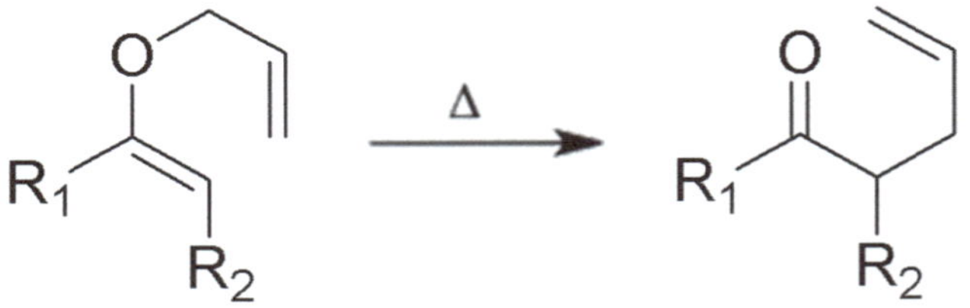

Based on the information provided, identify the expected product of the following reaction.

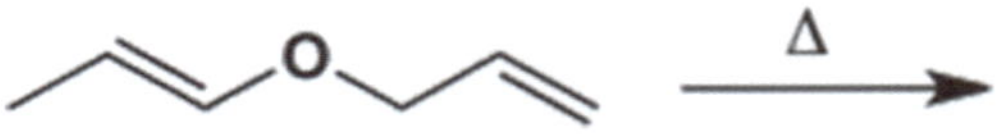

A.
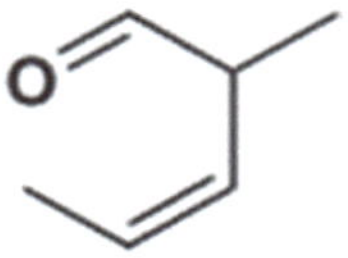

B.
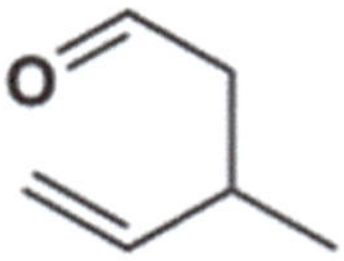

C.
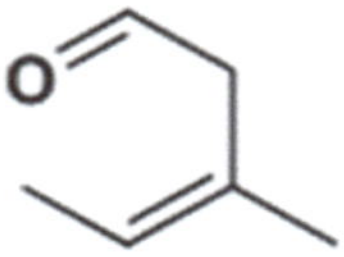

D.
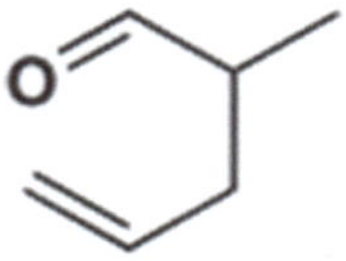

SPOILER ALERT

Gold Standard has cross-referenced the content in this chapter to examples from ACER's official GAMSAT practice materials. It is for you to decide when you want to explore these questions since you may want to preserve some of ACER's materials for timed mock-exam practice.

Examples – Oxidation of alcohols to aldehydes and ketones: Q53-55 of 2; focus on aldehydes to hemiacetals: Q57-59 of 3; Grignard reagent making aldehydes and ketones: Q95-99 of 4; oxidation of alcohols to aldehydes and ketones: Q69-72 of 5 (note that some units had a certain number of questions not counted towards this chapter but rather to related chapters for obvious reasons). Note that "Q" is followed by the question number, and, for example, "of 1" refers to booklet number 1 which is referenced in the Spoiler Alert table at the end of Chapter 1. The 15 full-length GAMSAT practice tests by Gold Standard, HEAPS-1 through HEAPS-15, contain specific cross-references to this chapter within the worked solutions. Note that the epic unit covering aldehydes and ketones with the production of acetals and ketals is from HEAPS-1; the iodoform-test unit is from HEAPS-3 (note that we explored the iodine number with an important calculation in Chapter 6, Alcohols).

High-level Importance

Chapter Checklist

- ☐ Access your online account to view answers, worked solutions and discussion boards.
- ☐ Reassess your 'learning objectives' for this chapter: Go back to the first page of this chapter and re-evaluate the top 3 boxes and the Introduction.
- ☐ Complete a maximum of 1 page of notes using symbols/abbreviations to represent the entire chapter based on your learning objectives. These are your Gold Notes.
- ☐ Consider your multimedia options based on your optimal way of learning:
  - ☐ Download the free Gold Standard GAMSAT app for your Android device or iPhone.
  - ☐ Create your own, tangible study cards or try the free app: Anki.
  - ☐ Record your voice reading your Gold Notes onto your smartphone (audio files, e.g., *memo* or MP3s) and listen during exercise, transportation, etc.
  - ☐ Try out the Gold Standard GAMSAT online videos at gamsat-prep.com, or you can try other options on YouTube like Khan Academy or Crash Course Organic Chemistry.
- ☐ Reassess your schedule for your full-length GAMSAT practice tests: ACER and/or HEAPS exams. Ensure that you have scheduled one full day to complete a practice test and 1-2 days for a thorough assessment of worked solutions while adding to your abbreviated Gold Notes.
- ☐ Reassess your progress in scheduling and/or evaluating stress reduction techniques such as regular exercise (sports), yoga, meditation and/or mindfulness exercises (*see* YouTube for suggestions).

CARBOXYLIC ACIDS

Chapter 8

Memorise	Understand	Importance
* IUPAC nomenclature	* Hydrogen bonding * Redox reactions * Relative acid strength * Resonance * Grignards, organometallic reagents	**Medium level: 6% of GAMSAT Organic Chemistry** questions released by ACER are related to content in this chapter (in our estimation). * Note that approximately 60% of the questions in GAMSAT Organic Chemistry are related to just 4 chapters: 2, 6, 7 and 12.

Introduction

Carboxylic acids are organic acids with a carboxyl group, which has the formula -C(=O)OH, usually written -COOH or $-CO_2H$. Carboxylic acids are Brønsted-Lowry acids (proton donors) that are actually, in the grand scheme of chemistry, weak acids. However, carboxylic acids are among the strongest *organic* acids. Salts and anions of carboxylic acids are called *carboxylates*.

Multimedia Resources at GAMSAT-Prep.com

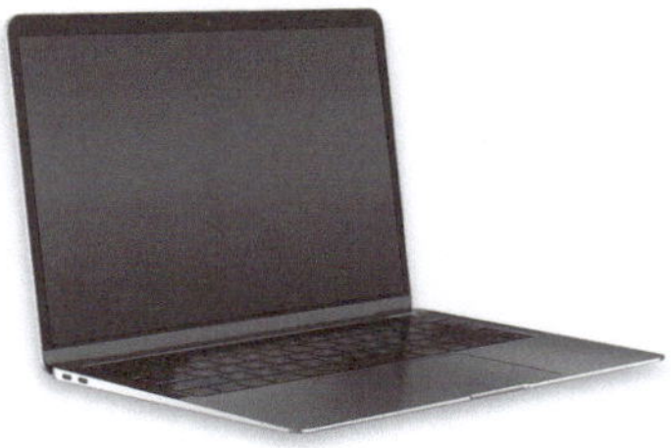

Open Discussion Boards
(*gamsat-prep.com/forum*)

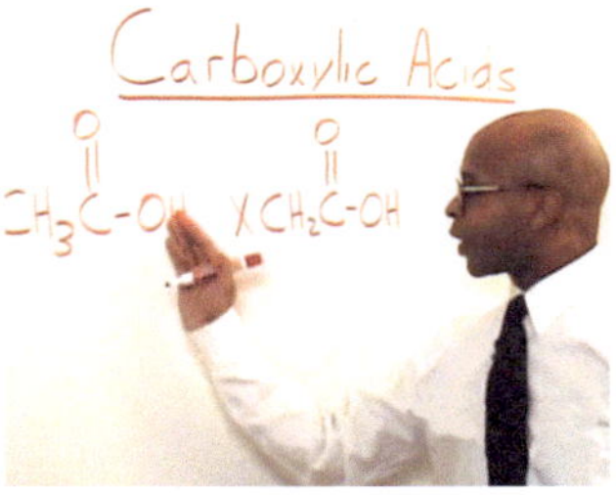

Science Preparation Videos

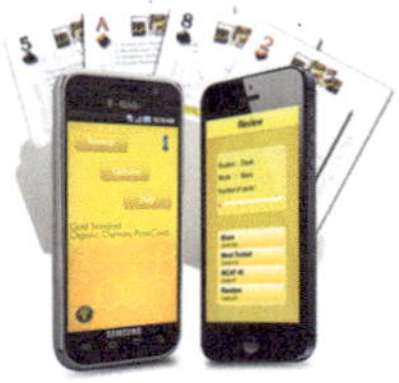

Flashcards

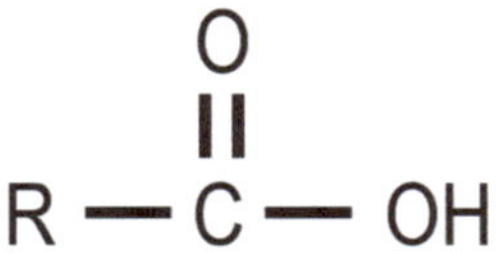

Special Guest

* The real GAMSAT may have advanced-level information presented (i.e. in a passage) but previous knowledge of said information is not required to answer the questions that would follow. Practice questions at the end of this chapter, as well as ACER and GS (HEAPS) practice GAMSATs can help you clarify this point.

8.1 Description and Nomenclature

Carboxylic acids are molecules containing the *carboxylic group* (carbonyl + hydroxyl), which is the basis for their chemistry. The general structure of a carboxylic acid is:

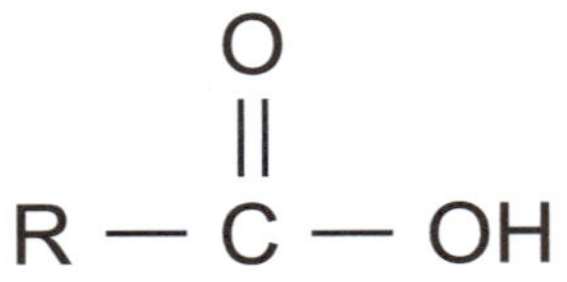

Systematic naming of these compounds is done by replacing the '–e' of the corresponding alkane with '–oic acid'. The molecule is numbered such that the carbonyl carbon is carbon number one. Many carboxylic acids have common names by which they are usually known (systematic names in italics):

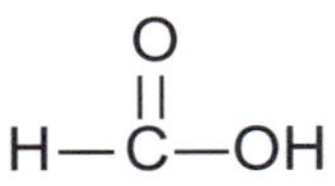

formic acid
methanoic acid

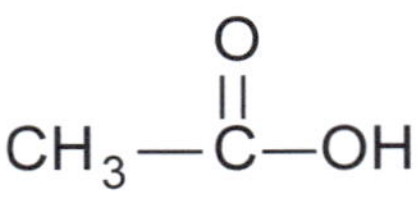

acetic acid
ethanoic acid

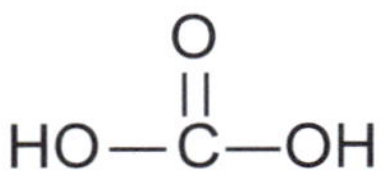

carbonic acid
hydroxymethanoic acid

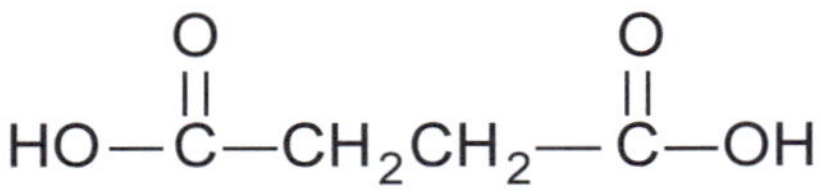

succinic acid
butanedioic acid

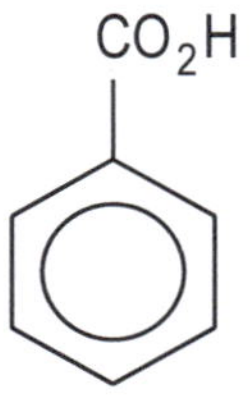

benzoic acid
same: *benzoic acid*

Low molecular weight carboxylic acids are liquids with strong odours and high boiling points. The high boiling point is due to the polarity and the hydrogen bonding capability of the molecule. Strong hydrogen bonding has a noticeable effect on boiling points and makes carboxylic acids boil at much higher temperatures than corresponding alcohols. Because of this hydrogen bonding, these molecules are water soluble. Carboxylic acids with more than 6 carbons are only slightly soluble in water, however, their alkali salts are quite soluble due to ionic properties. As well, carboxylic acids are soluble in dilute bases (NaOH or $NaHCO_3$), because of their acid properties.

The carboxyl group is the basis of carboxylic acid chemistry, and there are four important features to remember. Looking at a general carboxylic acid:

1. The hydrogen (H) is weakly acidic. This is due to its attachment to the oxygen atom, and because the carboxylate anion is resonance stabilised:

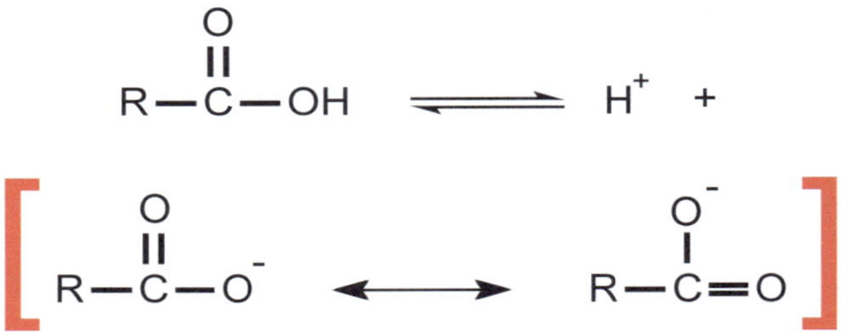

resonance forms

2. The carboxyl carbon is very susceptible to nucleophilic attack. This is due to the attached oxygen atom, and the carbonyl oxygen, both atoms being electronegative:

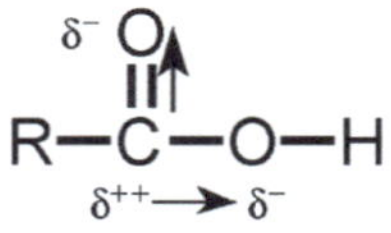

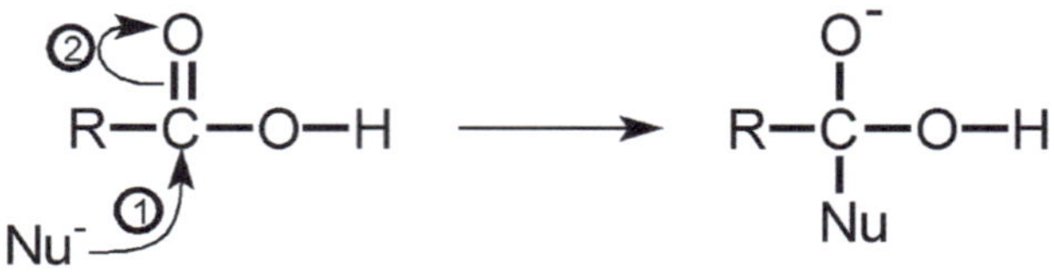

3. In basic conditions, the hydroxyl group, as is, is a good leaving group. In acidic conditions, the protonated hydroxyl (i.e. water) is an excellent leaving group. This promotes nucleophilic substitution:

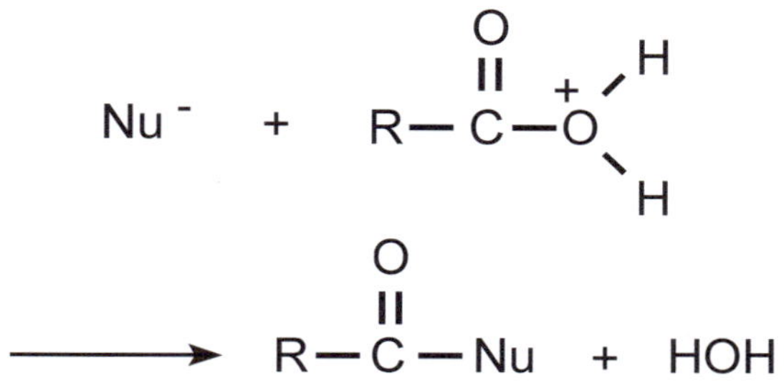

4. Because of the carbonyl and hydroxyl moieties (i.e. parts), hydrogen bonding is possible both inter- and intramolecularly:

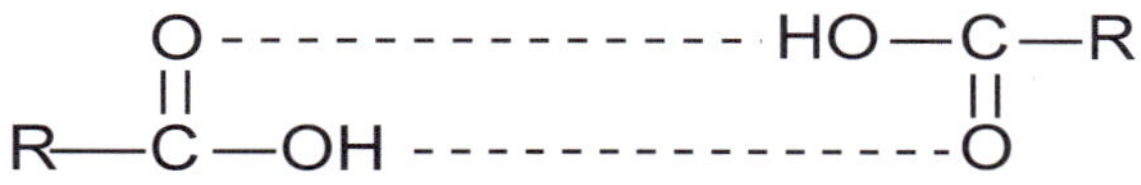

intermolecular (dimerization)

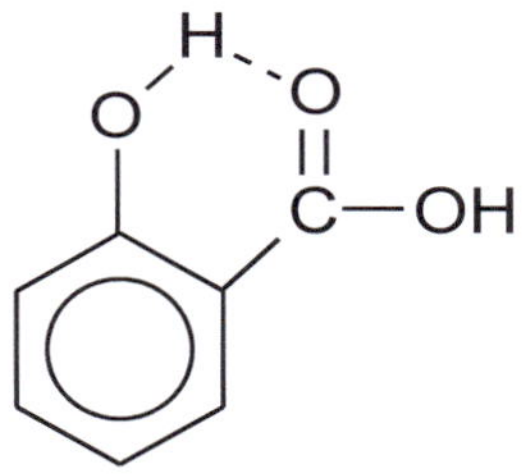

intramolecular

As implied by their name, carboxylic acids are acidic - the most common acid of all organic compounds. In fact, they are colloquially known as organic acids.

Organic classes of molecules in order of increasing acid strength are:

alkanes < ammonia < alkynes < alcohols < water < carboxylic acids.

In terms of substituents added to benzoic acid, electron-withdrawing groups such as $-Cl$ or $-NO_2$ inductively withdraw electrons and delocalise the negative charge, thereby stabilising the carboxylate anion and increasing acidity. Electron-donating groups such as $-NH_2$ or $-OCH_3$ donate electrons and concentrate the negative charge, thereby destabilising the carboxylate anion and decreasing acidity.

The relative acid strength among carboxylic acids depends on the <u>inductive effects</u> of the attached groups, and their proximity to the carboxyl. For example:

$CH_3CH_2{-}C(Cl)_2{-}COOH$ *is a stronger acid than* $CH_3CH_2{-}CH(Cl){-}COOH$.

The reason for this is that chlorine, which is electronegative, withdraws electron density and stabilises the carboxylate anion. Proximity is important, as:

$CH_3CH_2{-}C(Cl)_2{-}COOH$ *is a stronger acid than* $CH_3{-}C(Cl)_2{-}CH_2COOH$.

Thus the effect of halogen substitution decreases as the substituent moves further away from the carbonyl carbon atom (unsurprisingly, the effect of a charge decreases exponentially as distance increases; PHY 9.1).

Medium-level Importance

8.1.1 Foundational Nomenclature Exercises: Carboxylic Acids

Name the following ten compounds. If necessary, feel free to consult the nomenclature rules from ORG 3.1, 4.1 and 8.1. The answers are at the end of this chapter. Of course, it is more helpful to you in the long run to give a full effort first - rather than looking at the solutions before trying.

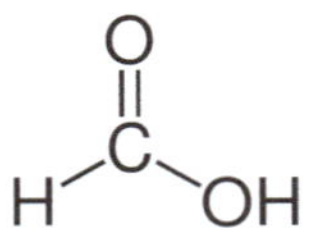

1) ____________________

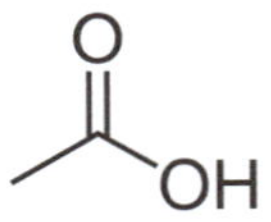

2) ____________________

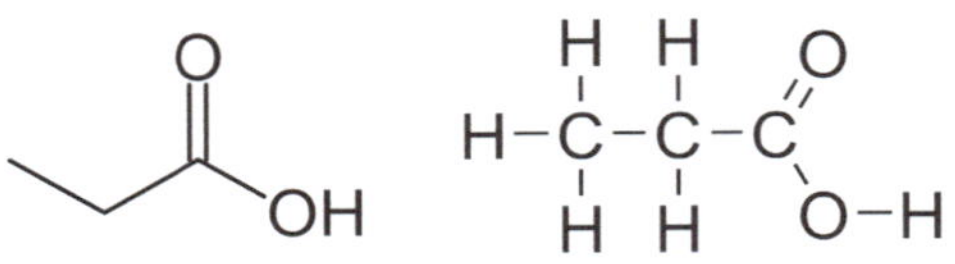

3) ____________________

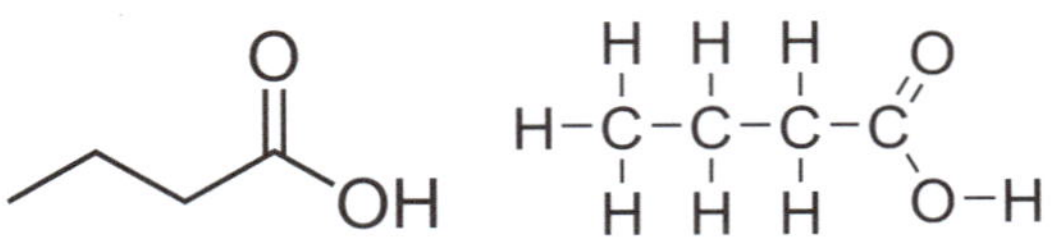

4) ____________________

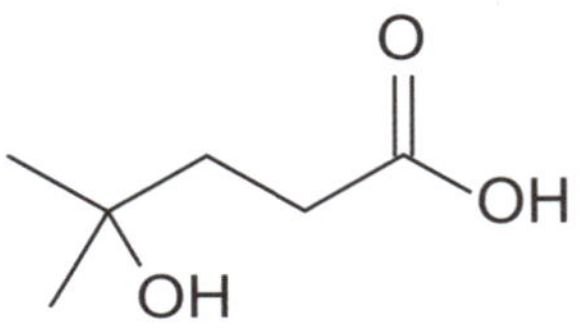

5) ____________________

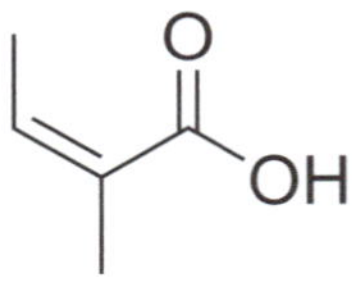

6) ____________________

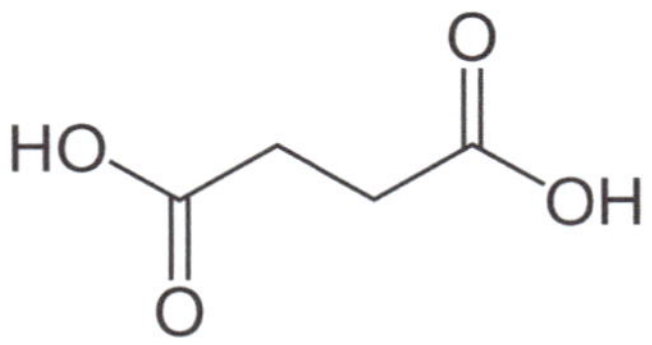

7) ____________________

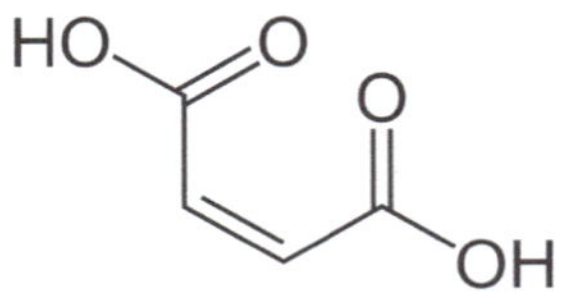

8) ____________________

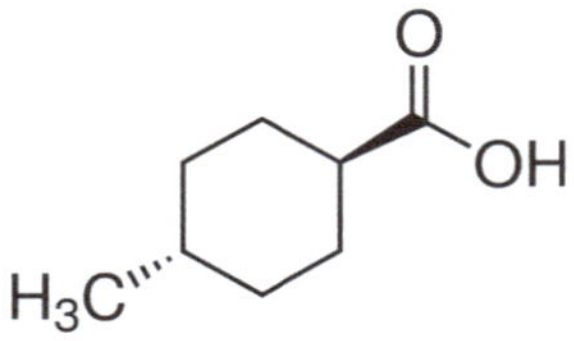

9) ____________________

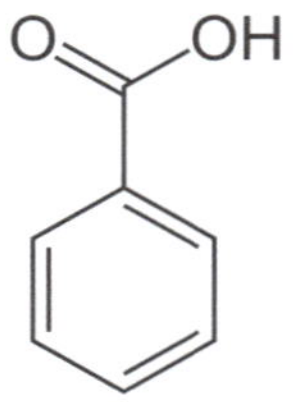

10) ____________________

Medium-level Importance

8.1.2 Carboxylic Acid Formation

A carboxylic acid can be formed by reacting a Grignard reagent with carbon dioxide, or by reacting an aldehyde with $KMnO_4$ (*see* ORG 6.2.2). Carboxylic acids are also formed by reacting a nitrile (in which nitrogen shares a triple bond with a carbon) with aqueous acid.

Mechanisms to synthesise carboxylic acids:

- Oxidative cleavage of alkenes/alkynes gives carboxylic acids in the presence of oxidising reagents such as $NaCr_2O_7$ or $KMnO_4$ or ozone.

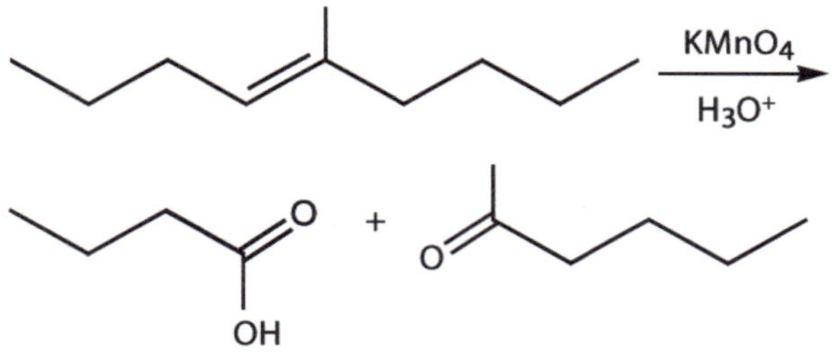

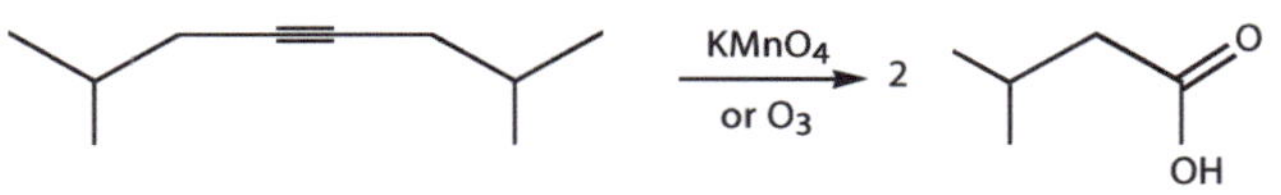

- Oxidation of primary alcohols and aldehydes gives carboxylic acids. Primary alcohols often react with an oxidant such as the Jones reagent (CrO_3, H_2SO_4). Aldehydes often react with oxidants such as the Jones reagent or Tollens' reagent $[Ag(NH_3)_2]^+$, also symbolised Ag_2O. Other reagents include: $K_2Cr_2O_7/H_2SO_4$ or CrO_3/H_2SO_4 or $KMnO_4$.

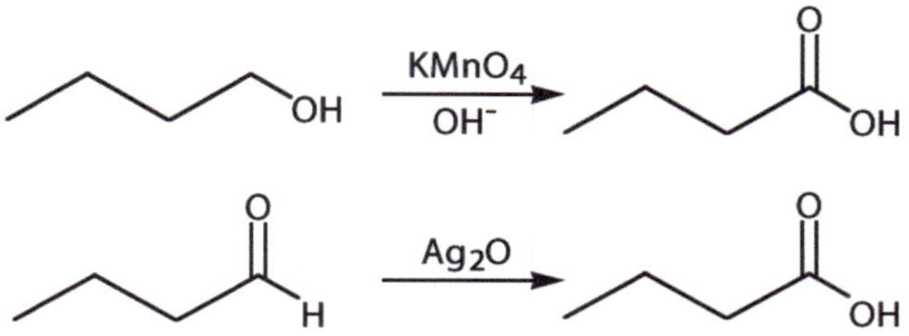

- Hydrolysis of nitriles, RCN, under either strong acid or base conditions can yield carboxylic acids and ammonia (or ammonium salts). Since cyanide anion CN^- is a good nucleophile in S_N2 reactions with primary and secondary alkyl halides, it allows the preparation of carboxylic acids from alkyl halides through cyanide displacement followed by hydrolysis of nitriles. Note that a nitrile hydrolysis reaction increases chain length by one carbon.

$$RCH_2X \xrightarrow{Na^{+}\,{}^{-}CN} RCH_2C\equiv N$$

$$\xrightarrow{H_3O^+} RCH_2COOH + NH_3$$

- Carboxylation of Grignards or other organometallic reagents react with carbon dioxide CO_2 to form carboxylic acids. Alkyl halides react with metal magnesium to form organomagnesium halide,

Medium-level Importance

which then reacts with carbon dioxide in a nucleophilic addition mechanism. Protonation of the carboxylate ion forms the final carboxylic acid product. Note that the carboxylation of a Grignard reagent increases chain length by one carbon.

Grignard reagents are particularly useful in converting tertiary alkyl halides into carboxylic acids, which otherwise is very difficult.

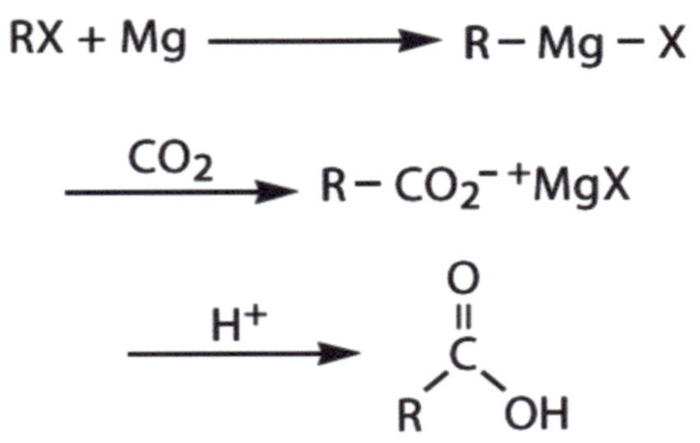

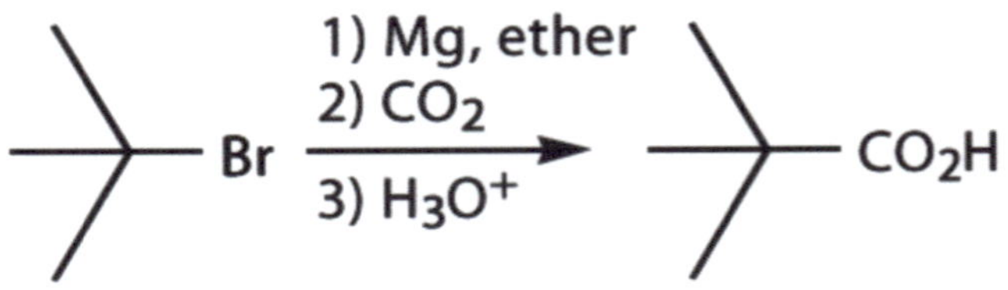

8.2 Important Reactions of Carboxylic Acids

Carboxylic acids undergo nucleophilic substitution reactions (ORG 6.2.3) with many different nucleophiles, under a variety of conditions:

$$Nu^- + R-\overset{O}{\overset{\|}{C}}-OH \longrightarrow R-\overset{O}{\overset{\|}{C}}-Nu + OH^-$$

If the nucleophile is –OR, the resulting compound is an ester. If it is $-NH_2$, the resulting compound is an amide. If it is Cl from $SOCl_2$, or PCl_5, the resulting compound is an acid chloride.

The typical esterification reaction may be summarised:

$$\underset{\text{alcohol}}{R'O^*H} + \underset{\text{acid}}{R-\overset{O}{\overset{\|}{C}}-OH} \longrightarrow \underset{\text{ester}}{R-\overset{O}{\overset{\|}{C}}-O^*R'} + H_2O$$

Notice that an asterisk* was added to the oxygen of the alcohol so that you can tell where that oxygen ended up in the product (i.e. the ester). In the lab, instead of an asterisk (!), an isotope (CHM 1.3; ORG 1.6) of oxygen is used as a tracer or label.

The <u>decarboxylation reaction</u> involves the loss of the carboxyl group as CO_2:

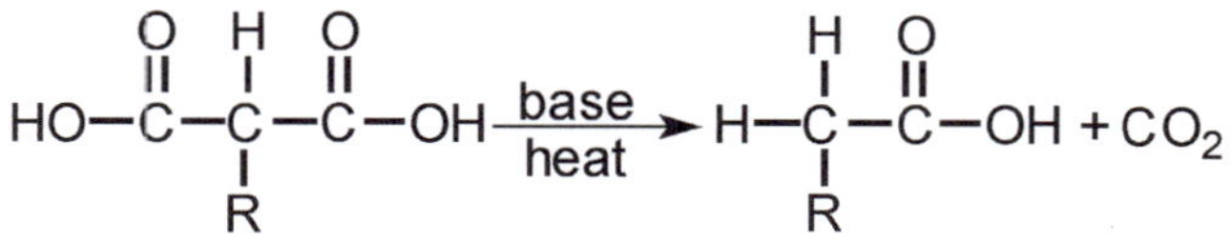

β – diacid

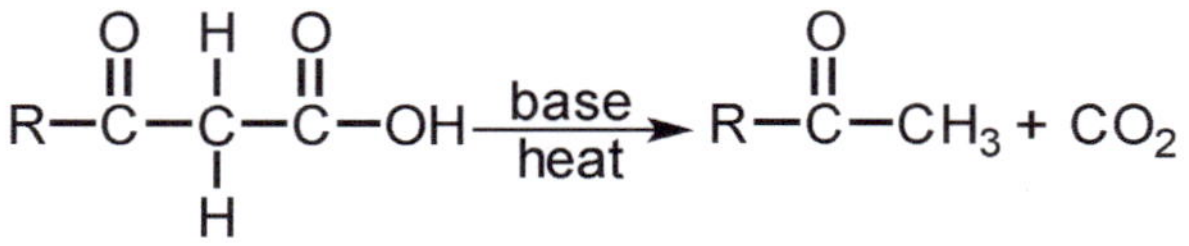

β – keto acid

This reaction is not important for most ordinary carboxylic acids. There are certain types of carboxylic acids that decarboxylate easily, mainly:

- Those which have a keto group at the β position, known as β-keto acids.
- Malonic acids and its derivatives (i.e. β-diacids: those with two carboxyl groups, separated by one carbon).
- Carbonic acid (CHM 1.5.1; ORG 8.1; BIO 12.4.1, 12.4.2) and its derivatives.

Carboxylic acids are reduced to alcohols with lithium aluminum hydride, $LiAlH_4$, or H_2/metals (*see* ORG 6.2.2).

$$LiAlH_4 + R-\overset{\overset{\large O}{\|}}{C}-OH \longrightarrow \underset{\text{alcohol}}{R-CH_2-OH}$$

Sodium borohydride, $NaBH_4$, being a milder reducing agent, only reduces aldehydes and ketones. Carboxylic acids may also be converted to esters or amides first, and then reduced (ORG 9.2, 9.3, 9.4).

Medium-level Importance

Solutions to Foundational Nomenclature Exercises: Carboxylic Acids

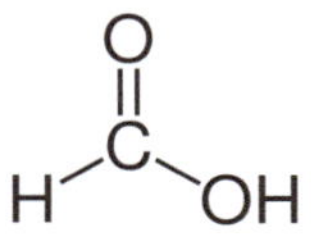 **1)** Preferred IUPAC name: formic acid; systematic IUPAC name: methanoic acid (usually, ACER uses *methanoic acid*, but that is not guaranteed)	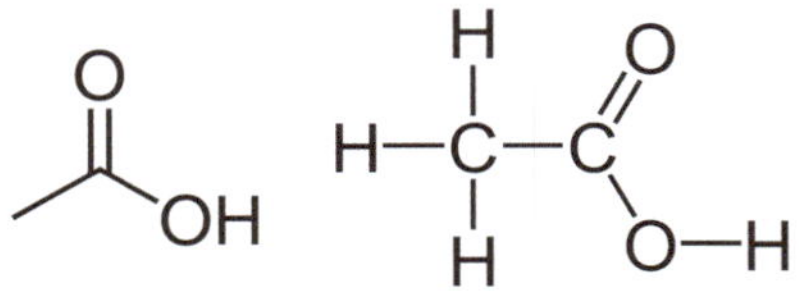 **2)** Preferred IUPAC name: acetic acid; systematic IUPAC name: ethanoic acid (ACER may use either name or both; the two structures are identical)

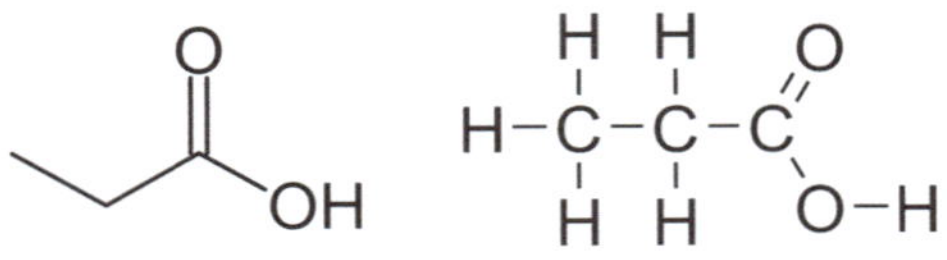

3) Preferred IUPAC name: propanoic acid; trivial name: propionic acid (usually, ACER uses *propanoic acid*; the two structures are identical)

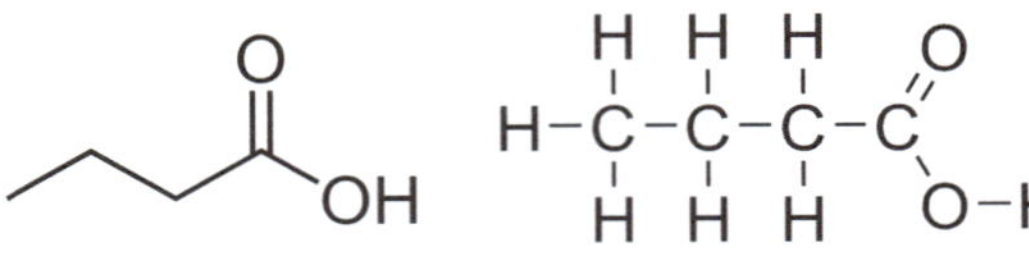

4) Preferred IUPAC name: butanoic acid; trivial name: butyric acid (ACER may use either name or both; the two structures are identical)

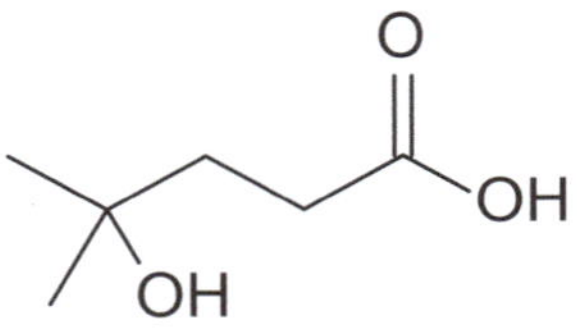

5) 4-hydroxy-4-methylpentanoic acid (note that you do not need to number the position of the carboxylic acid functional group since it must be carbon-1)

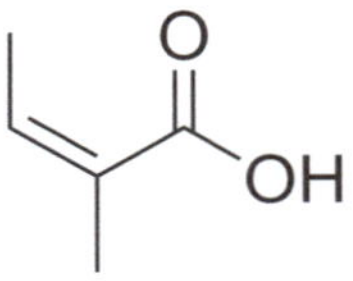

6) (2Z)-2-methylbut-2-enoic acid (it is a cis isomer)

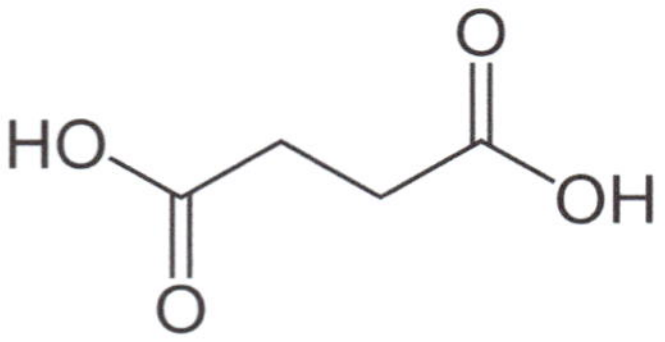

7) butanedioic acid [no need to number the COOH groups because they must be terminal; this molecule is the 'famous' metabolic intermediate *succinic acid*; $(CH_2)_2(CO_2H)_2$].

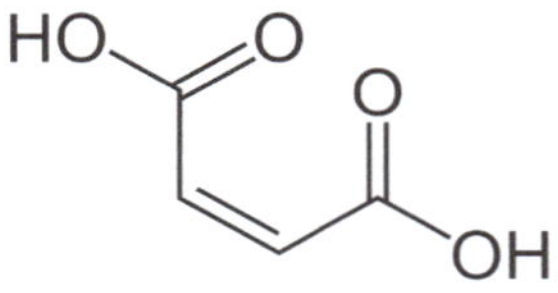

8) (2Z)-but-2-enedioic acid (cis-butenedioic acid; for your interest only: maleic acid)

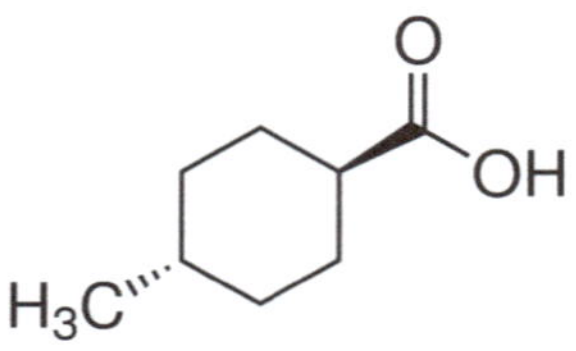

9) trans-4-methyl-1-cyclohexanecarboxylic acid (E)

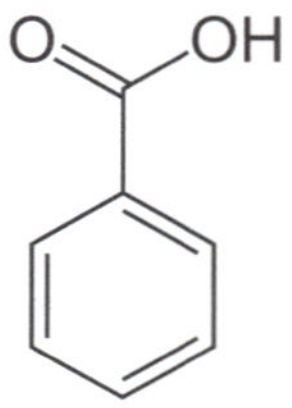

10) Preferred IUPAC name: benzoic acid; systematic IUPAC name: benzenecarboxylic acid

Questions or concerns? gamsat-prep.com/forum

Medium-level Importance

CHAPTER 8: Carboxylic Acids

GOLD STANDARD FOUNDATIONAL GAMSAT PRACTICE QUESTIONS

High-level Importance

11) Which of the following structures represents a carboxylic acid?

A. 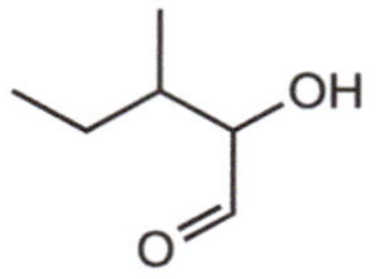

B. 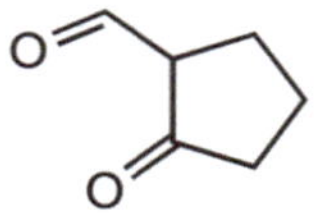

C. 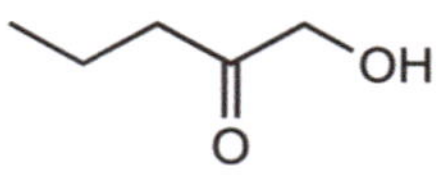

D. 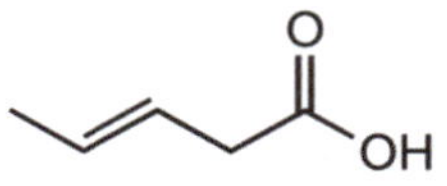

12) Acetic acid is also known as which of the following?

A. Formic acid
B. Acetone
C. Ethanoic acid
D. Acetaldehyde acid

GOLD STANDARD GAMSAT-LEVEL PRACTICE QUESTIONS

Note: You have already been exposed to GAMSAT-level practice questions related to carboxylic acids because of the overlap with respect to chemical reactions and other functional groups. For example, ozonolysis (ORG 8.1.2) was explored in an epic unit in Chapter 4, Questions 30-37, which is key to practicing the oxidation of alkenes to aldehydes, ketones and carboxylic acids. Hopefully, the 'famous' redox series of reactions from Chapter 6 (ORG 6.2.2), which includes carboxylic acids, has a comfortable place in your memory because it represents testable items. We will now approach carboxylic acids and practice questions from a different angle as compared to earlier chapters.

13) Oxidative cleavage of the double bond of an alkene is possible with heat and $KMnO_4$ as illustrated below.

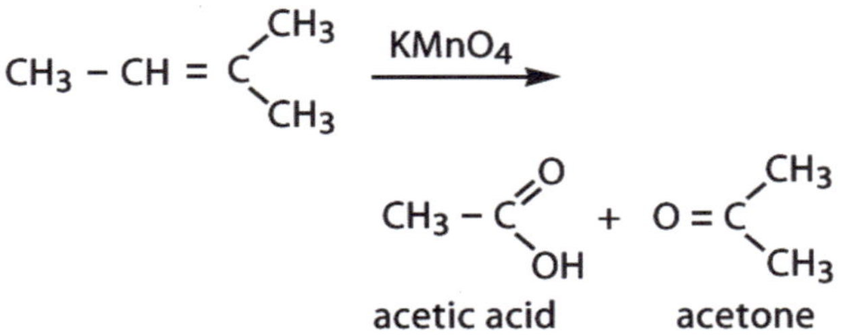

Given the application of heat, identify the expected product of the following reaction.

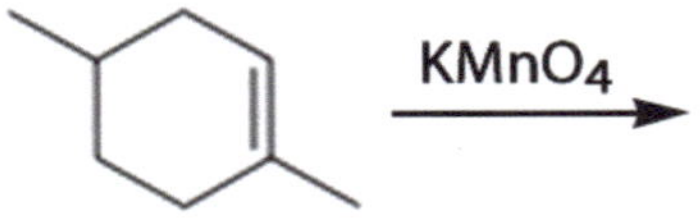

A. 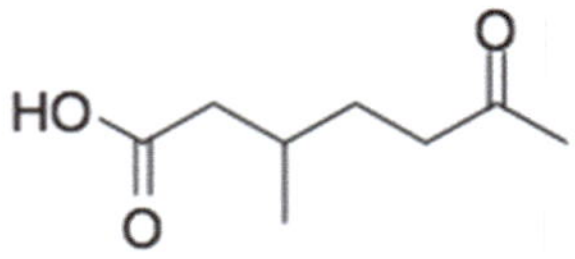

B. 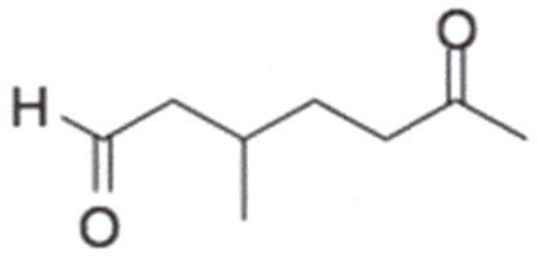

C. 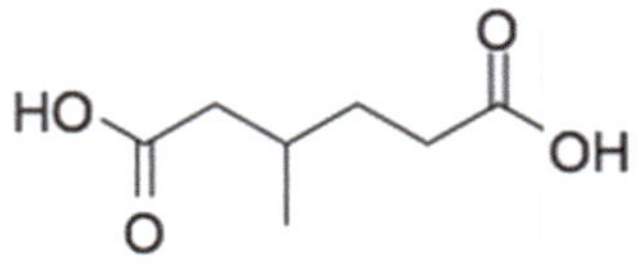

D. 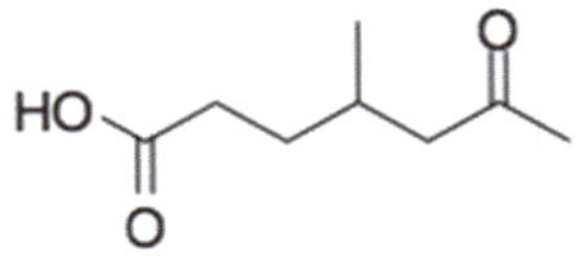

Questions 14–16

Figure 1 illustrates chemical methods often used by organic chemists for qualitative analysis of water soluble unknowns. Table 1 lists characteristic chemical tests of organic compounds. For instance, Fehling's tests that are positive are indicative of an aldehyde.

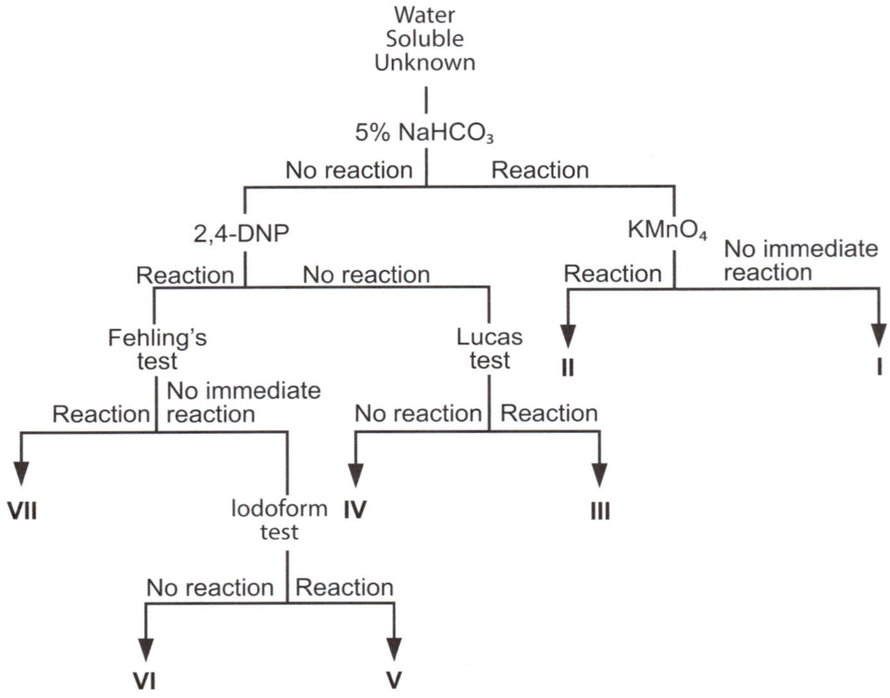

Figure 1

Chemical Test	Compounds
Sodium hydroxide	Organic acids: carboxylic acids and phenols
Lucas	Alcohols with 5 or less carbon atoms
Sodium bicarbonate	Carboxylic acids
2,4-Dinitro-phenylhy-drazine (DNP)	Aldehydes and ketones
Fehling's solution	Aldehydes
Iodine in sodium hydroxide (Iodoform)	Acetaldehydes and ketones with the CH_3-CO- group Alcohols with the $CH_3CH(OH)$- as a structural feature
Sulfuric acid	Alcohols, ethers, alkenes Soluble Lewis bases

Table 1

14) Cyclohexanol should fall into which of the following groups?

A. I
B. II
C. III
D. IV

15) A water soluble unknown is unreactive in the presence of sodium bicarbonate, gives a positive 2,4-DNP test and negative Fehling's and Iodoform tests. In which of the following classes should this compound be classified?

A. Aldehyde
B. Ketone
C. Carboxylic acid
D. Alcohol

16) Acetone should give positive test results for which of the following chemical tests?

- **A.** Lucas and sodium bicarbonate
- **B.** 2,4-DNP and Fehling's
- **C.** Iodoform and 2,4-DNP
- **D.** Iodoform and potassium permanganate

Questions 17–20

The carboxyl hydrogen (H) is weakly acidic. This is due to its attachment to the oxygen atom, and because the carboxylate anion, the conjugate base, is resonance stabilised:

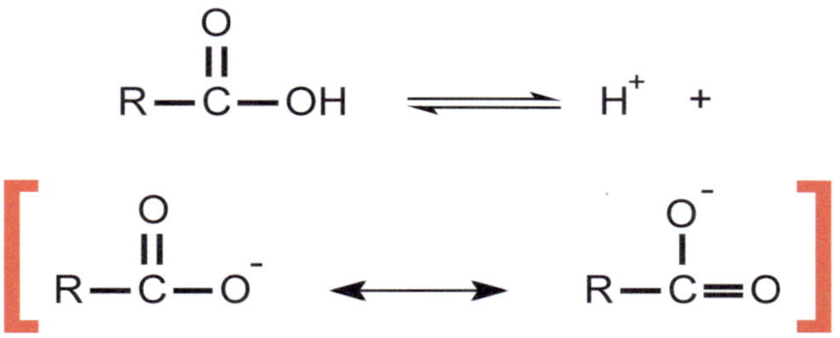

resonance forms

The relative acid strength among carboxylic acids depends on the inductive effects of the attached R group, and their proximity to the carboxyl.

For example:

CH_3CH_2-$C(Cl)_2$-COOH *is a stronger acid than* CH_3CH_2-CH(Cl)-COOH.

The reason for this is that chlorine, which is electronegative, withdraws electron density and stabilises the carboxylate anion.

Proximity is important, as:

CH_3CH_2-$C(Cl)_2$-COOH *is a stronger acid than* CH_3-$C(Cl)_2$-CH_2COOH.

17) Choose the molecule which is most acidic.

A.
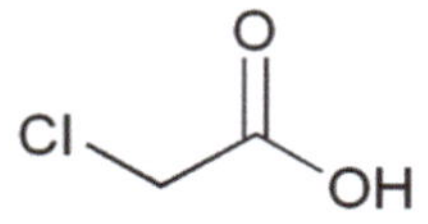

C.
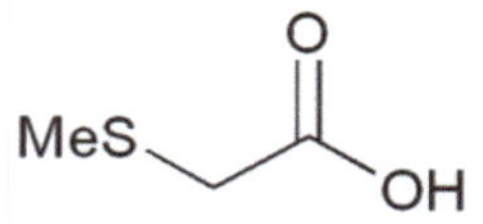

B.
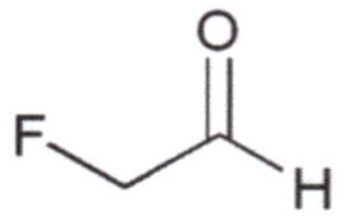

D.
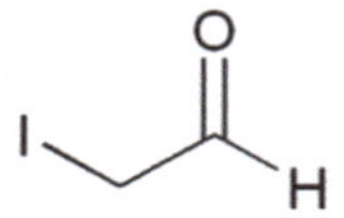

18) Which of the following acids has the largest pK_a?

- **A.** CH_3CO_2H
- **B.** FCH_2CO_2H
- **C.** CF_3CO_2H
- **D.** Cl_3CCO_2H

19) Which of the following organic compounds would have the strongest conjugate base?

A.
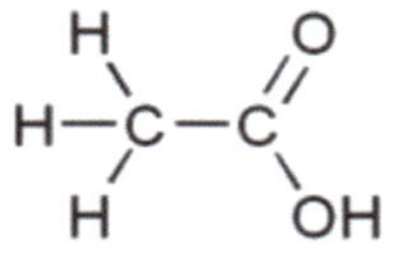

C.
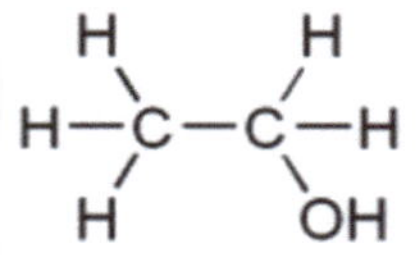

B.
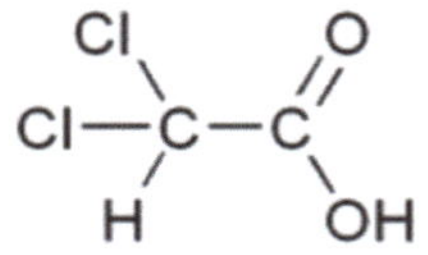

D.
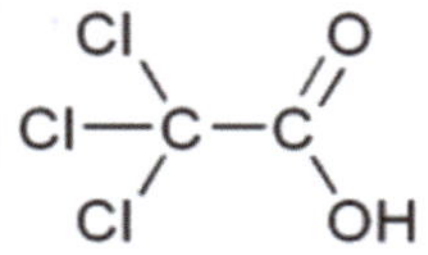

20) The pK_a of acetic acid in water is approximately 5. The pK_a of acetic acid in hexane would be expected to be which of the following?

- **A.** Less than 5
- **B.** Equal to 5
- **C.** More than 5
- **D.** Cannot be determined from the information provided.

High-level Importance

High-level Importance

SPOILER ALERT

Gold Standard has cross-referenced the content in this chapter to examples from ACER's official GAMSAT practice materials. It is for you to decide when you want to explore these questions since you may want to preserve some of ACER's materials for timed mock-exam practice.

Examples – EDG and EWG affect carboxylic acid strength (*note that ACER does expect that you know the relationship between pKa values and acid strength since they do not provide background information in this particular unit*): Q6-8 of 1; resonance structures with an example of the carboxylate anion, but most questions counted elsewhere: Q72-74 of 3; basic nomenclature of carboxylic acids, but otherwise, just reasoning: Q47-49 of 5. Note that "Q" is followed by the question number, and, for example, "of 1" refers to booklet number 1 which is referenced in the Spoiler Alert table at the end of Chapter 1. The 15 full-length GAMSAT practice tests by Gold Standard, HEAPS-1 through HEAPS-15, contain specific cross-references to this chapter within the worked solutions.

Chapter Checklist

- ☐ Access your online account to view answers, worked solutions and discussion boards.
- ☐ Reassess your 'learning objectives' for this chapter: Go back to the first page of this chapter and re-evaluate the top 3 boxes and the Introduction.
- ☐ Complete a maximum of 1 page of notes using symbols/abbreviations to represent the entire chapter based on your learning objectives. These are your Gold Notes.
- ☐ Consider your multimedia options based on your optimal way of learning:
  - ☐ Download the free Gold Standard GAMSAT app for your Android device or iPhone.
  - ☐ Create your own, tangible study cards or try the free app: Anki.
  - ☐ Record your voice reading your Gold Notes onto your smartphone (audio files, e.g., *memo* or MP3s) and listen during exercise, transportation, etc.
  - ☐ Try out the Gold Standard GAMSAT online videos at gamsat-prep.com, or you can try other options on YouTube like Khan Academy or Crash Course Organic Chemistry.
- ☐ Reassess your schedule for your full-length GAMSAT practice tests: ACER and/or HEAPS exams. Ensure that you have scheduled one full day to complete a practice test and 1-2 days for a thorough assessment of worked solutions while adding to your abbreviated Gold Notes.
- ☐ Reassess your progress in scheduling and/or evaluating stress reduction techniques such as regular exercise (sports), yoga, meditation and/or mindfulness exercises (*see* YouTube for suggestions).

CARBOXYLIC ACID DERIVATIVES
Chapter 9

Memorise

* IUPAC nomenclature

Understand

* Relative reactivity

Importance

Medium level: 6% of GAMSAT Organic Chemistry questions released by ACER are related to content in this chapter (in our estimation).
* Note that approximately 60% of the questions in GAMSAT Organic Chemistry are related to just 4 chapters: 2, 6, 7 and 12.

GAMSAT-Prep.com

Introduction

Carboxylic acid derivatives are a series of compounds that can be synthesised using carboxylic acids. For the GAMSAT, this includes acid chlorides, anhydrides, amides and esters.

Multimedia Resources at GAMSAT-Prep.com

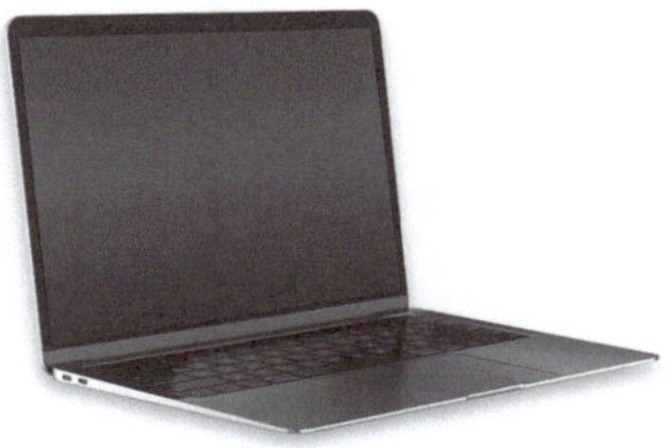

Open Discussion Boards
(*gamsat-prep.com/forum*)

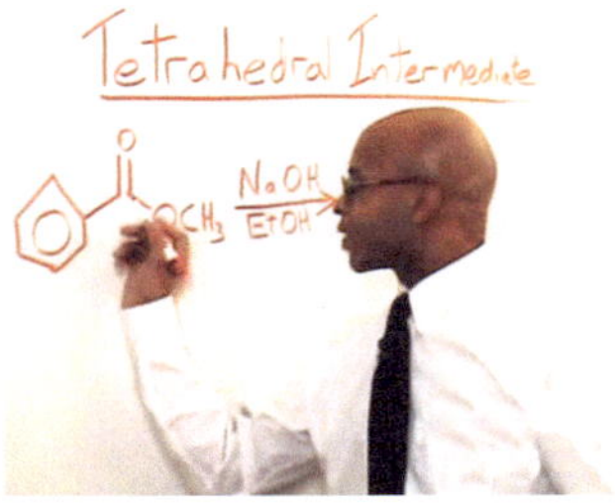

Science Preparation Videos

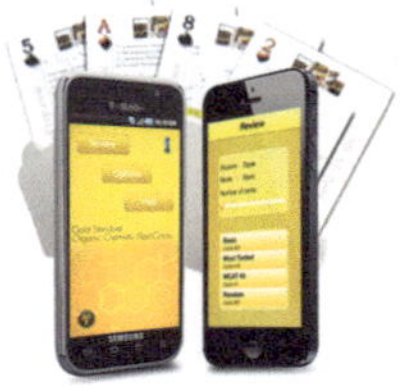

Flashcards

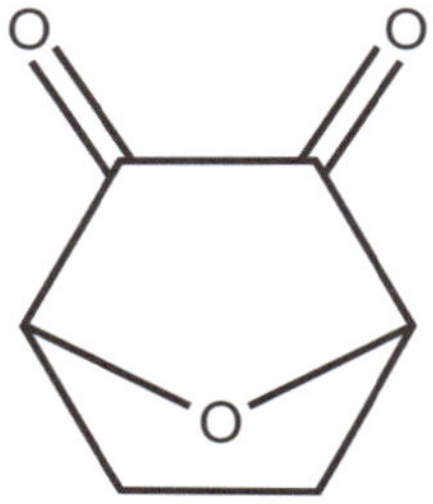

Special Guest

* The real GAMSAT may have advanced-level information presented (i.e. in a passage) but previous knowledge of said information is not required to answer the questions that would follow. Practice questions at the end of this chapter, as well as ACER and GS (HEAPS) practice GAMSATs can help you clarify this point.

9.1 Acid Halides (Acyl Halides)

Medium-level Importance

The general structure of an acid halide (= *acyl halide*) is:

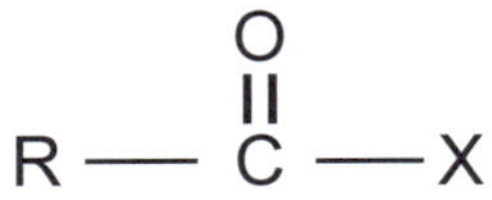

X = Halide

These are named by replacing the 'ic acid' of the parent carboxylic acid with the suffix 'yl halide.' For example:

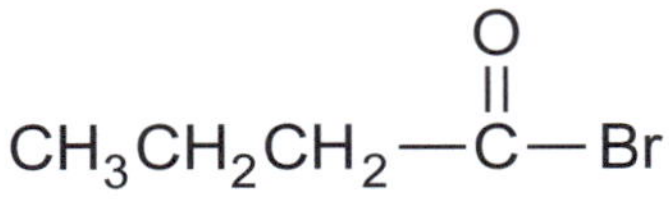

Butanoyl bromide

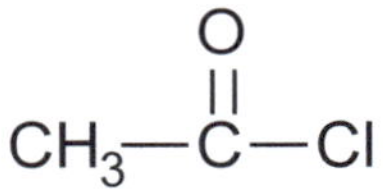

Acetyl chloride
(ethanoyl chloride)

An "acyl" group (IUPAC name: alkanoyl) refers to the functional group RCO-.

Acid chlorides are synthesised by reacting the parent carboxylic acid with PCl_5 or $SOCl_2$. Acid chlorides react with $NaBH_4$ to form alcohols. This can be done in one or two steps. In one step, the acid chloride reacts with $NaBH_4$ to immediately form an alcohol. In two steps, the acid chloride can react first with H_2/Pd/C to form a carboxylic acid; reaction of the carboxylic acid with $NaBH_4$ then produces an alcohol.

Acid halides can engage in nucleophilic reactions similar to carboxylic acids (*see* ORG 8.2); however, acid halides are more reactive (*see* ORG 9.6).

Acyl halides can be converted back to carboxylic acids through simple hydrolysis with H_2O. They can also be converted to esters by a reaction with alcohols. Lastly, acyl halides can be converted to amides ($RCONR_2$) by a reaction with amines.

9.1.1 Acid Anhydrides

The general structure of an acid anhydride is:

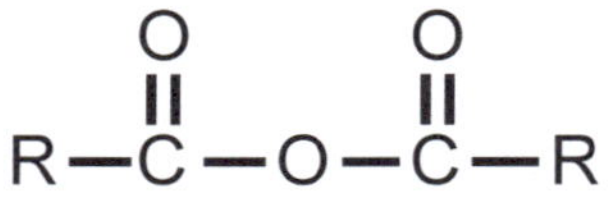

These are named by replacing the 'acid' of the parent carboxylic acid with the word 'anhydride.' For example:

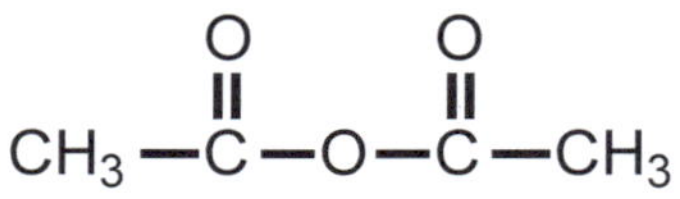

acetic anhydride
(ethanoic anhydride)

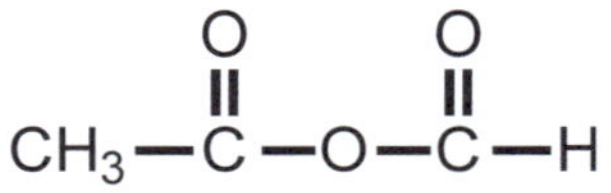

acetic formic anhydride
(ethanoic methanoic anhydride)

Anhydrides can be synthesised by the reaction of an acyl halide with a carboxylate salt and are a bit less reactive than acyl chlorides.

Both acid chlorides and acid anhydrides have boiling points comparable to esters of similar molecular weight.

9.2 Important Reactions of Carboxylic Acid Derivatives

- Nucleophilic acyl substitution reaction: Carboxylic acid derivatives undergo nucleophilic acyl substitution reactions in which a potential leaving group is substituted by the nucleophile, thereby generating a new carbonyl compound. Relative reactivity of carboxylic acid derivatives toward a nucleophilic acyl substitution reaction is amide < ester < acid anhydride < acid chloride. Note that it is possible to convert a more reactive carboxylic acid derivative to a less reactive one, but not the opposite.

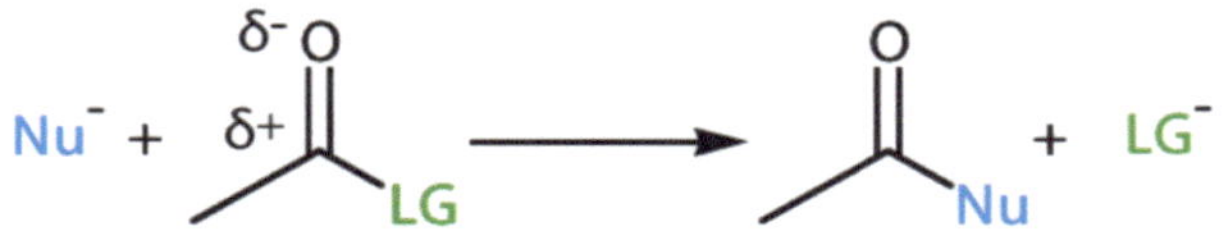

- Synthesis of acid halides: Acid halides are synthesised from carboxylic acids by the reaction with thionyl chloride ($SOCl_2$), phosphorus trichloride (PCl_3) or phosphorus pentachloride (PCl_5). Reaction with phosphorus tribromide PBr_3 produces an acid bromide.

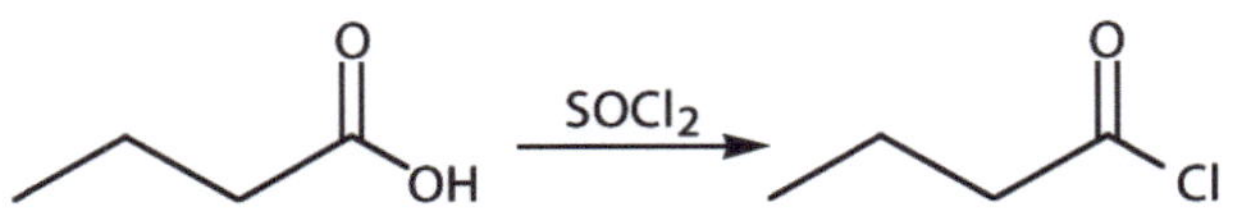

- Reactions of acid halides:

1. **Friedel-Crafts reaction:** A benzene ring attacks a carbocation electrophile -COR which is generated by the reaction with the $AlCl_3$ catalyst, yielding the final product Ar-COR.

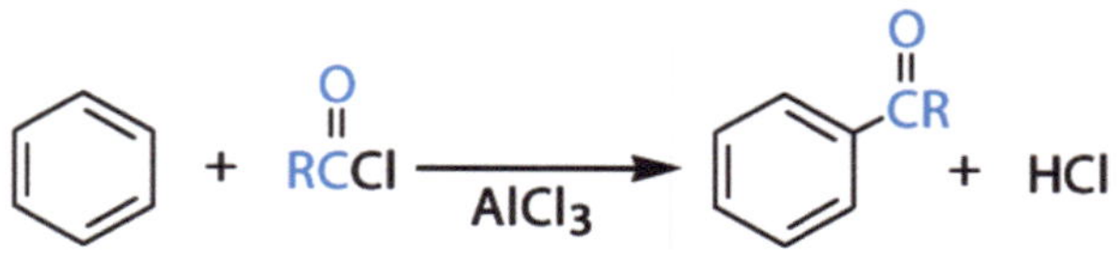

2. **Conversion into acids:** Acid chlorides react with water to yield carboxylic acids. The attack of the nucleophile water followed by elimination of the chloride ion gives the products carboxylic acid and HCl.

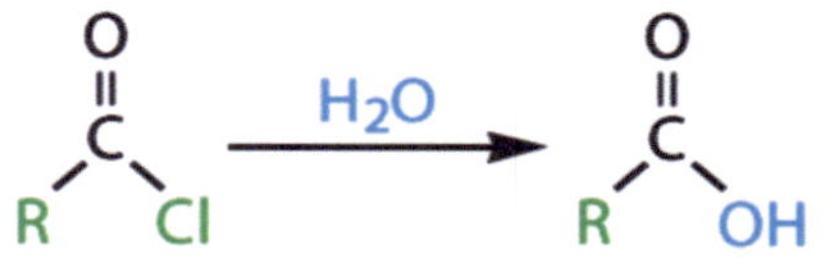

3. **Conversion into esters:** Acid chlorides react with alcohol to yield esters. The same type of nucleophilic acyl substitution mechanism is observed here. The alkoxide ion attacks the acid chloride while chloride is displaced.

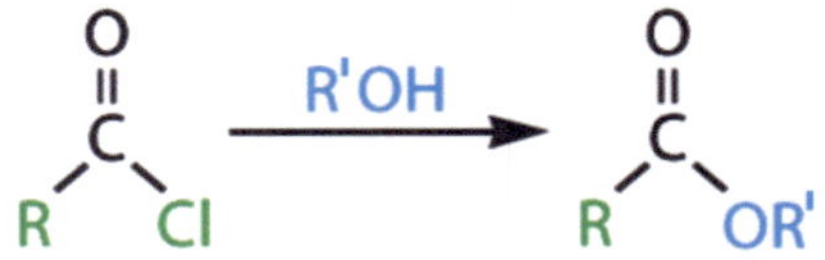

4. **Conversion into amides:** Acid chlorides react with ammonia or amines to yield amides. Both mono- and disubstituted amines react well with acid chlorides, but not trisubstituted amines. Two equivalents of ammonia or amine must be used: one reacting with the acid chloride while the other reacting with HCl to form the ammonium chloride salt.

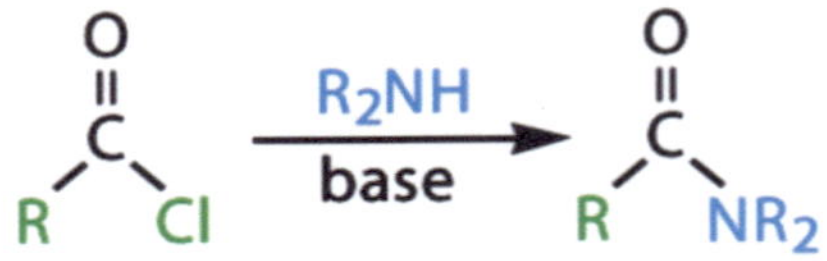

5. **Conversion into alcohols:** Acid chlorides are reduced by $LiAlH_4$ to yield primary alcohols. The reaction is a substitution reaction of -H for -Cl, which is then further reduced to yield the final product alcohol.

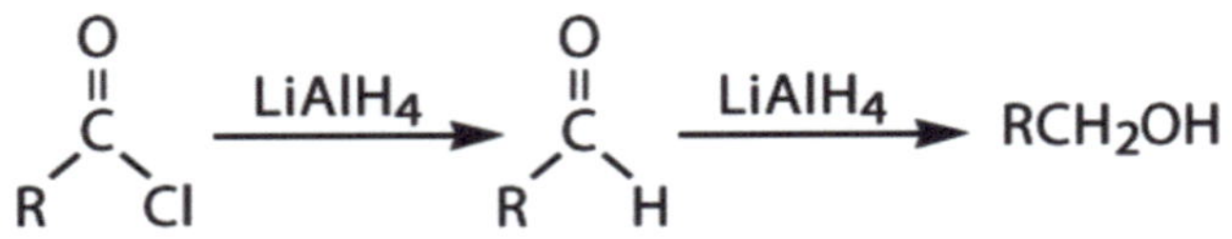

Acid chlorides react with Grignard reagents to yield tertiary alcohols. Two equivalents of the Grignard reagent attack the acid chloride yielding the final product, the tertiary alcohol.

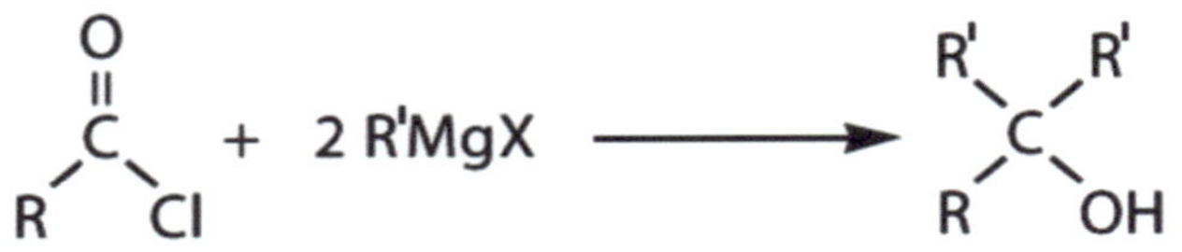

Acid chlorides also react with H_2 in the presence of Lindlar's catalyst ($Pd/BaSO_4$, quinoline) to yield an aldehyde intermediate which can then be further reduced to yield an alcohol.

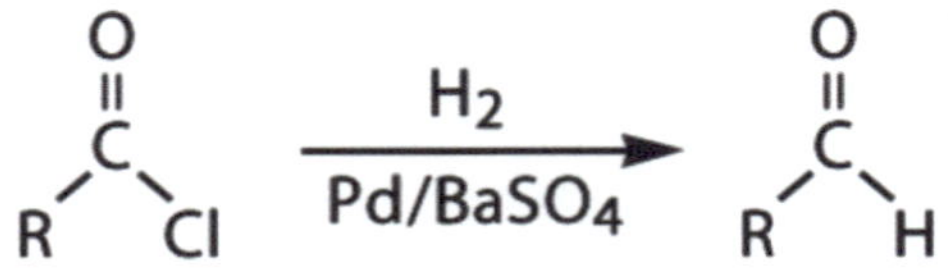

6. **Synthesis of acid anhydrides:** Acid anhydrides can be synthesised by a nucleophilic acyl substitution reaction of an acid chloride with a carboxylate anion.

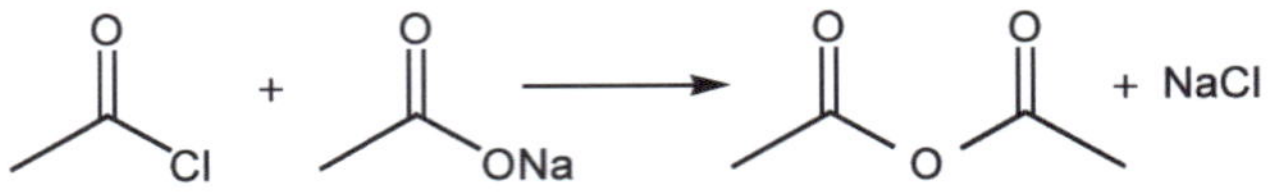

- Reactions of acid anhydrides: The chemistry of acid anhydrides is similar to that of acid chlorides. Since they are more stable due to resonance, acid anhydrides react more slowly.

1. **Conversion into acids:** Acid anhydrides react with water to yield carboxylic acids. The nucleophile in this reaction is water and the leaving group is a carboxylic acid.

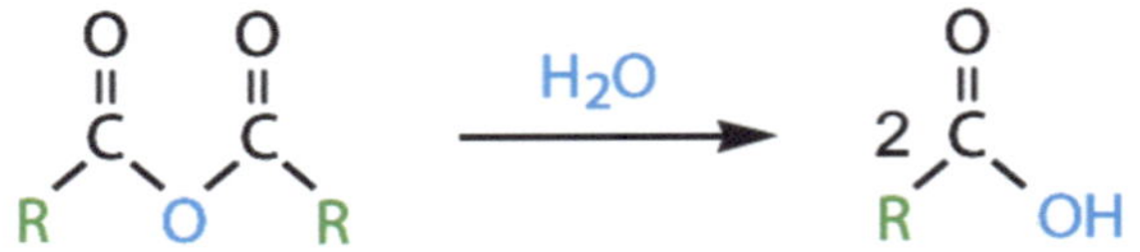

2. **Conversion into esters:** Acid anhydrides react with alcohols to form esters and acids as in the following example with ethanoic anhydride.

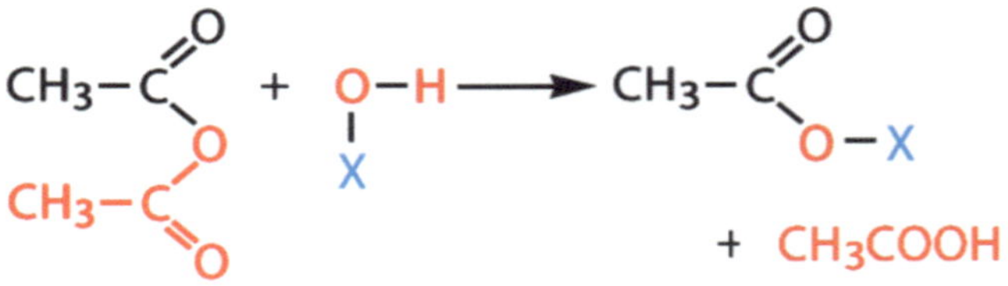

3. **Conversion into amides:** Ammonia (or an amine, ORG 11.1) attacks the acid anhydride, yielding an amide and the leaving group carboxylic acid, which is reacted with another molecule of ammonia to give the ammonium salt of the carboxylate anion.

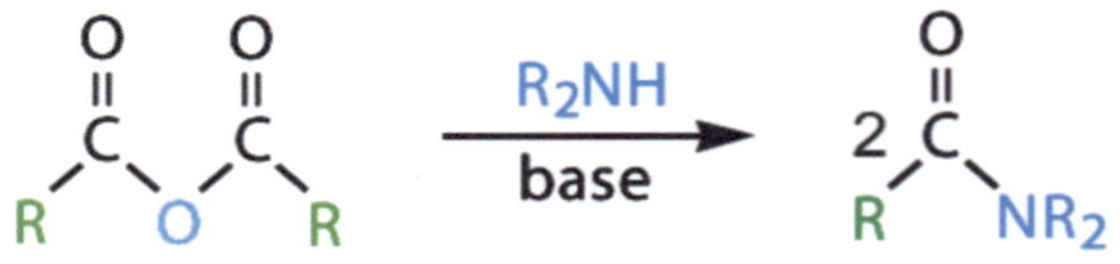

4. **Conversion into alcohols:** Acid anhydrides are reduced by $LiAlH_4$ "[H]" to yield primary alcohols.

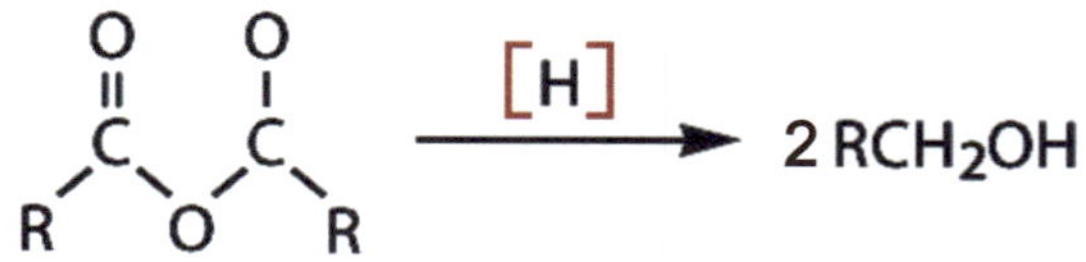

9.3 Amides

The general structure of an amide is:

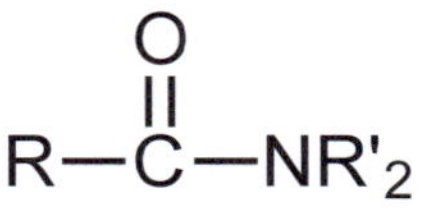

These are named by replacing the '-ic (oic) acid' of the parent anhydride with the suffix '-amide.' If there are alkyl groups attached to the nitrogen, they are named as substituents, and designated by the letter N. For example:

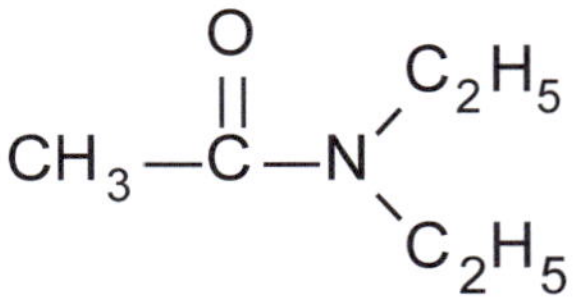
N,N-diethylacetamide

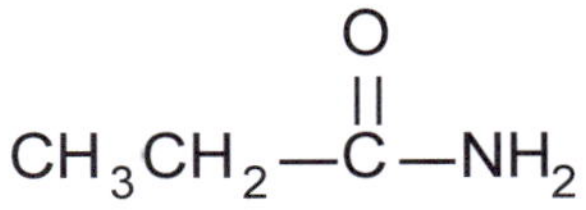
propanamide

Both unsubstituted and monosubstituted amides form very strong intermolecular hydrogen bonds, and as a result, they have very high boiling and melting points. The boiling points of disubstituted amides are similar to those of aldehydes and ketones. Amides are essentially neutral (no acidity, as compared to carboxylic acids, and no basicity, as compared to amines).

Amides may be prepared by reacting carboxylic acids (or other carboxylic acid derivatives) with ammonia:

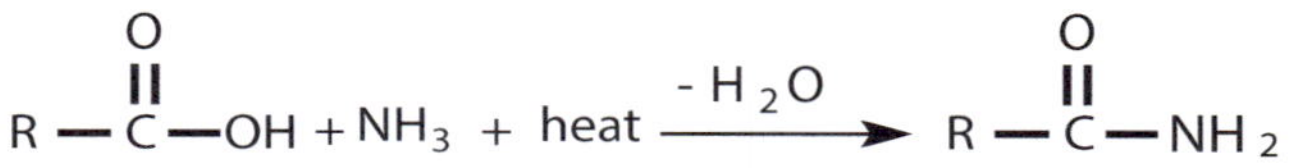

As well, amides undergo nucleophilic substitution reactions at the carbonyl carbon:

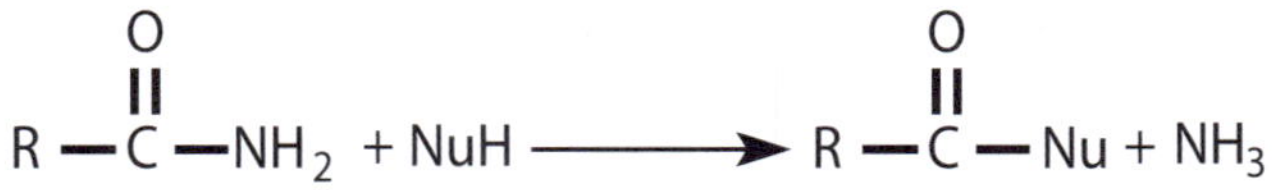

Amides can be hydrolysed to yield the parent carboxylic acid and amine. This reaction may take place under acidic or basic conditions:

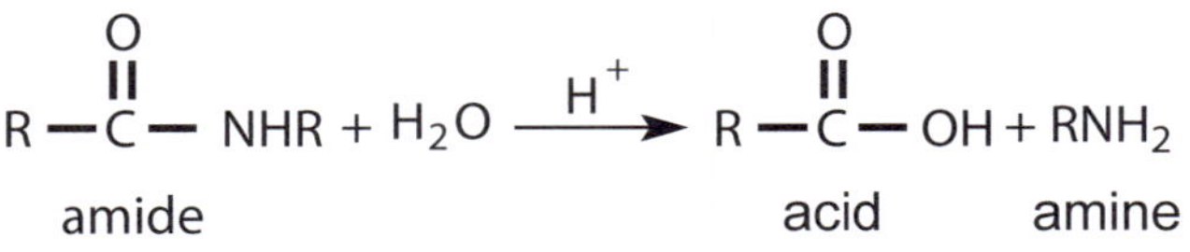

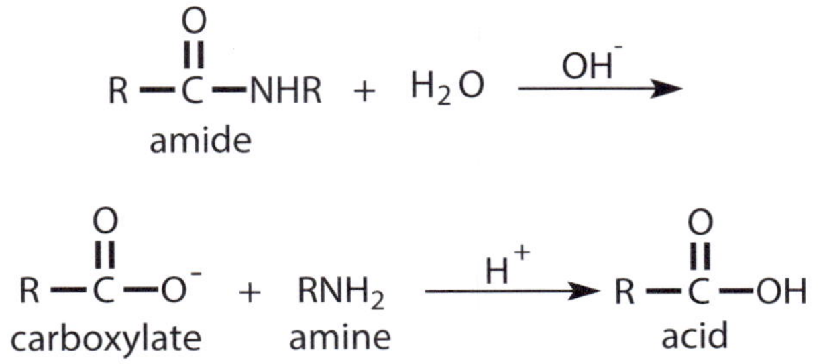

Amides can also form amines by reacting with $LiAlH_4$.

Amides can also be converted to primary amines with the loss of the carbonyl carbon. This is known as a Hofmann rearrangement:

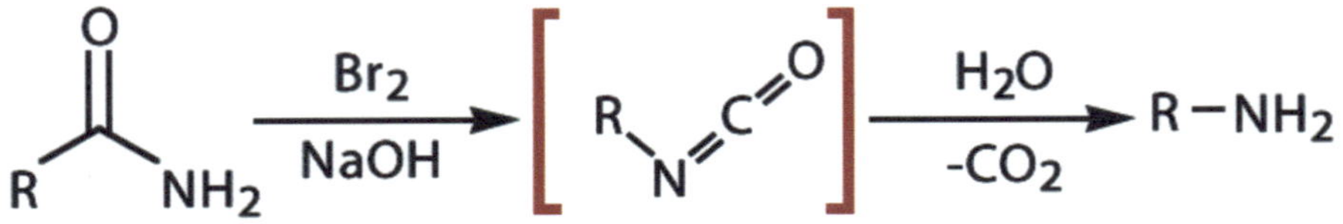

9.3.1 Important Reactions of Amides

Amides are much less reactive than acid chlorides, acid anhydrides or esters.

1. **Conversion into acids:** Amides react with water to yield carboxylic acids in acidic conditions or carboxylate anions in basic conditions.

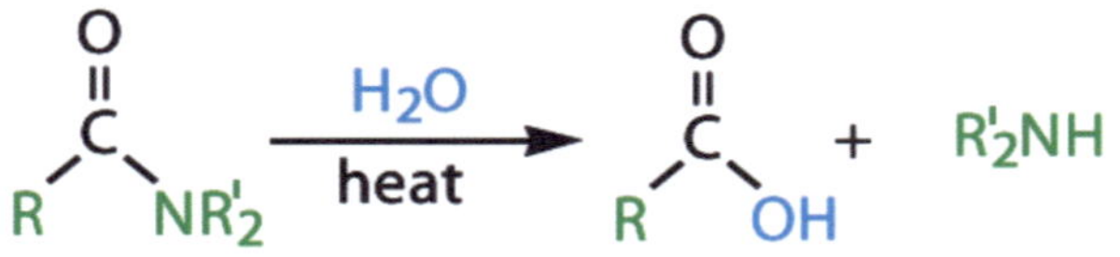

2. **Conversion into amines:** Amides can be reduced by $LiAlH_4$ to give amines. The net effect of this reaction is to convert an amide carbonyl group into a methylene group ($C{=}O \longrightarrow CH_2$).

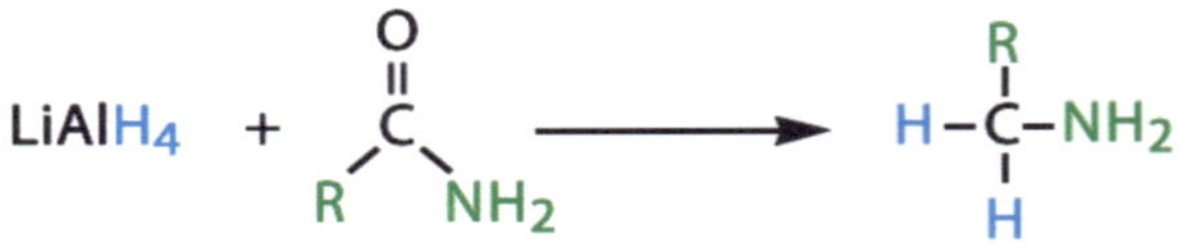

9.4 Esters

The general structure of an ester is:

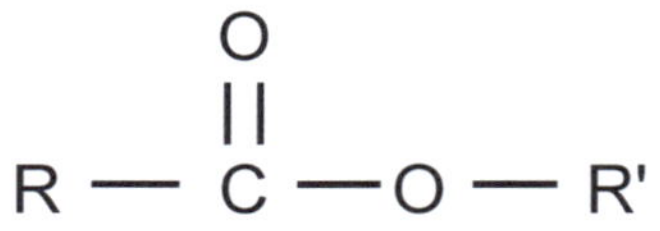

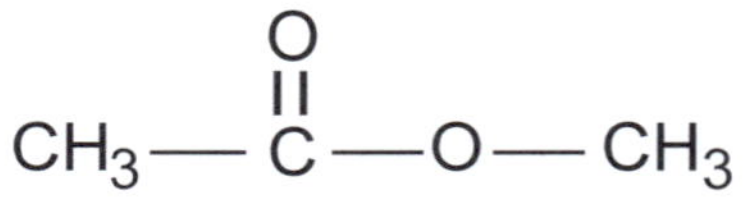

methyl acetate
(methyl ethanoate)

These are named by first citing the name of the alkyl group, followed by the parent acid, with the 'ic acid' replaced by 'ate.' For example:

The boiling points of esters are lower than those of comparable acids or alcohols, and similar to comparable aldehydes and ketones, because they are polar compounds, without hydrogens to form hydrogen bonds. Esters with longer side chains (R-groups) are more nonpolar than esters with shorter side chains (R-groups). Esters usually have pleasing, fruity odors.

Esters may be synthesised by reacting carboxylic acids or their derivatives with alcohols under either basic or acidic conditions:

$$\underset{\text{alcohol}}{R'O^{*}H} + \underset{\text{acid}}{R-\overset{\overset{O}{\|}}{C}-OH} \longrightarrow \underset{\text{ester}}{R-\overset{\overset{O}{\|}}{C}-O^{*}R'} + H_2O$$

As well, esters undergo nucleophilic substitution reactions at the carbonyl carbon:

$$R-\overset{\overset{O}{\|}}{C}-OR' + NuH \longrightarrow R-\overset{\overset{O}{\|}}{C}-Nu + R'OH$$

Esters may also be hydrolysed, to yield the parent carboxylic acid and alcohol. This reaction may take place under acidic or basic conditions.

$$\underset{\text{ester}}{R-\overset{\overset{O}{\|}}{C}-O^{*}R'} + H_2O \xrightarrow{H^+}$$

$$\underset{\text{acid}}{R-\overset{\overset{O}{\|}}{C}-OH} + \underset{\text{alcohol}}{R'O^{*}H}$$

Esters can be transformed from one ester into another by using alcohols as nucleophiles. This process is known as transesterification:

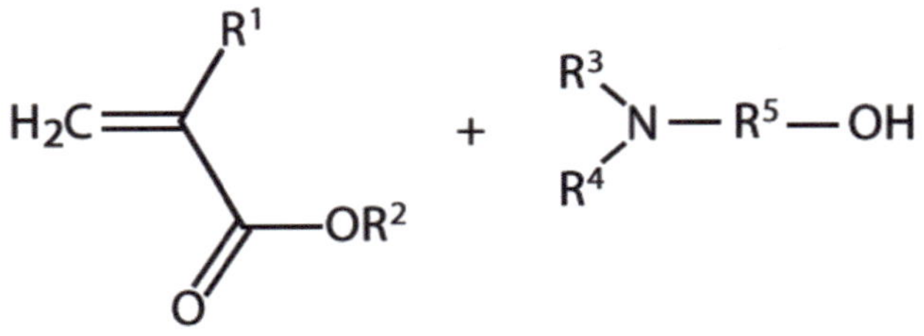

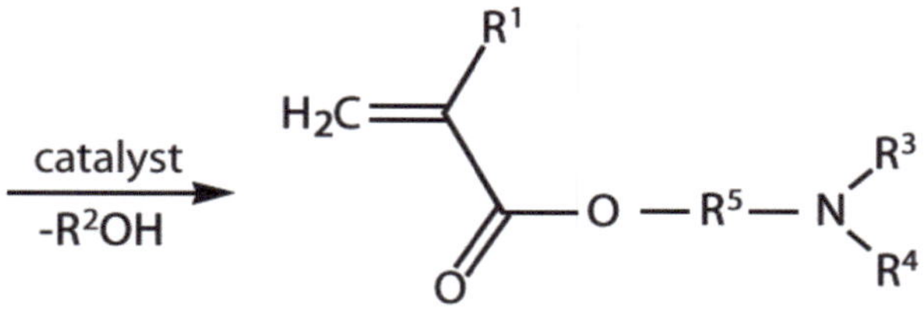

Another reaction type involves the formation of ketones using Grignard reagents. The ketone formed is usually only temporary and is further reduced to a tertiary alcohol due to the reactive nature of the newly formed ketone:

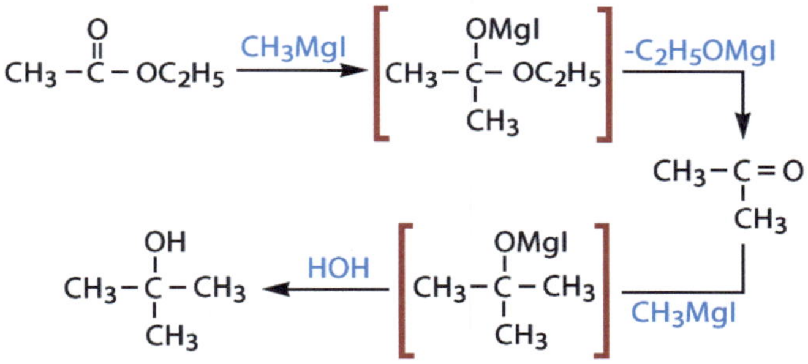

2-methylpropan-2-ol
(*tert*-butanol)

Medium-level Importance

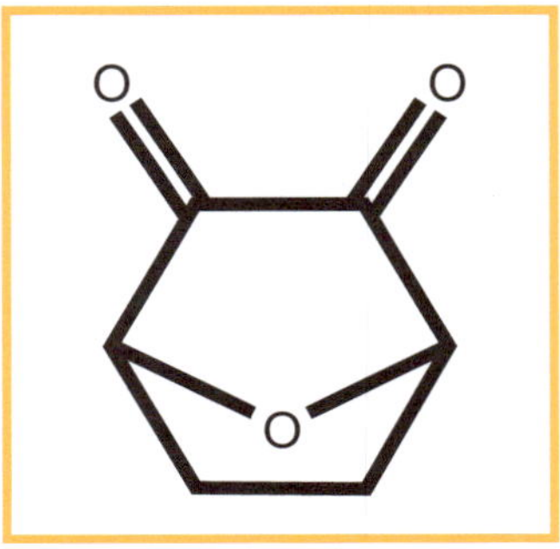

The Ester Bunny

NB: The Ester Bunny is NOT GAMSAT material. In fact for you super-keeners: is the Ester Bunny a real ester? Find out in our Forum!

An important reaction of esters involves the combination of two ester molecules to form an acetoacetic ester (when two moles of ethyl acetate are combined). This is known as the Claisen condensation and is similar to the aldol condensation seen in ORG 7.2.4:

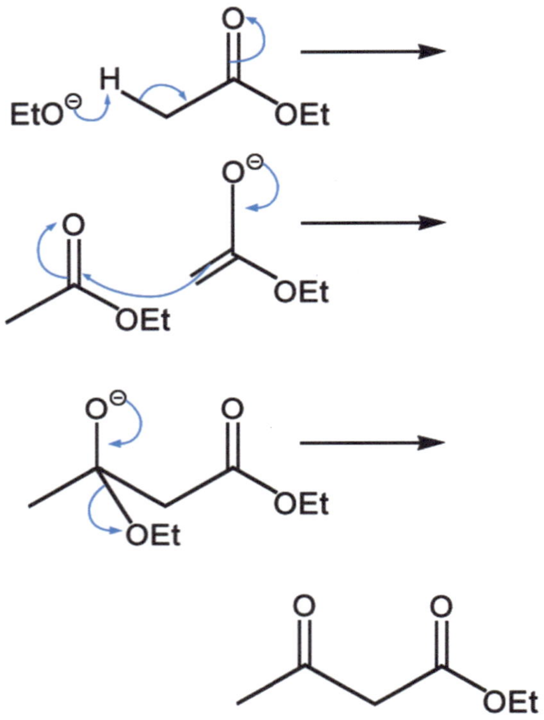

- More reactions with esters: Esters have similar chemistry to acid chlorides and acid anhydrides; however, they are less reactive toward nucleophilic substitution reactions.

1. **Conversion into amides:** Esters can react with ammonia or amines to give amides and an alcohol side product.

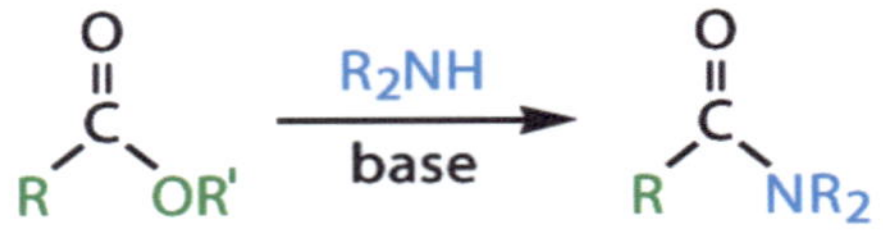

2. **Conversion into alcohols**: Esters can be easily reduced by $LiAlH_4$ to form primary alcohols. A hydride ion attacks the ester carbonyl carbon to form a tetrahedral intermediate. Loss of the alkoxide ion from the intermediate yields an aldehyde intermediate, which is further reduced by another hydride ion to give a primary alcohol final product.

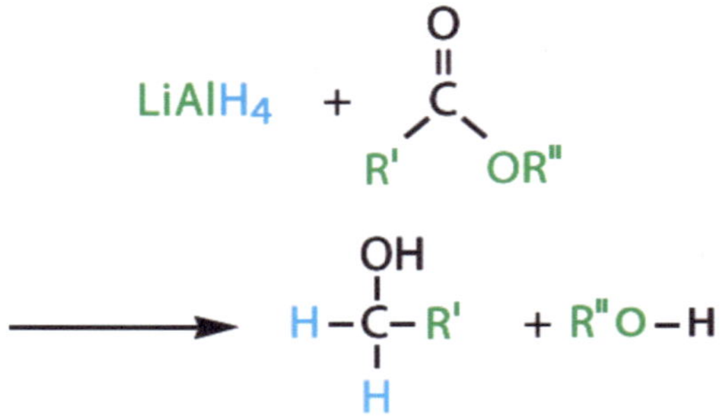

Esters can also be reduced to tertiary alcohols by reacting with a Grignard reagent (or alkyl lithium). Grignard reagents add to the ester carbonyl carbon to form ketone intermediates, which are further attacked by the next equivalent of the Grignard reagent. Thus two equivalents of the Grignard reagent (or alkyl lithium) are used to produce tertiary alcohols.

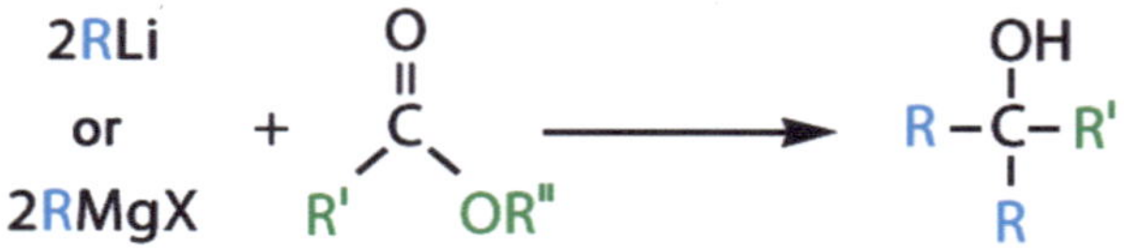

9.4.1 Fats, Glycerides and Saponification

A special class of esters is known as fats (i.e. mono-, di-, and triglycerides). These are biologically important molecules, and they are formed in the following reaction:

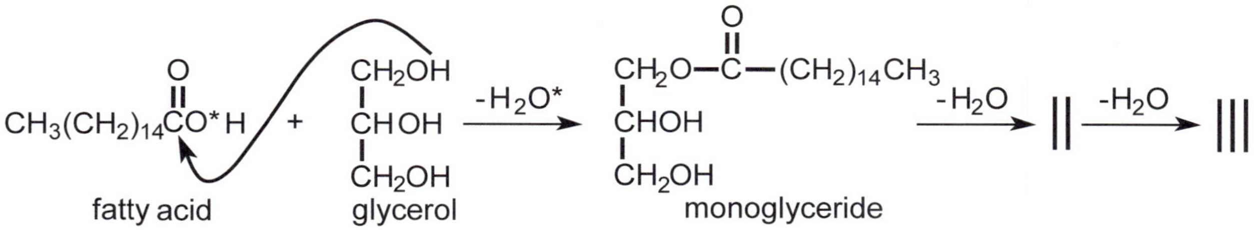

Fatty acids (= *long chain carboxylic acids*) are formed through the condensation of C2 units derived from acetate, and may be added to the monoglyceride formed in the above reaction, forming diglycerides, and triglycerides. Fats may be hydrolysed by a base to the components glycerol and the salt of the fatty acids. The salts of long chain carboxylic acids are called <u>soaps</u>. Thus this process is called *saponification*:

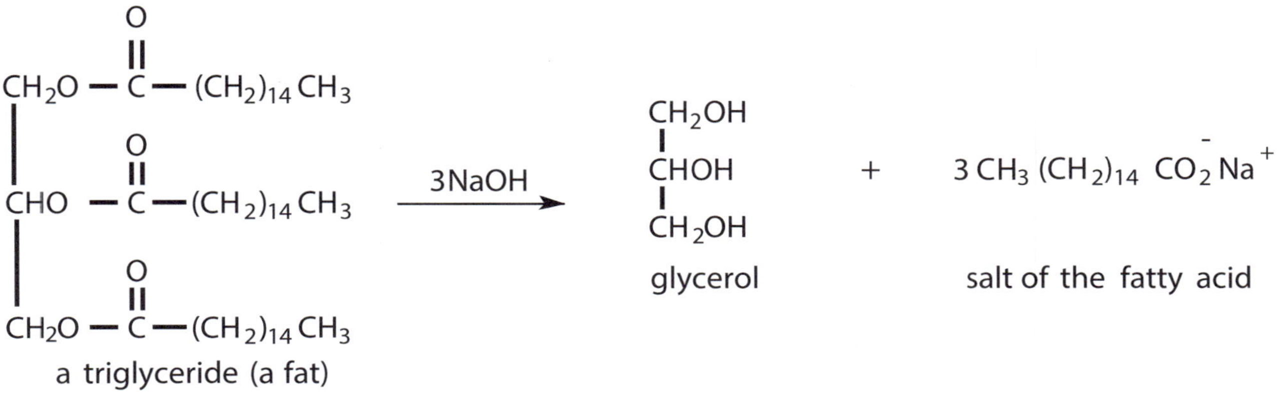

9.5 β-Keto Acids

β-keto acids are carboxylic acids with a keto group (i.e. *ketone*) at the β position. Thus it is an acid with a carbonyl group one carbon removed from a carboxylic acid group. Upon heating, the carboxyl group can be readily removed as CO_2. This process is called *decarboxylation*. For example:

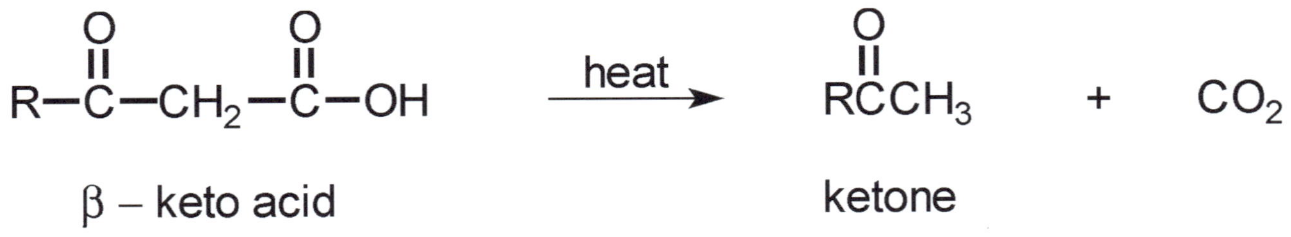

9.6 Relative Reactivity of Carboxylic Acid Derivatives

Medium-level Importance

Any factors that make the carbonyl group more easily attacked by nucleophiles favor the nucleophilic acyl substitution reaction. In terms of nucleophilic substitution, generally, carboxylic acid derivatives are more reactive than comparable non-carboxylic acid derivatives. One important reason for the preceding is that the carbon in carboxylic acids is also attached to the electronegative oxygen atom of the carbonyl group; therefore, carbon is more δ^+, thus being more attractive to a nucleophile. Hence an acid chloride (R-COCl) is more reactive than a comparable alkyl chloride (R-Cl); an ester (R-COOR') is more reactive than a comparable ether (R-OR'); and an amide (R-$CONH_2$) is more reactive than a comparable amine (R-NH_2).

Amongst carboxylic acid derivatives, the carbonyl reactivity in order from most to least reactive is:

acid chlorides > anhydrides >> esters
> acids > amides > nitriles

The reasons for this may be attributed to resonance effects and inductive effects. The resonance effect is the ability of the substituent to stabilise the carbocation intermediate by delocalisation of electrons. The inductive effect is the substituent group, by virtue of its electronegativity, to pull electrons away increasing the partial positivity of the carbonyl carbon.

Within each carboxylic acid derivative, steric or bulk effects also play an important role. The less the steric hindrance (ORG 2.4, 6.2.3), the more access a nucleophile will have to attack the carbonyl carbon, and vice versa.

9.7 Phosphate Esters

Phosphoric acid derivatives have similar features to those of carboxylic acid derivatives. Phosphoric acid and mono- or di-phosphoric esters are acidic. Under acidic conditions, these phosphoric esters can be converted to the parent acid H_3PO_4 and alcohols. To see the structure of phosphate esters, *see* ORG 12.5.

CHAPTER 9: Carboxylic Acid Derivatives

GOLD STANDARD FOUNDATIONAL GAMSAT PRACTICE QUESTIONS

1) Ethyl acetate is also known as which of the following?

A. Ethyl ethanoate
B. Ethanoic acid and ethanol
C. Acetic acid and ethanol
D. All of the above

2) Name the following compound.

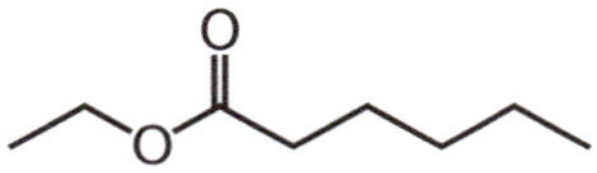

A. Methyl pentanoate
B. Ethyl pentanoate
C. Methyl hexanoate
D. Ethyl hexanoate

3) Name the following compound.

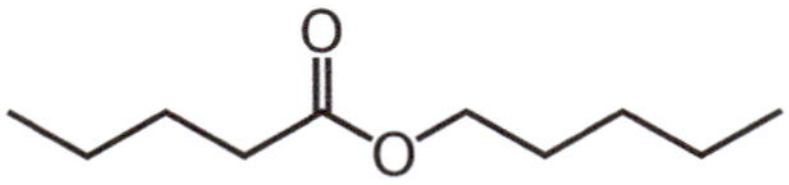

A. Pentyl pentanoate
B. Butyl butanoate
C. Pentyl butanoate
D. Dibutyl propanoate

4) Name the following compound.

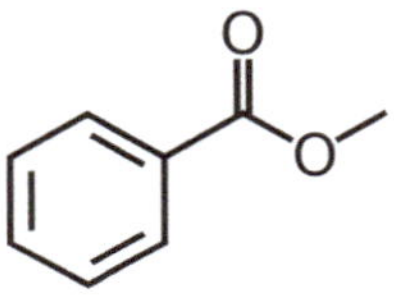

A. Benzyl methanoate
B. Methyl benzoate
C. Benzyl ethanoate
D. Ethyl benzoate

5) Name the following compound.

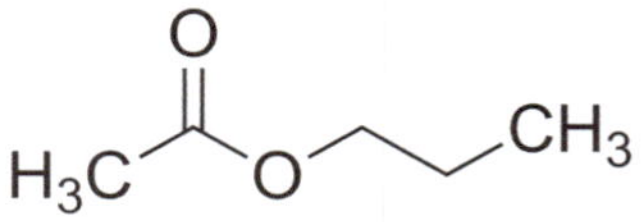

A. Acetyl methanoate
B. Methyl ethanoate
C. Ethyl propanoate
D. Propyl ethanoate

6) Name the following compound

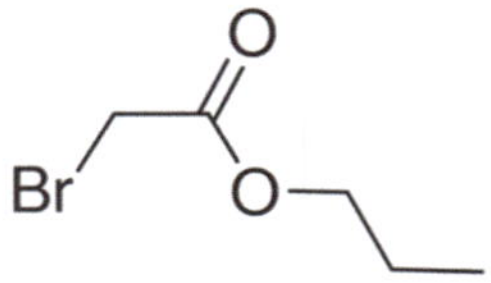

A. Bromoacetyl ethanoate
B. Ethyl bromoethanoate
C. Bromoethyl propanoate
D. Propyl bromoacetate

7) Which compound is an amide?

A.
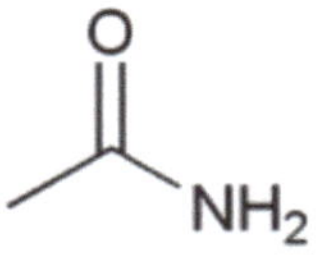

B.
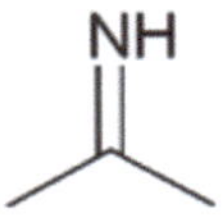

C.
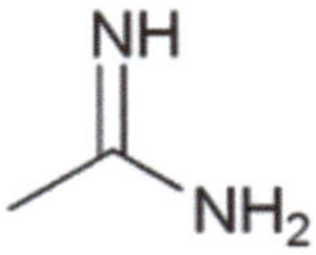

D.
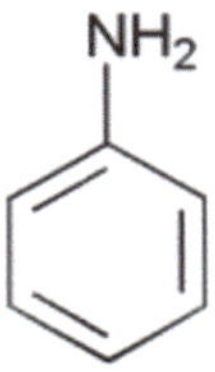

8) Which compound is a tertiary amide?

A. 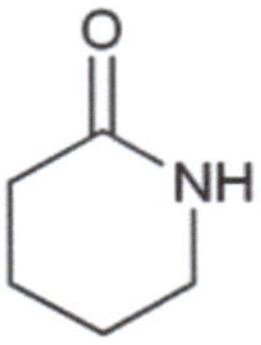

C. 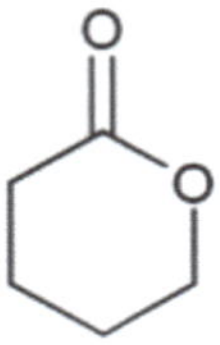

B. 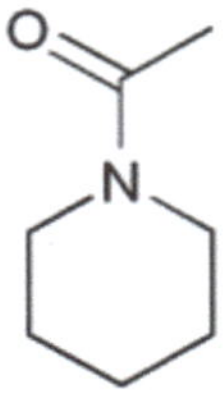

D. 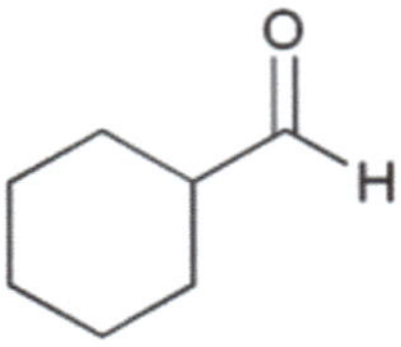

9) Which of the following is an amide?

A. 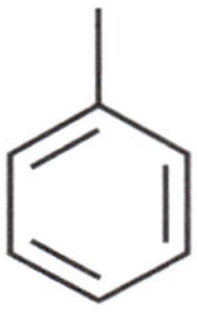

C. 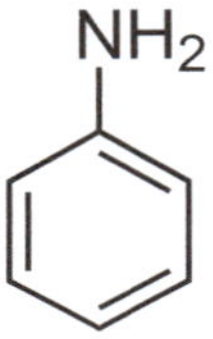

B. 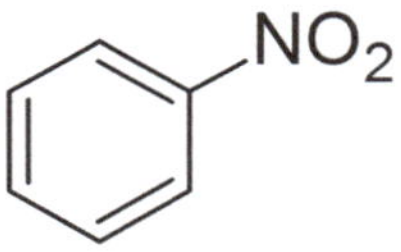

D. 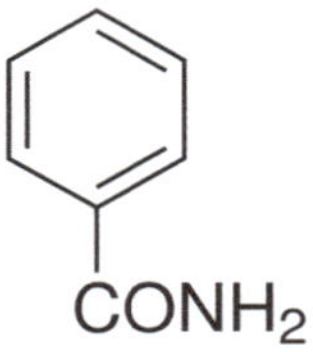

10) Which of the following is an anhydride?

A. 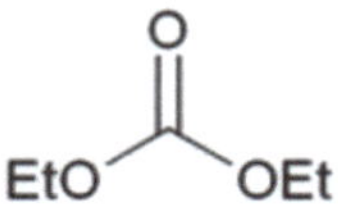

C. 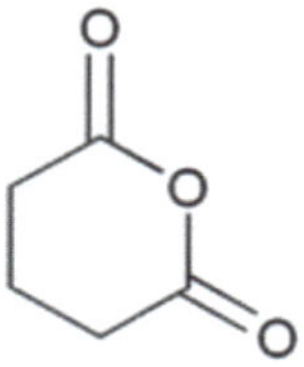

B. 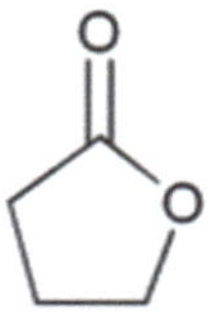

D. 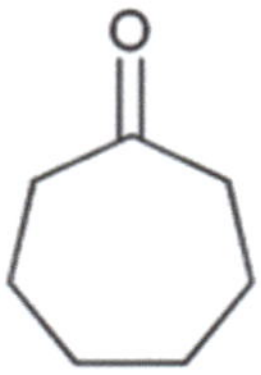

11) Which compound is an acyclic (*not* cyclic) ester?

A. 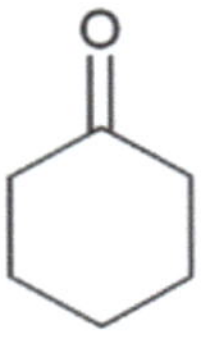

C. 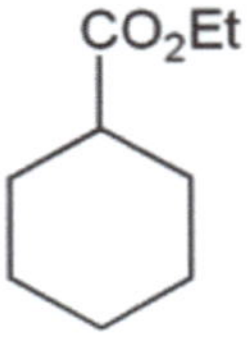

B. 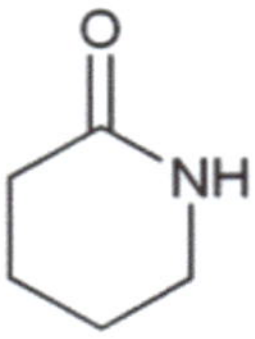

D. 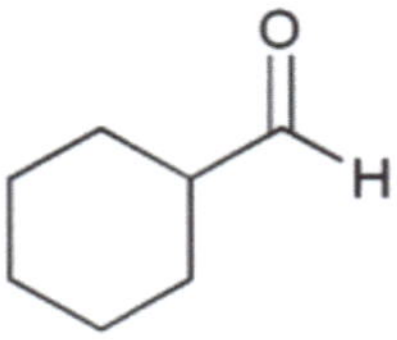

12) Which compound is a cyclic ester?

A. 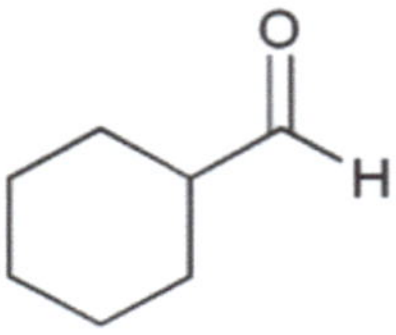

C. 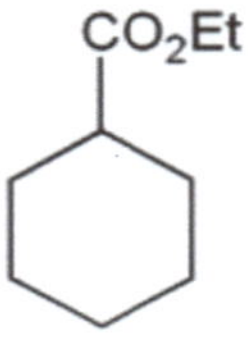

B. 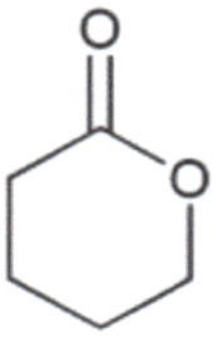

D. 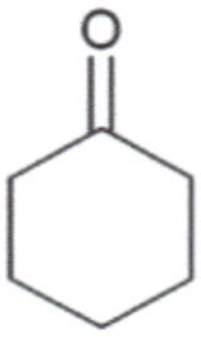

13) The transition shown below is an example of what type of chemical reaction?

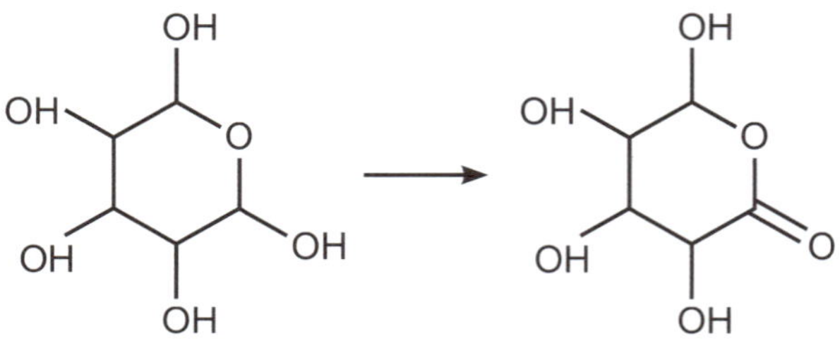

A. Reduction
B Oxidation
C. Dehydration
D. Sigmatropic rearrangement

GOLD STANDARD GAMSAT-LEVEL PRACTICE QUESTIONS

Questions 14–15

The **simplified molecular-input line-entry system** (SMILES) is a specification in the form of a line notation for describing the structure of chemical species using short ASCII strings. SMILES strings can be imported by most molecule editors for conversion back into two-dimensional drawings or three-dimensional models of the molecules.

Consider the structural formula and the SMILES notation below of acetylsalicylic acid, more commonly known as aspirin.

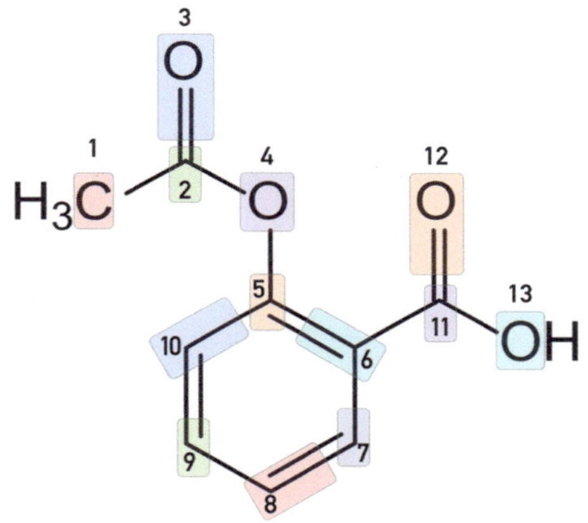

1 2 3 4 5 6 7 8 9 10 11 12 13

CC(=O)OC1=CC=CC=C1C(=O)O

Figure 1

Note that:

1) side chains are enclosed in parentheses;

2) double bonds are signified by the = (equality) symbol;

3) hydrogen atoms are not explicitly displayed as they can be inferred.

14) What is the SMILES notation for isobutanol (2-methylpropan-1-ol)?

A. CC(C)CO

B. CCCC(=O)

C. CC(C)COH

D. CC(=C)CO

15) Consider the ester tert-butyl formate.

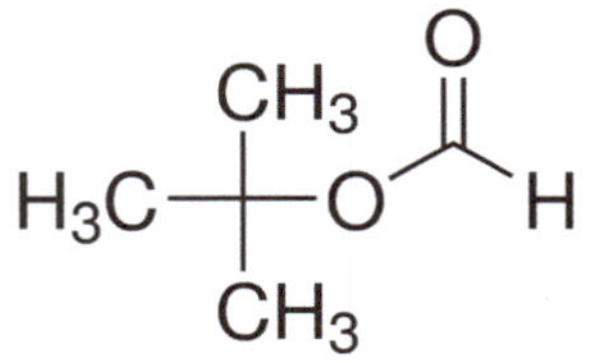

What is the SMILES notation for tert-butyl formate?

A. CC(C)(C)OC=O

B. (OC(C)(C)C)CO=C

C. CC(C)COC=OH

D. CCCOC=O

High-level Importance

Questions 16–24

Esters are often derived from a carboxylic acid and an alcohol with acid catalysis as follows:

$$\underset{\text{Hexanoic acid}}{CH_3(CH_2)_4CO_2H} + \underset{\text{Ethanol}}{CH_3CH_2OH} \xrightarrow{H^+} \underset{\text{Ethyl hexanoate}}{CH_3(CH_2)_4\overset{\overset{O}{\|}}{C}OCH_2CH_3}$$

The inorganic product that is not shown above is water.

The carbonyl carbon in a carboxylic acid is considered to be carbon-1. The adjacent carbon, carbon-2, is the alpha (α) carbon followed by the beta (β) carbon and the gamma (γ) carbon. Consider the structure of butanoic acid (i.e. butyric acid) with the carbons labelled appropriately.

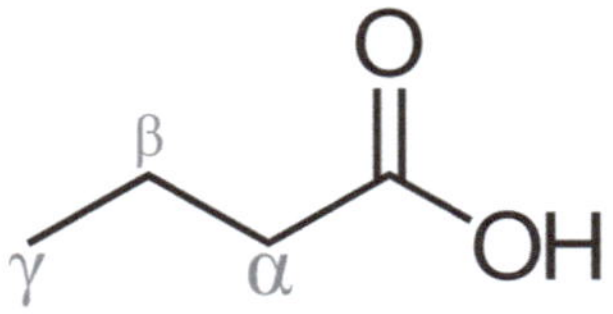

16) Lactone rings are cyclic esters that occur widely as building blocks in nature, such as in ascorbic acid and hormones, in addition to many medications. Lactones are formed by an intramolecular reaction. One of the ways to identify a lactone is to describe it based on the location of the hydroxy group which produced that lactone.

Based on this information, which of the following would be regarded as an alpha lactone?

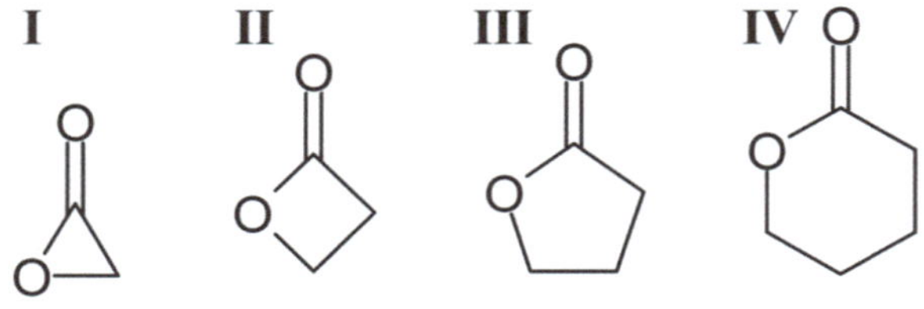

A. I
B. II
C. III
D. IV

17) Based on the information provided, which of the four preceding molecules would be the expected product of 4-hydroxybutanoic acid and an acid catalyst?

A. I
B. II
C. III
D. IV

18) Which of the following would be expected to produce a gamma-lactone?

A. 

B. 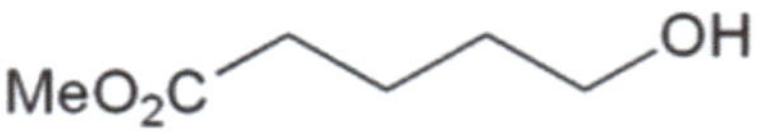

C. 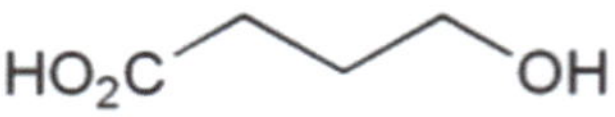

D. 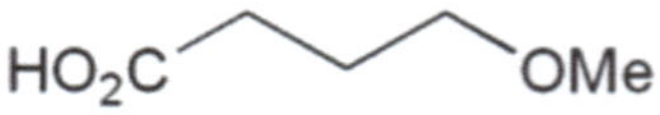

19) The monocyclic moiety of Lovastatin, a medication to lower cholesterol, is a hydroxylactone ("beta-hydroxy-delta-lactone"), and is shown below.

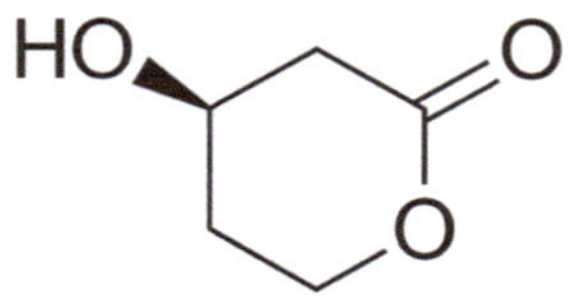

Which of the following with acid catalysis would be expected to produce the monocyclic moiety of Lovastatin and water?

A. 4-hydroxybutanoic acid
B. 3,4-dihydroxybutanoic acid
C. 5-hydroxypentanoic acid
D. 3,5-dihydroxypentanoic acid

20) Consider the following reaction which produces a lactone. Note the carbons in the reactant which are labelled 1, 2, 3 and 4.

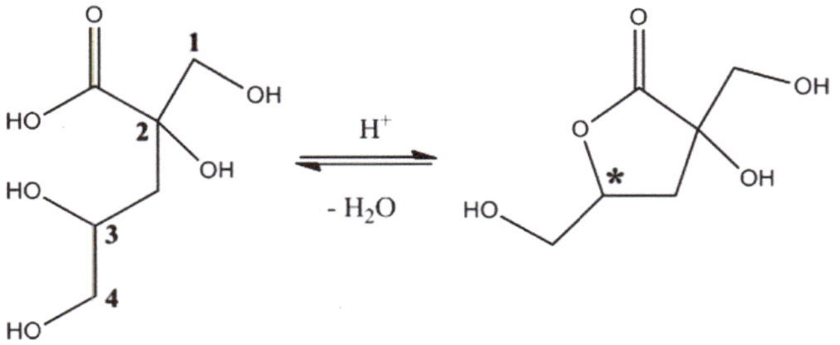

Identify the carbon in the reactant that is marked with the asterisk * in the lactone.

A. 1
B. 2
C. 3
D. 4

21) Based on the information provided, identify the product.

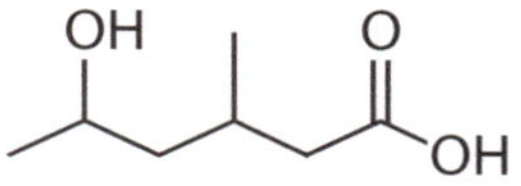

A. 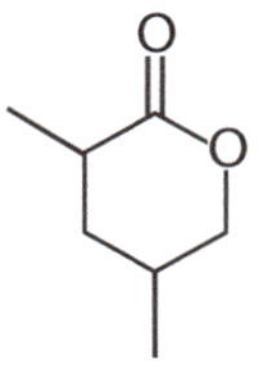

C. 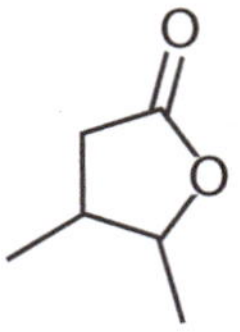

B. 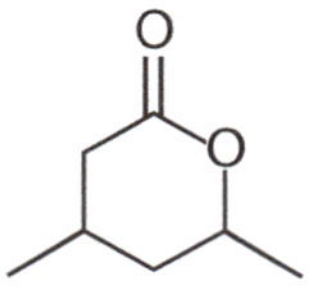

D. 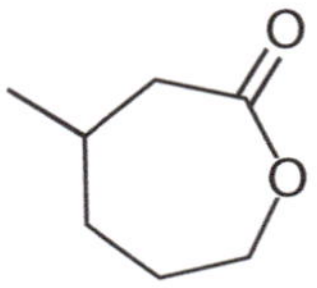

22) Consider the following additional information. A lactide is a lactone cyclic di-ester. Consider the following lactide.

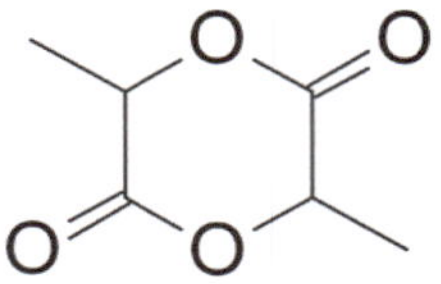

Which of the following molecules would likely make the lactide above after an acid-catalysed dehydration?

A. 1 x 2-hydroxyethanoic acid + 1 x ethanoic acid
B. 2 x 2-hydroxyethanoic acid
C. 1 x 2-hydroxyethanoic acid + 1 x 2-hydroxypropanoic acid
D. 2 x 2-hydroxypropanoic acid

23) Consider the molecule phthalic anhydride below.

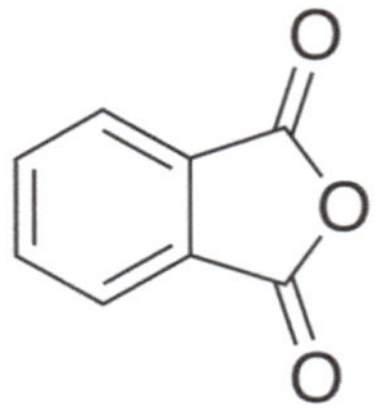

Phthalic anhydride can be produced using a similar sequence as lactone production. Which of the following molecules would likely be the reactant to produce phthalic anhydride?

A.

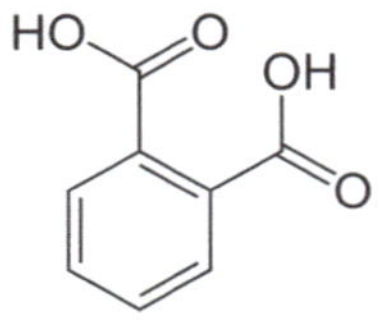

C.

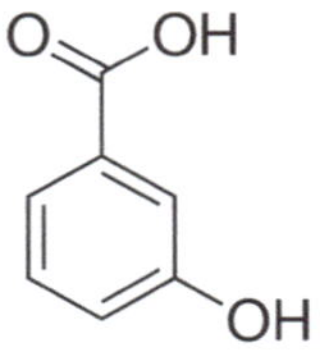

B.

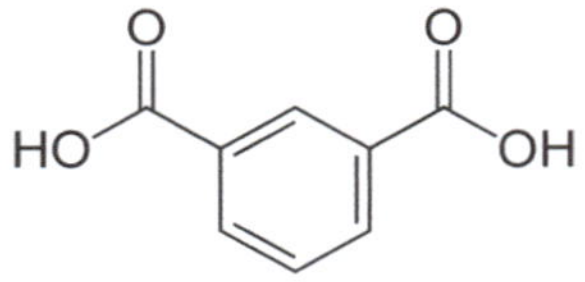

D.

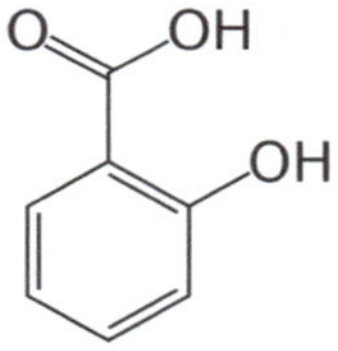

24) A lactam is a cyclic amide. The term combines portions of the words *lactone* + *amide*. Consider the following lactams.

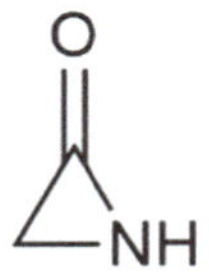

α-lactam

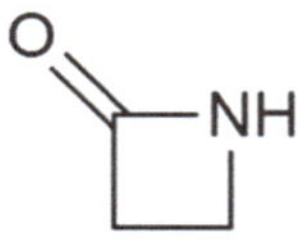

β-lactam

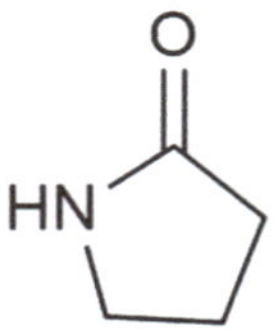

γ-lactam

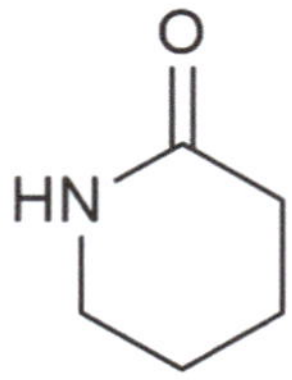

δ-lactam

Penicillin V is an antibiotic useful for the treatment of a number of bacterial infections. The structure of penicillin V is as follows:

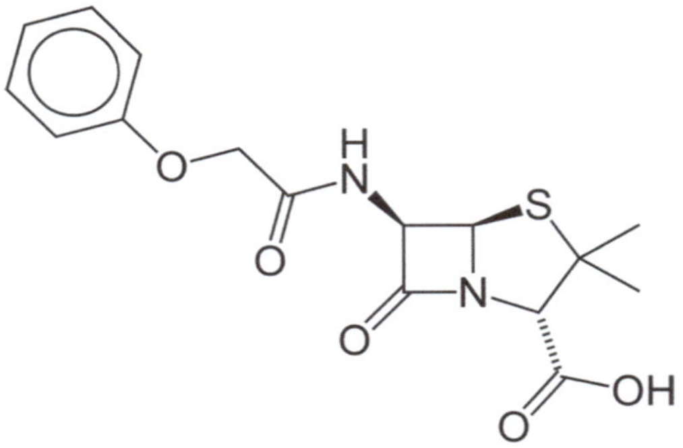

Note that: The maximum number of stereoisomers is given by 2^n where n is the number of stereocentres.

Penicillin V is best described as having a maximum of:

A. 2 stereoisomers and it is a γ-lactam.
B. 3 stereoisomers and it is a β-lactam.
C. 4 stereoisomers and it is a γ-lactam.
D. 8 stereoisomers and it is a β-lactam.

25) Enzymes are biological catalysts that typically have names related to their activity. Penicillin is a β-lactam antibiotic used in the treatment of bacterial infections caused by susceptible, usually Gram-positive, organisms. Beta-lactamases are enzymes produced by some bacteria that provide resistance to β-lactam antibiotics by breaking the antibiotic's structure.

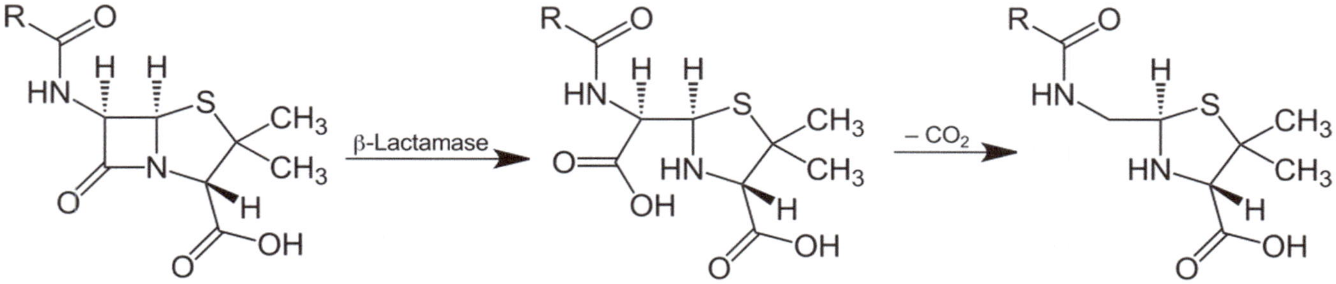

Beta-lactamase is best described as which of the following?

A. Reductase
B. Hydrolase
C. Decarboxylase
D. Oxidase

SPOILER ALERT

Gold Standard has cross-referenced the content in this chapter to examples from ACER's official GAMSAT practice materials. It is for you to decide when you want to explore these questions since you may want to preserve some of ACER's materials for timed mock-exam practice.

Examples – Bromo-esters including propyl bromoacetate (*without basic nomenclature, this mountain becomes impassable*) and hydroxycarboxylic acids: Q17-21 of 2; special mention, but not counted towards the importance of this chapter, is a unit where the focus is alcohol but ester nomenclature is helpful: Q40-42 of 5. Note that "Q" is followed by the question number, and, for example, "of 1" refers to booklet number 1 which is referenced in the Spoiler Alert table at the end of Chapter 1. The 15 full-length GAMSAT practice tests by Gold Standard, HEAPS-1 through HEAPS-15, contain specific cross-references to this chapter within the worked solutions. Note that lactides, lactones, and lactams is a unit from HEAPS-7 with some novel questions added to this chapter. Side note: Yes, we revealed β-lactam in Question 25 (ref. Q24), but you deserved a break!

High-level Importance

Chapter Checklist

- ☐ Access your online account to view answers, worked solutions and discussion boards.
- ☐ Reassess your 'learning objectives' for this chapter: Go back to the first page of this chapter and re-evaluate the top 3 boxes and the Introduction.
- ☐ Complete a maximum of 1 page of notes using symbols/abbreviations to represent the entire chapter based on your learning objectives. These are your Gold Notes.
- ☐ Consider your multimedia options based on your optimal way of learning:
    - ☐ Download the free Gold Standard GAMSAT app for your Android device or iPhone.
    - ☐ Create your own, tangible study cards or try the free app: Anki.
    - ☐ Record your voice reading your Gold Notes onto your smartphone (audio files, e.g., *memo* or MP3s) and listen during exercise, transportation, etc.
    - ☐ Try out the Gold Standard GAMSAT online videos at gamsat-prep.com, or you can try other options on YouTube like Khan Academy or Crash Course Organic Chemistry.
- ☐ Reassess your schedule for your full-length GAMSAT practice tests: ACER and/or HEAPS exams. Ensure that you have scheduled one full day to complete a practice test and 1-2 days for a thorough assessment of worked solutions while adding to your abbreviated Gold Notes.
- ☐ Reassess your progress in scheduling and/or evaluating stress reduction techniques such as regular exercise (sports), yoga, meditation and/or mindfulness exercises (*see* YouTube for suggestions).

ETHERS AND PHENOLS

Chapter 10

Memorise	Understand	Importance
* Basic nomenclature	* Electrophilic aromatic substitution	**Low level: 1% of GAMSAT Organic Chemistry** questions released by ACER are related to content in this chapter (in our estimation). * Note that approximately 60% of the questions in GAMSAT Organic Chemistry are related to just 4 chapters: 2, 6, 7 and 12.

GAMSAT-Prep.com

Introduction

Ethers are composed of an oxygen atom connected to two alkyl or aryl groups of the general formula R–O–R'. A classic example is the solvent and anesthetic diethyl ether, often just called "ether." Phenol is a toxic, white crystalline solid with a sweet tarry odor often referred to as a "hospital smell"! Its chemical formula is C_6H_5OH and its structure is that of a hydroxyl group (-OH) bonded to a phenyl ring thus it is an aromatic compound.

As you know by now, the Percent Importance relates to the assumed knowledge within the chapter, and is not related to the GAMSAT-level practice questions at the end of the chapter which should always be considered as being High-level Importance.

Multimedia Resources at GAMSAT-Prep.com

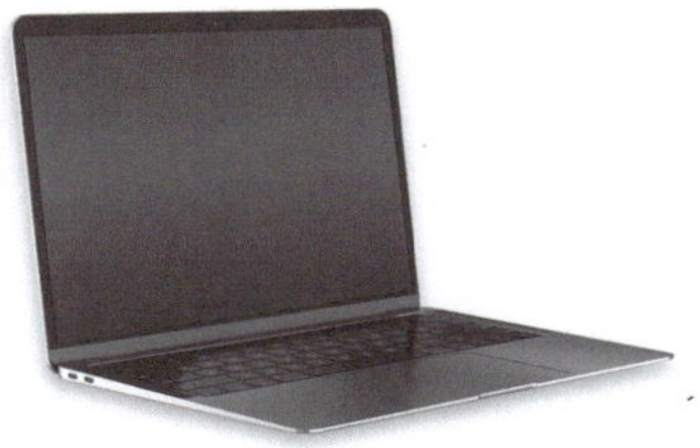

Open Discussion Boards
(*gamsat-prep.com/forum*)

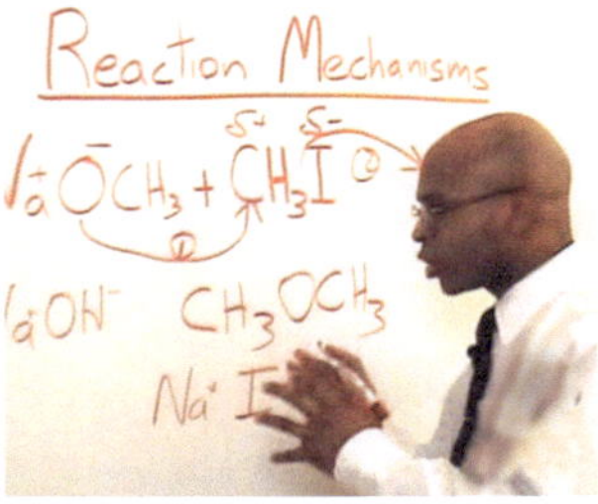

Science Preparation Videos

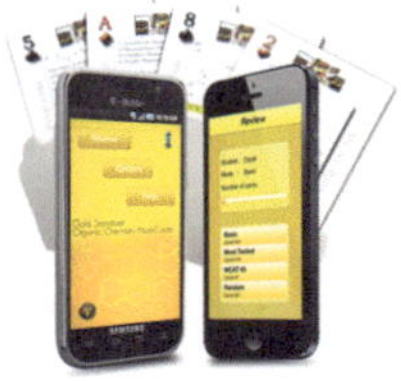

Flashcards

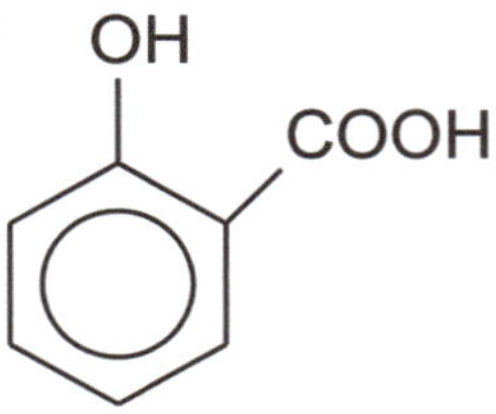

Special Guest

* The real GAMSAT may have advanced-level information presented (i.e. in a passage) but previous knowledge of said information is not required to answer the questions that would follow. Practice questions at the end of this chapter, as well as ACER and GS (HEAPS) practice GAMSATs can help you clarify this point.

10.1 Description and Nomenclature of Ethers

The general structure of an ether is R-O-R', where the R's may be either aromatic or aliphatic (= *non-aromatic hydrocarbon*). In the common system of nomenclature, the two groups on either side of the oxygen are named, followed by the word ether:

$CH_3 — O — CH_3$
dimethyl ether

$CH_3 — O — CH(CH_3)CH_3$
methyl isopropyl ether

In the systematic system of nomenclature, the alkoxy (RO-) groups are always named as substituents (note that the shorter alkyl group becomes the alkoxy substituent):

$CH_3—O—CH_3$
methoxy methane

$CH_3—O—CH(CH_3)CH_3$
methoxy isopropane

The boiling points of ethers are comparable to that of other hydrocarbons, which is regarded as relatively low temperatures when compared to alcohols. Ethers are more polar than other hydrocarbons, but are **not** capable of forming intermolecular hydrogen bonds (i.e., *those between two ether molecules because ethers are missing partially positive hydrogen atoms directly attached to F, O or N*). Ethers are only slightly soluble in water. However, they can form intermolecular hydrogen bonds between the ether and the water molecules.

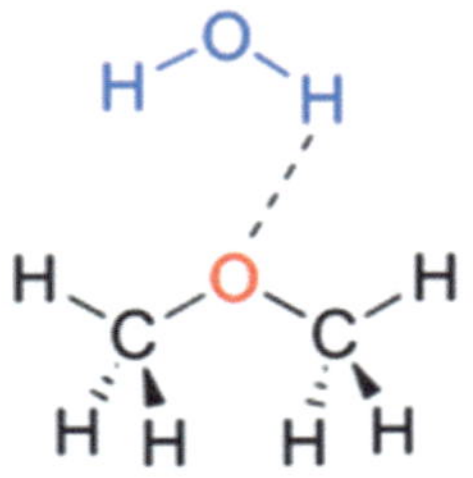

Ethers are good solvents, as the ether linkage is inert to many chemical reagents. Ethers are weak Lewis bases (CHM 3.4) and can be protonated to form positively charged conjugate acids (CHM 6.3). In the presence of a high concentration of a strong acid (especially HI or HBr), the ether linkage will be cleaved, to form an alcohol and an alkyl halide:

$$CH_3 — O — CH_3 + HI \longrightarrow CH_3 — OH + CH_3 — I$$

10.1.1 Important Reactions of Ethers

- Williamson ether synthesis: A metal alkoxide can react with a primary alkyl halide to yield an ether in an S_N2 mechanism. The alkoxide, which is prepared by the reaction of an alcohol with a strong base (ORG 6.2.4), acts as a nucleophile and displaces the halide. Since primary halides work best in an S_N2 mechanism, asymmetrical ethers will be synthesised by the reaction between unhindered halides and more hindered alkoxides. This reaction will not proceed with a hindered alkyl halide substrate:

$$Na^+ \, ^-OCH_3 + \, ^{\delta+}CH_3 - I^{\delta-} \longrightarrow CH_3 - O - CH_3 + Na^+ I^-$$

Low-level Importance

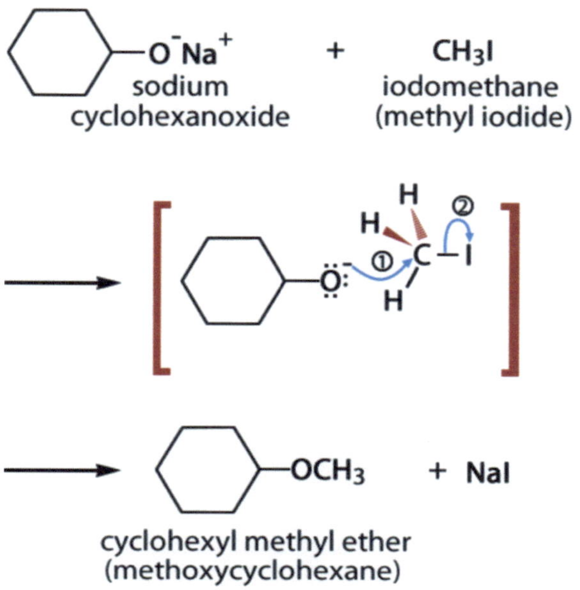

In a variant of the Williamson ether synthesis, an alkoxide ion displaces a chloride atom within the same molecule. The precursor compounds are called halohydrins (ORG 4.2.1). For example, with 2-chloropropanol, an intramolecular epoxide formation reaction is possible creating the cyclic ether called oxirane (C_2H_4O). Note that oxirane is a three-membered cyclic ether (= *epoxide*).

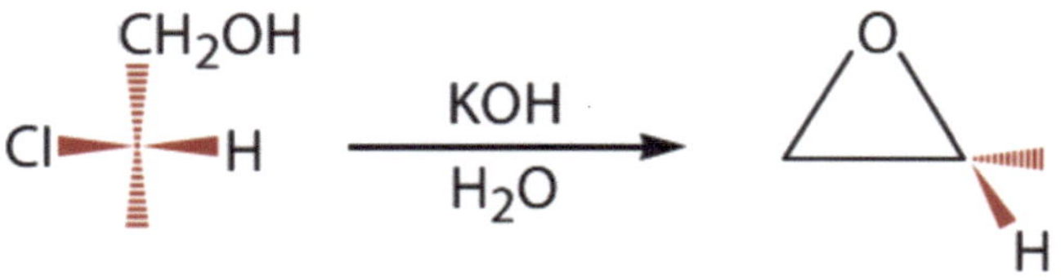

Cyclic ethers can also be prepared by reacting an alkene with m-CPBA (meta-chloroperoxybenzoic acid) which can also form an oxirane:

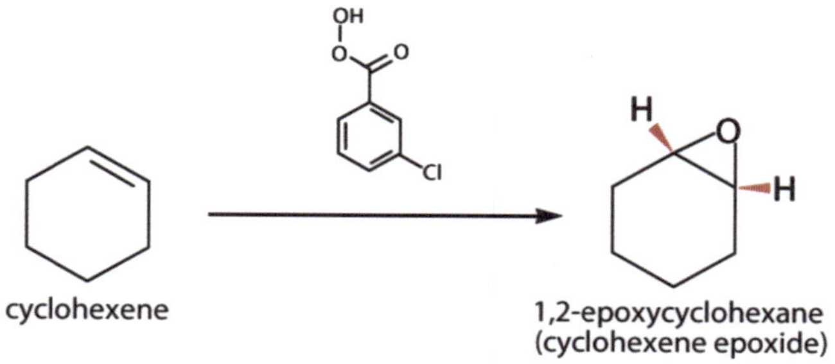

- <u>Acidic Cleavage</u>: Cleavage reactions of straight chain ethers takes place in the presence of HBr or HI (or even H_2SO_4) and is initiated by protonation of the ether oxygen.

Primary or secondary ethers react by an S_N2 mechanism in which I^- or Br^- attacks the protonated ether at the less hindered site. Tertiary, benzylic and allylic ethers react by an S_N1 or E1 mechanism because these substrates can produce stable intermediate carbocations. Consider the following S_N1 mechanism:

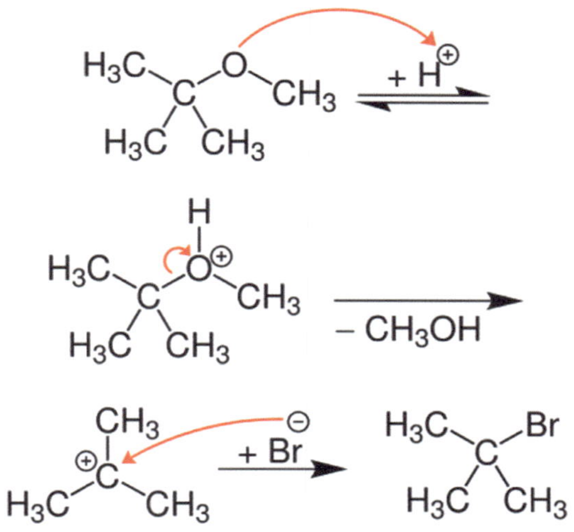

Consider the following S_N2 mechanism:

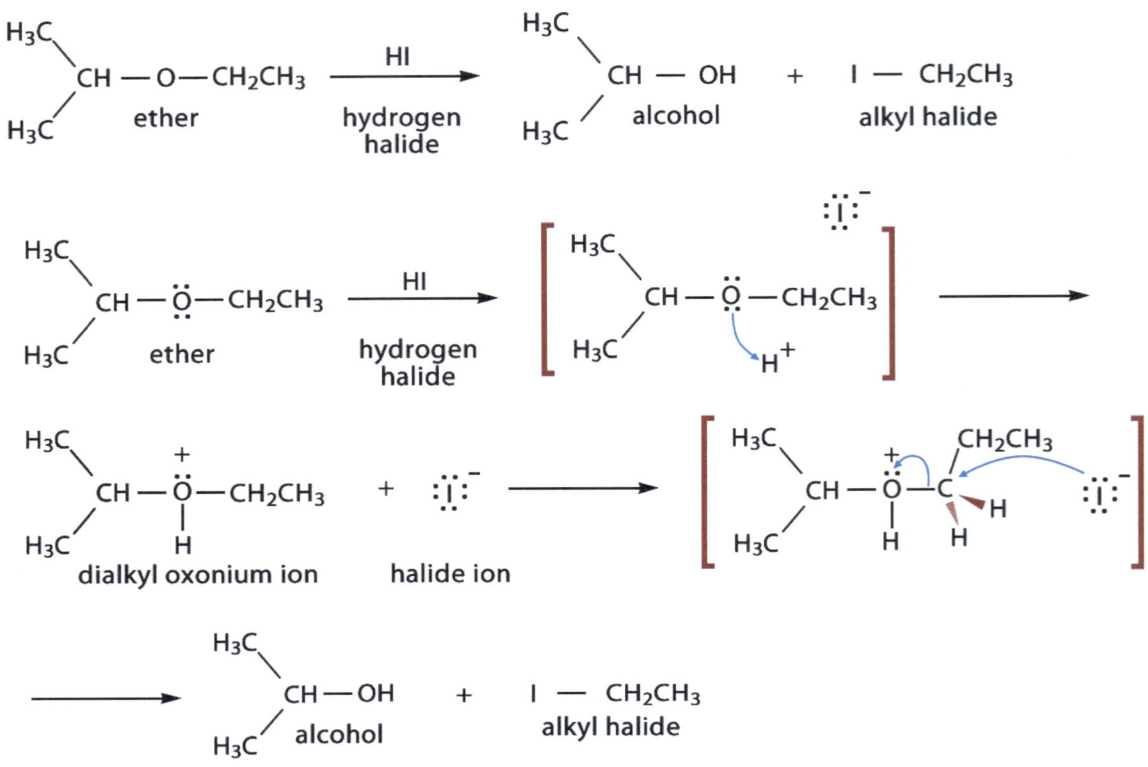

10.2 Phenols

A phenol is a molecule consisting of a hydroxyl (–OH) group attached to a benzene (aromatic) ring (ORG 5.1). The following are some phenols and derivatives which are important to biochemistry, medicine and nature:

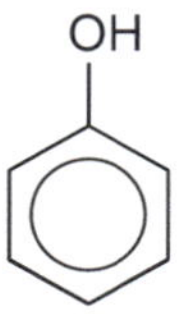

phenol

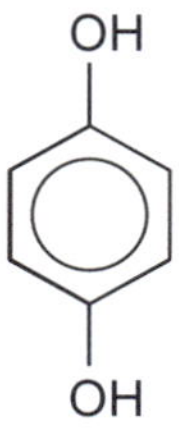

benzene-1,4-diol (hydroquinone)

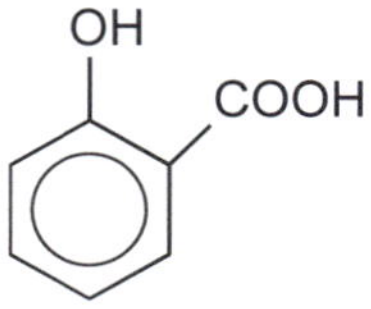

2-hydroxybenzoic acid (salicylic acid)

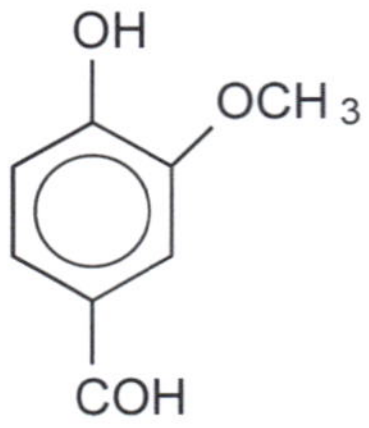

4-hydroxy-3-methoxybenzaldehyde (vanillin)

Phenols are more acidic than their corresponding alcohols. This is due mainly to the electron withdrawing and resonance stabilisation effects of the aromatic ring in the conjugate base anion (*the phenoxide ion*):

Low-level Importance

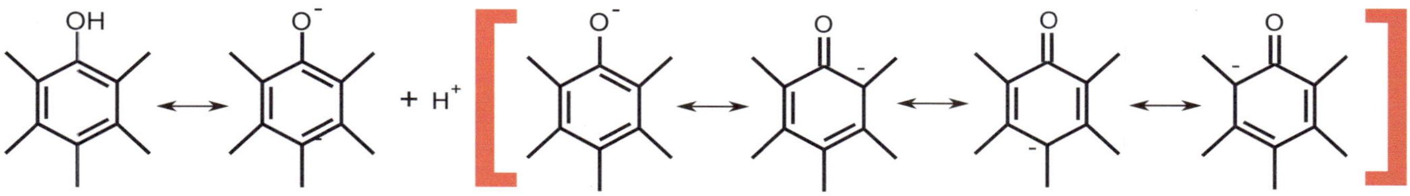

Substituent groups on the ring affect the acidity of phenols by both inductive effects (as with alcohols) and resonance effects. The resonance structures show that electron stabilising (*withdrawing* or *meta directing*) groups at the ortho or para positions should increase the acidity of the phenol. Examples of these groups include the nitro group ($-NO_2$), $-CN$, $-CO_2H$, and the weakly deactivating o-p directors - the halogens. Destabilising groups, such as alkyl groups, or other ortho-para directors, will make the compound less acidic. Phenols are ortho-para directors (*see* ORG Chapter 5).

Phenols can form hydrogen bonds, resulting in fairly high boiling points. Their solubility in water, however, is limited, because of the hydrophobic nature of the aromatic ring. Ortho phenols have lower boiling points than meta and para phenols, as they can form intramolecular hydrogen bonds. However, the para and even the ortho compounds can sometimes form intermolecular hydrogen bonds:

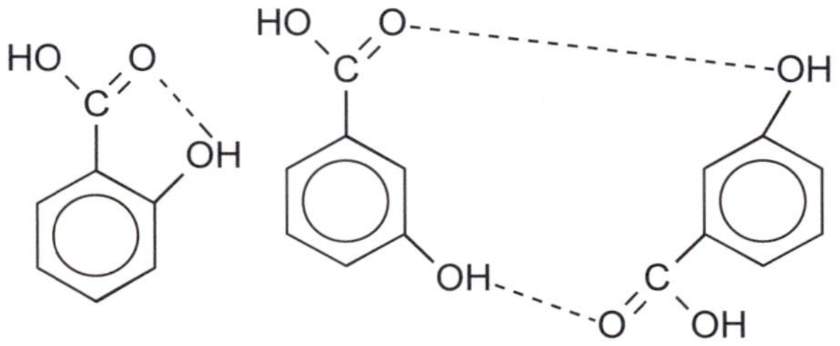

10.2.1 Electrophilic Aromatic Substitution for Phenols

The hydroxyl group is a powerful activating group and an ortho-para director in electrophilic substitutions. Thus phenols can brominate three times in bromine water as follows:

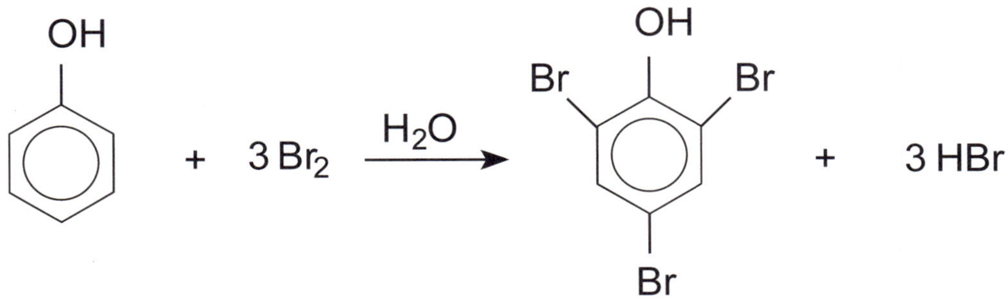

Low-level Importance

CHAPTER 10: Ethers and Phenols

GOLD STANDARD FOUNDATIONAL GAMSAT PRACTICE QUESTIONS

1) Which of the following compounds is an ether?

A. 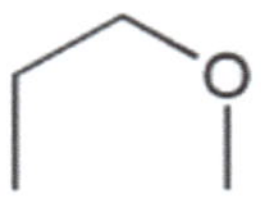

C. 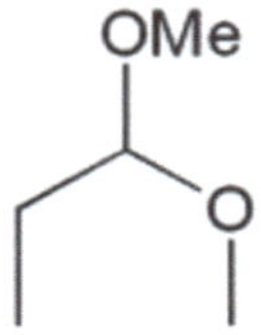

B. 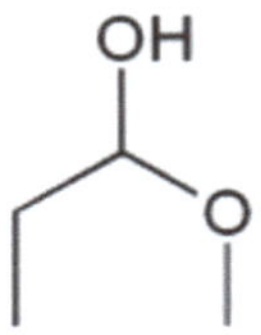

D. 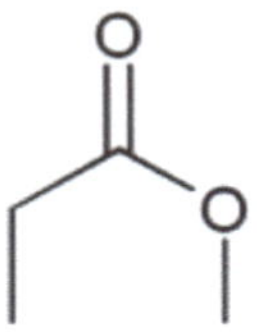

2) Identify the IUPAC name for $HOCH_2CH_2OC_2H_5$.
   - A. methoxypropanol
   - B. hydroxy-diethyl ether
   - C. 2-ethoxyethanol
   - D. 2-oxybutanol

3) Which of the following is **not** characteristic of hydrogen bonding?
   - A. The hydrogen atom involved must be covalently bonded to a very electronegative atom.
   - B. The hydrogen bonds are typically weaker than ionic or covalent bonds.
   - C. The other atom involved in the hydrogen bond (not the hydrogen atom) must be covalently bonded to a hydrogen atom.
   - D. The other atom involved in the hydrogen bond (not the hydrogen atom) must possess at least one lone pair of electrons.

4) Which of the following compounds has the highest boiling point?
   - A. Methane, CH_4
   - B. Ethane, CH_3CH_3
   - C. Ethanol, CH_3CH_2OH
   - D. Dimethyl ether, CH_3OCH_3

5) Which of the following molecules can be involved in hydrogen bond formation but cannot form hydrogen bonds with molecules of its own kind?
   - A. C_2H_5OH
   - B. HCOOH
   - C. CH_3OCH_3
   - D. HF

6) Which of the following compounds are phenols?

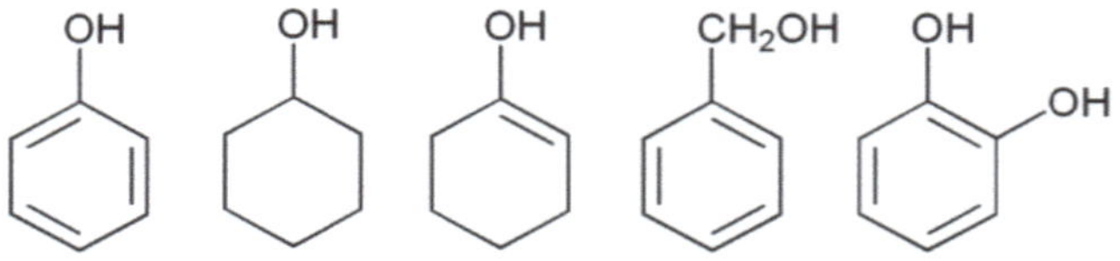

I II III IV V

   - A. **I** and **II**
   - B. **I** and **III**
   - C. **I** and **IV**
   - D. **I** and **V**

7) Identify the IUPAC name for the following molecule.

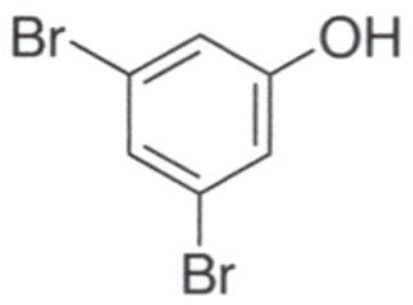

   - A. 1,5-dibromophenol
   - B. 1,3-dibromophenol
   - C. 2,4-dibromophenol
   - D. 3,5-dibromophenol

Low-level Importance

GOLD STANDARD GAMSAT-LEVEL PRACTICE QUESTIONS

Questions 8–10

A phenol is a molecule that consists of a phenyl group ($-C_6H_5$) bonded to a hydroxyl group (–OH). Positions that are ortho, meta and para to the –OH substituent are as shown in the diagram.

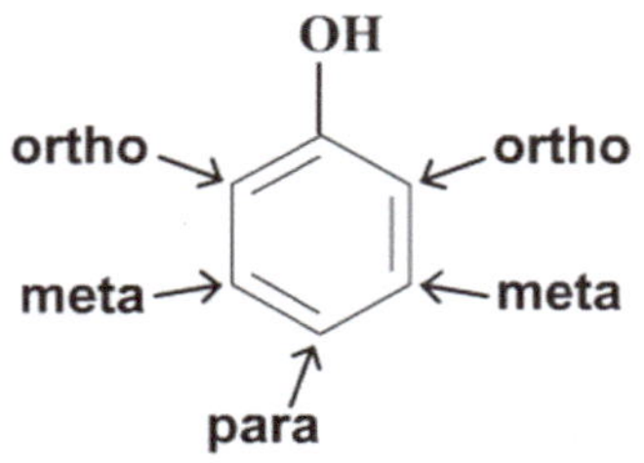

Substituents - especially at the ortho/para (O/P) positions - affect the acidity of phenols. Deactivating the phenyl ring results in a stronger acid while activating the ring weakens acid strength.

The following table summarises the effect of substituents attached to the ring where EDG = electron donating group, and EWG = electron withdrawing group.

EDG	EWG	EWG: Halogens
activates the ring	*deactivates the ring*	*weakly deactivating*
O/P Directing	Meta Directing	O/P Directing
i.e. alkyl groups	i.e. nitro ($-NO_2$)	i.e. bromine

8) The introduction of an ortho bromine atom into the phenol would have the effect of:

- **A.** lowering the pKa and thus decreasing the acidity of the phenol.
- **B.** lowering the pKa and thus increasing the acidity of the phenol.
- **C.** increasing the pKa and thus decreasing the acidity of the phenol.
- **D.** increasing the pKa and thus increasing the acidity of the phenol.

9) Rank the following from highest pKa to lowest pKa (Me = methyl).

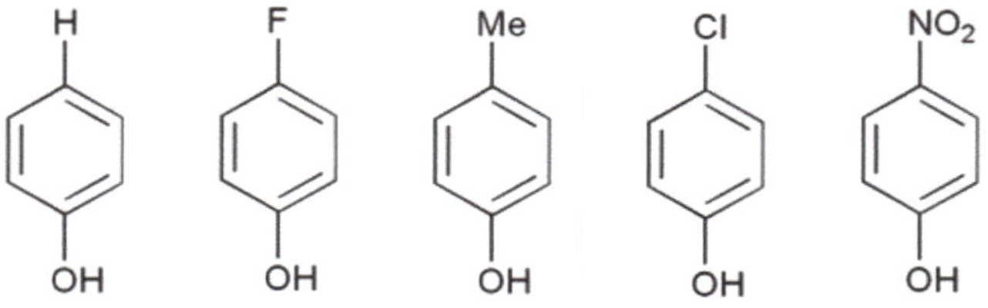

A B C D E

- **A.** C > A > B > E
- **B.** B > C > A > E
- **C.** E > A > C > D
- **D.** E > D > A > C

Question 10 relates to the following additional information.

Analogous to phenols, the relative acid strength among carboxylic acids depends on the inductive effects of the attached groups, but also to their proximity to the carboxyl group. For example, halogens are electronegative and thus can withdraw electron density and stabilise the carboxylate anion. Unsurprisingly, proximity is important as the effect of a charge decreases exponentially as distance increases.

10) What is the order of increasing acidity for the following compounds?

- **I.** 4-methylpentanoic acid
- **II.** 3-chloropentanoic acid
- **III.** 2-bromopentanoic acid
- **IV.** 2,2-dichloropentanoic acid

- **A.** **I < II < III < IV**
- **B.** **I < III < II < IV**
- **C.** **II < III < I < IV**
- **D.** **IV < III < II < I**

High-level Importance

Questions 11–14

Figure 1 illustrates a solubility based characterisation procedure, often used by organic chemists, for the qualitative analysis of monofunctional organic compounds. Table 1 lists the organic compounds comprising the various solubility classes of compounds from Figure 1.

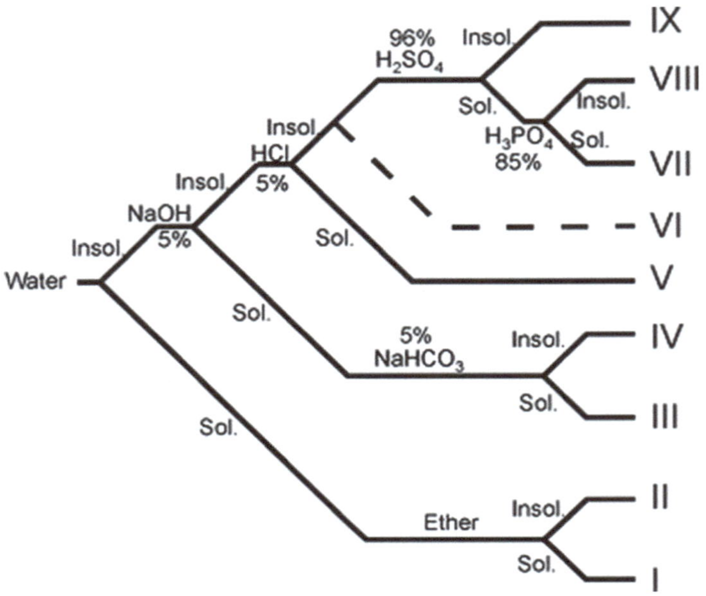

Figure 1: Solubility (Sol.) and insolubility (Insol.) of various compounds in different solvents.

Group	Compounds
I	Salts of organic acids, amino acids, amine chlorides Sugars (carbohydrates) and other polyfunctional compounds with hydrophilic substituents
II	Arenesulfonic acids Monofunctional carboxylic acids, alcohols, ketones, aldehydes, esters, amides and nitriles with 5 or less carbon atoms Monofunctional amines with 6 or less carbon atoms
III	Phenols with ortho- and/or para- electron withdrawing groups, beta-diketones Carboxylic acids with 6 or more carbon atoms
IV	Sulfonamides, nitro-compounds with alpha-hydrogens Phenols, oximes, enols, imides and thiophenols with 6 or more carbon atoms
V	Some oxy-ethers, anilines, aliphatic amines with 8 or more carbon atoms
VI	Neutral compounds containing sulfur or nitrogen with 6 or more carbon atoms

VII	Ethers with 7 or less carbon atoms Monofunctional esters, aldehydes, ketones, cyclic ketones, methyl ketones with between 6 and 8 carbon atoms; epoxides
VIII	Ethers, most other ketones Unsaturated hydrocarbons, aromatic compounds, particularly those which possess activating groups
IX	Alkanes, alkyl and aryl halides Aromatic compounds with electron withdrawing substituents, diaryl ethers

Table 1

11) The result from combining phenols and water can be explained by the fact that phenols:

A. can hydrogen bond.
B. cannot hydrogen bond.
C. are large compounds.
D. have an aromatic ring.

12) Benzoic acid should be soluble in which of the following solvent pairs?

A. Water and 5% HCl
B. 5% NaOH and 5% $NaHCO_3$
C. 5% HCl and 5% NaOH
D. 85% H_3PO_4 and 5% NaOH

13) The significance of the number of carbons present in compounds from Group VI is most consistent with which of the following statements?

A. Increasing the number of carbons increases the hydrophobic moiety.
B. Six carbon compounds are cyclical.
C. The number of carbons relates to the group number.
D. Compounds with six or more carbons are always amphoteric (*able to react both as a base and as an acid*).

14) According to the information provided, all of the following compounds would be included in the water soluble group EXCEPT:

A. 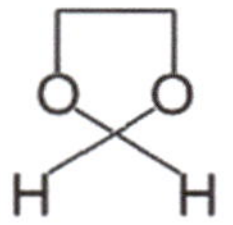

C. 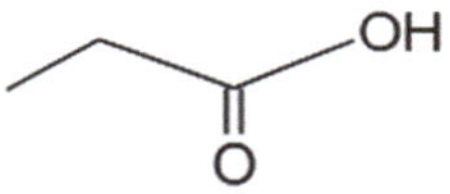

B. 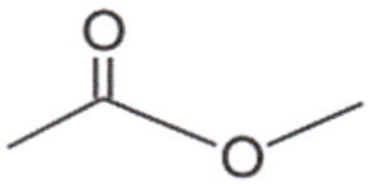

D. 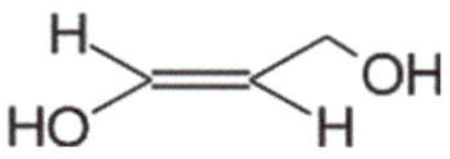

15) Which of the following is **not** a resonance structure of phenol?

A. 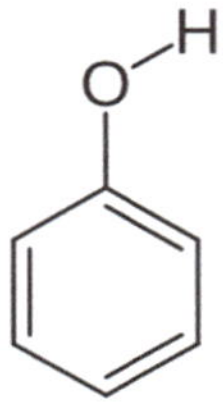

C. 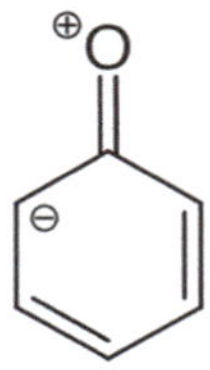

B. 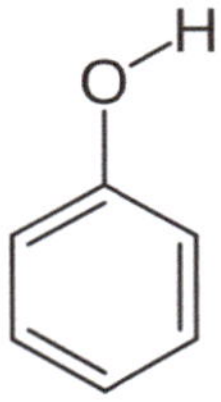

D. 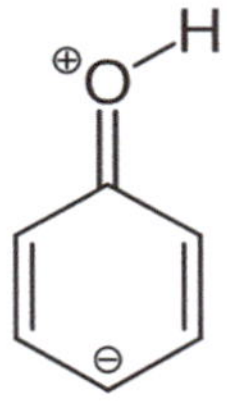

SPOILER ALERT

Gold Standard has cross-referenced the content in this chapter to examples from ACER's official GAMSAT practice materials. It is for you to decide when you want to explore these questions since you may want to preserve some of ACER's materials for timed mock-exam practice.

Examples – Special mention, as it relates to Question 15, carboxylic acid strength with attached halogens (*not counted for this chapter as it has already been counted for Chapter 8, Carboxylic Acids*): Q6-7 of 1; the phenoxide anion and charge delocalisation within the ring structure (*resonance*): Q74 of 3; also, special mention, relating pKa to ionisation (*not counted*): Q8-10 of 5. Note that "Q" is followed by the question number, and, for example, "of 1" refers to booklet number 1 which is referenced in the Spoiler Alert table at the end of Chapter 1. The 15 full-length GAMSAT practice tests by Gold Standard, HEAPS-1 through HEAPS-15, contain specific cross-references to this chapter within the worked solutions. Note that the unit with phenols, EWG, EDG and pKa is from HEAPS-5.

Chapter Checklist

- ☐ Access your online account to view answers, worked solutions and discussion boards.
- ☐ Reassess your 'learning objectives' for this chapter: Go back to the first page of this chapter and re-evaluate the top 3 boxes and the Introduction.
- ☐ Complete a maximum of 1 page of notes using symbols/abbreviations to represent the entire chapter based on your learning objectives. These are your Gold Notes.
- ☐ Consider your multimedia options based on your optimal way of learning:
    - ☐ Download the free Gold Standard GAMSAT app for your Android device or iPhone.
    - ☐ Create your own, tangible study cards or try the free app: Anki.
    - ☐ Record your voice reading your Gold Notes onto your smartphone (audio files, e.g., *memo* or MP3s) and listen during exercise, transportation, etc.
    - ☐ Try out the Gold Standard GAMSAT online videos at gamsat-prep.com, or you can try other options on YouTube like Khan Academy or Crash Course Organic Chemistry.
- ☐ Reassess your schedule for your full-length GAMSAT practice tests: ACER and/or HEAPS exams. Ensure that you have scheduled one full day to complete a practice test and 1-2 days for a thorough assessment of worked solutions while adding to your abbreviated Gold Notes.
- ☐ Reassess your progress in scheduling and/or evaluating stress reduction techniques such as regular exercise (sports), yoga, meditation and/or mindfulness exercises (*see* YouTube for suggestions).

High-level Importance

AMINES

Chapter 11

Memorise

* IUPAC nomenclature

Understand

* Effect of hydrogen bonds
* Resonance, delocalisation of electrons

Importance

Low level: 2% of GAMSAT Organic Chemistry
questions released by ACER are related to content in this chapter (in our estimation).
* Note that approximately 60% of the questions in GAMSAT Organic Chemistry are related to just 4 chapters: 2, 6, 7 and 12.

GAMSAT-Prep.com

Introduction

Amines are compounds and functional groups that contain a basic nitrogen atom with a lone pair. Amines are derivatives of ammonia (NH_3), where one or more hydrogen atoms are replaced by organic substituents such as alkyl and aryl groups (consider revising the functional groups presented in ORG 1.6).

As you know by now, the Percent Importance relates to the assumed knowledge within the chapter, and is not related to the GAMSAT-level practice questions at the end of the chapter which should always be considered as being High-level Importance.

Multimedia Resources at GAMSAT-Prep.com

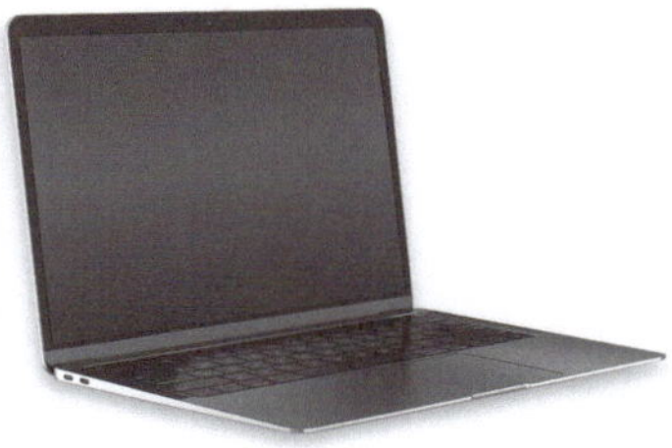

Open Discussion Boards
(*gamsat-prep.com/forum*)

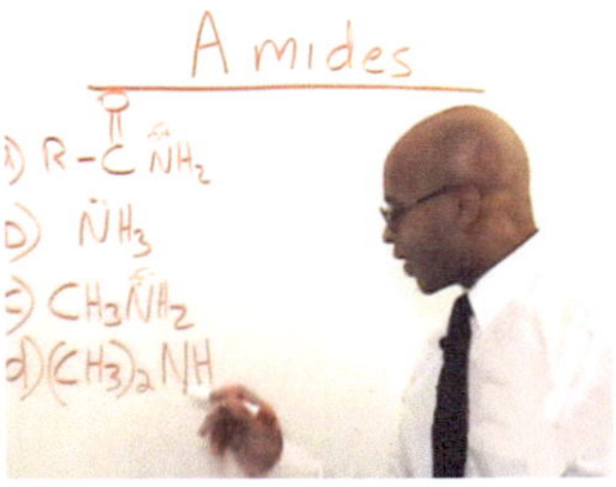

Science Preparation Videos

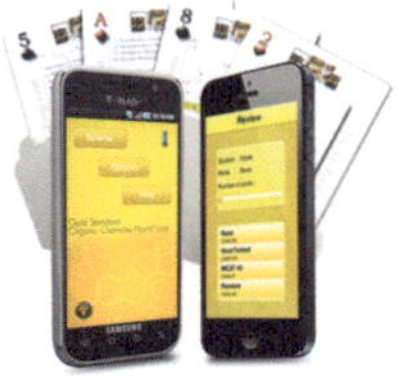

Flashcards

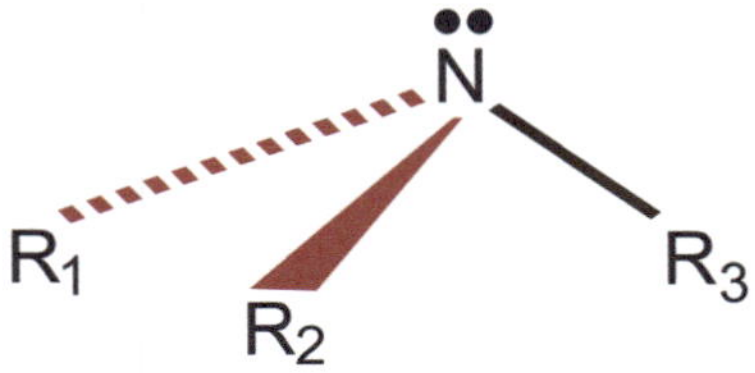

Special Guest

* The real GAMSAT may have advanced-level information presented (i.e. in a passage) but previous knowledge of said information is not required to answer the questions that would follow. Practice questions at the end of this chapter, as well as ACER and GS (HEAPS) practice GAMSATs can help you clarify this point.

11.1 Description and Nomenclature

Organic compounds with a trivalent nitrogen atom bonded to one or more carbon atoms are called amines. These are organic derivatives of ammonia. They may be classified depending on the number of carbon atoms bonded to the nitrogen:

Primary Amine:	RNH_2
Secondary Amine:	R_2NH
Tertiary Amine:	R_3N
Quaternary Salt:	$R_4N^+ X^-$

In the common system of nomenclature, amines are named by adding the suffix '-amine' to the name of the alkyl group. In a secondary or tertiary amine, where there is more than one alkyl group, the groups are named as N-substituted derivatives of the larger group:

$$CH_3 - \underset{}{\overset{CH_3}{\overset{|}{CH}}} - \overset{CH_3}{\overset{|}{N}} - CH_2 - CH_3$$

methyl ethyl isopropylamine

In the systematic system of nomenclature, amines are named analagous to alcohols, except the suffix '-amine' is used instead of the suffix '-ol'.

When amines are present with multiple asymmetric substituents, they are named by considering the largest group as the parent name and the other alkyl groups as N-substituents of the parent:

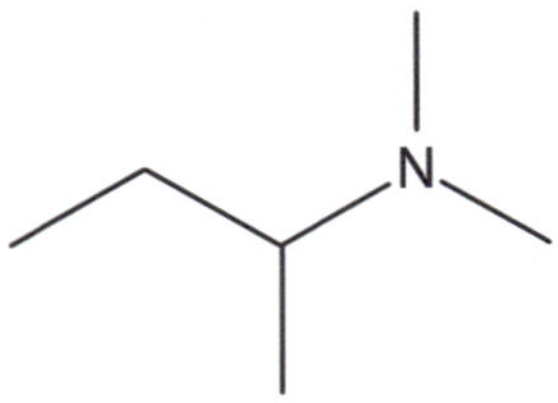

N, N-dimethyl-2-butanamine

The $-NH_2$ group is named as an amino substituent on a parent molecule when amines are present with more than one functional group:

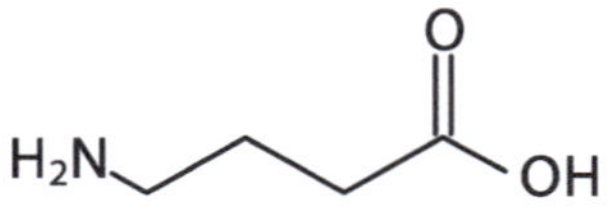

4-aminobutanoic acid

The bonding in amines is similar to the bonding in ammonia. The nitrogen atom is sp^3 hybridised (ORG 1.1, 1.2, CHM 3.5). Primary, secondary and tertiary amines have a trigonal pyramidal shape (CHM 3.5). The C-N-C bond angle is approximately 108°. Quaternary amines have a tetrahedral shape and a normal tetrahedral bond angle of 109.5°.

With its tetrahedral geometry, amines with three different substituents are considered chiral. Such amines are analogous to chiral alkanes in that the nitrogen atom will possess four different substituents - considering the lone pair of electrons to be the fourth substituent. However, unlike chiral alkanes, chiral amines do not exist in two separate enantiomers. Pyramidal nitrogen inversion between the two enantiomeric forms occurs so rapidly at room temperature that the two forms cannot be isolated.

11.1.1 The Basicity of Amines

Along with the three attached groups, amines have an unbonded electron pair. Most of the chemistry of amines depends on this unbonded electron pair:

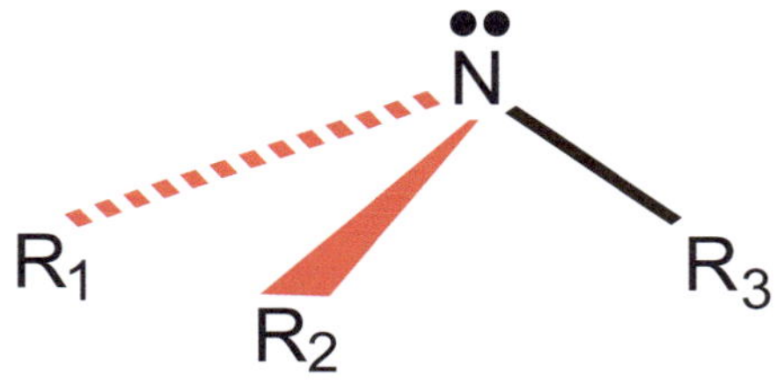

The electron pair is stabilised by the electron donating effects of alkyl groups. Thus the lone pair in tertiary amines is more stable than in secondary amines which, in turn, is more stable than in primary amines. As a result of this electron pair, amines are Lewis bases (*see* CHM 3.4), and good nucleophiles.

In aqueous solution, amines are weak bases, and can accept a proton:

$$R_3N + H_2O \longrightarrow R_3NH^+ + OH^-$$

The ammonium cation in the preceding reaction is stabilised, once again, by the electron donating effects of the alkyl groups. Conversely, should the nitrogen be adjacent to a carbocation, the lone pair can stabilise the carbocation by delocalising the charge.

The relative basicity of amines is determined by the following:

- If the free amine is stabilised relative to the cation, the amine is less basic.
- If the cation is stabilised relative to the free amine, the amine is more stable, thus the stronger base.

Groups that withdraw electron density (such as halides or aromatics) decrease the availability of the unbonded electron pair. Electron releasing groups (such as alkyl groups) increase the availability of the unbonded electron pair. The base strength then increases in the following series (where Ø represents a phenyl group):

$$NO_2{-}Ø{-}NH_2 < Ø{-}NH_2 < Ø{-}CH_2{-}NH_2 < NH_3 < CH_3{-}NH_2 < (CH_3)_2{-}N{-}H < (CH_3)_3{-}N$$

Note that a substituent attached to an aromatic ring can greatly affect the basicity of the amine. For example, electron withdrawing groups (i.e. $-NO_2$) withdraw electrons from the ring which, in turn, withdraws the lone electron pair (*delocalisation*) from nitrogen. Thus the lone pair is less available to bond with a proton; consequently, it is a weaker base. The opposite occurs with an electron donating group, making the amine, relatively, a better base (*see* ORG Chapter 5).

Low-level Importance

11.1.2 More Properties of Amines

- The nitrogen atom can hydrogen bond (using its electron pair) to hydrogens attached to other N's or O's. It can also form hydrogen bonds from hydrogens attached to it with electron pairs of N, O, F or Cl:

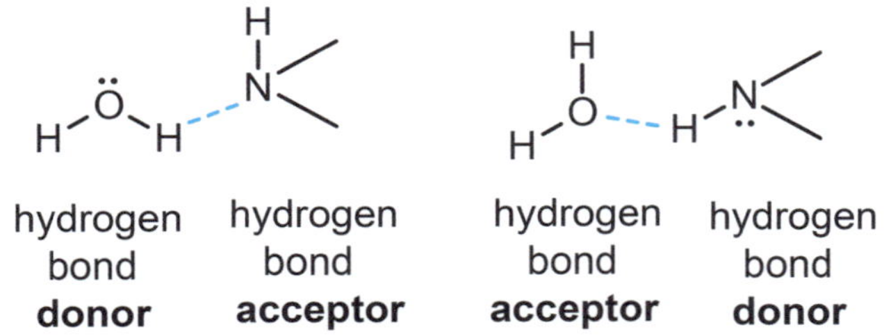

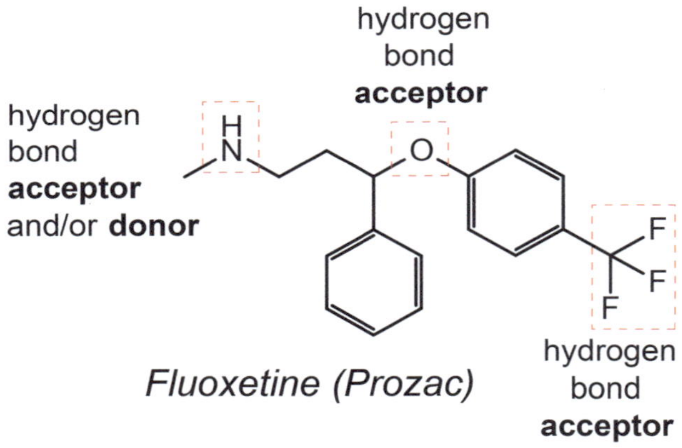

Fluoxetine (Prozac)

Note that primary or secondary amines can hydrogen bond with each other, but tertiary amines cannot. This leads to boiling points which are higher than would be expected for compounds of similar molecular weight, like alkanes, but lower than similar alcohols or carboxylic acids. The hydrogen bonding also renders low weight amines soluble in water.

- A dipole moment (ORG 1.5) is possible:

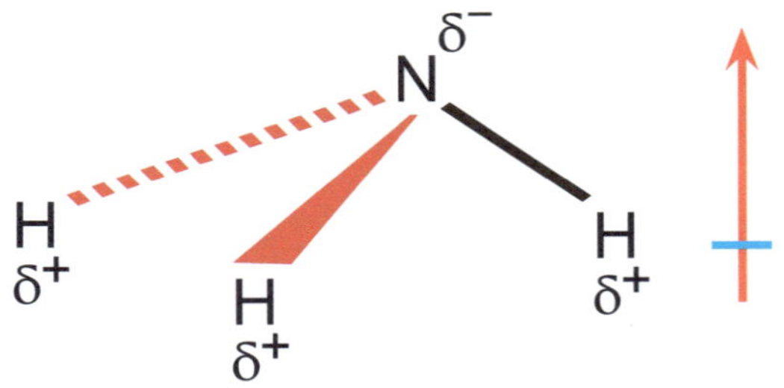

- The nitrogen in amines can contribute its lone pair electrons to activate a benzene ring. Thus amines are ortho-para directors (ORG 5.2.1).

- The solubility of quaternary salts decreases with increasing molecular weight. The quaternary structure has steric hindrance and the lone pair electrons on N is not available for H-bonding, thus their solubility is much less than other amines or even alkyl ammonium salts (i.e. $R\text{–}NH_3^+X^-$, $R_2\text{–}NH_2^+X^-$, $R_3\text{–}NH^+X^-$).

  Quaternary ammonium salts can be synthesised from ammonium hydroxides which are very strong bases.

$$\underset{\text{Quaternary hydroxide}}{(CH_3)_4N^+OH^-} + HCl \longrightarrow \underset{\text{Quaternary salt}}{(CH_3)_4N^+Cl^-} + H_2O$$

Low-level Importance

- **Amide formation** is an important reaction for protein synthesis. Primary and secondary amines will react with carboxylic acids and their derivatives to form *amides*:

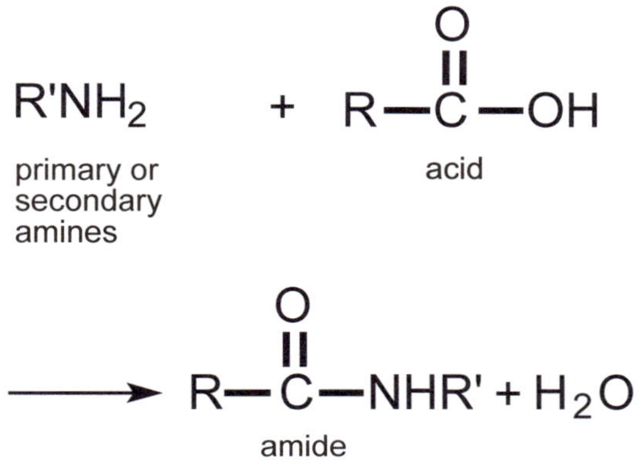

Amides can engage in resonance such that the lone pair electrons on the nitrogen is delocalised. Thus amides are by far less basic than amines.

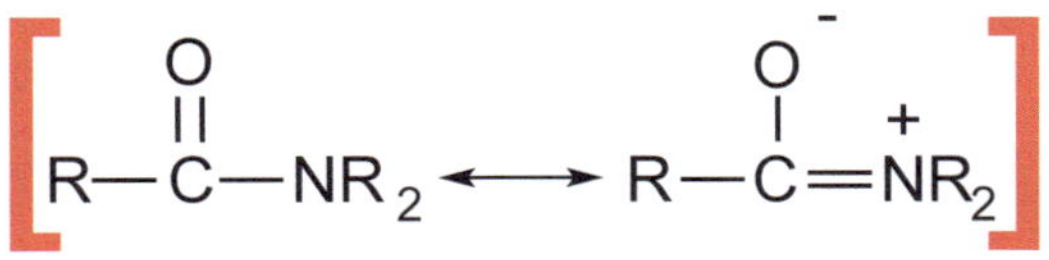

As can be seen, the C–N bond has a partial double bond character. Thus there is restricted rotation about the C–N bond.

- **Alkylation** is another important reaction which involves amines with alkyl halides:

$$RCH_2Cl + R'\,NH_2 \longrightarrow RCH_2NH\,R' + HCl$$

1°, 2° or 3° amine

Both amide formation and alkylation make use of the nucleophilic character of the electrons on nitrogen.

Thus ammonia or an alkyl amine reacts with an alkyl halide to yield an amine in an S_N2 mechanism. Ammonia produces a primary amine; a primary amine produces a secondary amine; a secondary amine produces a tertiary amine; and a tertiary amine produces a quaternary ammonium salt.

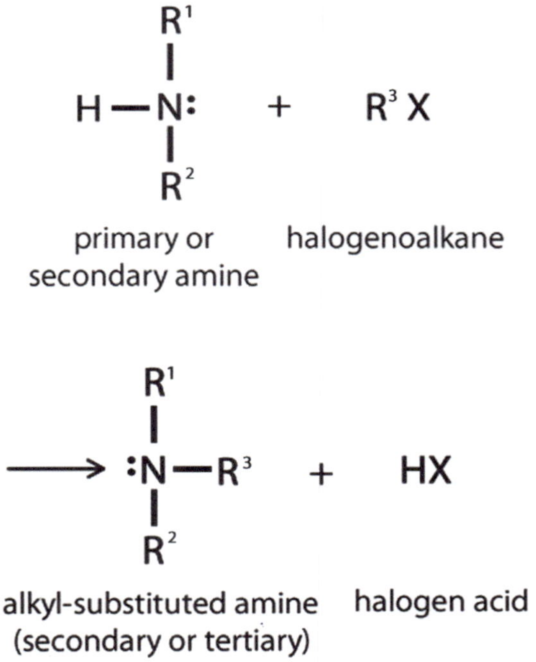

Note: Standard notation for R dictates that when you see a subscript (i.e. 2), just like for other atoms or groups, it means that 2 R groups are present. This has a different meaning than a superscript 2 (ORG 1.6) which means that there is only 1 R group at that position but it is different from any other R group with a different superscript. You will also notice on this page: the R prime notation (R') indicating a single R group different from R without the prime symbol (ORG 1.6). Any of the above notations could be used during the GAMSAT.

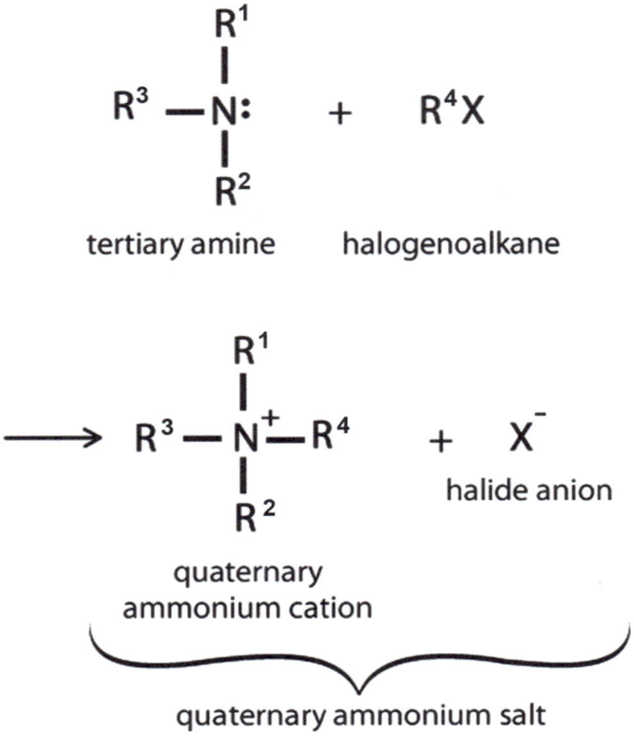

- **Gabriel synthesis:** Primary amines can also be obtained from azide synthesis and Gabriel synthesis in an S_N2 mechanism. The azide ion N_3^-, acting as a nucleophile, displaces the halide ion from the alkyl halide to form RN_3, which is then reduced by $LiAlH_4$ to form the desired primary amine.

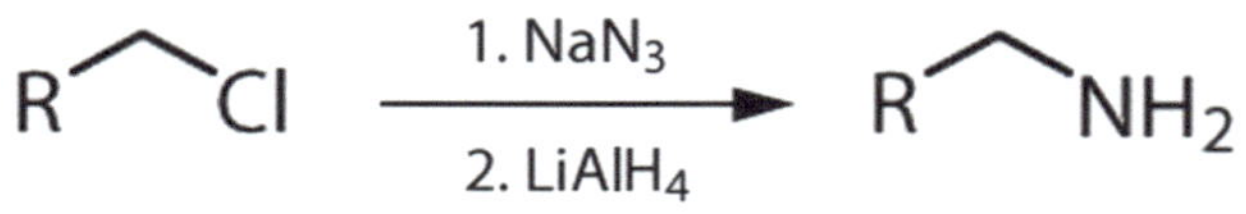

Gabriel amine synthesis occurs via a phthalimide ion displacing the halide from the alkyl halide followed by basic hydrolysis of the N-alkyl phthalimide yielding a primary amine.

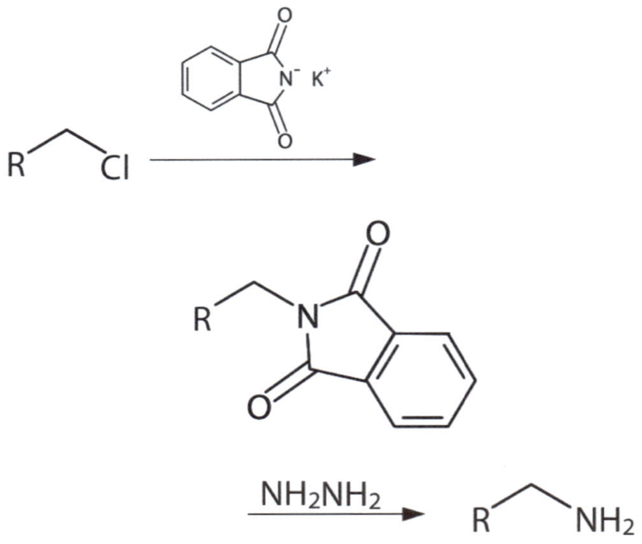

- **Reductive amination:** Amines can also be synthesised by reductive amination in which an aldehyde or ketone reacts with ammonia, a primary amine or a secondary amine to form a corresponding primary amine, secondary amine or tertiary amine.

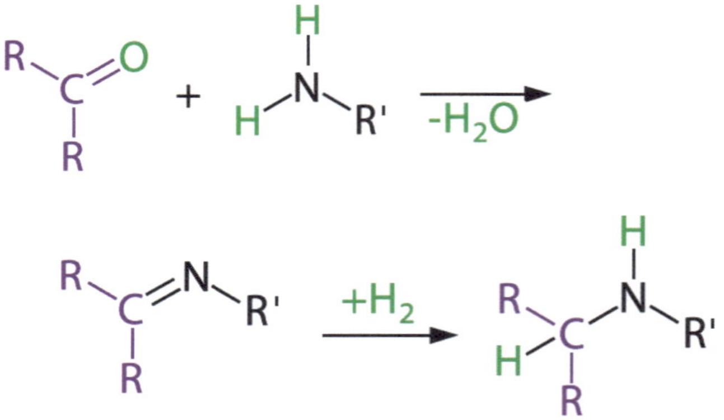

Low-level Importance

- **Reduction of nitriles**: Nitriles (−C≡N) can be reduced by $LiAlH_4$ to produce primary amines. This offers a way to convert alkyl halides into primary amines with one more carbon atom.

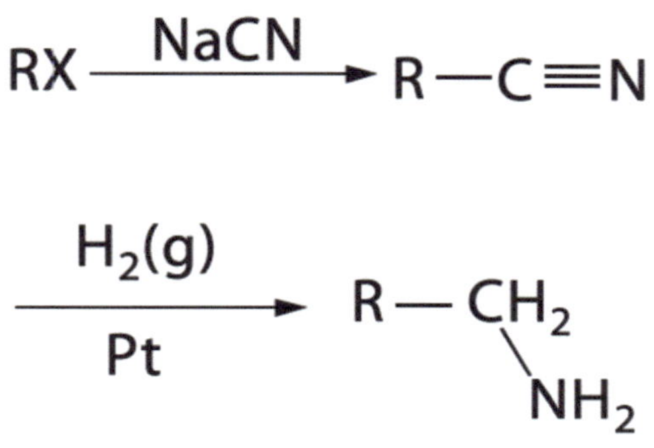

- **Reduction of amides**: Amides can also be reduced by $LiAlH_4$ to produce primary amines. Thus carboxylic acids can be converted into primary amines with the same number of carbon atoms.

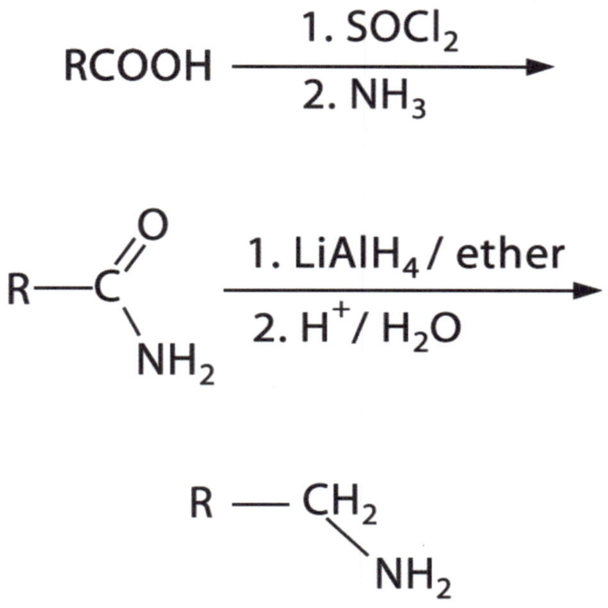

Free Gold Standard GAMSAT Organic Chemistry Reactions Summary
Yes, it's online, it's free and it summarises the most important reactions. You can find the link on the Members home page when you log into your gamsat-prep.com account or you can google it. You can choose to print the page and work through examples changing the different R groups to H's, secondary alkyl groups, aryl groups, etc. to see if you are really following what is happening and that you can name the products. Our Summary page also includes a free YouTube video by Dr. Ferdinand explaining each reaction. Each reaction is also cross-referenced (at the bottom of the page) to a specific section of this textbook for further reading should you wish.

CHAPTER 11: Amines

GOLD STANDARD FOUNDATIONAL GAMSAT PRACTICE QUESTIONS

1) The compound $CH_3–CH_2–NH–CH_3$ is an example of a:

A. primary amine.
B. secondary amine.
C. tertiary amine.
D. primary amide.

2) Which compound is a primary amine with the formula $C_5H_{13}N$?

A. 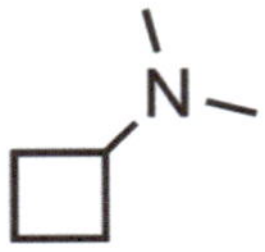

C. 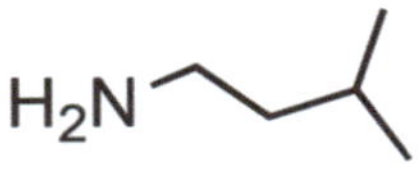

B. 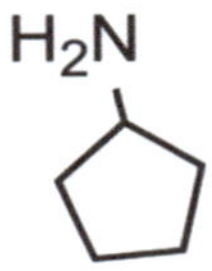

D. 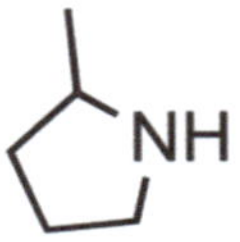

3) Which compound is a tertiary amine?

A. 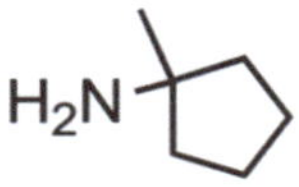

C. 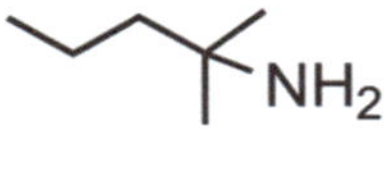

B. 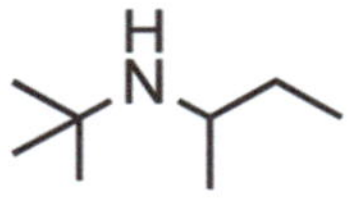

D. 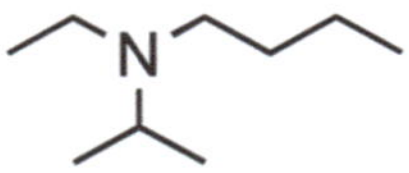

4) Which compound would you expect to have the lowest boiling point?

A. 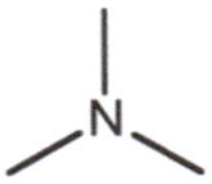

C. 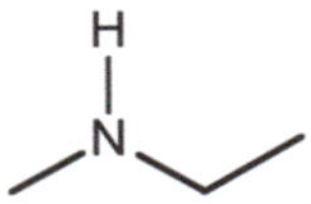

B. 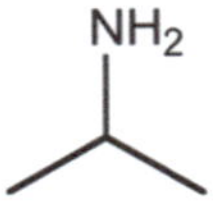

D. 

5) Consider the structure of the medication that can be used to decrease saliva production during surgery: *atropine*. (note: the wavy line from carbon to OH is a bond that only indicates that there is a mixture of isomers)

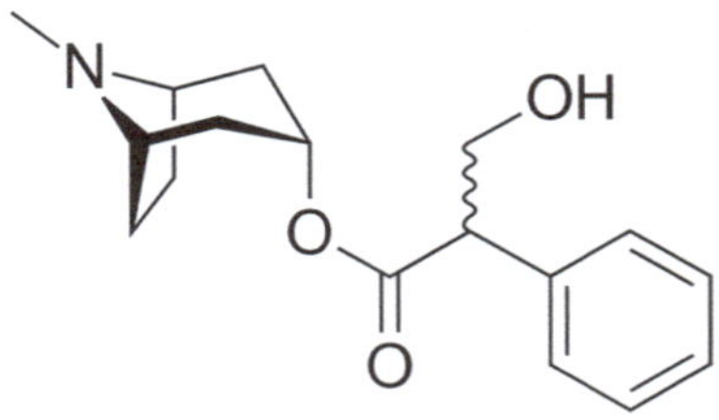

Which of the following functional groups is **not** in atropine?

A. Ketone
B. Amine
C. Alcohol
D. Ester

Low-level Importance

6) There are 6 dashed red lines below. How many of the 6 correctly represent a hydrogen bond?

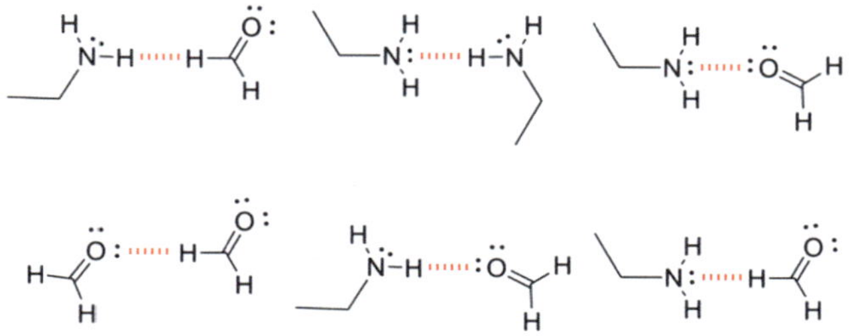

A. Less than 3
B. 3
C. 4
D. More the 4

Questions 7–10

Feel free to consult the nomenclature rules for the next 3 questions (ORG 11.1). ACER is very unlikely to ask a nomenclature question involving amines, but if they would, they would begin by reminding you of the rules.

7) Identify the IUPAC name for the following compound.

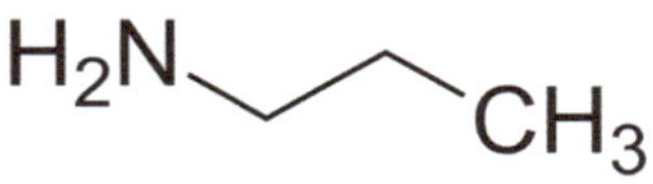

A. Propan-1-amine
B. *N*-isopropylamine
C. Aminobutane
D. *N*-aminoisopropane

8) Identify the IUPAC name for the following compound.

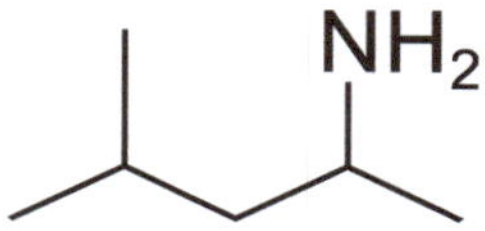

A. 2-methylbutanamine
B. 4-methylhexanamine
C. 2-methylpentan-4-amine
D. 4-methylpentan-2-amine

9) Which of the following amines is paired with an *incorrect* IUPAC name?

A. 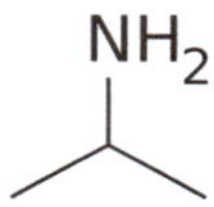

1-methylethanamine

B. 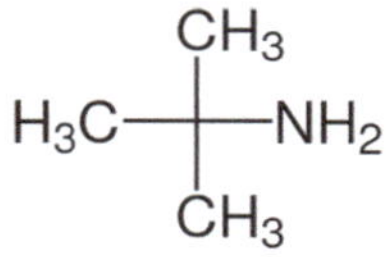

2-methylpropan-2-amine

C. 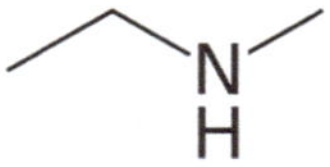

N-methylethan-1-amine

D. More than one of the above is paired with an incorrect IUPAC name.

10) Identify the correct IUPAC name for $CH_2{=}CHCH_2NHCH_3$.

A. 2-Amino-4-pentene
B. 4-Aminopent-1-ene
C. Allylmethylamine
D. *N*-methylprop-2-en-1-amine

Low-level Importance

High-level Importance

GOLD STANDARD GAMSAT-LEVEL PRACTICE QUESTIONS

Questions 11–16

Consider the following 3 structures below.

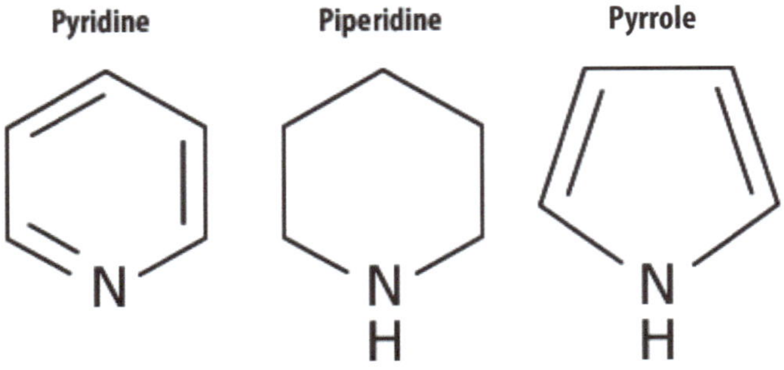

Figure 1: Pyridine, piperidine and pyrrole: 3 organic compounds with similar molecular structures.

Pyridine is a basic heterocyclic organic compound with the chemical formula C_5H_5N. It is structurally related to benzene, with one C-H group replaced by a nitrogen atom.

Piperidine is an organic compound with the molecular formula $(CH_2)_5NH$. This heterocyclic amine consists of a six-membered ring containing five methylene units and one nitrogen atom bonded to a hydrogen atom. It is a colourless fuming liquid with an odor described as ammoniacal, pepper-like.

Pyrrole is a heterocyclic aromatic organic compound, a five-membered ring with the formula C_4H_4NH. It is a colourless volatile liquid that darkens readily upon exposure to air.

Many molecules have dipole moments which are due to a non-uniform distribution of positive and negative charges. The size of the dipole moment for the 3 molecules above is listed as follows in units called "debye", respectively:

$$\mu = 2.25 \text{ D}, \mu = 1.17 \text{ D}, \mu = 1.06 \text{ D}.$$

11) In the context of the passage, "methylene" is most consistent with which of the following?

A. $-CH_2$
B. $=CH_2$
C. $=CH_2=$
D. $CH_2=CH_2$

12) In the absence of any change in intermolecular forces, the lower the molecular mass, the greater the vapor pressure, and thus the lower the boiling point. Ignoring any changes to intermolecular forces, which of the following would be expected to have the highest boiling point?

A. Pyridine
B. Piperidine
C. Pyrrole
D. Cannot be determined from the information provided.

13) Ignoring any effect based on molecular weight, only considering intermolecular forces (except for hydrogen bonding) and the information provided in the passage, which of the following would be expected to have the highest boiling point?

A. Pyridine
B. Piperidine
C. Pyrrole
D. Cannot be determined from the information provided.

14) Studies have confirmed that pyridine actually has a boiling point less than pyrrole. What does pyridine lack which could best account for this relative boiling point difference?

A. Sufficiently high molecular weight
B. Dipole-dipole forces
C. Hydrogen bonds
D. Resonance

15) Consider the structure of pyrrolidine (C_4H_9N) below.

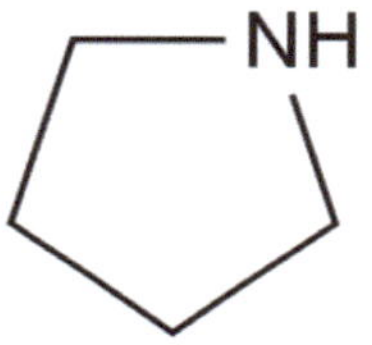

Which of the following would provide the simplest description of a method to produce pyrrolidine?

A. The oxidation of piperidine
B. The oxidation of pyrrole
C. The reduction of piperidine
D. The reduction of pyrrole

16) Heme is an iron-containing component of hemoglobin. Consider the structure of heme below.

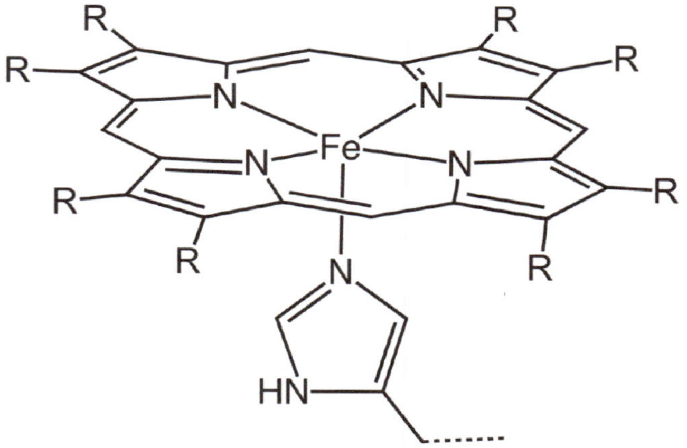

Which of the following best approximates subunits (monomers) contained in heme?

A. 4 pyrrole subunits
B. 4 pyridine subunits
C. 4 piperidine subunits
D. 1 pyridine subunit 'below' the iron atom

High-level Importance

High-level Importance

Questions 17–22

Opioids are substances that act on opioid receptors to produce morphine-like effects. Opioids are primarily used for pain relief (analgesic). Consider the structure of morphine below.

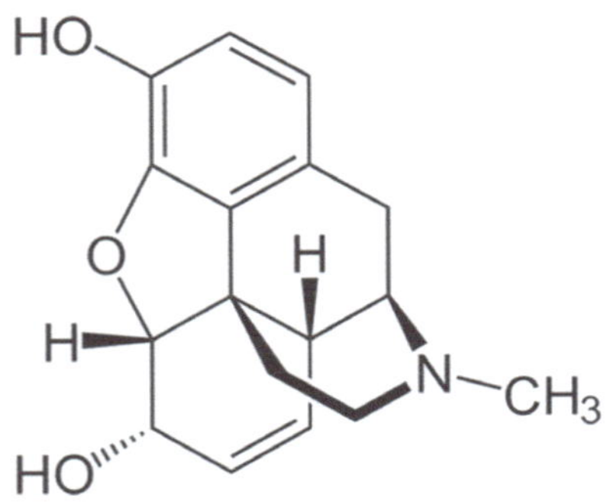

Morphine and other opioids share a characteristic set of four features called the 'morphine rule':

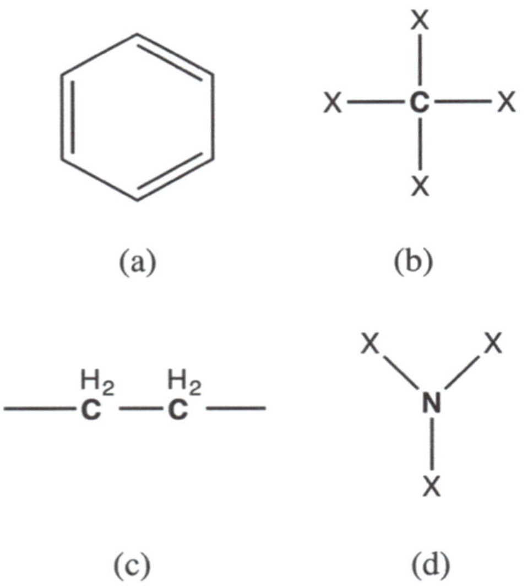

(a) a benzene ring;

(b) structure (a) linked to a quaternary carbon atom;

(c) two adjacent CH_2 groups ('linker') between (b) and (d), and

(d) a tertiary nitrogen atom.

Note that:

- A primary position is where the atom is attached to one carbon.
- A secondary position is where the atom is attached to two carbons.
- A tertiary position is where the atom is attached to three carbons.
- A quaternary position is where the atom is attached to four carbons.

17) Based on the information provided, which of the following is most consistent with the morphine rules?

A. X cannot be hydrogen.
B. An opioid must have at least 15 carbons.
C. Additional functional groups are essential for morphine-like effects.
D. The 2 carbons in the linker must both be secondary positions.

18) Consider the molecule trimethyldiphenylpropylamine below.

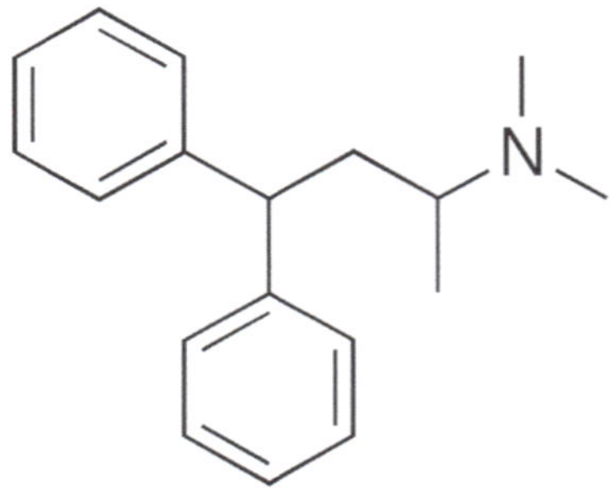

How many of the 4 morphine rules can be found in the structure of trimethyldiphenylpropylamine?

A. 4
B. 3
C. 2
D. 1

The next 2 questions refer to the following additional information.

Consider the structures of the molecules below.

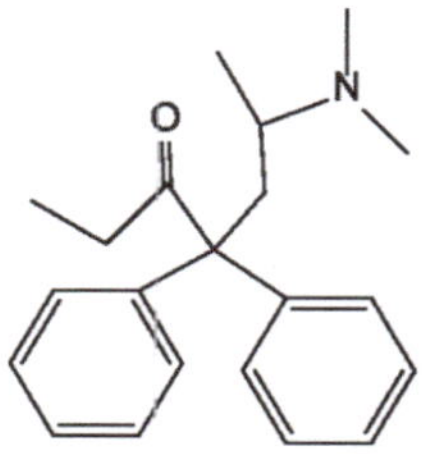

Methadone

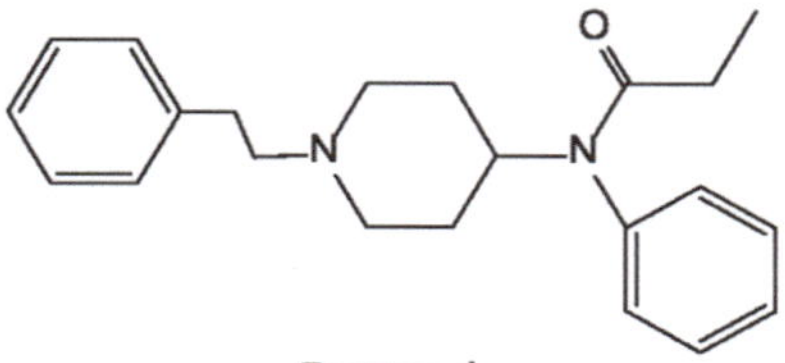

Fentanyl

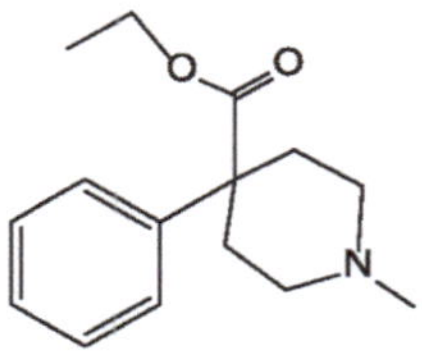

Meperidine

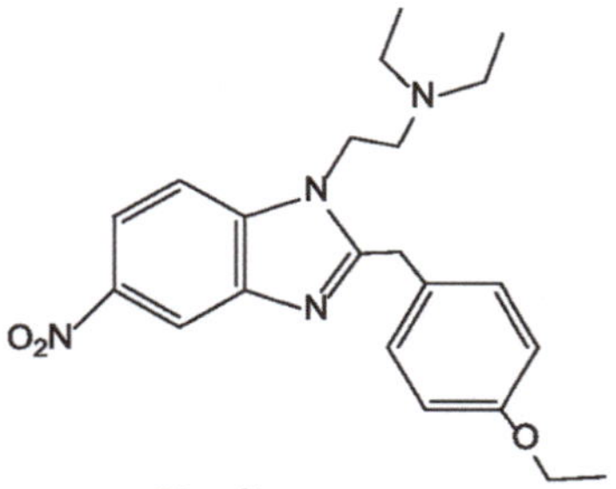

Etonitazene

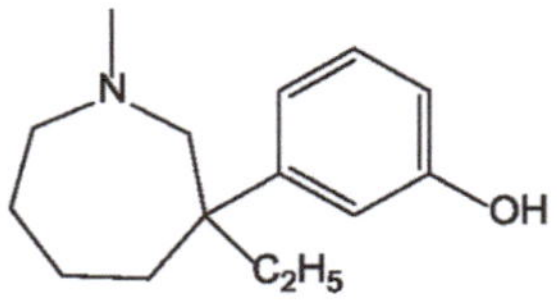

Meptazinol

19) How many of the 5 preceding molecules do **not** obey the morphine rule?

A. All
B. 3-4
C. 1-2
D. 0

20) Based on the structures provided, at standard temperature and pressure, which of the following would be expected to have the greatest solubility in water?

A. Methadone
B. Morphine
C. Fentanyl
D. Meptazinol

21) The general structure for codeine is as follows:

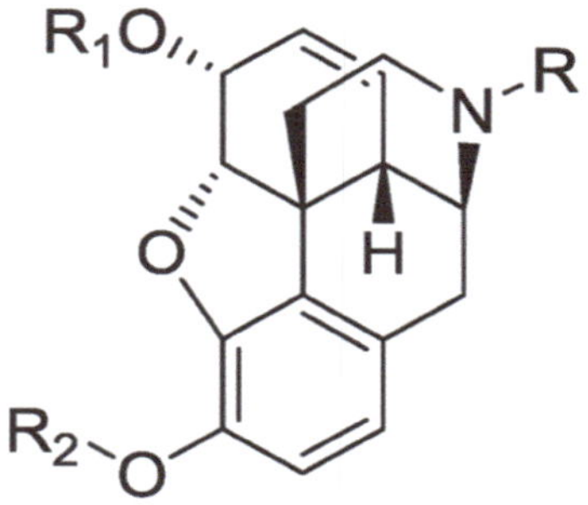

Which of the following would most clearly point to the fact that codeine follows the morphine rule?

A. $R_1 = R_2 = H$
B. $R = R_1 = H$
C. $R_1 = R_2 = CH_3$
D. $R = R_2 = CH_3$

22) Consider the structure of morphine provided in the passage. How many stereocentres does morphine have?

A. More than 5
B. 5
C. 4
D. Less than 4

High-level Importance

23) In chemistry, resonance is a way of representing delocalised electrons within certain molecules where the bonding cannot be expressed by one single Lewis formula. A molecule with delocalised electrons can be represented by several contributing structures. Each of the following structures is a resonance form of the molecule shown below EXCEPT one. Which one is the EXCEPTION?

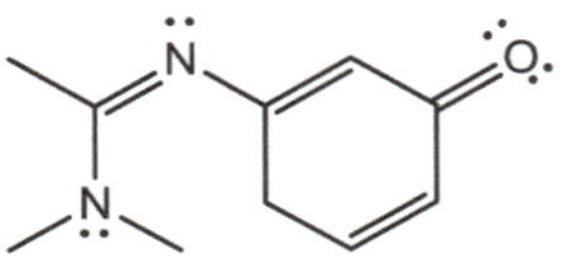

A. 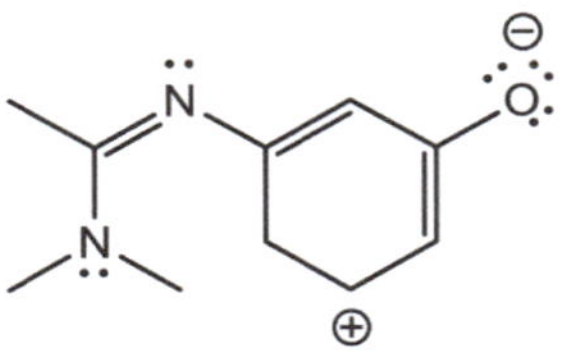

C. 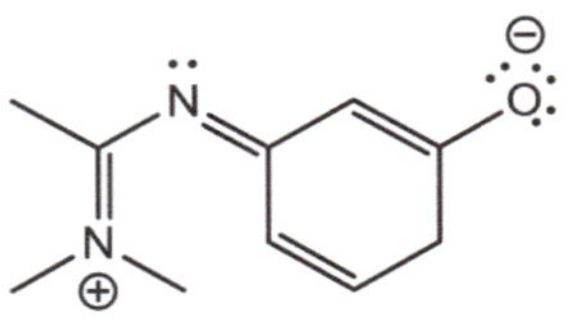

B. 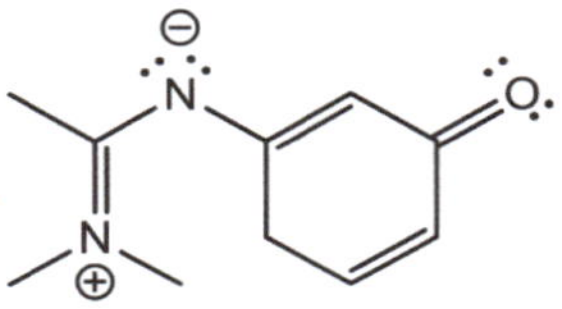

D. 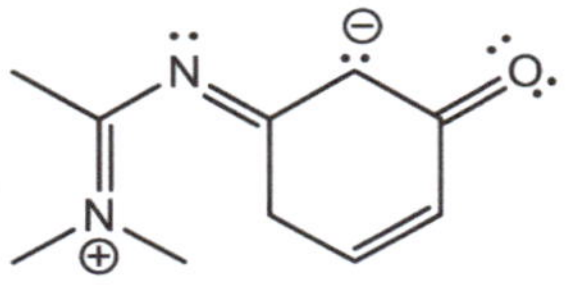

Questions 24–25

Molecular rearrangements in which a sigma-bonded atom or group, flanked by one or more pi-electron systems, shifts to a new location with a corresponding reorganisation of the pi-bonds, are called *sigmatropic reactions.*

The aza-Cope rearrangements are examples of heteroatom versions of the Cope rearrangement, which is a [3,3]-sigmatropic rearrangement that shifts single and double bonds between two allylic components. Aza-Cope rearrangements are generally classified as follows:

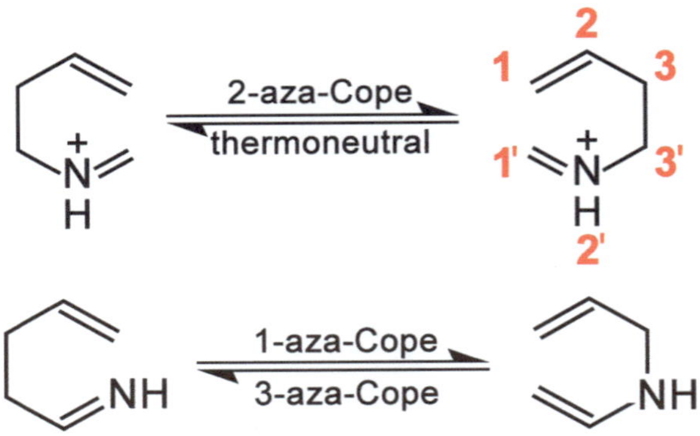

Figure 1

Note the directions of the equilibrium arrows. For example, the first forward reaction in Figure 1 is indicated as 2-aza-Cope, while the reverse reaction is indicated as thermoneutral.

Consider the following aza-Cope sigmatropic reaction.

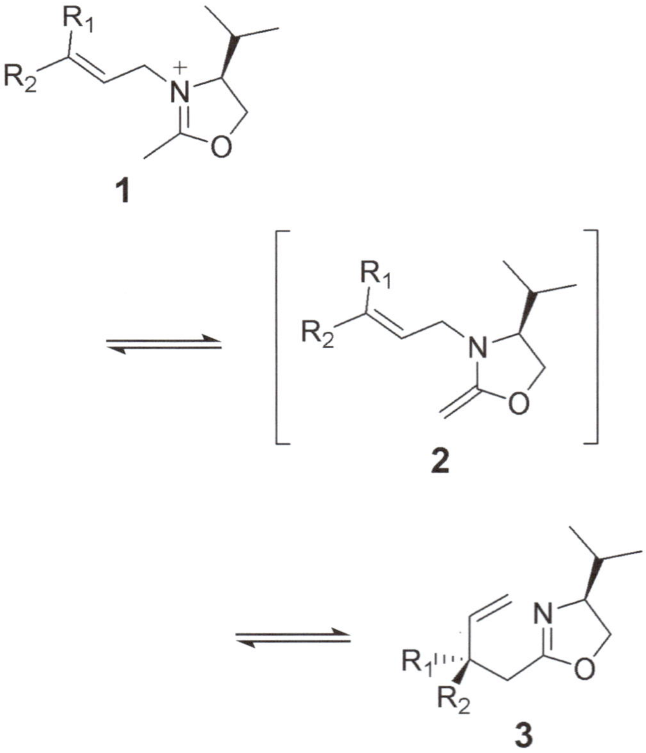

Figure 2

24) Based on the information provided, which of the following is true regarding the numbered compounds in Figure 2?

A. The transformation from **1** to **2** is a 1-aza-Cope.

B. The transformation from **2** to **1** is a 2-aza-Cope.

C. The transformation from **2** to **3** is a 3-aza-Cope.

D. Neither **A** nor **B** nor **C** is correct.

25) The quaternary ammonium ion *N*-allyl-*N*,*N*-dimethylanilinium ion is illustrated below.

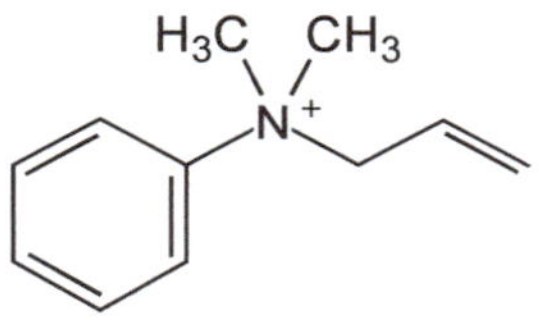

In a similar reaction to aza-Cope, if the *N*-allyl-*N*,*N*-dimethylanilinium ion underwent a [3,3]-sigmatropic rearrangement, which of the following would be most likely?

A.
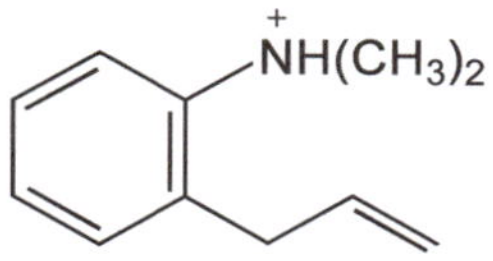

B.
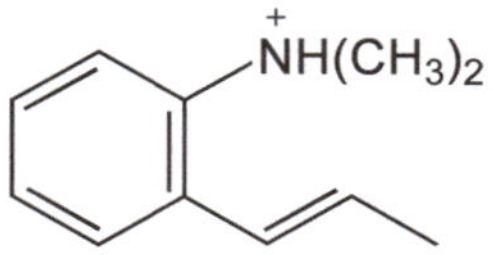

C.
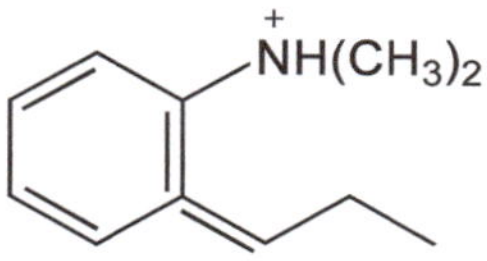

D.
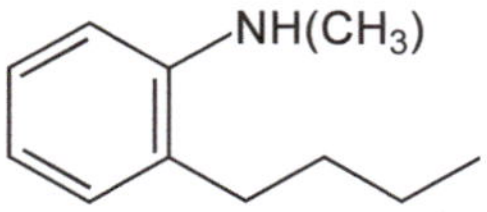

SPOILER ALERT

Gold Standard has cross-referenced the content in this chapter to examples from ACER's official GAMSAT practice materials. It is for you to decide when you want to explore these questions since you may want to preserve some of ACER's materials for timed mock-exam practice.

Examples – Correct representation of a hydrogen bond (*which we put in Foundational; not counted for this chapter since it was ascribed to general chemistry*): Q8 of 3; quaternary ammonium ion and piperidine with reactions based on substituents: Q95-98 of 3. Note that "Q" is followed by the question number, and, for example, "of 1" refers to booklet number 1 which is referenced in the Spoiler Alert table at the end of Chapter 1. The 15 full-length GAMSAT practice tests by Gold Standard, HEAPS-1 through HEAPS-15, contain specific cross-references to this chapter within the worked solutions. Note that 2 units are from the Gold Standard virtual reality (VR) mock exams: the unit with the secondary amine piperidine, as well as pyridine, and pyrrole are from VR-1; the unit exploring the morphine rule is from VR-2. ACER loves to give rules to see if you can apply them 'on the go' with novel situations.

Chapter Checklist

- ☐ Access your online account to view answers, worked solutions and discussion boards.
- ☐ Reassess your 'learning objectives' for this chapter: Go back to the first page of this chapter and re-evaluate the top 3 boxes and the Introduction.
- ☐ Complete a maximum of 1 page of notes using symbols/abbreviations to represent the entire chapter based on your learning objectives. These are your Gold Notes.
- ☐ Consider your multimedia options based on your optimal way of learning:
  - ☐ Download the free Gold Standard GAMSAT app for your Android device or iPhone.
  - ☐ Create your own, tangible study cards or try the free app: Anki.
  - ☐ Record your voice reading your Gold Notes onto your smartphone (audio files, e.g., *memo* or MP3s) and listen during exercise, transportation, etc.
  - ☐ Try out the Gold Standard GAMSAT online videos at gamsat-prep.com, or you can try other options on YouTube like Khan Academy or Crash Course Organic Chemistry.
- ☐ Reassess your schedule for your full-length GAMSAT practice tests: ACER and/or HEAPS exams. Ensure that you have scheduled one full day to complete a practice test and 1-2 days for a thorough assessment of worked solutions while adding to your abbreviated Gold Notes.
- ☐ Reassess your progress in scheduling and/or evaluating stress reduction techniques such as regular exercise (sports), yoga, meditation and/or mindfulness exercises (*see* YouTube for suggestions).

BIOLOGICAL MOLECULES

Chapter 12

Memorise

* Basic structures

Understand

* Effect of H, S, hydrophobic bonds
* Effect of pH, isoelectric point
* Different ways of drawing structures
* Identify a peptide bond
* Condensation, hydrolysis
* Hydration, dehydration

Importance

High level: 15% of GAMSAT Organic Chemistry

questions released by ACER are related to content in this chapter (in our estimation).

* Note that approximately 60% of the questions in GAMSAT Organic Chemistry are related to just 4 chapters: 2, 6, 7 and 12.

GAMSAT-Prep.com

Introduction

Biological molecules truly involve the chemistry of life. Such molecules include amino acids and proteins, carbohydrates (glucose, disaccharides, polysaccharides), lipids (triglycerides, steroids) and nucleic acids (DNA, RNA).

Multimedia Resources at GAMSAT-Prep.com

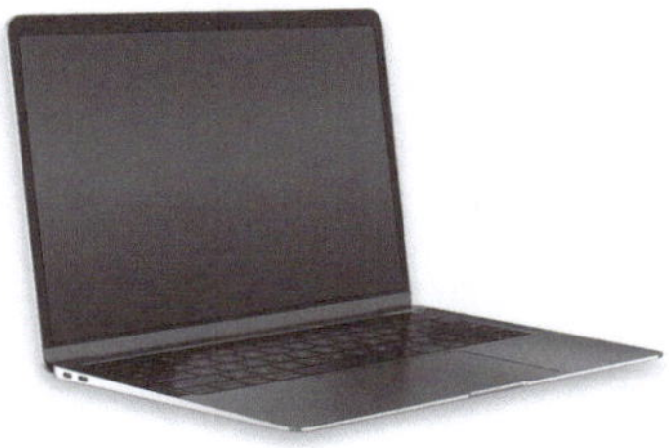

Open Discussion Boards
(*gamsat-prep.com/forum*)

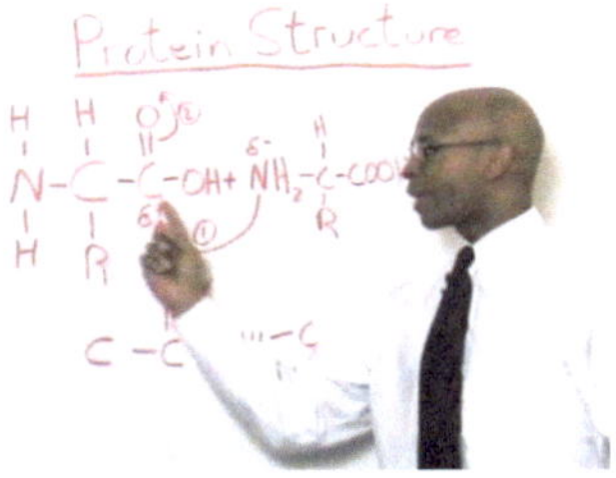

Science Preparation Videos

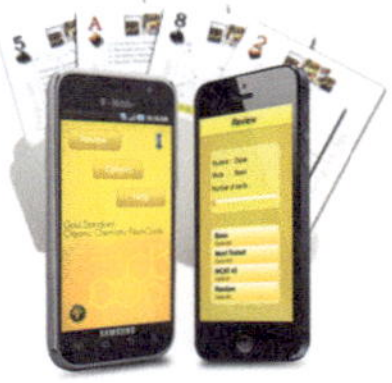

Flashcards

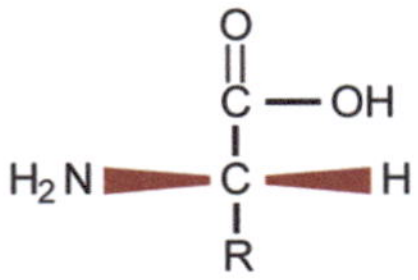

Special Guest

* The real GAMSAT may have advanced-level information presented (i.e. in a passage) but previous knowledge of said information is not required to answer the questions that would follow. Practice questions at the end of this chapter, as well as ACER and GS (HEAPS) practice GAMSATs can help you clarify this point.

12.1 Amino Acids

High-level Importance

Protein-building amino acids are molecules that contain a side chain (*R*), a carboxylic acid, and an amino group at the α carbon. Thus the general structure of α-amino acids is:

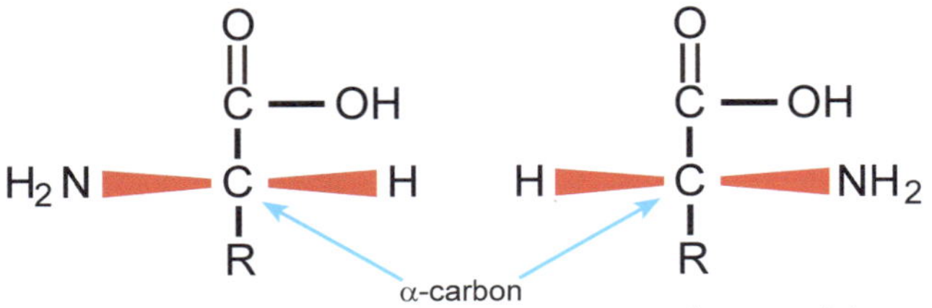

L - amino acid "left-handed" isomer   D - amino acid "right-handed" isomer

From your GAMSAT Organic Chemistry revision, you should remember that the carbonyl carbon (C=O) in a carboxylic acid is carbon-1 (ORG 8.1), and the adjacent carbon (carbon-2) is the alpha position, carbon-3 is the beta position (ORG 7.1), and carbon-4 is thus the gamma position.

Amino acids may be named systematically as substituted carboxylic acids; however, there are 20 important α-amino acids that are known by common names. These are naturally occurring and they form the building blocks of most proteins found in humans. The following are a few examples of α-amino acids:

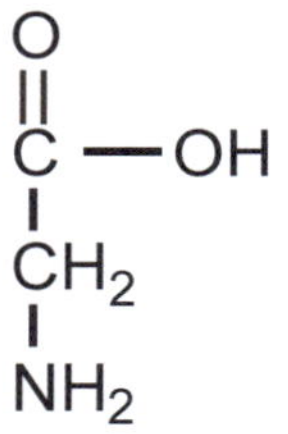

Glycine

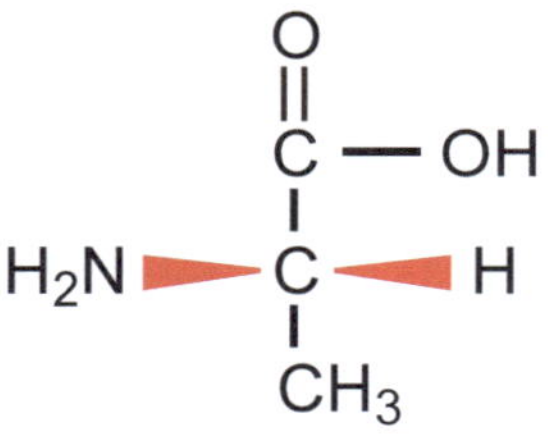

Alanine

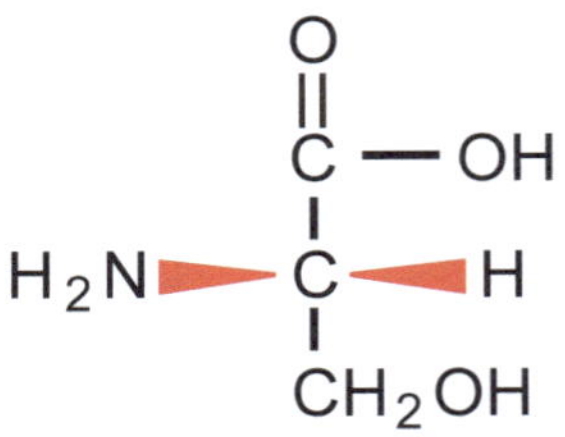

Serine

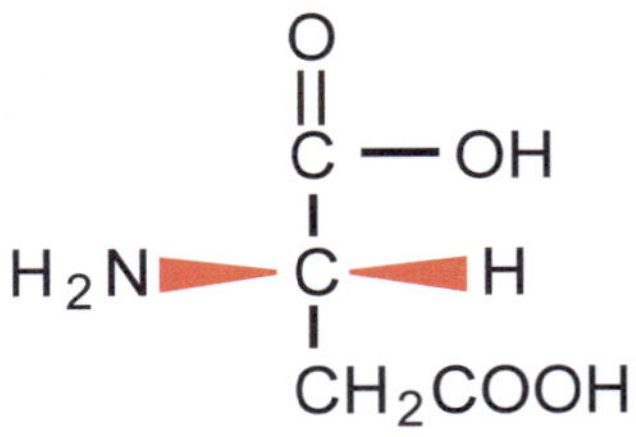

Aspartic acid

Note that the D/L system is commonly used for amino acid and carbohydrate chemistry. The reason is that naturally occurring amino acids have the same relative configuration, the L-configuration, while naturally occurring carbohydrates are nearly all D-configuration. However, the absolute configuration (i.e. R/S) depends on the priority assigned to the side group (*see* ORG 2.3.1 *for rules*).

The illustrations of the preceding amino acids are all in the L configuration and they also correspond to the S absolute stereochemistry (*except glycine which cannot be assigned any configuration since it is not chiral*).

The following mnemonic is helpful for determining the D/L isomeric form of an amino acid: the "CORN" rule. The substituents **CO**OH, **R**, **N**H_2, and H are arranged around the chiral centre. Starting with H away from the viewer, if these groups are arranged clockwise around the chiral carbon, then it is the D-form. If counter-clockwise, it is the L-form. Of course, if hydrogen is pointing towards the viewer - like the structures on this page - then the pattern is reversed.

Also note that, except for glycine, the α-carbon of all amino acids are chiral indicating that there must be at least two different enantiomeric forms. Notice in the preceding illustrations that the alpha carbon in glycine is not bonded to 4 different substituents since it is bonded to hydrogen twice; however, the alpha carbon in alanine, serine and aspartic acid has 4 different substituents in each case meaning that carbon is chiral. Notice that chirality of carbon hinges on its attachment to 4 different substituents (i.e. groups/ligands) and NOT necessarily 4 different atoms. A chiral carbon is sometimes referred to as a stereocentre or as a stereogenic or asymmetric carbon (ORG 2.2, 2.3).

Many important amino acids can play critical non-protein roles within the body. For example, glutamate and gamma-aminobutyric acid ("GABA", a non-standard gamma-amino acid) are, respectively, the main excitatory and inhibitory neurotransmitters in the human brain (BIO 5.1).

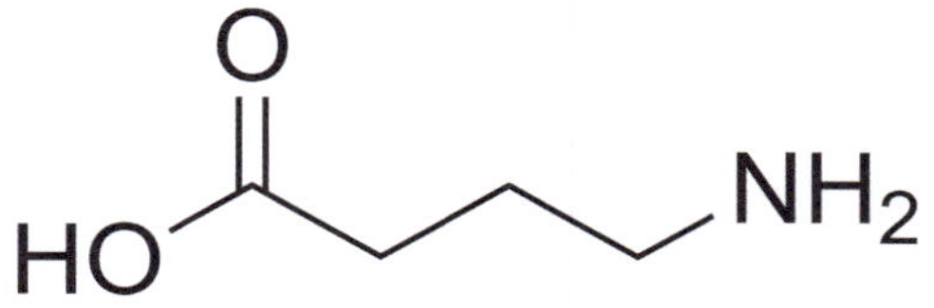

GABA: A gamma-amino acid.
Notice that the amino group is attached to the 3rd carbon from the carbonyl carbon (C=O).

Unless specified otherwise, the following sections will be exploring features of alpha-amino acids.

12.1.1 Hydrophilic vs. Hydrophobic

Different types of amino acids tend to be found in different areas of the proteins that they make up. Amino acids which are ionic and/or polar are hydrophilic, and tend to be found on the exterior of proteins (i.e. *exposed to water*). These include aspartic acid and its amide, glutamic acid and its amide, lysine, arginine and histidine. Certain other polar amino acids are found on either the interior or exterior of proteins. These include serine, threonine, and tyrosine. Hydrophobic ('water-fearing") amino acids which may be found on the interior of proteins include methionine, leucine, tryptophan, valine and phenylalanine. Hydrophobic molecules tend to cluster in aqueous solutions (= *hydrophobic bonding*). Alanine is a nonpolar amino acid which is unusual because it is less hydrophobic than most nonpolar amino acids. This is because its nonpolar side chain is very short.

Glycine is the smallest amino acid, and the only one that is not optically active. It is often found at the 'corners' of proteins. Alanine is small and, although hydrophobic, is found on the surface of proteins.

12.1.2 Acidic vs. Basic

High-level Importance

Amino acids have both acid and base components (= *amphoteric*). The amino acids with the R group containing an amino ($-NH_2$) group are basic. The two basic amino acids are lysine and arginine. Amino acids with an R group containing a carboxyl ($-COOH$) group are acidic. The two acidic amino acids are aspartic acid and glutamic acid. One amino acid, histidine, may act as either an acid or a base, depending upon the pH of the resident solution. This makes histidine a very good physiologic buffer. The rest of the amino acids are considered to be neutral.

The basic $-NH_2$ group in an amino acid is present as an ammonium ion, $-NH_3^+$. The acidic carboxyl $-COOH$ group is present as a carboxylate ion, $-COO^-$. As a result, amino acids are dipolar ions, or *zwitterions*. In an aqueous solution, there is an equilibrium present between the dipolar, the anionic, and the cationic forms of the amino acid (*see* below). Also note that the way amino acids are presented in ORG 12.1 is a simplification since, at any pH, some part of an amino acid will *always* bear a charge due to the presence of both acidic and basic functional groups.

Therefore, the charge on the amino acid will vary with the pH of the solution, and with the isoelectric point. This point is the pH where a given amino acid will be neutral (i.e. have no net charge). This isoelectric point is the average of the two pK_a values (CHM 6.1, 6.3) of an amino acid (*depending on the dissociated group*):

$$\text{isoelectric point} = pI = (pK_{a1} + pK_{a2})/2$$

Since this is a commonly tested GAMSAT concept, let's further summarise for the average amino acid: When in a relatively acidic solution, the amino acid is fully protonated and exists as a cation, that is, it has two protons available for dissociation, one from the carboxyl group and one from the amino group. When in a relatively basic solution, the amino acid is fully deprotonated and exists as an anion, that is, it has two proton accepting groups, the carboxyl group and the amino group.

At the isoelectric point (pI), although the amino acid is overall neutral, it is a dipolar zwitterion. This means that the carboxyl group is deprotonated forming a carboxylate anion, and the amino group is protonated forming an ammonium cation. At their pI, amino acids (and proteins) have minimum solubility in water or salt solutions and often precipitate out of solution. With no net charge, they tend to remain (and interact) together, as opposed to when they have an overall, identical (repulsive) charge which increases interaction with a polar solvent (e.g., water; *'like dissolves like'*).

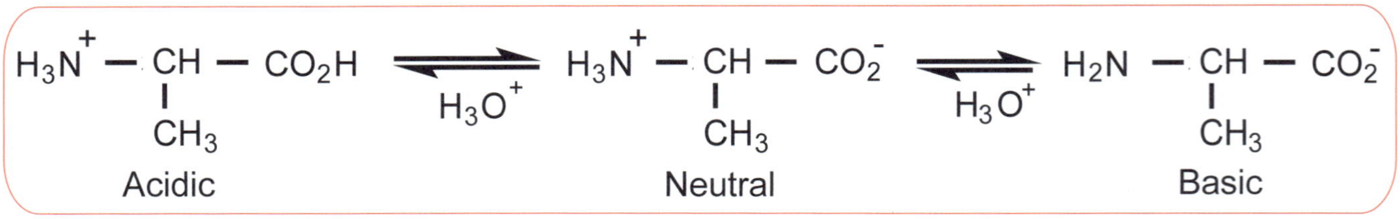

12.1.3 The 20 Alpha-Amino Acids

Approximately 500 amino acids are known - of these, only 22 are proteinogenic ("protein building") amino acids. Of these, 20 amino acids are known as "standard" and are found in human beings and other eukaryotes, and are encoded directly by the universal genetic code (BIO 3). The 2 exceptions are the "non-standard" pyrrolysine — found only in some methanogenic organisms but not humans — and selenocysteine which is present in humans and a wide range of other organisms.

Of the 20 standard amino acids, 9 are called "essential" for humans because they cannot be created from other compounds by the human body, and so must be taken in as food.

The following categorises amino acids based on side chains, pK_a and charges at human, physiological pH (~7.4):

1. Nonpolar amino acids: R groups are hydrophobic and thus decrease solubility. These amino acids are usually found within the interior of the protein molecule.

2. Polar amino acids: R groups are hydrophilic and thus increase the solubility. These amino acids are usually found on the protein's surface.

3. Acidic amino acids: R groups contain an additional carboxyl group. These amino acids have a negative charge at physiological pH.

4. Basic amino acids: R groups contain an additional amine group. These amino acids have a positive charge at physiological pH. Note that asparagine and glutamine have amide side chains and are thus not considered basic (*see* ORG 9.3).

Table IV.A.1.1: Basic Nomenclature for Biological Molecules. The exception to the monomer/polymer rule is lipids since lipid base units are not generally considered monomers.

Building block	Polymerises to form...	Chemical bonds	Macromolecule
Monomers	Dimer, trimer, tetramer, oligomers, etc.	Covalent* bonds	Polymer
Amino acids	Dipeptide, tripeptide, tetra/oligopeptide, etc	Peptide bonds	Polypeptide, protein (e.g. insulin, hemoglobin)
Monosaccharides ('simple sugars'**)	Disaccharide, tri/tetra/ oligosaccharide, etc.	Glycosidic bonds	Polysaccharide (e.g. starch, glycogen)
Nucleotides	Nucleotide dimer, tri/tetra/oligomer, etc.	Phosphodiester bonds	Polynucleotides, nucleic acids (e.g. DNA, RNA)

*There are exceptions. For example, in certain circumstances polypeptides are considered monomers and they may bond non-covalently to form dimers (i.e. higher orders of protein structure which will be discussed in following sections).

**Note that disaccharides are also sugars (i.e. sucrose is a glucose-fructose dimer known as 'table sugar'; lactose is a glucose-galactose dimer known as 'milk sugar').

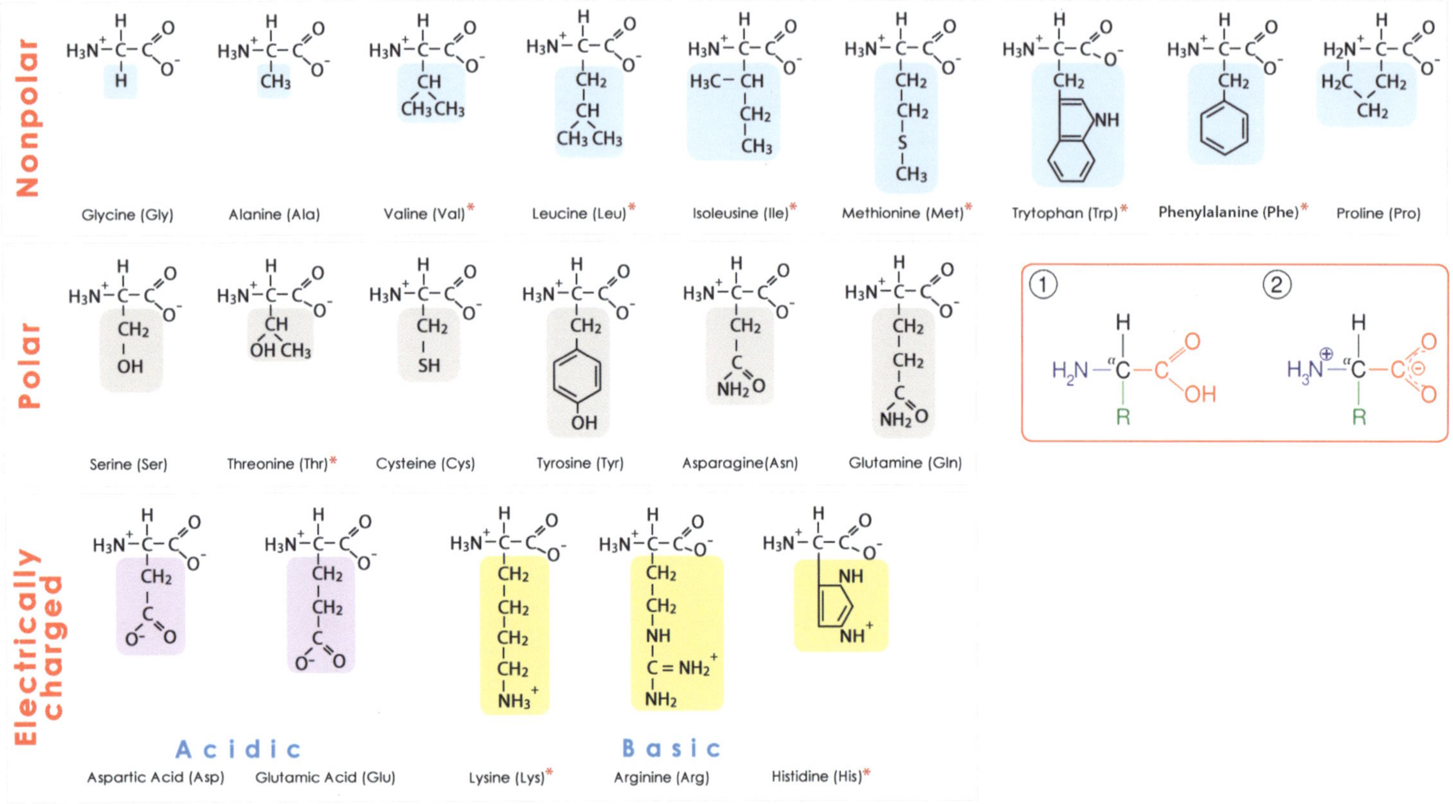

Figure IV.A.1.1: The 20 Standard Amino Acids. A red asterisk * is used to indicate the 9 essential amino acids.
Notice that if the acidic electrically charged amino acids are fully protonated, the overall charge would be +1 but if fully deprotonated, the overall charge would be -2. The opposite being true for basic amino acids: If fully protonated, the overall charge would be +2 but if fully deprotonated, the overall charge would be -1. These cases are different than for the average amino acid described at the end of section ORG 12.1.2. Skim through the names and structures of the 20 standard amino acids but please do not memorise.

Note the inset (in the red box) which shows the general structure for an amino acid in both the (1) unionised and (2) zwitterionic forms. For the latter, note the resonance stabilised carboxylate anion in red, the primary ammonium ion in blue, and the variable R group in green.

High-level Importance

12.2 Proteins

12.2.1 General Principles

An oligopeptide consists of between 2 and 20 amino acids joined together by amide *(peptide)* bonds. Oligopeptides include dipeptides (2 amino acids), tripeptides (3), tetrapeptides (4), pentapeptides (5), etc. Polypeptides - generally regarded to be between the size of oligopeptides and proteins - are polymers of up to 100 or even 1000 α-amino acids (depending on the molecule and the reference). Proteins are long chain polypeptides which often form higher order structures. These peptide bonds are derived from the amino group of one amino acid, and the acid group of another. When a peptide bond is formed, a molecule of water is released (*condensation = dehydration = water loss*). The bond can be broken by adding water (*hydrolysis = water lyses = water 'breaks apart' another molecule*).

Since proteins are polymers of amino acids, they also have isoelectric points. Classification as to the acidity or basicity of a protein depends on the numbers of acidic and basic amino acids it contains. If there is an excess of acidic amino acids, the isoelectric point will be at a pH of less than 7. At pH = 7, these proteins will have a net negative charge. Similarly, those with an excess of basic amino acids will have an isoelectric point at a pH of greater than 7. Therefore, at pH = 7, these proteins will have a net positive charge. Proteins can be separated according to their isoelectric point on a polyacrylamide gel (*electrophoresis*; ORG 13). We will be discussing protein synthesis in Biology Chapter 3.

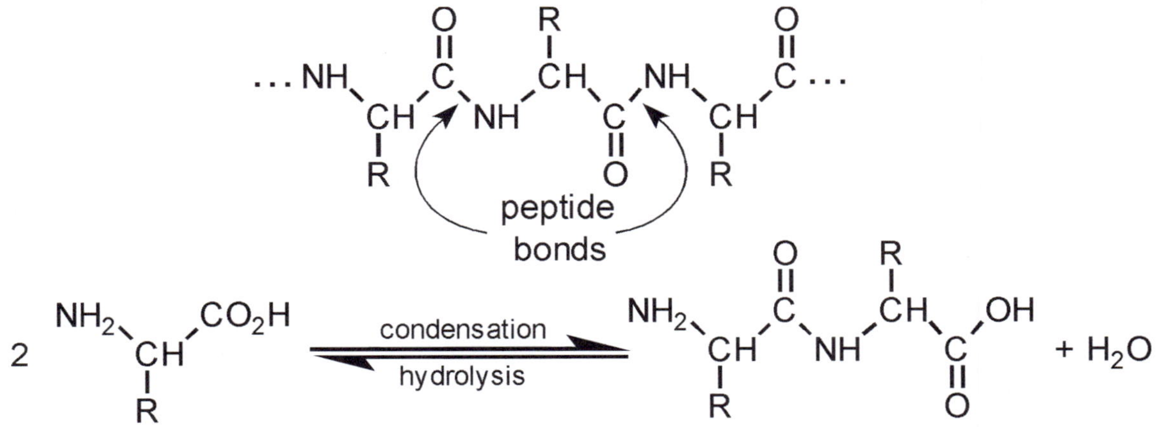

Figure IV.A.1.2: Condensation and hydrolysis. Note that the forward reaction shows 2 moles of amino acid producing a dipeptide and water. The dipeptide is composed of 2 amino acid 'residues' (i.e. what is left over once water is removed). By convention, the amino group (N-terminus) is on the left and the carboxyl group (C-terminus) is on the right.

12.2.2 Protein Structure

High-level Importance

Protein structure may be divided into primary, secondary, tertiary and quaternary structures. The primary structure is the sequence of amino acids as determined by the DNA and the location of covalent bonds (*including disulfide bonds*). This structure determines the higher order structures.

The primary structure is usually shown using 3-letter abbreviations for the amino acid residues as shown in Fig IV.A.1.1. By convention, the amino group (N-terminus) is on the left and the carboxyl group (C-terminus) on the right. For example, insulin (BIO 6.3.4) is composed of 51 amino acids in 2 chains. One chain has 30 amino acids, and the other has 21 amino acids with the following primary structure: GLY-ILE-VAL-GLU-GLN-CYS-CYS-THR-SER-ILE-CYS-SER-LEU-TYR-GLN-LEU-GLU-ASN-TYR-CYS-ASN.

The secondary structure is the orderly inter- or intramolecular *hydrogen bonding* of the protein chain. The resultant structure may be the more stable α-helix (e.g. keratin), or β-strands forming a β-pleated sheet (e.g. silk). Proline is an amino acid which cannot participate in the regular array of H-bonding in an α-helix. Proline disrupts the α-helix, thus it is usually found at the beginning or end of a molecule (i.e. hemoglobin).

The tertiary structure is the further folding of the protein molecule onto itself. This is the 3D shape (spatial organisation) of an entire protein molecule. Protein folding is largely self-organising mainly based on the protein's primary structure. The tertiary structure is maintained by *noncovalent bonds* like hydrogen bonding, Van der Waals forces, hydrophobic bonding and electrostatic bonding (CHM 4.2). The resultant structure is a globular protein with a hydrophobic interior and hydrophilic exterior. Enzymes are classic examples of such a structure. In fact, enzyme activity often depends on tertiary structure.

The covalent bonding of cysteine (*disulfide bonds or bridge*) helps to stabilise the tertiary structure of proteins. Cysteine will form sulfur-sulfur covalent bonds with itself, producing *cystine*. For example, insulin is composed of 2 polypeptide chains, an A-chain and a B-chain (2 = a dimer), which are linked together by disulfide bonds.

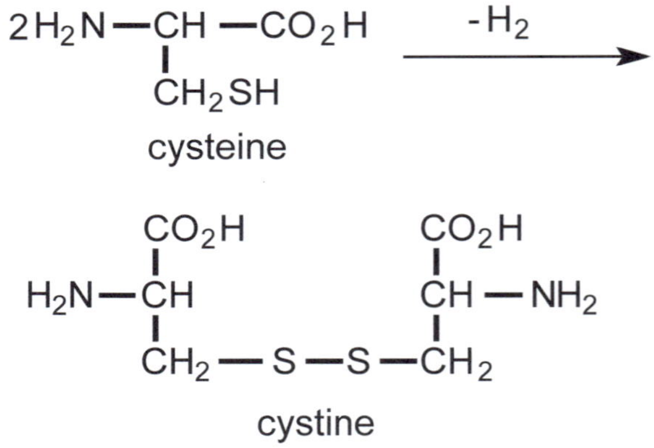

The quaternary structure is when there are two or more protein chains bonded together by noncovalent bonds. For example, hemoglobin (BIO 7.5.1) consists of four polypeptide subunits (*globin*) held together by hydrophobic bonds forming a globular almost tetrahedryl arrangement.

The secondary, tertiary, and quaternary structures of a protein may be destroyed in a number of ways (= *denaturation*). For example, heating (cooking) can break hydrogen bonds. Altering the pH can protonate or deprotonate the molecule and interrupt ionic interactions. Reducing agents can break disulfide bonds. Depending on the conditions, denaturation may be reversible.

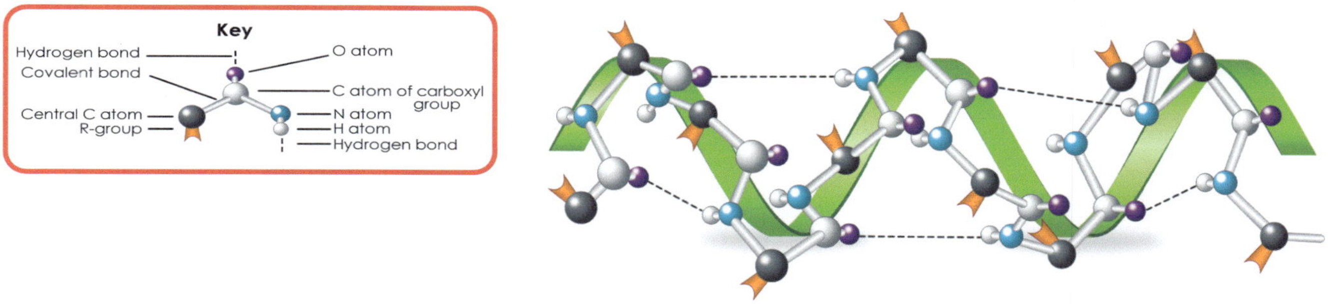

Figure IV.A.1.3: Secondary Structure: α-helix; note the peptide chain is coiled into a helical structure around a central axis. This helix is stabilised by hydrogen bonding between the N-H group and C=O group four residues away. A typical example with this secondary structure is keratin. Keratin is a fibrous, structural protein found in skin, hair and nails (BIO 13.2, 13.3.1). Seen in green above, a spiral ribbon can symbolise an α-helix.

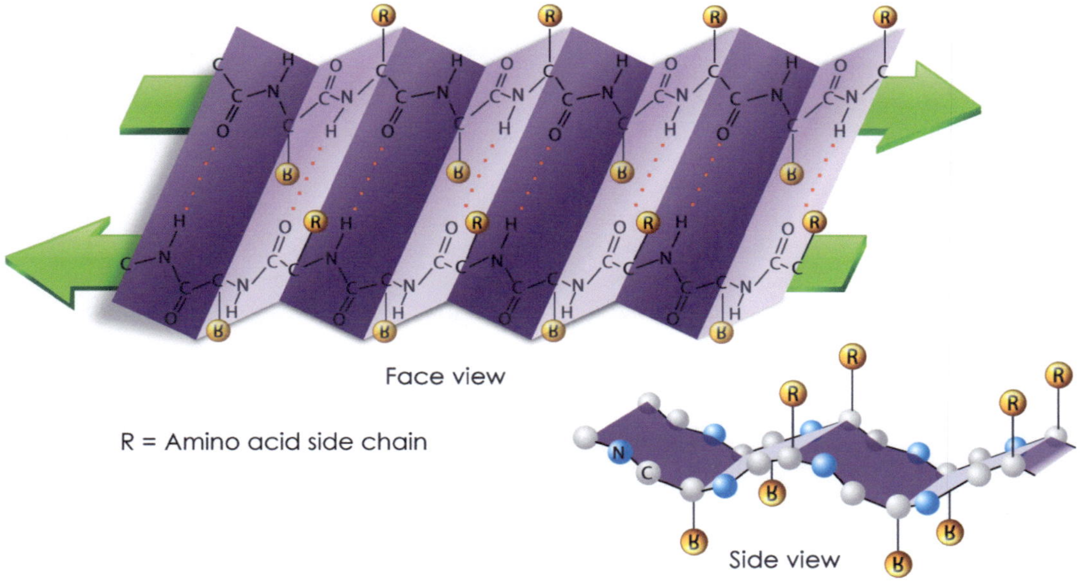

Figure IV.A.1.4: Secondary Structure: 2 β-strands (green arrows) forming a β-pleated sheet. Peptide chains lie alongside each other in a parallel manner. This structure is stabilised by hydrogen bonding between the N-H group on one β-strand and C=O group on another. A typical example with this secondary structure is produced by some insect larvae: the protein fiber "silk" which is mostly composed of fibroin.

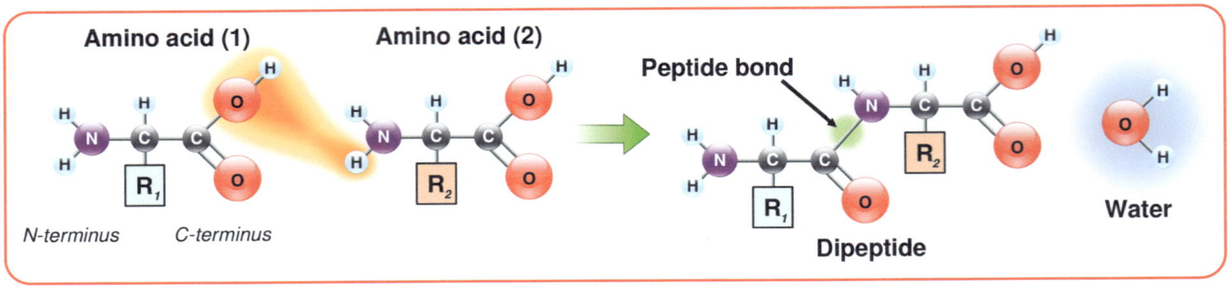

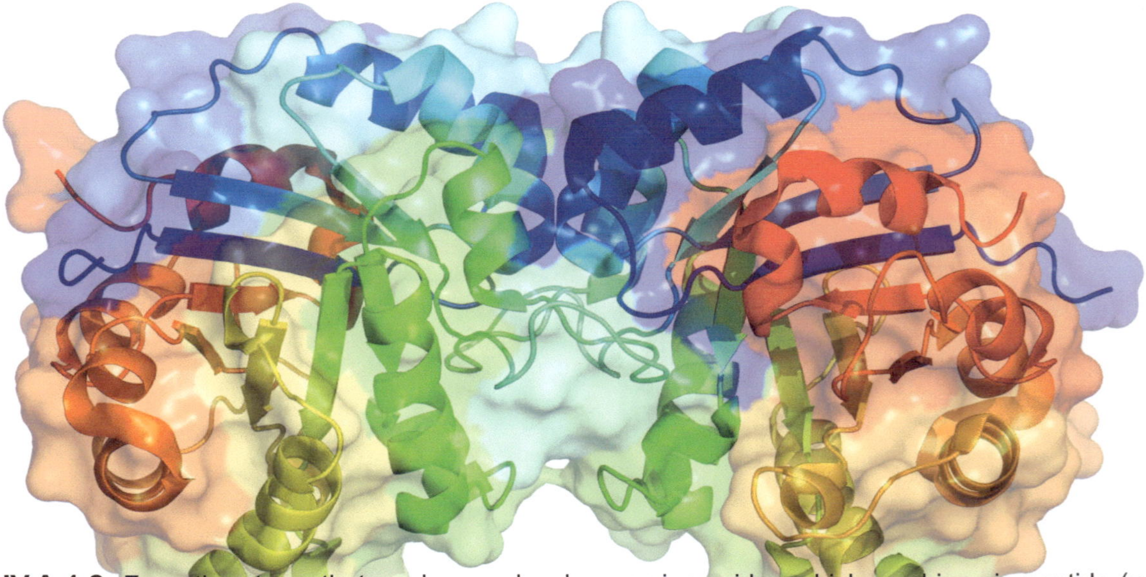

Figure IV.A.1.2: From the atoms that produce molecules - amino acids - which combine via peptide (= *amide*) bonds in a specific order (= **primary structure**), to the level of organisation of these same molecules which conglomerate in a specified way based on the primary structure to produce higher-order structures resulting in the protein above. Approximately 250 amino acid residues combine to produce each of the 2 identical subunits (= *dimer*; notice the similarity between the left and right sides of the main image above). **Secondary structure:** The curled (helical, cylindrical, spiral) ribbons indicate α-helices. Arrows with thickness show the direction and twist of β-strands from amino to the carboxyl end forming parallel β-sheets. Aside from the preceding, note the strands (like rope or spaghetti) which can be coils, loops or turns relatively high in glycine (the smallest amino acid) and proline (with its unique, cyclic secondary amine R group). **Tertiary structure:** The overall 3D shape (globular structure), which is central to the function of the protein, can be seen - in part - as the 'surface contour' of the actual structure (based on a space-filling model). The 3D structure of each of the 2 subunits contains eight α-helices on the outside and eight parallel β-strands on the inside. In the illustration, the ribbon backbone of each subunit is coloured in blue to red from N-terminus to C-terminus. **Quaternary structure:** 2 subunits (left-right in the image) forming a dimer held together by various noncovalent bonds.

The protein above is the enzyme (= catalyst) triose phosphate isomerase (TPI). TPI catalyses a reaction in glycolysis (= the lysis or breakdown of glucose to produce energy, BIO 4.5) thus is essential for efficient energy production. TPI is a highly efficient enzyme, performing the reaction billions of times faster than it would occur naturally in solution. The reaction is so efficient that it is said to be 'catalytically perfect': It is limited only by the rate the substrate can diffuse into and out of the enzyme's active site.

In the GAMSAT Biology Masters Series, we will be exploring many of the specific functions of proteins. Suffice to say for now that proteins are involved in virtually every process within cells. Proteins include the enzymes that accelerate the rate of (= catalyse) biochemical reactions. Proteins also have both structural (cytoskeleton) and mechanical functions (muscle: actin and myosin). Other protein functions include cell signaling, immune responses, cell adhesion and the cell cycle. Proteins are a necessary component of our diets since we cannot synthesise all the amino acids we need and thus must obtain essential amino acids from food.

During the GAMSAT, it is likely that you will read passages that describe various methods in which proteins can be purified from other cellular components. These techniques include ultracentrifugation, precipitation, electrophoresis and chromatography (ORG 13). Protein structure and function are often studied using immunohistochemistry (BIO 1.5.1), nuclear magnetic resonance (NMR) and mass spectrometry (ORG 14).

12.3 Carbohydrates

12.3.1 Description and Nomenclature

In general, the names of most carbohydrates are recognisable by an -ose suffix. Carbohydrates are sugars and their derivatives. Formally they are 'carbon hydrates,' that is, they have the general formula $C_m(H_2O)_n$. Usually they are defined as polyhydroxy aldehydes and ketones, or substances that hydrolyse to yield polyhydroxy aldehydes and ketones. The basic units of carbohydrates are monosaccharides (sugars; *see* table in ORG 12.1.3).

There are two ways to classify sugars. One way is to classify the molecule based on the type of carbonyl group it contains: one with an aldehyde carbonyl group is an *aldose*; one with a ketone carbonyl group is a *ketose*. The second method of classification depends on the number of carbons in the molecule: those with 6 carbons are hexoses, with 5 carbons are pentoses, with 4 carbons are tetroses, and with 3 carbons are trioses. Sugars may exist in either the ring form, as hemiacetals, or in the straight chain form, as polyhydroxy aldehydes. *Pyranoses* are 6 carbon sugars in the ring form; *furanoses* are 5 carbon sugars in the ring form.

In the ring form, there is the possibility of α or β *anomers*. Anomers occur when 2 cyclic forms of the molecule differ in conformation only at the hemiacetal carbon (carbon 1). Generally, pyranoses take the 'chair' conformation, as it is very stable, with all (usually) hydroxyl groups at the equatorial position. *Epimers* are diastereomers that differ in the

High-level Importance

configuration of only one stereogenic centre. For carbohydrates, epimers are 2 monosaccharides which differ in the conformation of one OH group.

To determine the number of possible optical isomers, one need only know the number of asymmetric carbons, normally 4 for hexoses and 3 for pentoses, designated as n. The number of optical isomers is then 2^n, where n is the number of asymmetric carbons (ORG 2.2.2).

Most of the naturally occurring aldoses have the D-configuration. Thus they have the same *relative* configuration as D-glyceraldehyde. The configuration (D or L) is *only* assigned to the highest numbered chiral carbon. The *absolute* configuration can be determined for any chiral carbon. For example, assessing its image (end of ORG 12.3.1), it can be determined that the absolute configuration of D-glyceraldehyde is the R-configuration.

Most carbohydrates contain one or more chiral carbons. For this reason, they are optically active. The names and structures of some common sugars are shown in Figure IV.A.1.5.

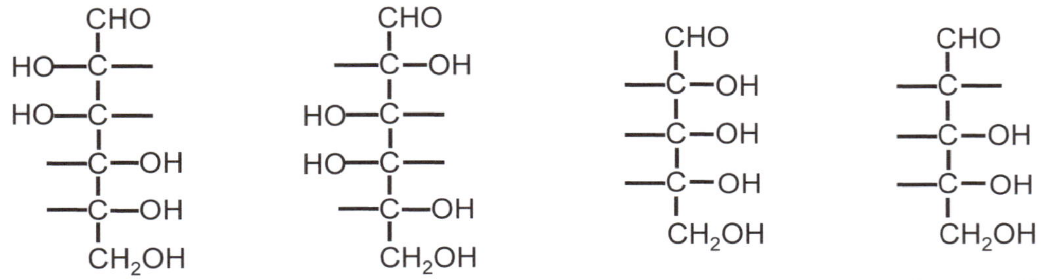

D - Mannose (C_2 epimer of glucose) | D - Galactose (C_4 epimer of glucose) | D - Ribose (in RNA) | 2 - Deoxy - D - ribose (in DNA)

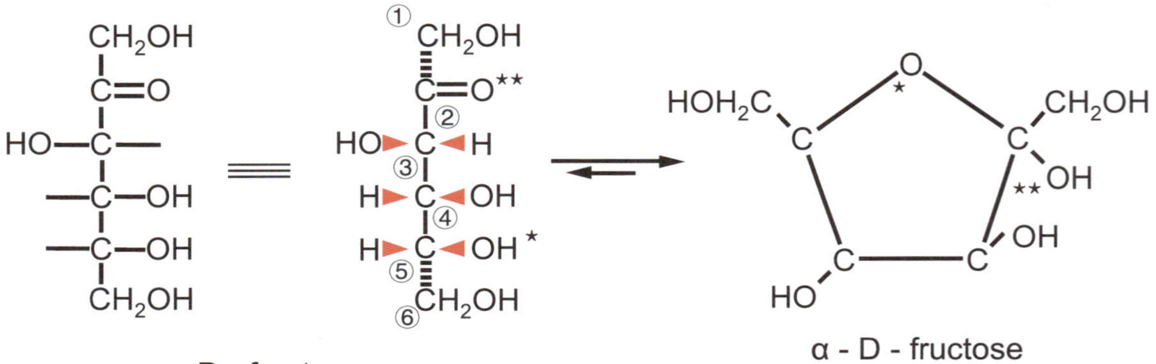

D - fructose (1,3,4,5,6-pentahydroxy-2-hexanone)

α - D - fructose (a furanose)

Figure IV.A.1.5 Part I: Names and configurations of common sugars. Notice that the asterisk * and ** allow you to follow a specific oxygen atom. Following atoms through a reaction is a common GAMSAT-type question. An asterisk, a prime symbol (') or a labelled isotope (ORG 1.6) are examples of techniques that may be used to identify the atom that you must follow. *See* ORG 12.3.2 for another example of a sugar 'folding' to become cyclic. Note that 3 parallel lines (≡) indicates: 'identical to'.

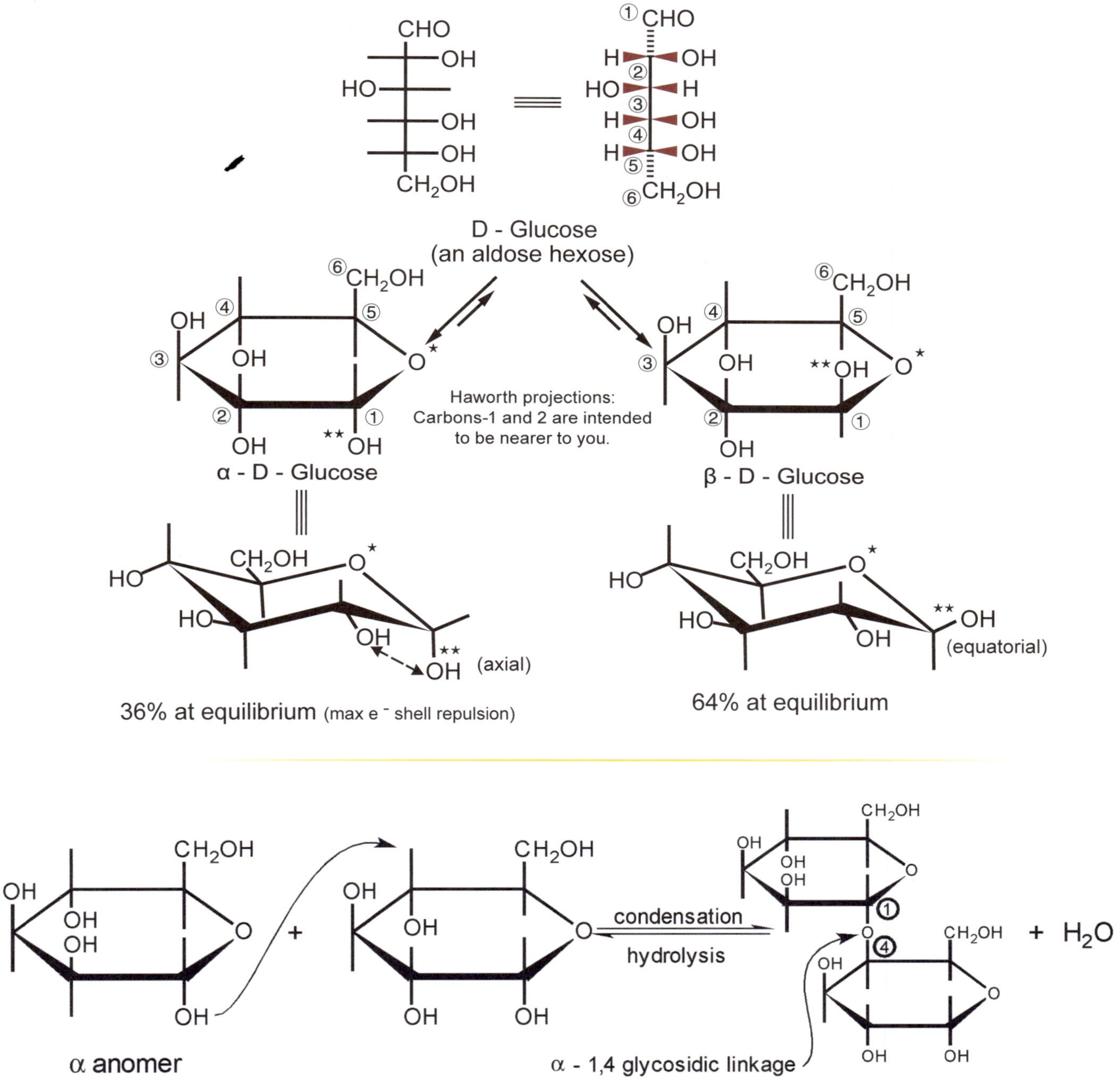

Figure IV.A.1.5 Part II: Names, structures and configurations of common sugars. Though not by convention, H belongs to the end of all empty bonds in the diagrams above. Note the following equivalent positions for substituents with glucose as an example: Right on Fischer = down on Hawthorne = alpha configuration = axial in the chair confirmation, and the opposite if on the left for a Fischer projection. The images below the yellow line show 2 monosaccharides engaging in a glycosidic bond (= linkage) to form a disaccharide (ORG 12.3.2, ORG 12.1.3 table).

High-level Importance

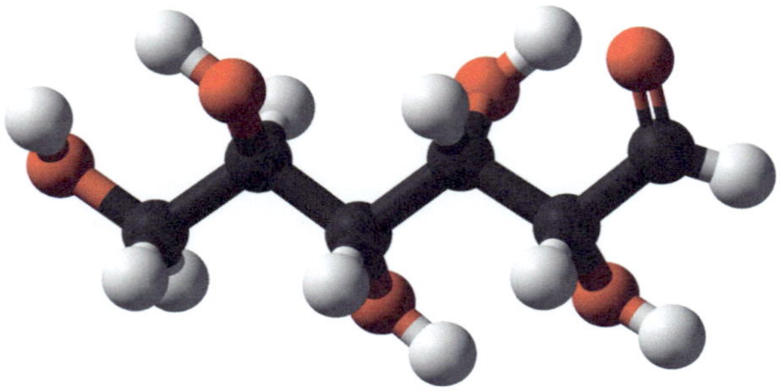

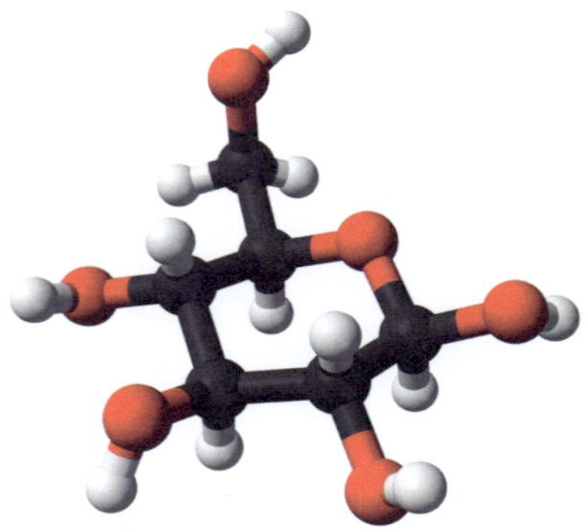

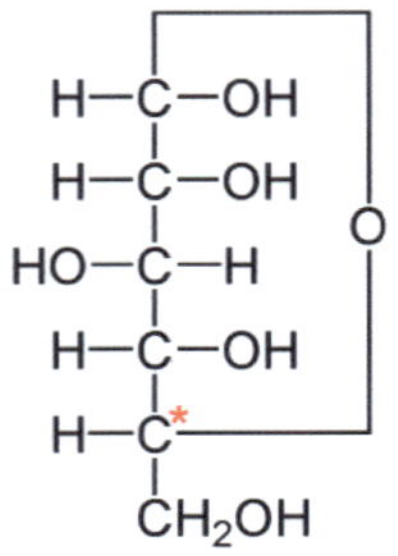

1

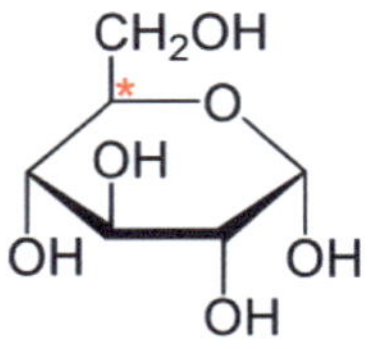

2

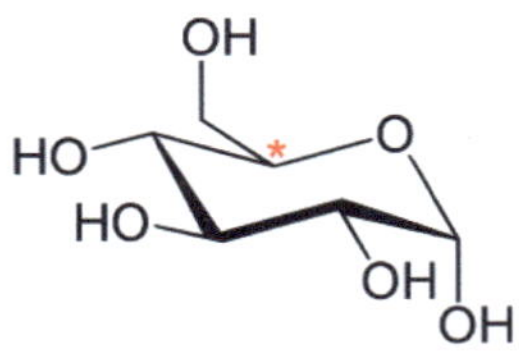

3

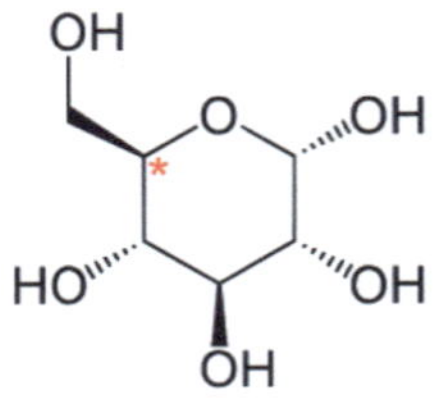

4

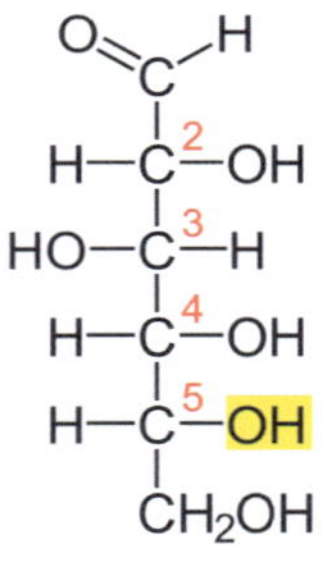

D-Glucose

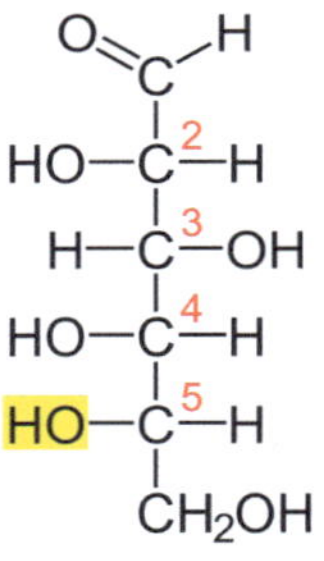

L-Glucose

Equivalent Positions in Different Structures			
Any Chiral Carbon (ORG 2.2)		Anomeric Carbon (ORG 12.3.2)	
Fischer Projection	Haworth Projection	Configuration	Chair Conformation
right	down	α	axial (ORG 3.3)
left	up	β	equatorial

Figure IV.A.1.5 Part III: Different ways to represent glucose, $C_6H_{12}O_6$. The 3D ball-and-stick model of the linear D-glucose and the cyclic β-D-glucose (or more specifically, β-D-glucopyranose), are presented at the top where carbon is grey, oxygen is red, and hydrogen is white. The images in the middle row reflect 4 different illustrations of α-D-glucopyranose (1 carbon atom is followed with a red asterisk but, ideally, you should be able to identify the presence and orientation of each atom across all images on this page): **(1)** modified Fischer projection; **(2)** Haworth projection; **(3)** chair conformation; **(4)** structural formula showing the absolute stereochemistry. In the last row of images, notice that the carbon atoms numbered 2, 3, 4, and 5 each have four different groups attached to them, whereas carbon atoms 1 and 6 have only three different substituents each. Thus, there are four chiral carbon atoms in the linear form of glucose. The bottommost chiral carbon determines D/L: if OH is on the right, D; if on the left, L. The ring-closing reaction makes carbon C-1 chiral since its four bonds lead to -H, to -OH, to carbon C-2, and to the ring oxygen. Note that the information in the table above is not meant to be memorised. It should make sense after observing the structures carefully. Spatial reasoning with carbohydrates is helpful for ACER's Red Booklet 'GAMSAT Practice Questions', Unit 8, Q19-21. Go to the Video section of gamsat-prep.com for the worked solutions.

In the diagram that follows, you will notice a Fischer projection to the far left (*see* ORG 2.3.1). You will also find Fischer projections throughout this chapter since they are a common way to represent carbohydrates. Recall that the horizontal lines in a Fischer projection are projecting towards you.

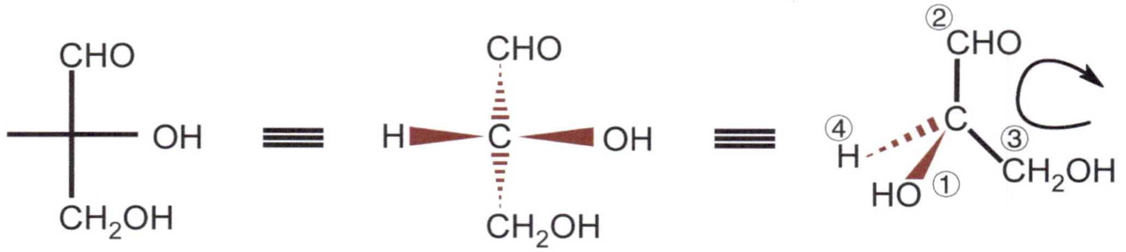

Fischer projection and 3D representation of D-glyceraldehyde, R-glyceraldehyde (*see* ORG 2.1, 2.2, 2.3 for rules). D/L can be determined by looking ONLY at the bottommost asymmetric (chiral) carbon in a Fischer projection: if the OH is on the right, D, on the left, L. Consider looking at the various sugars in this chapter to confirm that they are indeed in the D-configuration. For amino acids (*see* ORG 12.1), the amino group determines D/L.

12.3.2 Important Reactions of Carbohydrates

Hemiacetal Reaction

Monosaccharides can undergo an intramolecular nucleophilic addition reaction to form cyclic hemiacetals (*see* ORG 7.2.2). For example, the hydroxyl group on C4 of ribose attacks the aldehyde group on C1 forming a five-membered ring called furanose.

Diastereomers differing in configuration at this newly formed chiral carbon (= C1 where the straight chain monosaccharide converted into a furanose or pyranose) are known as anomers. This newly chiral carbon, which used to be a carbonyl carbon, is known as the

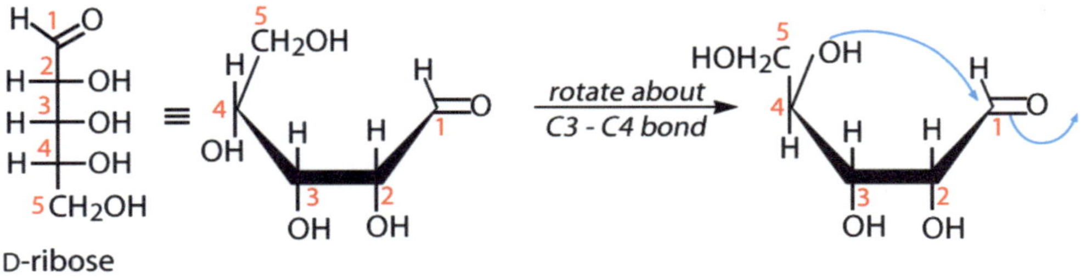

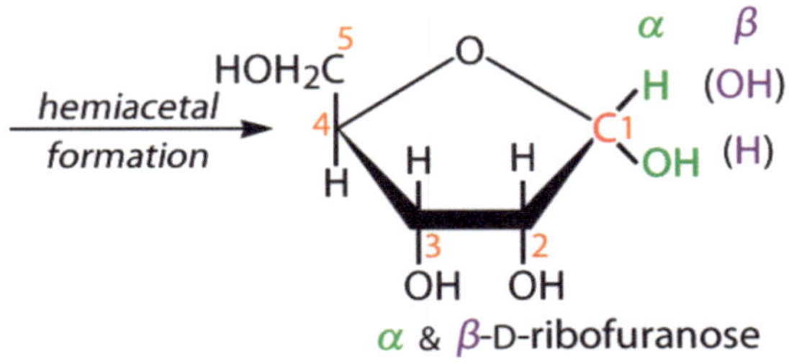

Note: It is not necessary to memorise the names of products in this section (ORG 12.3.2). However, you are expected to be able to follow what goes where. Of course during the real exam, there will be no colour and it is unlikely that they would politely number all the carbons to make it easy for you to follow! ACER practice materials have several passages based on carbohydrates including the "Red" booklet ('GAMSAT Practice Questions') current units 8 (Q19-21) and 14 (Q36-39).

High-level Importance

anomeric centre. When the OH group on C1 is *trans* to CH_2OH, it is called an α anomer. When the OH group on C1 is *cis* to CH_2OH, it is called a β anomer. {Mnemonic: α looks like an underwater fish, so the OH is down; β = birds so the OH is up.}

Mutarotation is the formation of both anomers into an equilibrium mixture when exposed to water.

Glycosidic Bonds

A disaccharide is a molecule made up of two monosaccharides, joined by a *glycosidic bond* between the hemiacetal carbon of one molecule, and the hydroxyl group of another. The glycosidic bond forms an α-1,4-glycosidic linkage if the reactant is an α anomer. A β-1,4-glycosidic linkage is formed if the reactant is a β anomer. When the bond is formed, one molecule of water is released (condensation). In order to break the bond, water must be added (hydrolysis). *See* Fig. IV.A.1.5 Part II for the preceding reactions and see below for common disaccharides and their component monomers.

- Sucrose (common sugar or table sugar) = glucose + fructose
- Lactose (milk sugar) = glucose + galactose
- Maltose (α-1,4 bond) = glucose + glucose
- Cellobiose (β-1,4 bond) = glucose + glucose

Ester Formation

Monosaccharides react with acid chloride or acid anhydride to form esters (*see* ORG 9.4, 9.4.1). All of the hydroxyl groups can be esterified.

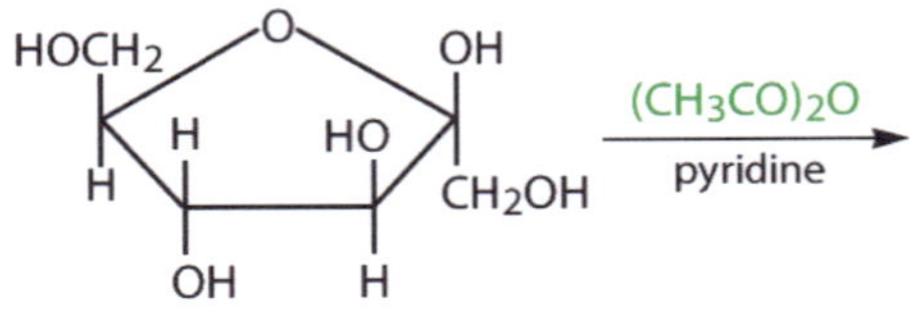

β-D-fructofuranose

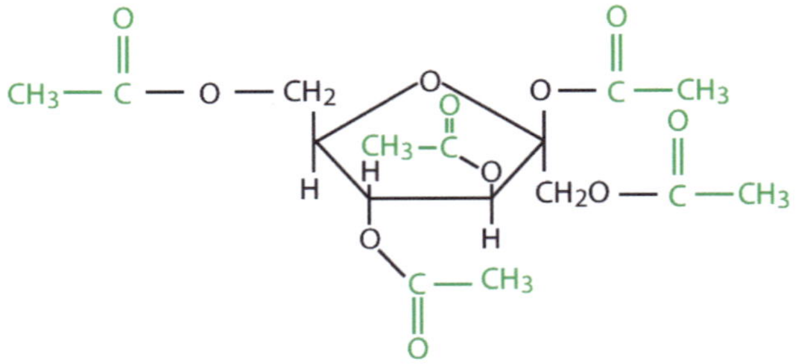

penta-*O*-acetyl-*β*-D-fructofuranoside

Ether Formation

Monosaccharides react with alkyl halide in the presence of silver oxide to form ethers. All of the hydroxyl groups are converted to -OR groups.

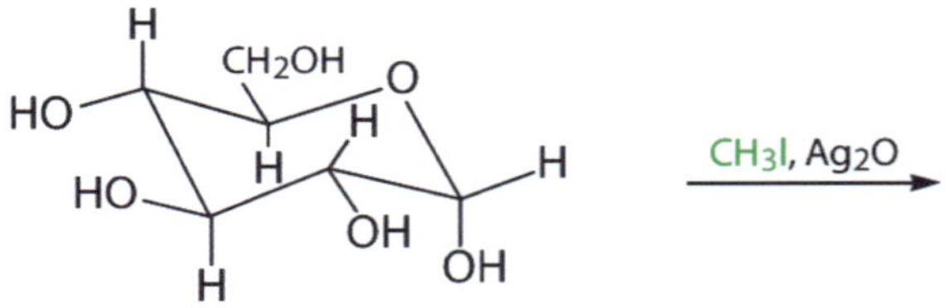

α-D-glucopyranose

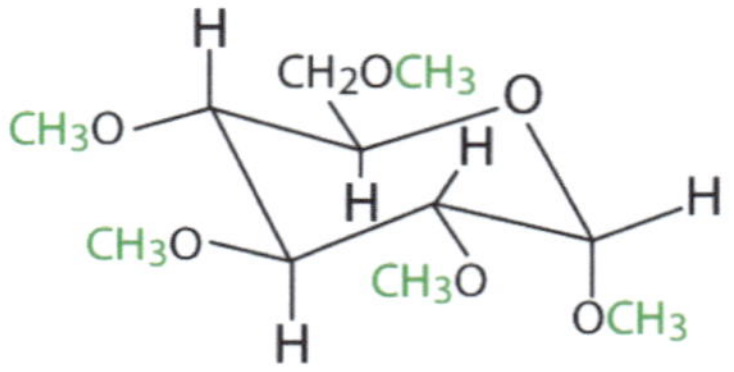

methyl-2, 3, 4, 6-tetra-*O*-methyl-α-D-glucopyranoside

Ether synthesis can also proceed using alcohols (*see* ORG 10.1):

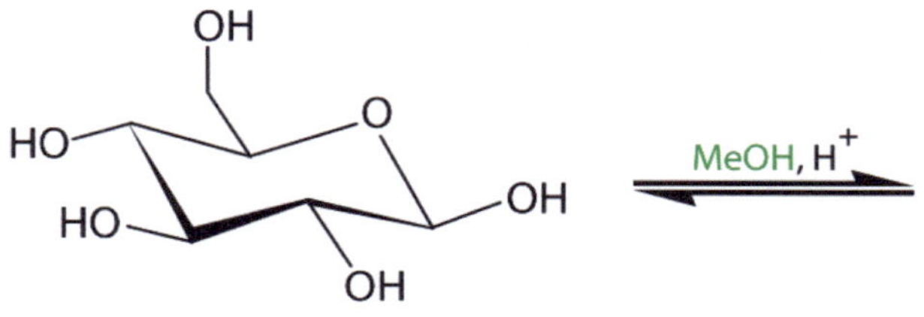

β-D-glucopyranose

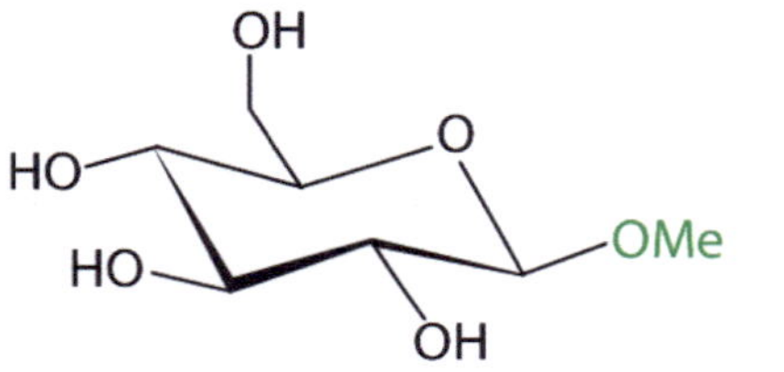

methyl-*β*-D-glucopyranoside

Reduction Reaction

Open chain monosaccharides are present in equilibrium between the aldehyde/ ketone and the hemiacetal form. Therefore, monosaccharides can be reduced by $NaBH_4$ to form polyalcohols (*see* ORG 6.2.2).

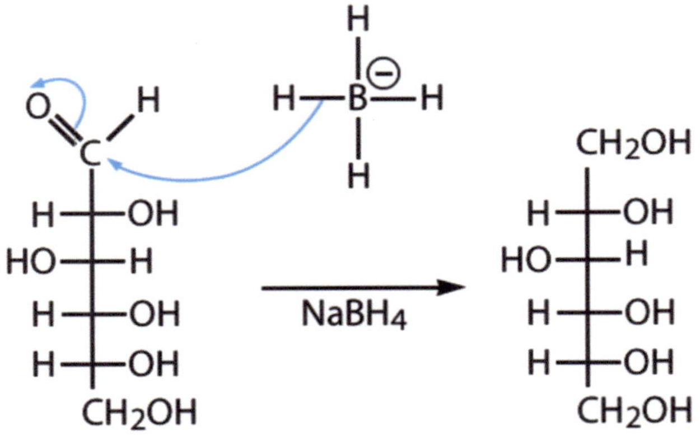

D-glucose **D-sorbitol**

Oxidation Reaction

Again, the hemiacetal ring form is in equilibrium with the open chain aldehyde/ ketone form. Aldoses can be oxidised by the Tollens' reagent $[Ag(NH_3)_2]^+$, Fehling's reagent ($Cu^{2+}/Na_2C_4H_4O_6$), and Benedict's reagent ($Cu^{2+}/Na_3C_6H_5O_7$) to yield carboxylic acids. If the Tollens' reagent is used, metallic silver is produced as a shiny mirror. If the Fehling's reagent or Benedict's reagent is used, cuprous oxide is produced as a reddish precipitate.

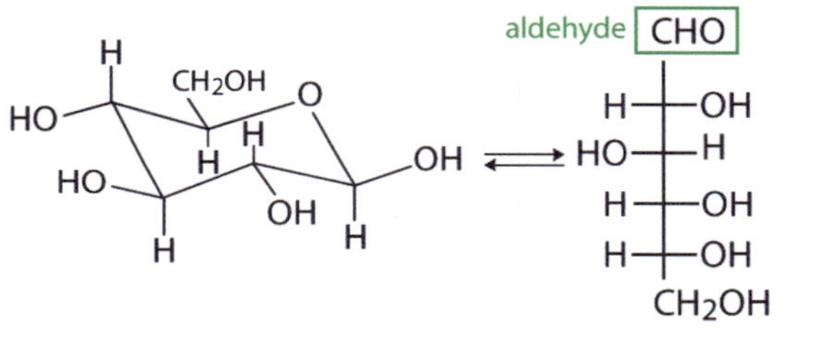

β-D-glucose open-chain form

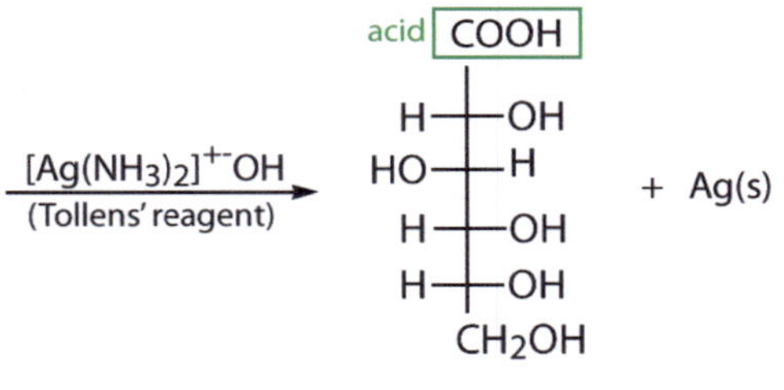

D-gluconic acid
(+ side products)

Redox (reduction/oxidation) and chain extending GAMSAT questions are usually easily solved by noticing that the stereochemistry of groups that are not directly involved in the reaction remain unchanged. For these substituents, the integrity of the Fischer projection is intact (in other words, whether the H or OH is on the left or right of the structure does not change).

When aldoses are treated with bromine water, the aldehyde is oxidised to a carboxylic acid group, resulting in a product known as an *aldonic acid*:

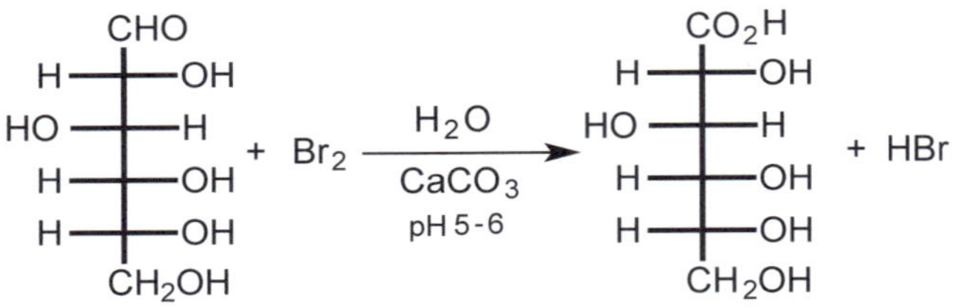

D - glucose (an aldose) D-Gluconic acid (an aldonic acid)

Aldoses treated with dilute nitric acid will have both the primary alcohol and aldehyde groups oxidise to carboxylic acid groups, resulting in a product known as an *aldaric acid*:

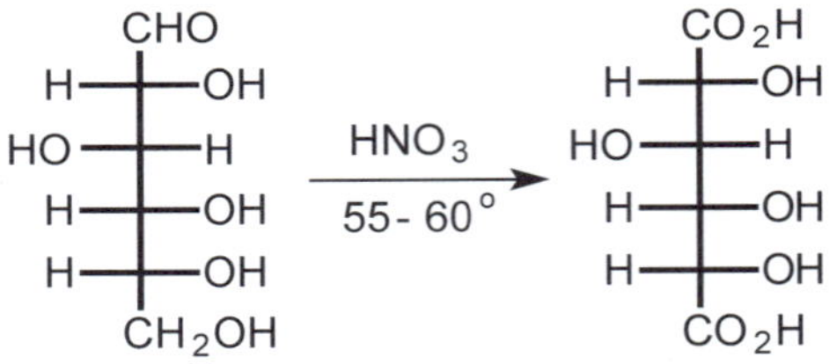

D-glucose (an aldose) D-Glucaric acid (an aldaric acid)

Reducing Sugars/Non-reducing Sugars

All aldoses are reducing sugars because they contain an aldehyde carbonyl group. Some ketoses such as fructose are reducing sugars as well. They can be isomerised through keto-enol tautomerisation (ORG 7.1) to an aldose, which can be oxidised normally. Glycosides are non-reducing sugars because the acetal group cannot be hydrolysed to aldehydes. Thus they do not react with the Tollens' reagent.

12.3.3 Polysaccharides

Polymers of many monosaccharides are called polysaccharides. As in disaccharides, they are joined by glycosidic linkages. They may be straight chains, or branched chains. Some common polysaccharides are:

- Starch (plant energy storage)
- Cellulose (plant structural component)
- Glycocalyx (associated with the plasma membrane)
- Glycogen (animal energy storage in the form of glucose)
- Chitin (structural component found in shells or arthropods)

Carbohydrates are the most abundant organic constituents of plants. They are the source of chemical energy in living organisms, and, in plants, they are used in making the support structures. Cellulose consists of $\beta(1\rightarrow4)$ linked D-glucose. Starch and glycogen are mostly $\alpha(1\rightarrow4)$ glycosidic linkages of D-glucose.

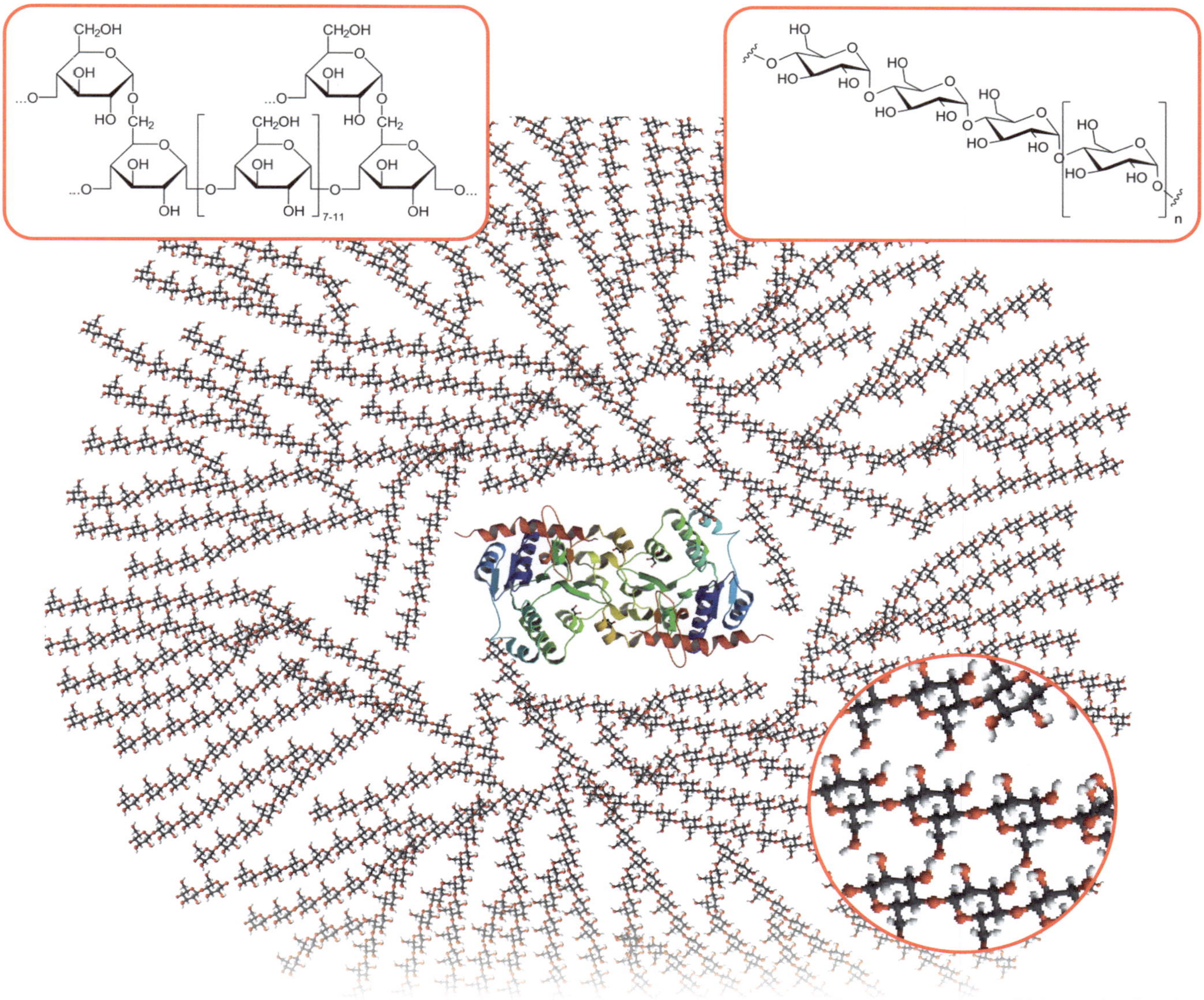

Figure IV.A.1.5 Part III A matter of perspective: The structure of glycogen. Glycogen is a multi-branched polysaccharide of glucose that serves as a form of energy storage in animals, fungi, and bacteria. As humans, it is our main form of energy storage and it is found primarily in liver and muscle. In the left inset, repeating subunits (residues) of glucose can be seen as a linear chain (horizontally, note that '7-11' signifies 7 to 11 subunits) linked together by α(1→4) glycosidic bonds (that identical bonding pattern is also symbolised in the top right inset from a different perspective; you should be able to match carbons from the 2 insets). Branches are linked to the horizontal chains by α(1→6) glycosidic bonds (indicated by the vertical bonding in the left inset). The main image above is glycogen in a schematic 2D cross-sectional view (like cutting an orange down the middle and looking at one cut half). In the centre is the core protein glycogenin and it is surrounded by chains and branches of glucose residues. The protein displays structural elements that we have already discussed (ORG 12.2.2), and the ball-and-stick model of the glucose polymer (magnified in the lower, right inset) follows the same rules we have seen before: O: red, C: grey, H: white. The entire globular granule may contain around 30 000 glucose residues. Central image: Häggström, Mikael (2014).

12.4 Lipids

High-level Importance

Lipids are a class of organic molecules containing many different types of substances, such as fatty acids, fats, waxes, triacyl glycerols, terpenes and steroids. The main biological functions of lipids include storing energy, signaling and acting as structural components of cell membranes (BIO 1.1).

Lipids are relatively water-insoluble or nonpolar (e.g. oil floating on water). Lipids can be linear or cyclic in structure, and may or may not be aromatic. In general, the bulk of lipid structure is nonpolar or hydrophobic; however, often a part of their structure is polar or hydrophilic. This duality makes many lipids amphipathic (= amphiphilic) molecules (having both hydrophobic and hydrophilic portions).

Triacyl glycerols are oils and fats of either animal or plant origin. In general, fats are solid at room temperature, and oils are liquid at room temperature.

Triacyl glycerols are also commonly referred to as triglycerides (= triacylglycerides) and are, by definition, fatty acid triesters of the trihydroxy alcohol glycerol. {Note: "triacyl" refers to the presence of 3 acyl substituents (RCO-, ORG 9.1)}

Glycerol + 3 Fatty acids = Triglyceride

The general structure of a triacyl glycerol is:

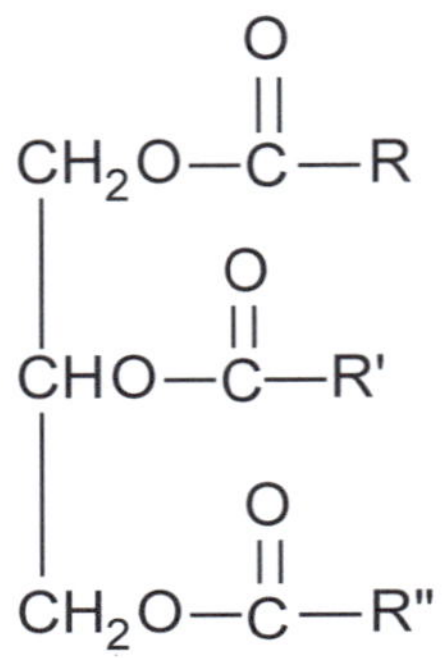

The R groups may be the same or different, and are usually long chain alkyl groups. Upon hydrolysis of a triacyl glycerol, the products are three fatty acids and glycerol. The fatty acids may be saturated (= no multiple bonds, i.e. *palmitic acid*) or unsaturated (= containing double or triple bonds, i.e. *oleic acid*). Unsaturated fatty acids are usually in the cis configuration. Saturated fatty acids have a higher melting point than unsaturated fatty acids. Some common fatty acids are:

$$CH_3(CH_2)_{14}COOH$$

palmitic acid

$$CH_3(CH_2)_{16}COOH$$

stearic acid

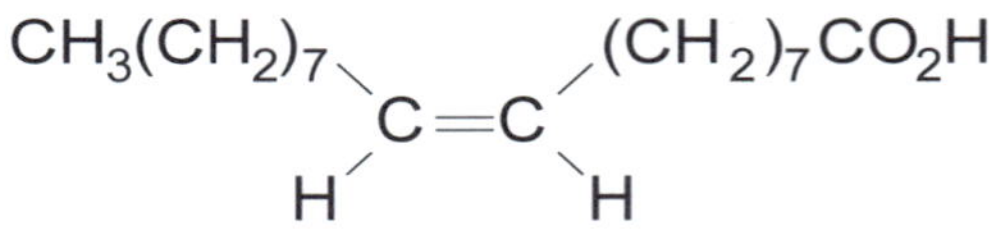

oleic acid

The water is blue, the hydrophilic layer is purple and the hydrophobic area is orange-yellow.

General formula for a saturated fatty acid = $C_nH_{2n+1}COOH = CH_3(CH_2)_nCOOH$

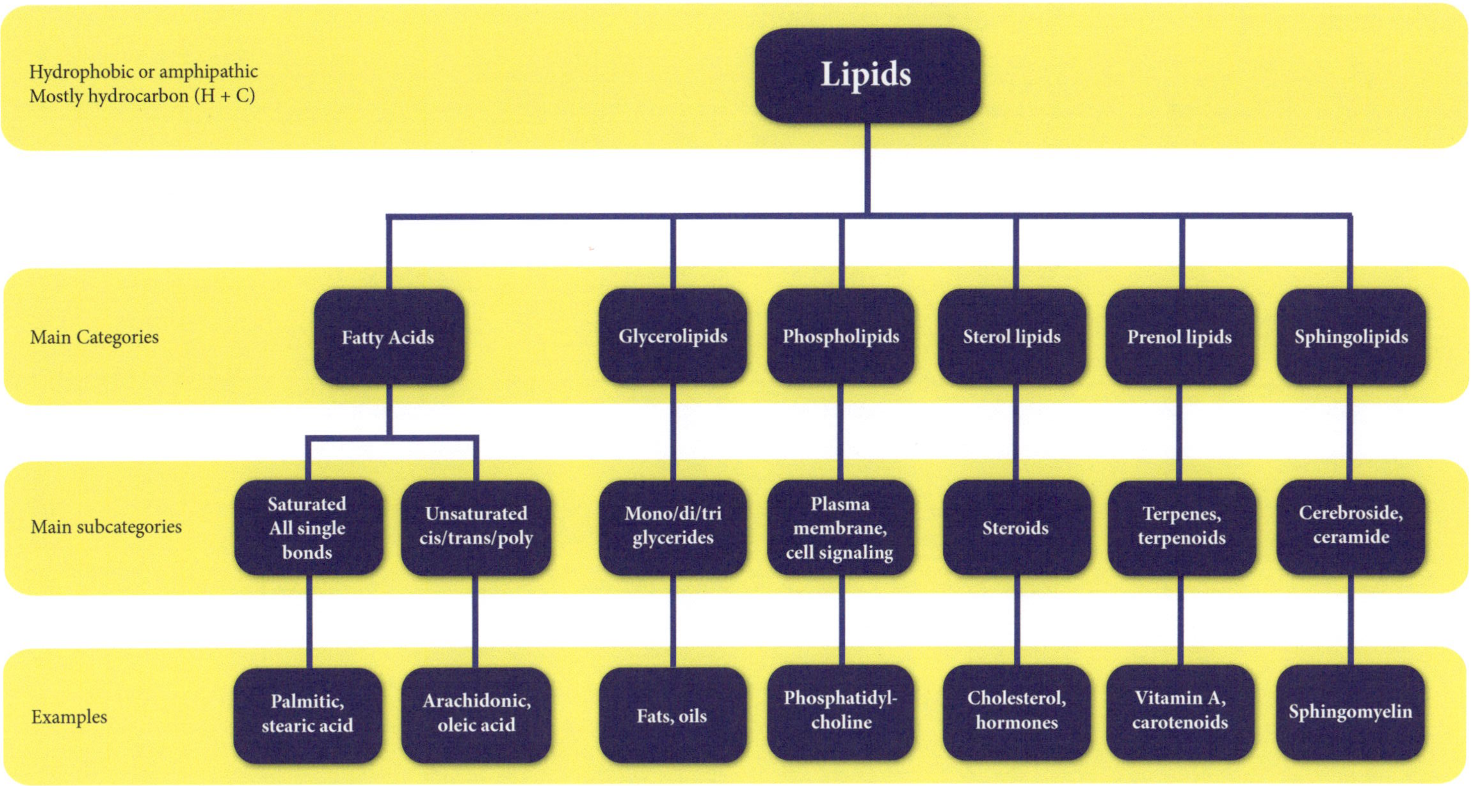

Figure A.1.6: Categories of lipids. Note that prostaglandins - hormone-like lipids - are derived from unsaturated fatty acids. Waxes, like oils and fats, are lipids. However, oils and fats are esters of glycerol whereas waxes may contain esters of carboxylic acids and long chain alcohols or combinations of long chain fatty acids and primary alcohols. The chart above is meant to give you an overview of lipids but please do not memorise.

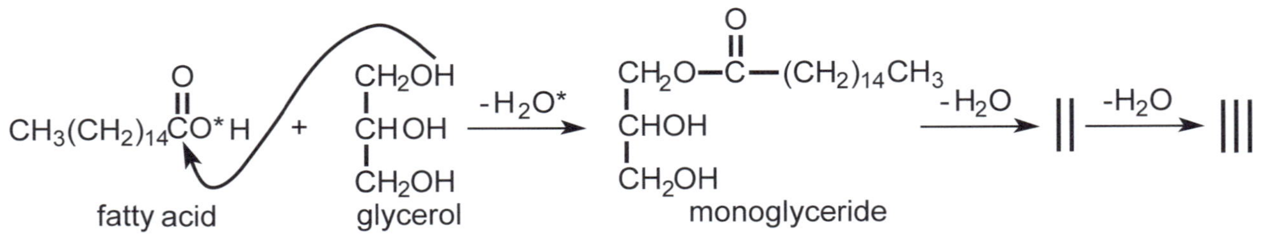

Biosynthesis of fats and oils. Fats and oils are a special class of esters (i.e. mono-, di-, and triglycerides). Fatty acids (= long chain carboxylic acids) may be added to the monoglyceride formed in the above reaction, forming diglycerides, and triglycerides.

"Essential" fatty acids are fatty acids that humans - and other animals - must ingest because the body requires them but cannot synthesise them. Only two are known in humans: alpha-linolenic acid and linoleic acid. Because they have multiple double bonds that begin near the methyl end, they are both known as polyunsaturated omega fatty acids (omega is the last letter of the Greek alphabet thus signifying the methyl end).

A wax is a simple ester of a fatty acid and a long-chain alcohol. In general, a wax, such as the wax in your ears, serves as a protective coating.

Soap is a mixture of salts of long chain fatty acids formed by the hydrolysis of fat. This process is called saponification. Soap possesses both a nonpolar hydrocarbon tail and a polar carboxylate head. When soaps are dispersed in aqueous solution, the long nonpolar tails are inside the sphere while the polar heads face outward. Recall that a sphere is the shape that minimises surface tension (i.e. the smallest surface area relative to volume; CHM 4.2).

Soaps are surfactants (BIO 12.3). They are compounds that lower the surface tension of a liquid because of their amphipathic nature

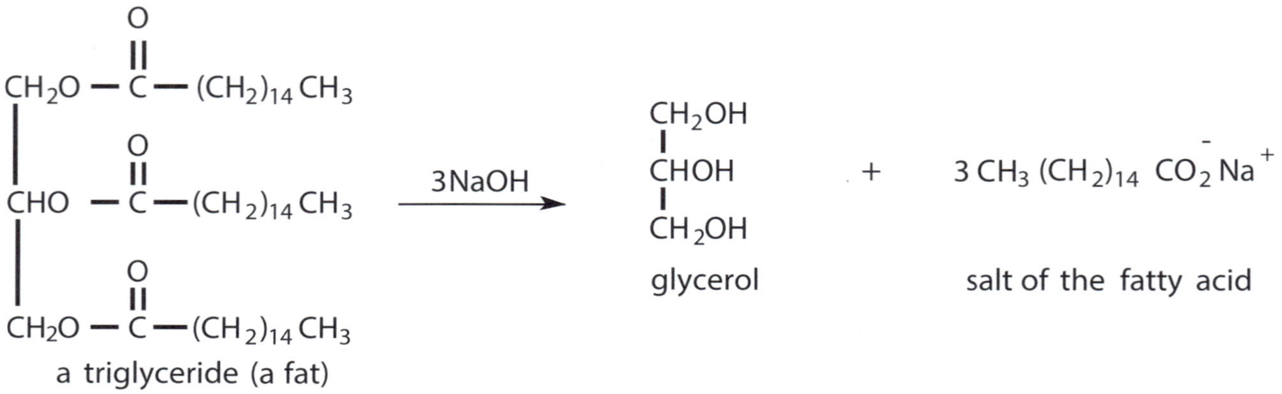

Saponification. Fats may be hydrolysed by a base to the components glycerol and the salt of the fatty acids. The salts of long chain carboxylic acids are called soaps. Thus this process is called saponification.

(i.e. they contain both hydrophobic tails and hydrophilic heads; *see* BIO 1.1).

Of course, the cellular membrane is a lipid bilayer (Biology Chapter 1). The polar heads of the lipids align towards the aqueous environment, while the hydrophobic tails minimise their contact with water and tend to cluster together. Depending on the concentration of the lipid, this interaction may result in micelles (spherical), liposomes (spherical) or other lipid bilayers.

Micelles are closed lipid monolayers with a fatty acid core and polar surface. The main function of bile (BIO 9.4.1) is to facilitate the formation of micelles, which promotes the processing or emulsification of dietary fat and fat-soluble vitamins.

Liposomes are composed of a lipid bilayer separating an aqueous internal compartment from the bulk aqueous environment. Liposomes can be used as a vehicle for the administration of nutrients or pharmaceutical drugs.

The dual solubility nature of soap is why it removes oil or grease from skin or clothes. The soap forms a micelle that surrounds the nonpolar oil/grease in the nonpolar 'centre' of the micelle. The polar end of the soap micelle is soluble in water, allowing the oil/grease to be removed during rinsing.

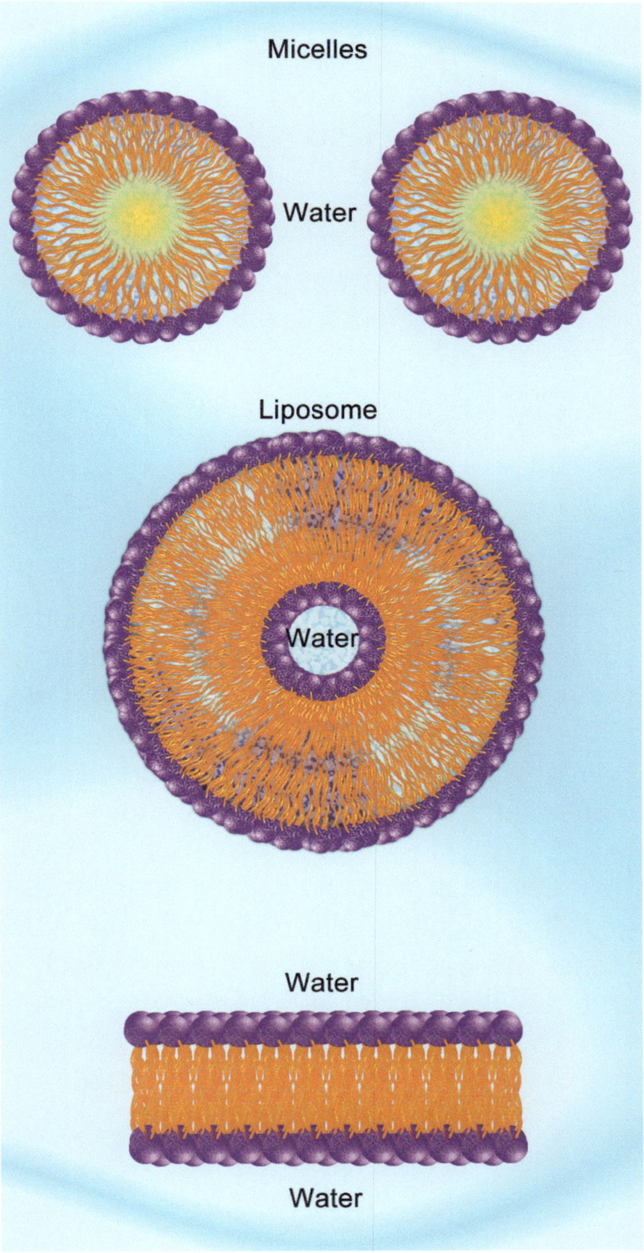

Figure IV.A.1.7. Amphipathic molecules arranged in micelles, a liposome and a bilipid layer.

High-level Importance

High-level Importance

12.4.1 Steroids

Steroids are a class of lipids which are derivatives of the basic ring structure:

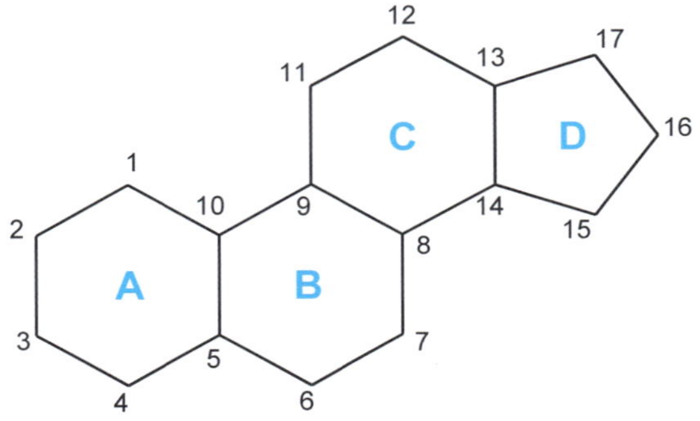

The IUPAC-recommended ring-lettering and the carbon atoms are numbered as shown. Many important substances are steroids, some examples include: cholesterol, D vitamins, bile acids, adrenocortical hormones, and male and female sex hormones.

Cholesterol is the most abundant steroid. It is a component of the plasma membrane and can serve as a building block to produce other steroids (including hormones) and related molecules. Cholesterol comes from the diet, but may be synthesised by the liver if necessary.

The rate-limiting step in the production of steroids (= *steroidogenesis*) in humans is the conversion of cholesterol to pregnenolone, which is in the same family as progesterone. This occurs inside mitochondria (BIO 1.2.1) and serves as the precursor for all human steroids.

Since such a significant portion of a steroid contains hydrocarbons, which are hydrophobic, steroids can dissolve through the hydrophobic interior of a cell's plasma membrane (BIO 1.1, 6.3). Furthermore, steroid hormones contain polar side groups which allow the hormone to easily dissolve in water. Thus steroid hormones are well designed to be transported through the vascular space, to cross the plasma membranes of cells, and to have an effect either in the cell's cytosol or, as is usually the case, in the nucleus.

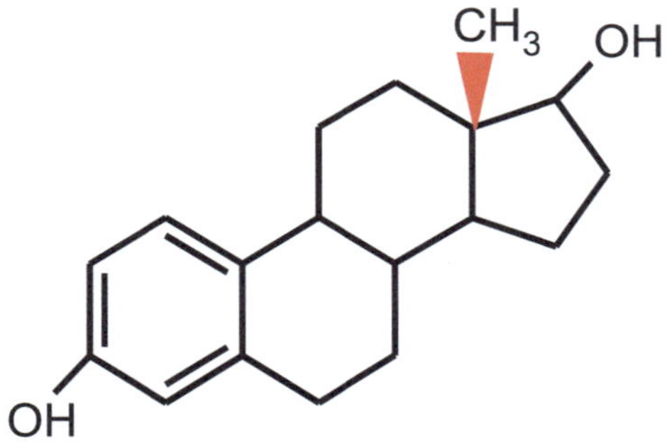

Estradiol
(an estrogen)

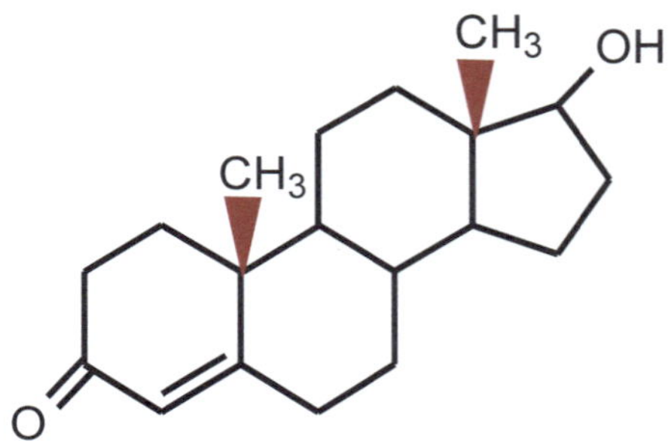

Testosterone
(an androgen)

12.4.2 Lipoproteins

Most biological molecules are proteins, followed by lipids. In fact, proteins and lipids by far dominate the biological molecules in the human body. Lipoproteins comprise unique biochemical assemblies (aggregates) containing both proteins and lipids, bound to the proteins, which allow lipids to move through hydrophilic intracellular and extracellular spaces. Many enzymes, structural proteins, transporters, antigens and toxins are lipoproteins.

Using electrophoresis and ultracentrifugation, lipoproteins can be classified according to size and density. Lipoproteins are larger and less dense when the fat to protein ratio is increased. Thus there are four major classes of plasma lipoproteins which enable lipids to be carried in the blood stream: **(1)** chylomicrons carry triglycerides from the intestines to the liver, to skeletal muscle, and to adipose tissue ("body fat"); **(2)** very low-density lipoproteins (VLDL) carry liver-synthesised triglycerides to adipose tissue; **(3)** low-density lipoproteins (LDL = "bad cholesterol") carry cholesterol from the liver to cells of the body; **(4)** and high-density lipoproteins (HDL = "good cholesterol") collect cholesterol from the body's tissues, and take it back to the liver.

12.5 Phosphorous in Biological Molecules

Phosphorous is an essential component of various biological molecules including adenosine triphosphate (ATP), phospholipids in cell membranes (BIO 1.1), and the nucleic acids which form DNA (BIO 1.2.2). Phosphorus can also form phosphoric acid (key to making the phosphate buffer in plasma; CHM 6.8), and several phosphate esters.

A phospholipid is produced from three ester linkages to glycerol. Phosphoric acid is ester linked to the terminal hydroxyl group and two fatty acids are ester linked to the two remaining hydroxyl groups of glycerol (*see Biology Section 1.1 for a schematic view of a phospholipid*).

ATP is critical for life since it transports chemical energy within cells. The components ADP and P_i (= *inorganic phosphate*) combine using the energy generated from a coupled reaction to produce ATP. We will be discussing

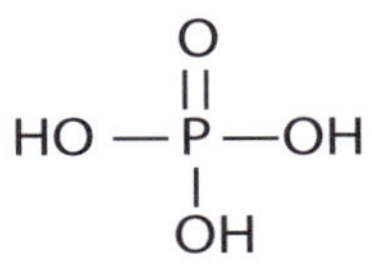

phosphoric acid

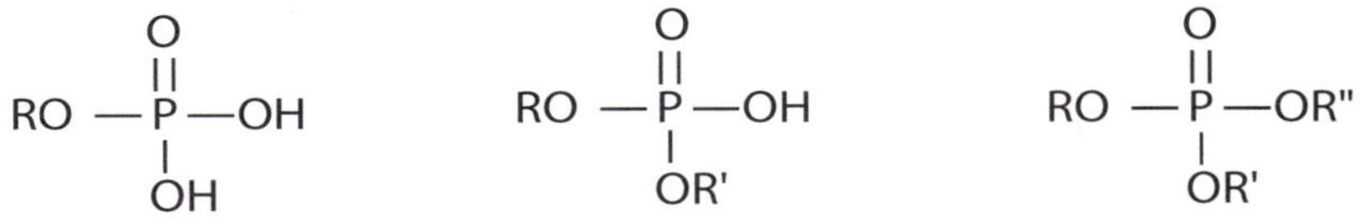

phosphate esters

High-level Importance

the bioenergetics of ATP in Biology Chapter 4. The linkage between the phosphate groups are via *anhydride bonds*:

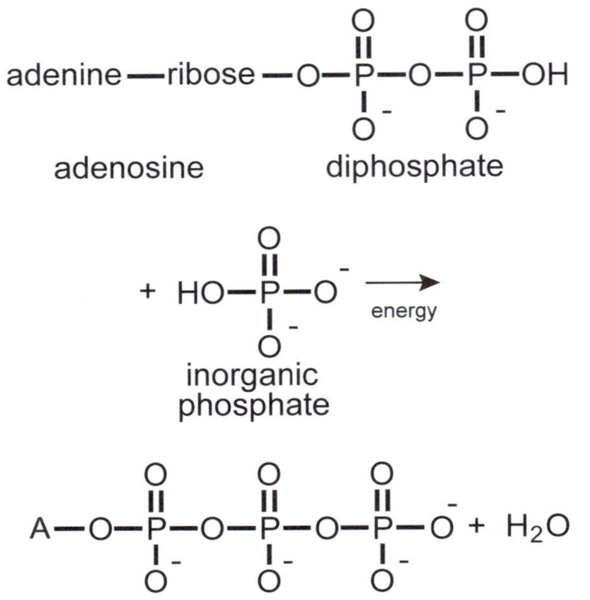

adenosine triphosphate, $C_{10}H_{16}N_5O_{13}P_3$

ATP is shown as shorthand above, the skeletal structure below, and the ball-and-stick model at the top of the next column with P: orange, O: red, N: blue, C: grey, H: white.

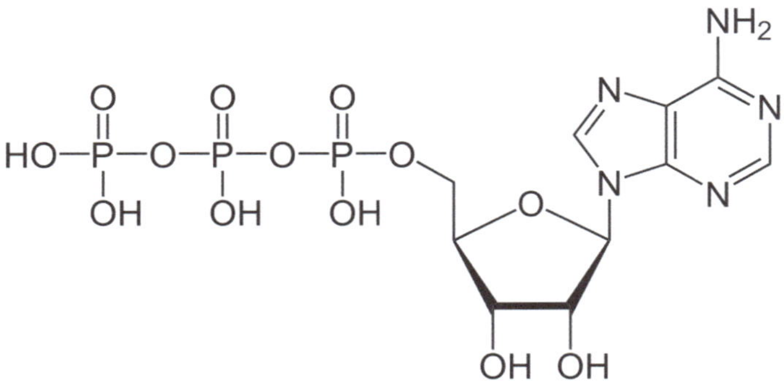

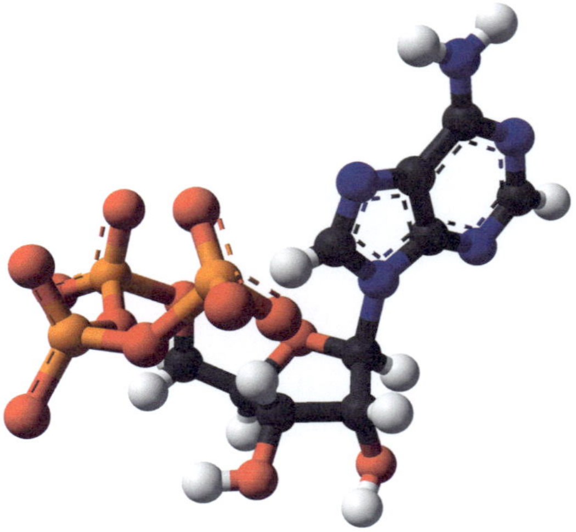

In DNA, the phosphate groups engage in two ester linkages creating phosphodiester bonds. It is the 5' phosphorylated position of one pentose ring which is linked to the 3' position of the next pentose ring (*see* BIO 1.2.2):

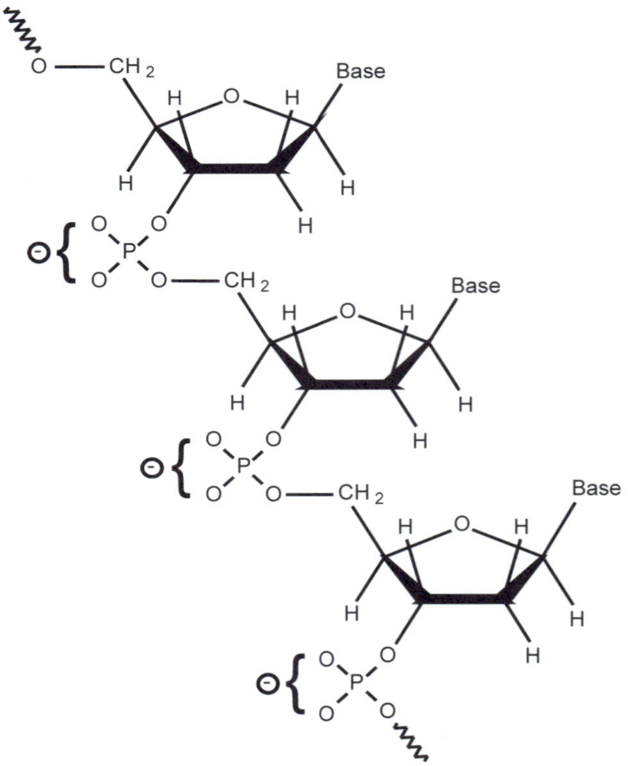

CHAPTER 12: Biological Molecules

GOLD STANDARD GAMSAT-LEVEL PRACTICE QUESTIONS

Questions 1–10

Amino acids are biologically important organic compounds containing amine and carboxylic acid functional groups, usually along with a side-chain specific to each amino acid. Twenty of the proteinogenic amino acids are known as "standard" amino acids (*see* Figure 2).

Amino acids in a polypeptide chain or protein are linked by peptide bonds and it is standard for the sequence, or primary structure, to run from the amino end (N-terminal) to the carboxyl end (C-terminal), which is the way that peptides are named. Proteases are able to perform proteolysis, a process that involves the hydrolysis of the peptide bond between specific amino acids in a polypeptide chain.

Depending on the enzyme, the specificity of proteases ranges significantly but all proteases cleave peptide bonds at specific locations. Some require a specific amino acid sequence or motif, while others will cleave indiscriminately at certain residues - trypsin, for example, targets exposed lysines and arginines.

Table 1 shows a list of proteases commonly used in the laboratory. Each cleavage site is marked with the symbol •. Different cleavage sites are separated by commas (,), while continuous sequences are marked by hyphens (-). "X" denotes any amino acid.

Protease	Cleavage Sites
Chymotrypsin	Trp•-X, Tyr•-X, Phe•-X, Leu•-X
Cyanogen bromide	Met•-X
Papain	[Hydrophobic]-[Arg OR Lys] •-[Any amino acid except Val]
Thrombin	Arg•-Gly
Trypsin	Lys•-X, Arg•-X

Table 1: Common proteases and their associated cleavage sites

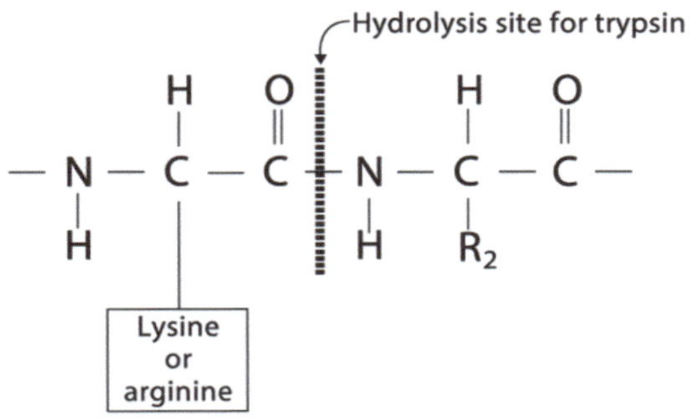

Figure 1: Hydrolysis of a polypeptide by trypsin

High-level Importance

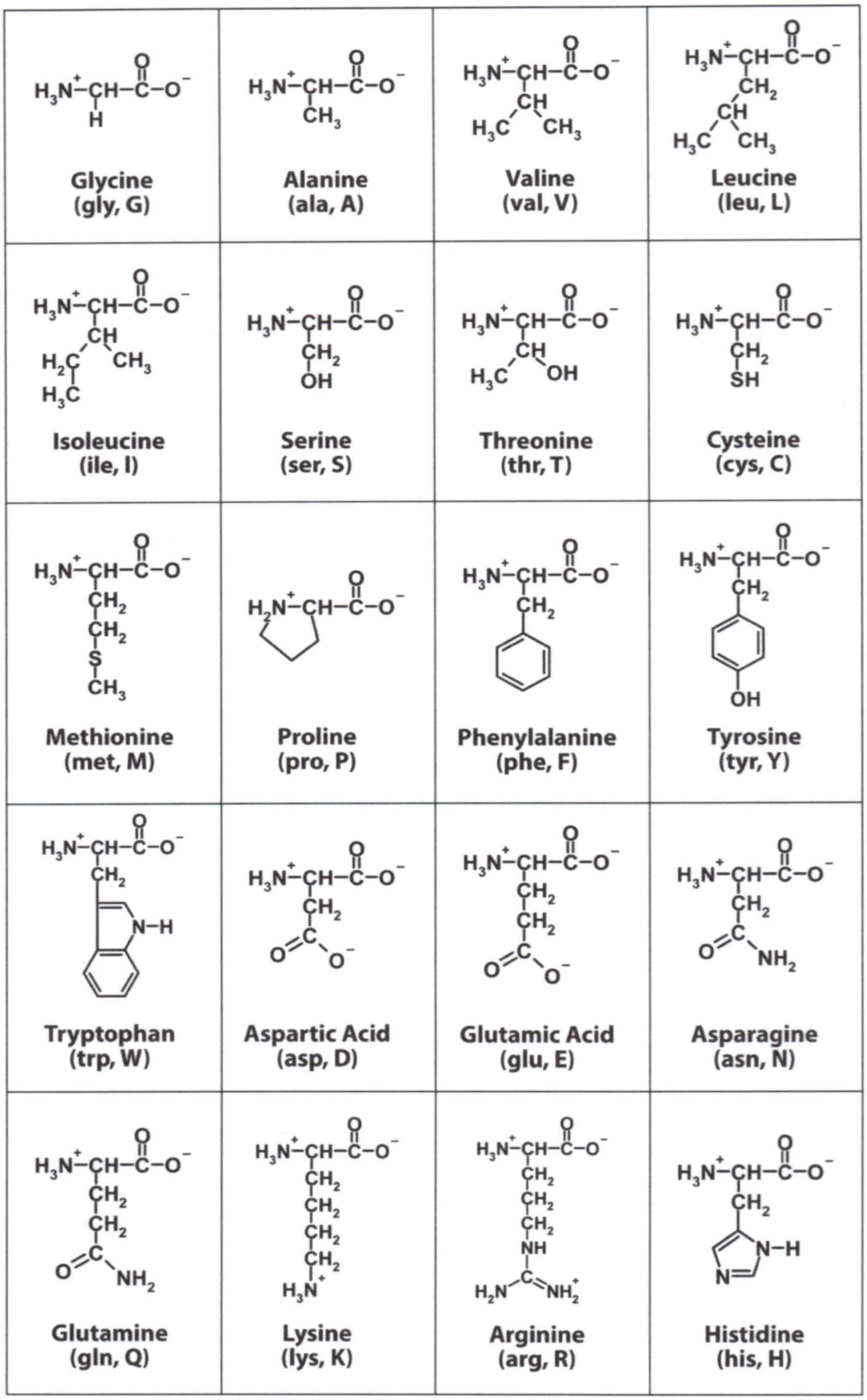

Figure 2: The 20 standard amino acids, at neutral pH, with their 1- and 3-letter abbreviations

1) Figure 2 presents the 1- and 3-letter abbreviations of the 20 standard amino acids.

Bradykinin is a peptide that causes blood vessels to dilate. Its amino acid sequence is as follows:

Arg-Pro-Pro-Gly-Phe-Ser-Pro-Phe-Arg

If bradykinin would be fragmented in all possible ways to form tetrapeptides, then six tetrapeptides would be possible: beginning from the left and moving to the right, Arg-Pro-Pro-Gly, Pro-Pro-Gly-Phe, ... , Ser-Pro-Phe-Arg. Consider that length is measured as the number of amino acids attached in a row. Using bradykinin as an example to generate a rule, and considering other peptides that also have no repeated sequences, given a peptide of length n, how many shorter peptides of length *x* can be produced?

A. 2^n
B. $2^n - x$
C. $(n - x) - 1$
D. $1 + (n - x)$

2) Proteases must function by:

A. dehydrating a peptide bond.
B. attacking hydrogen bonds.
C. adding a water molecule to the carbon in a peptide bond.
D. separating hydroxyls.

3) At a pH of 12, which of the following dipeptides, indicated by the 1-letter abbreviations, would have the most negative charge?

A. G-D
B. W-K
C. Q-N
D. P-G

4) Which of the following sequences would be digested by papain?

A. Ala-Lys-Val
B. Val-Lys-Val
C. Phe-Arg-Trp
D. Lys-Arg-Trp

5) The following peptide is digested with both cyanogen bromide and trypsin:

Ala-Phe-Ile-Met-Gln-Gln-Met-Arg-Val-Lys-Ser-Thr-Arg-Glu-Asn-Cys-Gly

How many fragments will result?

A. 3
B. 4
C. 5
D. More than 5

6) An octopeptide was analysed and found to contain the following amino acids: 2 Arg, 1 Glu, 1 Ser, 1 Met, 1 Trp, 1 Lys, 1 Gly.

The native octopeptide was first digested with papain, which resulted in a pentapeptide and a tripeptide. UV analysis showed that the pentapeptide was the only fragment that contained an aromatic ring. Another test, which specifically stains for carboxylic acids, shows that only the tripeptide contains an additional carboxylic acid functional group, and analysis demonstrated that glycine was in the third position of the tripeptide. Further digestion with trypsin yielded four fragments of varying sizes: 2 monopeptides, 1 dipeptide, and 1 tetrapeptide. Finally, all fragments were digested with cyanogen bromide, which resulted in 5 total fragments: 2 monopeptides and 3 dipeptides. The native sequence would be most consistent with which of the following?

A. Met-Arg-Ser-Trp-Lys-Glu-Gly-Arg
B. Arg-Ser-Met-Trp-Lys-Glu-Arg-Gly
C. Arg-Arg-Gly-Lys-Glu-Met-Ser-Trp
D. Trp-Arg-Gly-Met-Ser-Trp-Lys-Arg

High-level Importance

7) Morphiceptin, illustrated below, is a tetrapeptide with the end-hydroxyl group replaced by an amino group. It is an opioid with analgesic effects like opium which are reversed by naloxone.

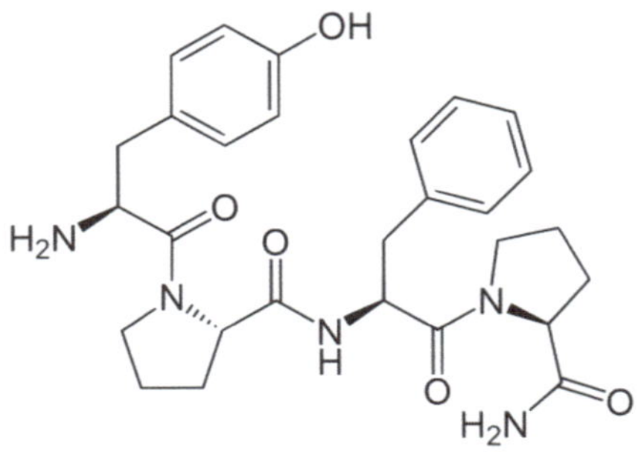

Which of the following is the most accurate description of morphiceptin?

A. Tyr-Pro-Pro-Phe-NH_2
B. Phe-Pro-Tyr-Pro-NH_2
C. Tyr-Pro-Phe-Pro-NH_2
D. Pro-Phe-Pro-Tyr-NH_2

8) Cholecystokinin (CCK) is a family of peptide hormones, with varying numbers of amino acids, that stimulate the digestion of fat and protein in the GI system. A sulfated form of CCK, illustrated below, can activate the CCK receptor.

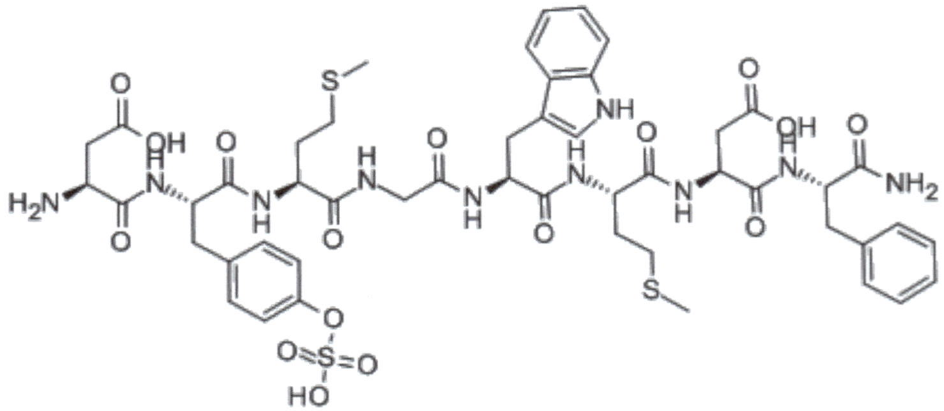

Given the structure of the sulfated form of CCK in the preceding image, which of the following is the most accurate descriptor?

A. Pentapeptide
B. Hexapeptide
C. Heptapeptide
D. Octapeptide

9) How many different tripeptides can be produced with the amino acid combination of one each of Phe, Pro and Asp?

A. 2
B. 4
C. 6
D. 8

Question 10 refers to the following additional information.

The isoelectronic point is the pH at which the amino acid does not migrate in an electric field. This means it is the pH at which the amino acid is neutral, *i.e.* the zwitterion form is dominant.

There are 3 cases to consider:

- **Neutral side chains**

  These amino acids are characterised by two pKas: pKa_1 and pKa_2 for the carboxylic acid and the amine, respectively. The isoelectronic point will be the average of these two pKas, *i.e.* $pI = 1/2\ (pKa_1 + pKa_2)$.

- **Acidic side chains**

  The pI will be at a lower pH because the acidic side chain introduces an "extra" negative charge. So the neutral form exists under more **acidic** conditions when the extra negative charge has been neutralised.

- **Basic side chains**

  The pI will be at a higher pH because the basic side chain introduces an "extra" positive charge. So the neutral form exists under more **basic** conditions when the extra positive charge has been neutralised.

10) The following is a list of the acid/base properties of some amino acids with ionisable side chains. Which amino acid has the greatest isoelectric point?

Amino acid	pKa_1	pKa_2	pKa_3
Aspartic acid	1.88	3.65	9.60
Glutamic acid	2.19	4.25	9.67
Tyrosine	2.20	9.11	10.07
Cysteine	1.96	8.18	10.28

A. Aspartic acid
B. Glutamic acid
C. Tyrosine
D. Cysteine

11) Which of the following is **not** consistent with the β anomer of D-glucose? (Note: If you need a hint, you can look at the bottom of the page, it is upside down.)

A.
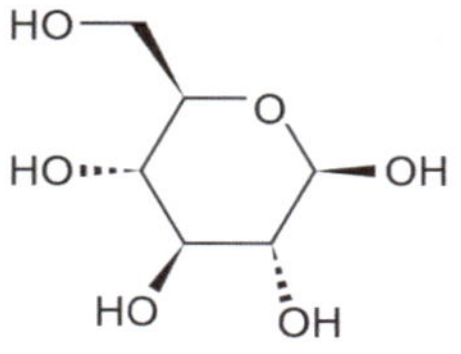

C.
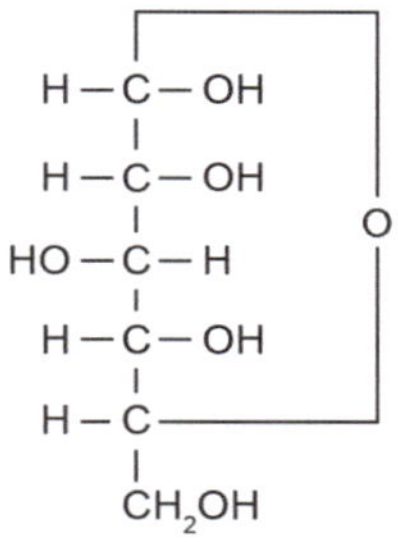

B.
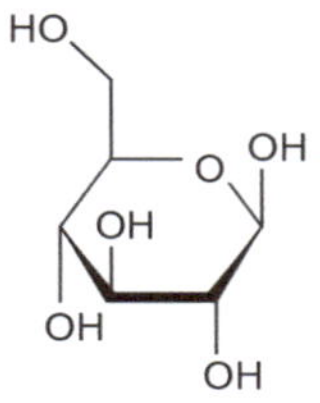

D.
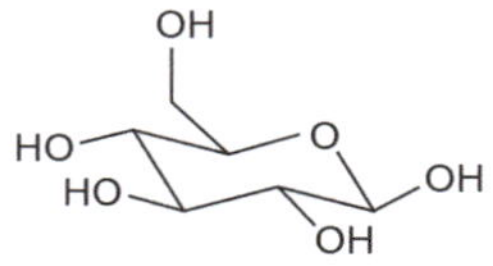

Hint: It is definitely not required to have memorised the structure by name, but rather it is expected that you can identify which structure is not like the other 3 structures.

High-level Importance

Questions 12–17

A fatty acid is a carboxylic acid (-COOH) with a long hydrocarbon chain, which is either saturated or unsaturated. Fatty acids without double bonds are known as saturated. Fatty acids that have one or more carbon–carbon double bonds are known as unsaturated. Consider the two following tables.

Formula	Common Name	Melting Point
$CH_3(CH_2)_{10}CO_2H$	lauric acid	45 °C
$CH_3(CH_2)_{12}CO_2H$	myristic acid	55 °C
$CH_3(CH_2)_{14}CO_2H$	palmitic acid	63 °C
$CH_3(CH_2)_{16}CO_2H$	stearic acid	69 °C
$CH_3(CH_2)_{18}CO_2H$	arachidic acid	76 °C

Table 1: Saturated Fatty Acids

Formula	Common Name	Melting Point
$CH_3(CH_2)_5CH{=}CH(CH_2)_7CO_2H$	palmitoleic acid	0 °C
$CH_3(CH_2)_7CH{=}CH(CH_2)_7CO_2H$	oleic acid	13 °C
$CH_3(CH_2)_4CH{=}CHCH_2CH{=}CH(CH_2)_7CO_2H$	linoleic acid	–5 °C
$CH_3CH_2CH{=}CHCH_2CH{=}CHCH_2CH{=}CH(CH_2)_7CO_2H$	linolenic acid	–11 °C
$CH_3(CH_2)_4(CH{=}CHCH_2)_4(CH_2)_2CO_2H$	arachidonic acid	–49 °C

Table 2: Unsaturated Fatty Acids

The position of the carbon atoms in a fatty acid can be indicated from the -COOH (or carboxy) end, or from the $–CH_3$ (or methyl) end (AKA, the omega or ω end). If indicated from the -COOH end, then the C-1, C-2, C-3, ...(etc.) notation is used (the numerals just below the structure in the diagram below, where C-1 is the –COOH carbon). If the position is counted to the first carbon with a double bond from the omega end, then the position is indicated by the ω-n notation (the numeral n just above the structure in the diagram below, where ω-1 refers to the methyl carbon).

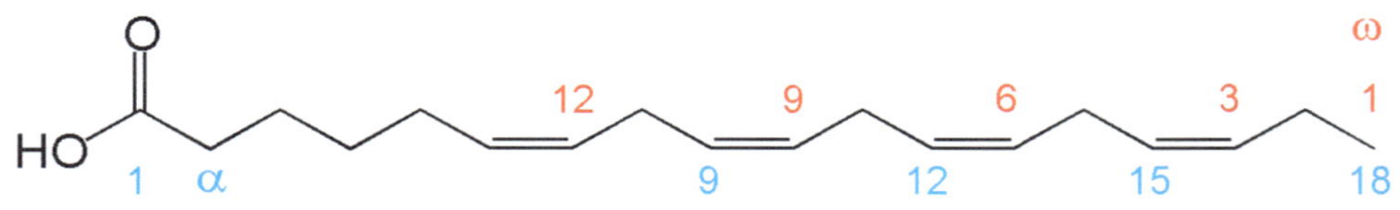

12) According to the information provided, decreasing melting point is most associated with an increase in:

A. Molecular weight
B. Unsaturation
C. Saturation
D. More than one of the above

13) How many omega-6 fatty acids are listed in the tables provided?

A. One
B. Two
C. Three
D. More than three

14) Stearidonic acid ($C_{18}H_{28}O_2$) has how many double bonds in its hydrocarbon chain?

A. One
B. Two
C. Three
D. Four

15) Saponification value is expressed by the amount of potassium hydroxide in mg required to saponify one (1) gram of fat. The longer chain fatty acids found in fats have low saponification values because they have a relatively fewer number of carboxylic functional groups per unit mass of the fat as compared to shorter chain fatty acids.

Identify the fatty acid with the highest saponification value.

A. Palmitic acid
B. Palmitoleic acid
C. Arachidic acid
D. Arachidonic acid

The next 2 questions use the following additional information.

The iodine value is a measure of the degree of unsaturation in a fatty acid. One molecule of iodine (I_2, molecular weight: 254) reacts with one double bond. The iodine value is given by the mass (in grams) of iodine that reacts with 100 g of a particular fatty acid.

Note the following relative atomic masses which may be of use: H = 1.0, C = 12.0, O = 16.0.

16) As compared to arachidonic acid, the iodine value of clupanodonic acid ($C_{22}H_{34}O_2$) can be best described as which of the following?

A. More than twice as great
B. Greater but less than twice as great
C. The same
D. Less

17) Which of the following is the best estimate for the iodine value of linoleic acid?

A. 508
B. 340
C. 170
D. 85

Questions 18–20

A steroid is an organic compound with four rings arranged in a specific configuration. Terpenes are major biosynthetic building blocks. Steroids are derivatives of the terpene squalene and the terpenoid lanosterol. The difference between terpenes and terpenoids is that terpenes are hydrocarbons, whereas terpenoids contain additional functional groups.

Terpenes are derived biosynthetically from units of isoprene, which has the molecular formula C_5H_8. Isoprene units can be linked together "head to tail" (i.e., from one end of the longest chain to the other end from another molecule) to form linear chains, or they may be arranged to form rings. The isoprene unit is thus one of nature's common building blocks.

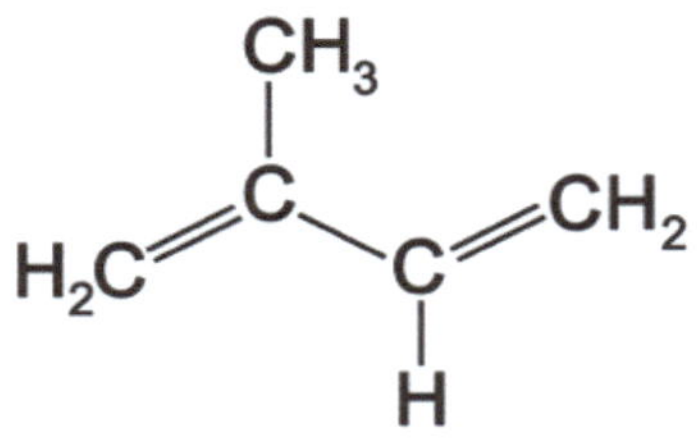

Isoprene (methylbuta-1,3-diene, a hemiterpene)

Table 1: Classification of Terpenes

Terpenes	Isoprene units
Monoterpenes	2
Sesquiterpenes	3
Diterpenes	4
Sesterterpenes	5
Triterpenes	6
Carotenoids	8

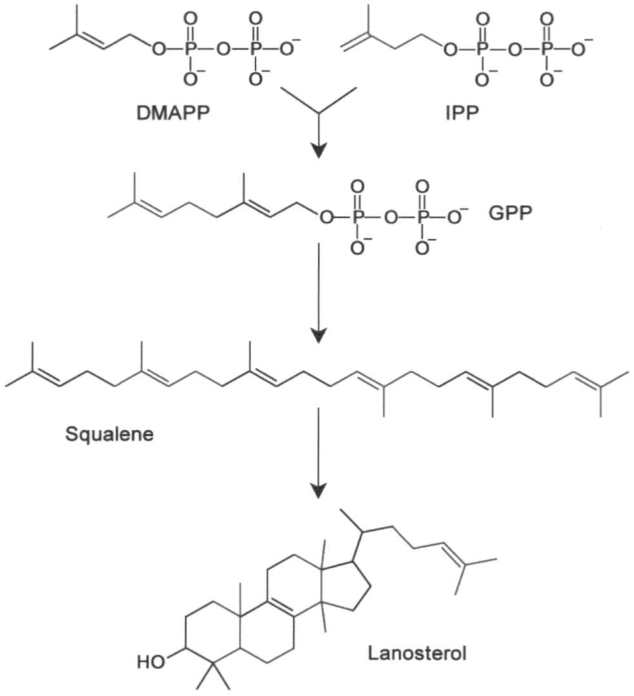

Figure 1: Summary of lanosterol synthesis with intermediates isopentenyl pyrophosphate (IPP), dimethylallyl pyrophosphate (DMAPP), geranyl pyrophosphate (GPP), and squalene shown. Some intermediates are omitted.

18) Consider the structure of geranylfarnesol.

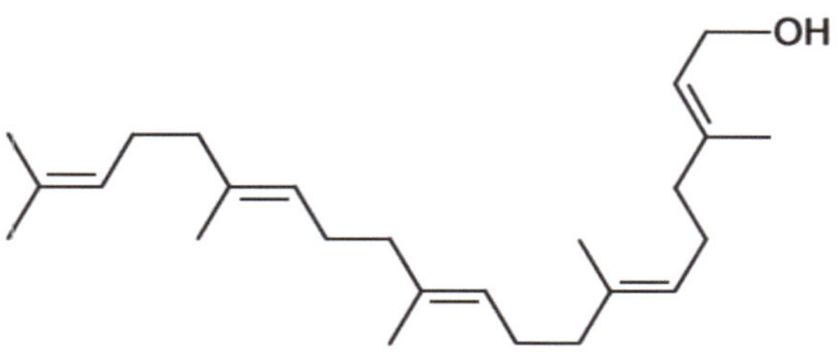

Geranylfarnesol is best classified, based on the number of carbon atoms in its structure, as which of the following?

A. Sesquiterpenoid
B. Diterpenoid
C. Sesterterpenoid
D. Triterpenoid

19) Consider the following image.

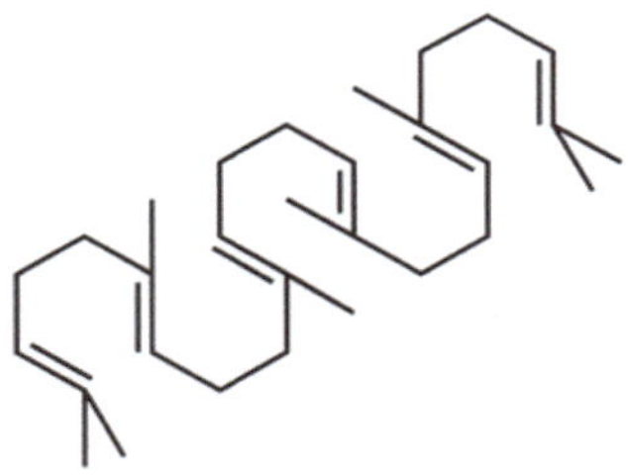

The molecule above is best categorised as:

A. a sesterterpene.
B. a steroid.
C. an all *Z* hydrocarbon.
D. squalene.

20) From the pathway illustrated in Figure 1, which of the following could NOT have reasonably occurred?

A. $NADPH + H^+ \longrightarrow NADP^+$
B. Condensation reaction
C. Oxidation
D. All the above could have reasonably occurred.

21) Consider the following image of a short segment of DNA.

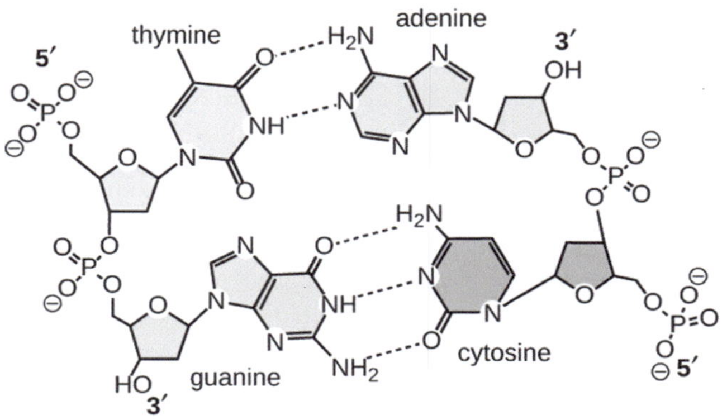

Normal intracellular pH ranges from 6.8 to 7.4. Which of the following represents a likely explanation as to why DNA denatures (*changes shape*) when the pH is raised above 9?

A. Protons dissociate from the phosphate groups in the backbone, which disrupts the hydrogen-bonding pattern between strands.
B. Protons bind to guanine residues giving them additional positive charges which disrupt the hydrogen bonding to the other strand.
C. Protons dissociate from guanine bases disrupting the hydrogen bonding to the other strand.
D. Protons bind to functional groups that serve as hydrogen-bond acceptors, thus disrupting the hydrogen bonding to the other strand.

High-level Importance

Questions 22–24

An elevated concentration of plasma LDL cholesterol is a major risk factor for the development of coronary heart disease. Cholesterol is biosynthesised in a series of 25 separate enzymatic reactions that initially involves 2 successive condensations of three acetyl-CoA units to form the compound HMG-CoA. This is reduced and then converted in a series of reactions to the isoprenes that are building-blocks of squalene (a terpene) - the immediate precursor to sterols - which cyclises and is further metabolised to cholesterol.

Lovastatin is a cholesterol-lowering agent isolated from the fungus *Aspergillus terreus*. Its metabolite is an inhibitor of HMG-CoA reductase which catalyses an early and rate-limiting step in the biosynthesis of cholesterol.

Consider the structure of lovastatin below.

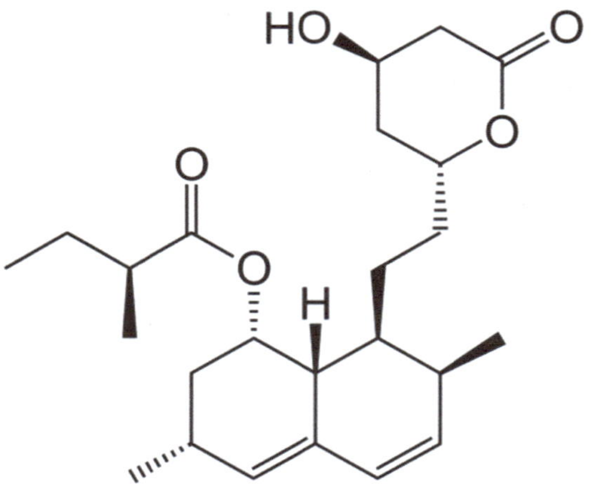

Note that the bicyclic moiety (e.g. part) of lovastatin is referred to as the hexahydro-naphthalene ring (i.e. the portion of the lovastatin molecule with 2 cyclic components).

Also note that assigning a stereochemical configuration at each asymmetric (chiral) carbon in a molecule can be done by using the following CIP priority rules:

1. Identify the chiral carbon, and the four attached groups.
2. Assign priorities to the four groups, using the following rules:
   i. Atoms of higher atomic number have higher priority.
   ii. The higher priority is assigned to the group with the atom of higher atomic number or mass at the first point of difference.
   iii. If the difference between the two groups is due to the number of otherwise identical atoms, the higher priority is assigned to the group with the greater number of atoms of higher atomic number or mass.
   iv. To assign priority of double or triple bonded groups, multiple-bonded atoms are considered as equivalent number of single bonded atoms, thus:

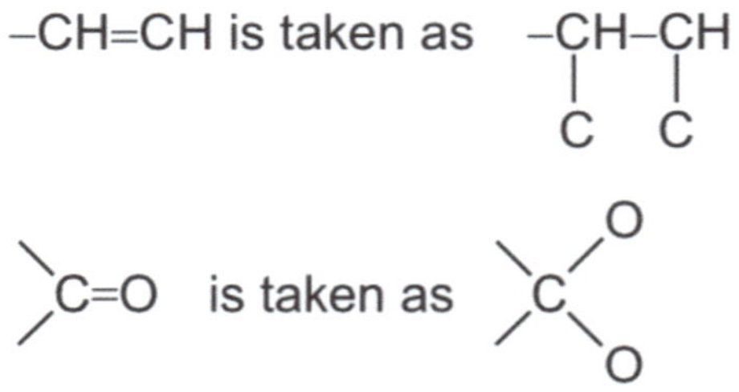

3. The chiral carbon is then evaluated from the side opposite the atom or group with the lowest priority. If the order of the other three atoms or groups in decreasing priorities is clockwise, the arrangement is designated *R*; if counterclockwise, the arrangement is designated *S*.

If two groups with the higher priorities are on opposite sides of a double bond, then it is an *E*- isomer, and if on the same side of the double bond, then it is a *Z*-isomer.

22) The HMG moiety in the molecule HMG-CoA has how many carbons?

A. 4
B. 6
C. 9
D. 18

23) Lovastatin has 2 double bonds in the hexahydro-naphthalene moiety. From left to right, applying the CIP rules, which of the following is consistent with the configuration at the 2 double bonds?

A. *E, E*
B. *E, Z*
C. *Z, E*
D. *Z, Z*

24) In the segments of lovastatin that are outside of the hexahydro-naphthalene moiety, as compared to *R* configuration chiral centres, lovastatin has:

A. one more *S* configuration chiral centre.
B. one fewer *S* configuration chiral centre.
C. the same number of *S* chiral centres.
D. None of the above since Lovastatin has no *S* chiral centres.

25) Which of the following represents two structures that are equivalent?

A.

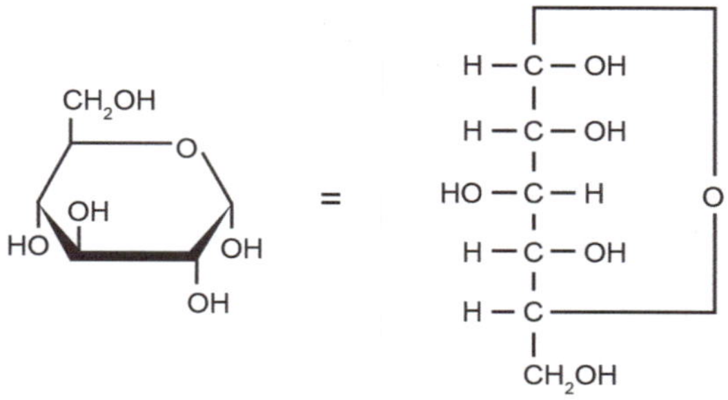

B.

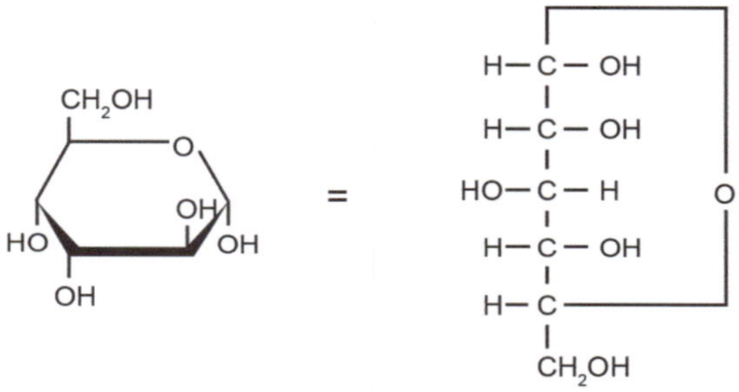

C.

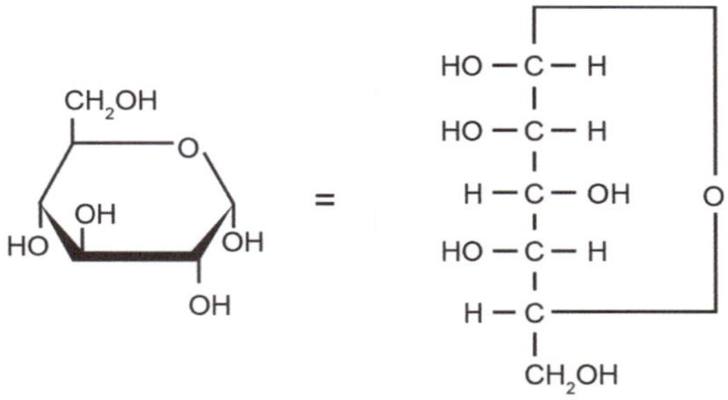

D.

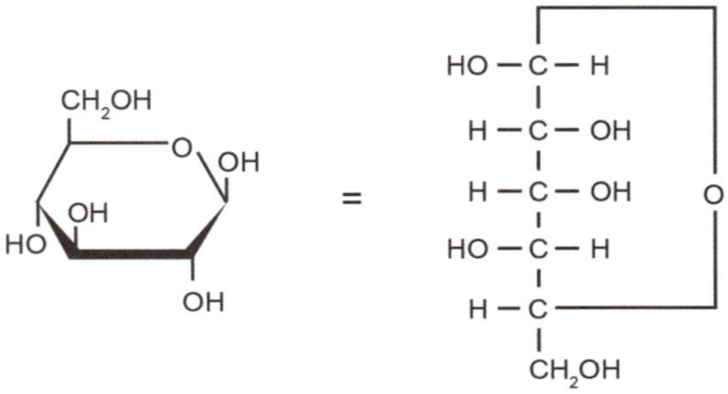

High-level Importance

Questions 26–30

Local anaesthetics prevent or relieve pain by interrupting nerve conduction. All local anaesthetics are membrane stabilising drugs; they reversibly decrease the rate of depolarisation and repolarisation of excitable membranes. They bind to specific receptor sites on the sodium channels in nerves and block the movement of ions through these pores. Structural features of local anaesthetics are shown in Figure 1.

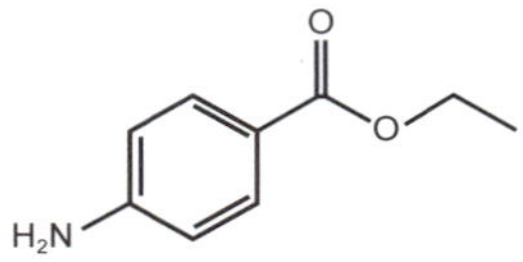

BENZOCAINE

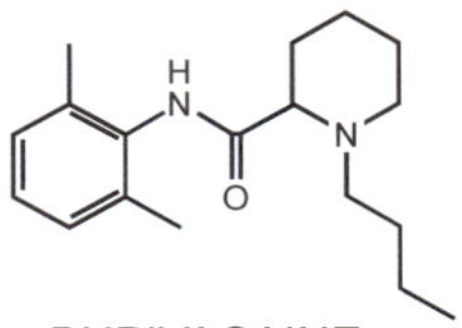

BUPIVACAINE

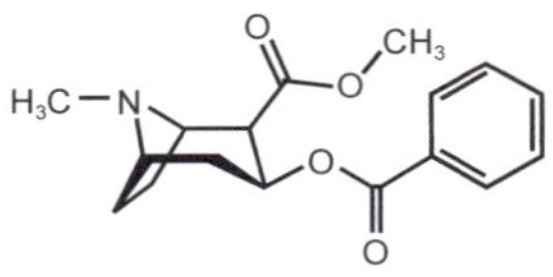

COCAINE

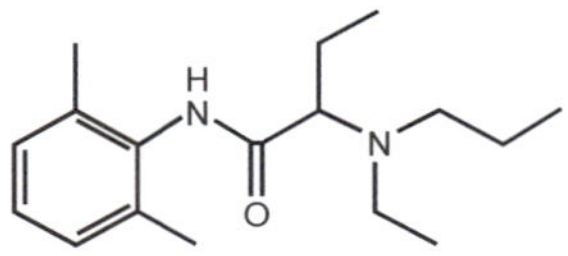

ETIDOCAINE

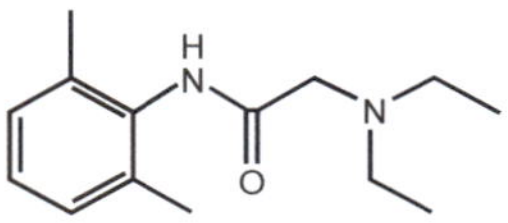

LIDOCAINE

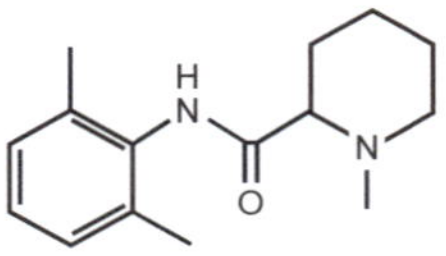

MEPIVACAINE

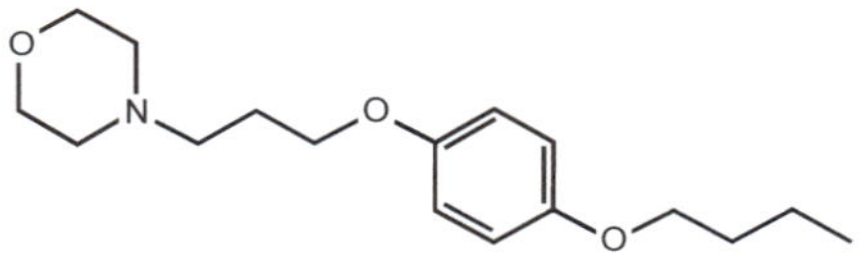

PRAMOXINE

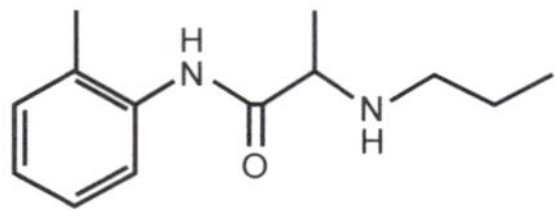

PRILOCAINE

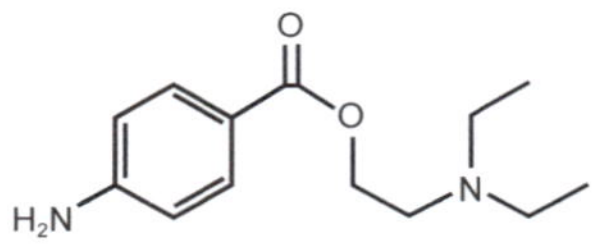

PROCAINE

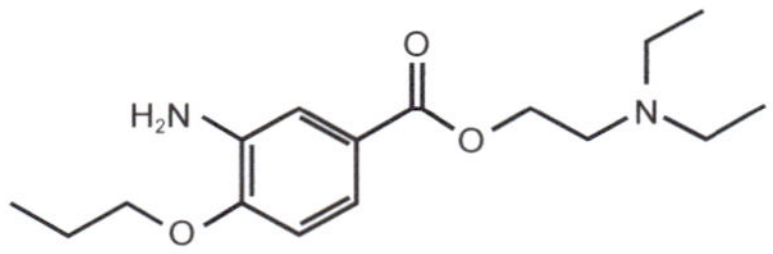

PROPARACAINE

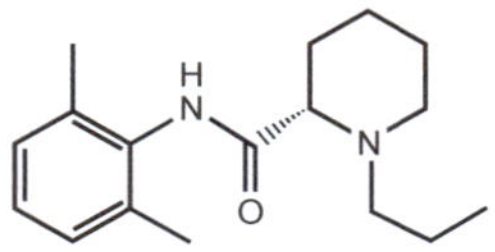

ROPIVACAINE

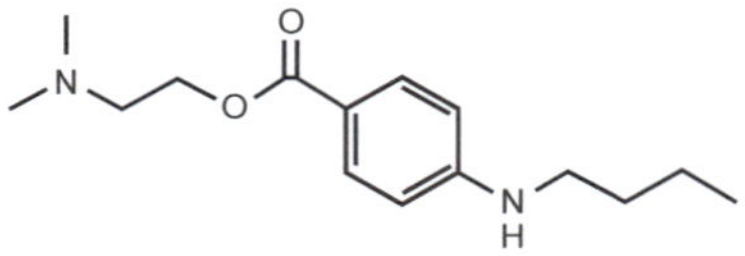

TETRACAINE

Figure 1: Structures of 12 of the most commonly used local anaesthetics

Both the chemical and pharmacologic properties of local anaesthetic drugs determine their clinical properties. Local anaesthetic agents are weak bases, and exist in ionised and unionised forms.

During manufacture they are precipitated as powdered solids which are relatively insoluble. For this reason, they are produced as water-soluble salts to allow them to be injected. These are usually hydrochloride salts which produce a mildly acidic solution that is stable and can be injected. Sodium bicarbonate ($NaHCO_3$) is often added to local anaesthetics as part of their manufacture.

Anaesthetic	pKa
Mepivacaine	7.6
Etidocaine	7.7
Articaine	7.8
Lidocaine	7.9
Prilocaine	7.9
Bupivacaine	8.1
Procaine	9.1

Table 1: The pKa of several local anaesthetic agents

Local anaesthetics must pass through the nerve membrane in a non-ionised lipid-soluble base form, and once they are within the nerve, they must equilibrate into an ionic form to be active (Figure 2). The fraction of the base form is inversely related to how long it takes these anaesthetics to act (onset time). The pH of normal body tissue is 7.4, but active infections can increase the acidity of surrounding tissues considerably.

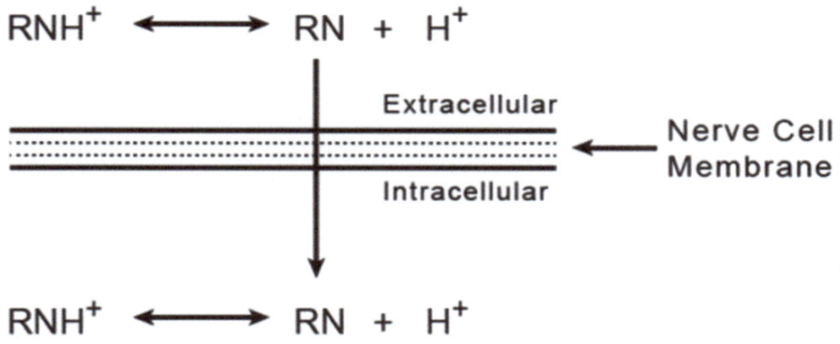

Figure 2: Movement of local anaesthetic ions through the cell membrane of a nerve cell which leads to local analgesia. The receptor site for activity is thought to be located at the cytoplasmic (inner) portion of the sodium channel.

26) Of the 12 local anaesthetics illustrated in Figure 1, how many are **not** chiral?

A. More than half
B. Half
C. Less than half
D. The structures are not drawn in a way as to determine their chirality.

27) At normal tissue pH of 7.4, which of the anaesthetics in Table 1 would have the highest percentage of diffusible form available to penetrate the cell membrane?

A. Procaine
B. Mepivacaine
C. Bupivacaine
D. Either lidocaine or prilocaine

28) Why would sodium bicarbonate be added to local anaesthetics?

- **A.** To inhibit the formation of the base form so they take longer to work.
- **B.** To increase the amount of the base form which shortens the time it takes to work.
- **C.** To increase the amount of cationic form present and so it becomes less painful to inject.
- **D.** To equilibrate the amounts of cationic and base form present.

29) Amide-linked local anaesthetics such as lidocaine are metabolised by amine dealkylation in the liver by the cytochrome P450 system. Which of the following is likely to be a metabolite of lidocaine?

A.

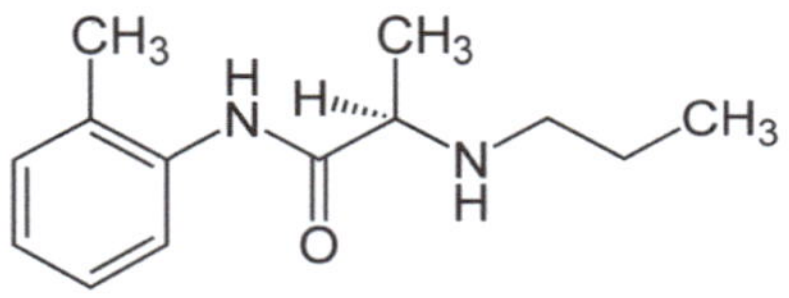

B.

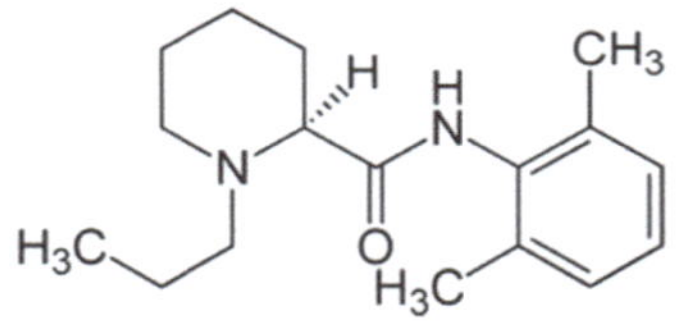

C.

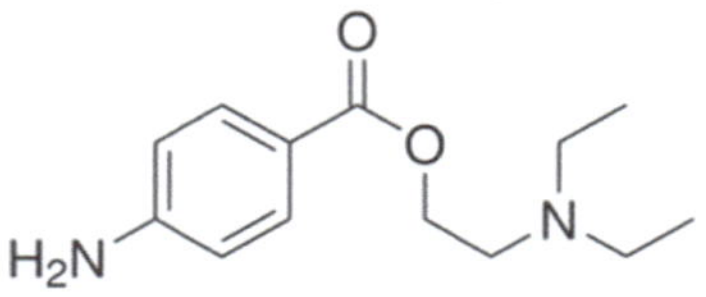

D.

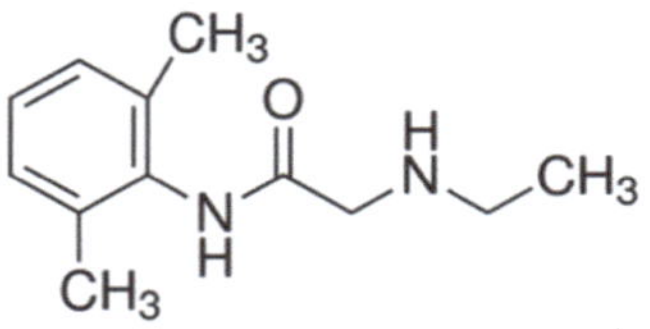

30) What effect would injecting lidocaine into an infected site have on the onset time of analgesia?

- **A.** It would decrease it.
- **B.** It would have no effect.
- **C.** It would increase it.
- **D.** It would have a result more like mepivacaine.

31) The structure of β-D-glucose is shown below in two different projection systems. The circled hydroxyl group in Fig. 1 would be located at which position in the modified Fischer projection depicted in Fig. 2?

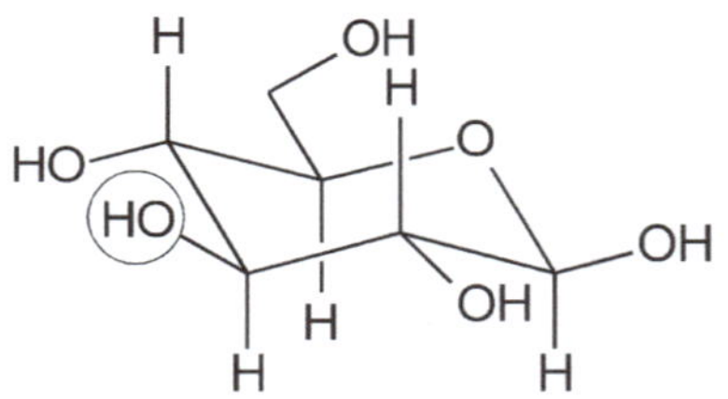

Figure 1

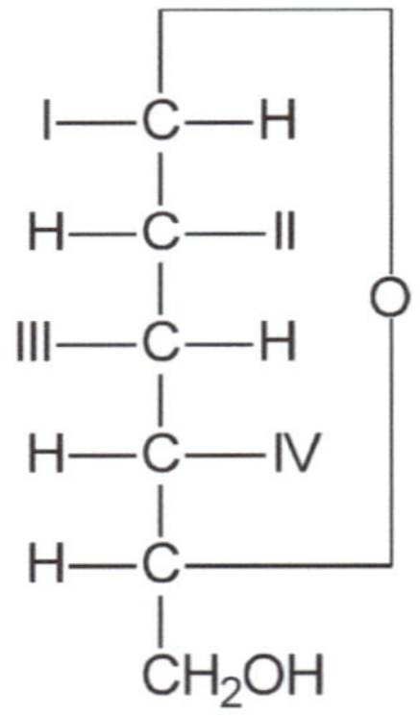

Figure 2

- **A.** I
- **B.** II
- **C.** III
- **D.** IV

Questions 32–33

Amino acids are carboxylic acids that contain an amine functional group. Table 1 lists the twenty amino acids which are normally present in proteins, including their abbreviations.

Full Name	Abbreviation (3 letter)	Abbreviation (1 letter)
Alanine	Ala	A
Arginine	Arg	R
Asparagine	Asn	N
Aspartate	Asp	D
Cysteine	Cys	C
Glutamate	Glu	E
Glutamine	Gln	Q
Glycine	Gly	G
Histidine	His	H
Isoleucine	Ile	I
Leucine	Leu	L
Lysine	Lys	K
Methionine	Met	M
Phenylalanine	Phe	F
Proline	Pro	P
Serine	Ser	S
Threonine	Thr	T
Tryptophan	Trp	W
Tyrosine	Tyr	Y
Valine	Val	V

Table 1

Under certain conditions, the amine group of one amino acid and the carboxyl group of a second can react, uniting the two amino acids by an amide bond, also known as a *peptide* bond. At a pH of 7.4, an amino acid may be neutral, or possess a charge of plus or minus 1.

The feature that differentiates one amino acid from another is the side chain attached to the α-carbon.

The side chains directly impact the categorisation of amino acids.

The most important properties of amino acids are illustrated in Figure 1. For example, at a pH of 7.4, amino acid K (*lysine* in Table 1) has a positive charge.

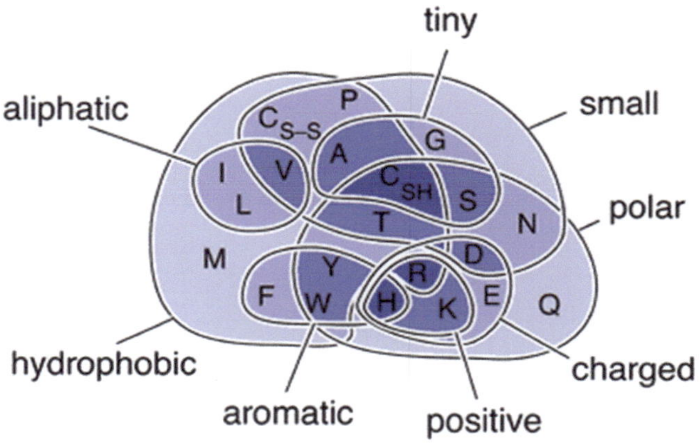

Figure 1: Euler/Venn diagram displaying properties of amino acids at pH 7.4.

32) According to Figure 1, which of the following is **not** accurate?

A. Valine is small and aliphatic.
B. Asparagine is polar and small.
C. Threonine is small and polar.
D. Arginine is positive and aromatic.

33) According to the information provided, at a pH of 7.4, what is the net charge of the following polypeptide?

Ala-Phe-Glu-Lys-Asp-Pro-Asp

A. −2
B. −1
C. 0
D. +1

Questions 34–35

The structure of an amino acid can be transposed into a mathematical matrix as illustrated in Figure 1.

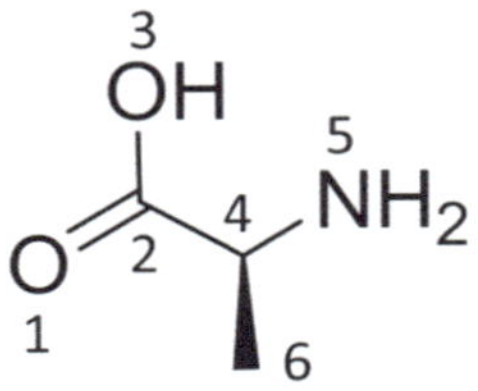

A	1	2	3	4	5	6
1	-	**1**	0	0	0	0
2	**1**	-	**1**	Y	0	0
3	0	**1**	-	0	0	0
4	0	X	0	-	**1**	**1**
5	0	0	0	**1**	-	0
6	0	0	0	**1**	0	-

D	1	2	3	4	5	6
1	0	1	2	2	3	3
2	1	0	1	1	2	2
3	2	1	0	R	Q	3
4	2	1	S	0	1	1
5	3	2	T	1	0	2
6	3	2	3	1	2	0

Figure 1: Adjacency **A** and distance **D** matrices of L-alanine structured by row *i* and column *j*. In the adjacency matrix, an entry a *i,j* is 1 if atoms *i* and *j* are connected with a bond, and 0 otherwise. An entry d *i,j* in the distance matrix is the topological distance of atoms *i* and *j*. (ref. Bajusz, Rácz, Héberger; Reference Module in Chemistry, 2017)

Note that some numerical entries in Figure 1 have been replaced by **green** letters.

34) Based on the information provided and Figure 1, identify the correct equivalences.

A. **X** = 0, **Y** = 1
B. **X** = 1, **Y** = 0
C. **X** = **Y** = 0
D. **X** = **Y** = 1

35) Based on the information provided and Figure 1, identify the correct equivalence.

A. **Q** = 3
B. **R** = 3
C. **S** = 1
D. **T** = 1

SPOILER ALERT ⚠

Gold Standard has cross-referenced the content in this chapter to examples from ACER's official GAMSAT practice materials. It is for you to decide when you want to explore these questions since you may want to preserve some of ACER's materials for timed mock-exam practice.

Examples – Carbohydrates, the structure of monosaccharides with Fischer and Haworth representations: Q19-21 of 1; cellular respiration, oxidation of glucose, structural isomers, empirical formula and oxidation vs. hydration: Q36-39 of 1; table of fatty acids, assessment of saturation vs. unsaturation, and the iodine value: Q32-35 of 3; biological molecules and assessing stereocentres: Q59-60 of 4; DNA, solubility and hydrogen bonds: Q66 of 5; carbohydrates and assessing stereocentres: Q76-78 of 5; beta-carotene and counting conjugations: Q83 of 5. Note that "Q" is followed by the question number, and, for example, "of 1" refers to booklet number 1 which is referenced in the Spoiler Alert table at the end of Chapter 1. The 15 full-length GAMSAT practice tests by Gold Standard, HEAPS-1 through HEAPS-15, contain specific cross-references to this chapter within the worked solutions. Note that the epic unit discussing the cleavage of proteins and peptides into amino acid sequences is from HEAPS-1; the table of fatty acids with assessment of saturation vs. unsaturation, and the iodine value comes from HEAPS-3; some independent carbohydrate-structural units (Fischer, Hawthorne, etc.) are from HEAPS-6 and 8; the cholesterol-lowering drug Lovastatin is from HEAPS-6. Special mention: Chapter 7 Aldehydes and Ketones explored a recurrent GAMSAT theme of acetals, hemiacetals, ketals and hemiketals, including some carbohydrates, in the GAMSAT-level practice questions at the end of that chapter.

High-level Importance

Chapter Checklist

- ☐ Access your online account to view answers, worked solutions and discussion boards.
- ☐ Reassess your 'learning objectives' for this chapter: Go back to the first page of this chapter and re-evaluate the top 3 boxes and the Introduction.
- ☐ Complete a maximum of 1 page of notes using symbols/abbreviations to represent the entire chapter based on your learning objectives. These are your Gold Notes.
- ☐ Consider your multimedia options based on your optimal way of learning:
    - ☐ Download the free Gold Standard GAMSAT app for your Android device or iPhone.
    - ☐ Create your own, tangible study cards or try the free app: Anki.
    - ☐ Record your voice reading your Gold Notes onto your smartphone (audio files, e.g., *memo* or MP3s) and listen during exercise, transportation, etc.
    - ☐ Try out the Gold Standard GAMSAT online videos at gamsat-prep.com, or you can try other options on YouTube like Khan Academy or Crash Course Organic Chemistry.
- ☐ Reassess your schedule for your full-length GAMSAT practice tests: ACER and/or HEAPS exams. Ensure that you have scheduled one full day to complete a practice test and 1-2 days for a thorough assessment of worked solutions while adding to your abbreviated Gold Notes.
- ☐ Reassess your progress in scheduling and/or evaluating stress reduction techniques such as regular exercise (sports), yoga, meditation and/or mindfulness exercises (*see* YouTube for suggestions).

SEPARATIONS AND PURIFICATIONS
Chapter 13

Memorise

* Interactions between organic molecules

Understand

* Different phases in the various techniques
* How to improve separation, purification
* How to avoid overheating (distillation)

Importance

Medium level: 5% of GAMSAT Organic Chemistry questions released by ACER are related to content in this chapter (in our estimation).
* Note that approximately 60% of the questions in GAMSAT Organic Chemistry are related to just 4 chapters: 2, 6, 7 and 12.

GAMSAT-Prep.com

Introduction

Separation techniques are used to transform a mixture of substances into two or more distinct products. The separated products may be different in chemical properties or some physical property (i.e. size). Purification in organic chemistry is the physical separation of a chemical substance of interest from foreign or contaminating substances.

Multimedia Resources at GAMSAT-Prep.com

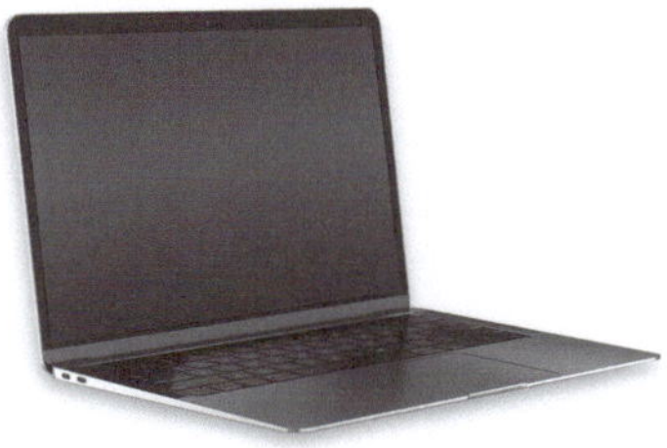

Open Discussion Boards
(*gamsat-prep.com/forum*)

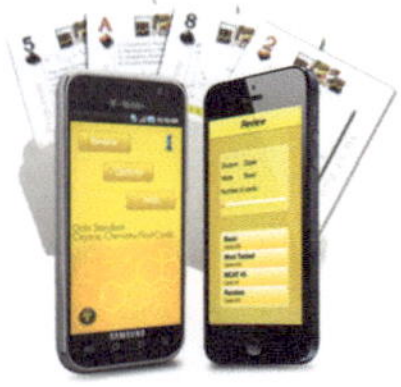

Flashcards

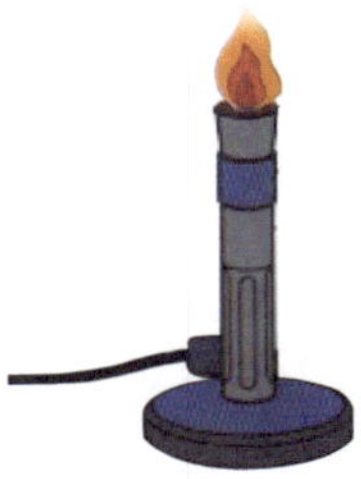

Special Guest

* The real GAMSAT may have advanced-level information presented (i.e. in a passage) but previous knowledge of said information is not required to answer the questions that would follow. Practice questions at the end of this chapter, as well as ACER and GS (HEAPS) practice GAMSATs can help you clarify this point.

13.1 Separation Techniques

Extraction is the process by which a solute is transferred (*extracted*) from one solvent and placed in another. This procedure is possible if the two solvents used cannot mix (= *immiscible*) and if the solute is more soluble in the solvent used for the extraction.

For example, consider the extraction of solute A which is dissolved in solvent X. We choose solvent Y for the extraction since solute A is highly soluble in it and because solvent Y is immiscible with solvent X. We now add solvent Y to the solution involving solute A and solvent X. The container is agitated. Solute A begins to dissolve in the solvent where it is most soluble, solvent Y. The container is left to stand, thus the two immiscible solvents separate. The phase containing solute A can now be removed.

In practice, solvent Y would be chosen such that it would be sufficiently easy to evaporate (= *volatile*) after the extraction so solute A can be easily recovered. Also, it is more efficient to perform several extractions using a small amount of solvent each time, rather than one extraction using a large amount of solvent.

The main purpose of **filtration** is to isolate a solid from a liquid. There are two basic types of filtration: gravity filtration and vacuum filtration. In gravity filtration the solution containing the substance of interest is poured through the filter paper with the solvent's own weight responsible for pulling it through. This is often done using a hot solvent to ensure that the product remains dissolved (e.g. filter used in a coffee maker).

In vacuum filtration the solvent is forced through the filter with a vacuum on the other side. This is helpful when it is necessary to isolate large quantities of solid.

Sublimation is a process which goes from a heated solid directly into the gas phase without passing through the intermediate liquid phase (CHM 4.3.1). Low pressure reduces the temperature required for sublimation. The substance in question is heated and then condensed on a cool surface ('cold finger'), leaving the non-volatile impurities behind.

Centrifugation is a separation process that involves the use of centrifugal forces for the sedimentation of mixtures. Particles settle at different rates depending on their size, viscosity, density and shape. Compounds of greater mass and density settle toward the bottom while compounds of lighter mass and density remain on top. This process is most useful in separating polymeric materials such as biological macromolecules.

Distillation is the process by which compounds are separated based on differences in boiling points. Compounds with a lower boiling point are preferentially vaporised, condensed on a water cooler, and are separated from compounds with higher boiling points.

For instance, a classic example of simple distillation is the separation of salt from water. The solution is heated. Water will boil and vaporise at a far lower temperature than salt. Hence the water boils away leaving salt behind. Water vapor can now be condensed into pure liquid water (*distilled water*).

As long as one compound is more volatile (CHM 4.4.2, 5.1.1), the distillation process is quite simple. If the difference between the two boiling points is low, it will be more difficult to separate the compounds by this method. Here are 3 standard ways to separate compounds using distillation:

1. **Simple distillation** is used to separate liquids whose boiling points differ by at least 25 °C and that boil below 150 °C. The composition of the distillate depends on the composition of the vapors at a given temperature and pressure.
2. **Vacuum distillation** is used to separate liquids whose boiling points differ by at least 25 °C and that boil above 150 °C. The vacuum environment prevents compounds from decomposition because the low pressure reduces the temperature required for distillation.
3. **Fractional distillation** is used to separate liquids whose boiling points are less than 25 °C apart. The repeated vaporisation-condensation cycle of compounds will eventually yield vapors that contain a greater and greater proportion of the lower boiling point component.

The fractional distillation apparatus can include a column filled with glass beads which is placed between the distillation flask and the condenser (*see* Figure IV.B.13.0). The glass beads increase the surface area over which the less volatile compound can condense and drip back down to the distillation (distilling) flask below. The more volatile compound boils away and condenses. Thus the two compounds are separated.

The efficiency of the distillation process in producing a pure product is improved by repeating the distillation process, increasing the length of the fractionating column and avoiding overheating. Overheating may destroy the pure compounds or increase the percent of impurities. Some of the methods which are used to prevent overheating include boiling slowly, the use of boiling chips (= *ebulliator*, which makes bubbles) and the use of a vacuum which decreases the vapor pressure and thus the boiling point.

Medium-level Importance

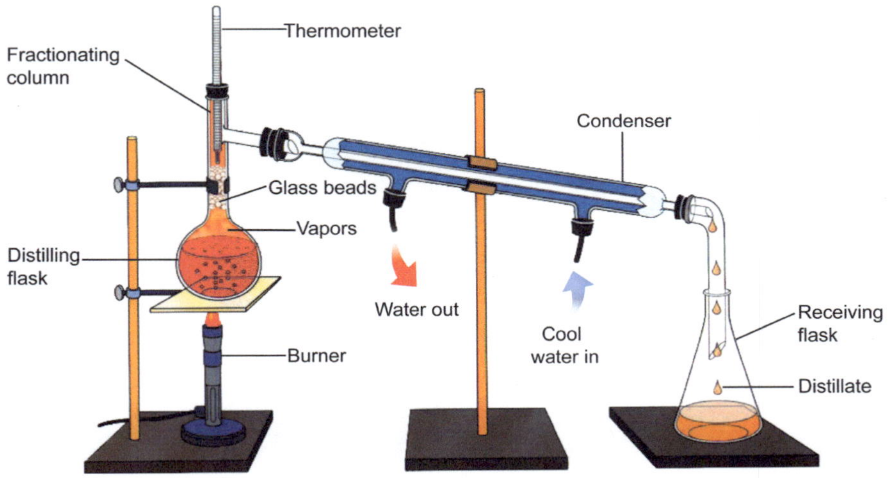

Figure IV.B.13.0: Standard fractional distillation apparatus heated with a Bunsen burner.

13.2 Chromatography

Chromatography is the separation of a mixture of compounds by their distribution between two phases: one stationary and one moving. The mobile phase is run through the stationary phase. Different substances distribute themselves according to their relative affinities for the two phases. This causes the separation of the different compounds. Molecules are separated based on differences in polarity and molecular weight.

13.2.1 Gas-Liquid Chromatography

In **gas-liquid chromatography**, the *stationary phase* is a liquid absorbed to an inert solid. The liquid can be polyethylene glycol, squalene, or others, depending on the polarity of the substances being separated.

The mobile phase is a gas (i.e. He, N_2) which is unreactive both to the stationary phase and to the substances being separated. The sample being analysed can be injected in the direction of gas flow into one end of a column packed with the stationary phase. As the sample migrates through the column, certain molecules will move faster than others. As mentioned, the separation of the different types of molecules is dependent on size (*molecular weight*) and charge (*polarity*). Once the molecules reach the end of the column, special detectors signal their arrival.

13.2.2 Thin-Layer Chromatography

Thin-layer chromatography (TLC) is a solid-liquid technique, based on adsorptivity and solubility. The *stationary phase* is a type of finely divided polar material, usually silica gel or alumina, which is thinly coated onto a glass plate. *Adsorption* is the *ad*hesion of atoms, ions or molecules from a gas, liquid or dissolved solid to a surface.

A mixture of compounds is placed on the stationary phase, as mentioned, either a thin layer of silica gel or alumina on a glass sheet. Silica gel is a very polar and hydrophobic substance. The mobile phase is usually of low polarity and moves by capillary action. Therefore, if silica gel is used as the stationary phase, nonpolar compounds move quickly while polar compounds have a strong interaction with the gel and are stuck tightly to it. In reverse-phase chromatography, the stationary phase is nonpolar and the mobile phase is polar; as a result, polar compounds move quickly while nonpolar compounds stick more tightly to the adsorbant.

There are several types of interactions that may occur between the organic molecules

Medium-level Importance

in the sample and the silica gel, in order from weakest to strongest (*see* CHM 3.4, 4.2):

- Van der Waals force (nonpolar molecules)
- Dipole-dipole interaction (polar molecules)
- Hydrogen bonding (hydroxylic compounds)
- Coordination (Lewis bases)

Molecules with functional groups with the greatest polarity will bind more strongly to the stationary phase and thus will not rise as high on the glass plate.

Organic molecules will also interact with the *mobile phase* (= a solvent), or *eluent*, used in the process. The more polar the solvent, the more easily it will dissolve polar molecules. The mobile phase usually contains organic solvents like ethanol, benzene, chloroform, acetone, etc.

As a result of the interactions of the organic molecules with the stationary and moving phases, for any adsorbed compound, there is a dynamic distribution equilibrium between these phases. The different molecules will rise to different heights on the plate. Their presence can be detected using special stains (i.e. pH indicators, $KMnO_4$) or UV light (*if the compound can fluoresce; CHM 11.6*).

Each spot from the TLC can be objectively assessed by its retardation factor (R_f) which is equal to the distance migrated over the total distance covered by the solvent.

$$R_f = \frac{\text{(distance traveled by sample)}}{\text{(distance traveled by solvent)}}$$

An R_f value will always be in the range of 0 to 1; if the substance moves, it can only move in the direction of the solvent flow, and cannot move faster than the solvent. For example, if a particular substance in an unknown mixture travels 3.0 cm and the solvent front travels 5.0 cm, the retardation factor would be 3.0/5.0 = 0.6.

In the following diagram, what formula would you use to describe the R_f values of the blue and yellow dots, respectively?

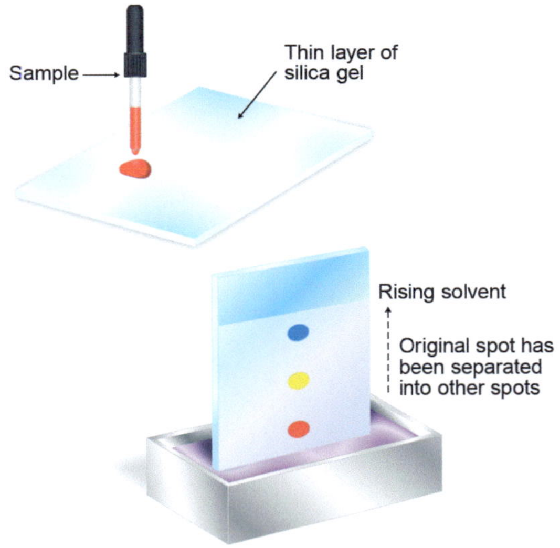

Figure IV.B.13.1 Part I: Thin-layer Chromatography.

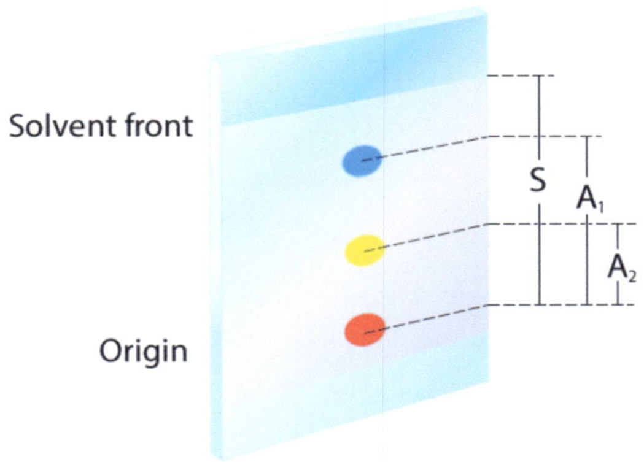

Figure IV.B.13.1 Part II: Calculating the retardation factor from the point of origin of the mixed sample from Fig. IV.B.13.1 Part I.

Medium-level Importance

Using the equation provided, the retardation factors would be:

blue: $R_{f1} = A_1/S$; yellow: $R_{f2} = A_2/S$.

13.2.3 Paper Chromatography: Conventional and 2D

Conventional, **paper chromatography** has been largely replaced by TLC. The former's mobile phase is a solution that travels up the stationary phase, due to capillary action. The mobile phase is generally an alcohol-solvent mixture, while the stationary phase is a strip of chromatography paper, also called a *chromatogram*.

A more useful variant is 2D (two-dimensional) chromatography. This technique involves using two solvents and rotating the paper 90° between trials. This is more helpful for separating complex mixtures of compounds having similar polarity, for example, amino acids. {Note: 2D chromatography is used in ACER's *GAMSAT Practice Test 1*, questions 20-26 (unit 7). Go to the Video section of gamsat-prep.com for the worked solutions.}

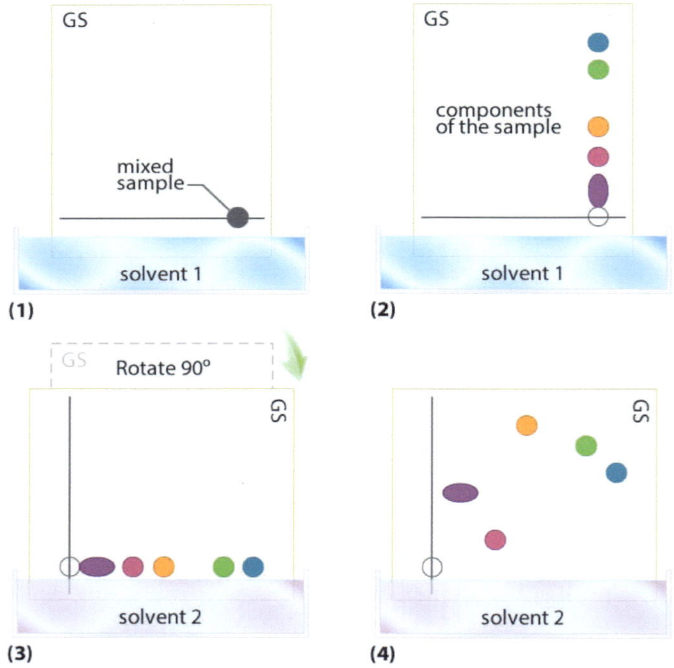

Figure IV.B.13.2: 2D Paper Chromatography. Regarding the 4 images: **(1)** a mixed sample can be placed in either the bottom left or bottom right corner to begin; **(2)** the initial chromatogram (conventional, 1D) is complete; **(3)** rotation into a different solvent; **(4)** the final 2D chromatogram is complete. R_f values can be calculated for each solvent separately and can provide unique information for each of the components of the sample in the illustration.

13.2.4 Column Chromatography

Column chromatography is similar to TLC in principle; however, column chromatography uses silica gel or alumina as an adsorbant in the form of a column rather than TLC which uses paper in a layer-like form. The solvent and compounds move down the column (by gravity) allowing much more separation. The solvent drips out into a waiting flask where fractions containing bands corresponding to the different compounds are collected. After the solvent has evaporated, the compounds can then be isolated. Often the desired compounds are proteins or nucleic acids for which several techniques exist:

1. Ion exchange chromatography – Beads coated with charged substances are placed in the column so that they will attract compounds with an opposing charge.
2. Size exclusion chromatography – The column contains beads with tiny pores which allow small substances to enter, leaving larger molecules to pass through the column faster.
3. Affinity chromatography – Columns are customised to bind a substance of interest (e.g. a receptor or antibody) which allows it to bind very tightly.

13.3 Gel Electrophoresis

Gel electrophoresis is an important method to separate biological macromolecules (i.e. protein and DNA) based on size and charge of molecules. Molecules are made to move through a gel which is placed in an electrophoresis chamber. When an electric current is applied, molecules move at different velocities. These molecules will move towards either the cathode or anode depending on their size and charge (**an**ions move towards the **an**ode while **cat**ions move towards the **cat**hode). The migration velocity is proportional to the net charge on the molecule and inversely proportional to a coefficient dependent on the size of the molecule. Highly charged, small molecules will move the quickest with size being the most important factor.

There are three main types of electrophoresis:

1. Agarose gel electrophoresis – Used to separate pieces of negatively charged nucleic acids based on their size.

2. SDS-polyacrylamide gel electrophoresis (SDS-PAGE) – Separates proteins on the basis of mass and not charge. The SDS (sodium dodecyl sulfate) binds to

proteins and creates a large negative charge such that the only variable affecting their movement is the frictional coefficient which is solely dependent on mass.

3. Isoelectric focusing – The isoelectric point is the pH at which the net charge of a protein is zero (ORG 12.1.2). A mixture of proteins can be separated by placing them in an electric field with a pH gradient. The proteins will lose their charge and come to a stop when the pH is equal to their isoelectric point.

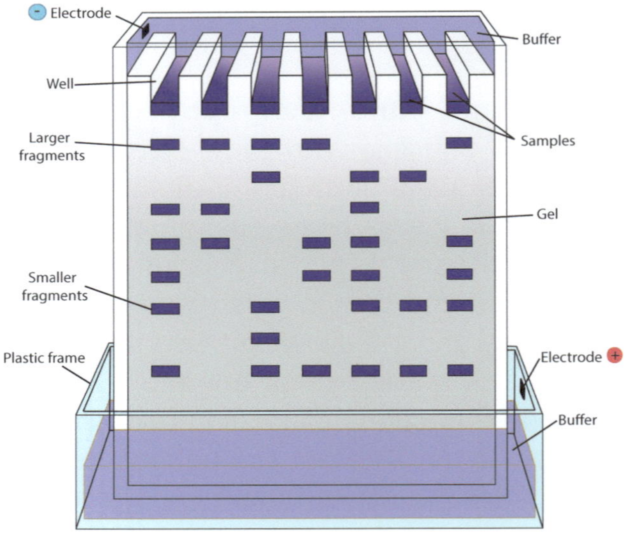

Figure IV.B.13.3: Gel Electrophoresis.

Medium-level Importance

13.4 Recrystallisation

Recrystallisation is a useful purification technique. A solid organic compound with some impurity is dissolved in a hot solvent, and then the solvent is slowly cooled to allow the pure compound to reform or *recrystallise*, while leaving the impurities behind in the solvent. This is possible because the impurities do not normally fit within the crystal structure of the compound.

In choosing a solvent, solubility data (e.g. K_{sp} at various temperatures, etc.) regarding both the compound to be purified and the impurities should be known. The data should be analysed such that the solvent would:

- have the capability to dissolve alot of the compound (to be purified) at or near the boiling point of the solvent, while being able to dissolve little of the compound at room temperature. As well, the impurities should be soluble in the cold solvent.
- have a low boiling point, so as to be easily removed from the solid in a drying process.
- not react with the solid.

Practice questions, answers and worked solutions for this chapter and Chapter 14 are accessible through your online account.

SPOILER ALERT

Gold Standard has cross-referenced the content in this chapter to examples from ACER's official GAMSAT practice materials. It is for you to decide when you want to explore these questions since you may want to preserve some of ACER's materials for timed mock-exam practice.

Examples – 2D chromatography (ORG 13.2.3) explored in a relatively long unit: Q20-26 of 3. Note that "Q" is followed by the question number, and, for example, "of 1" refers to booklet number 1 which is referenced in the Spoiler Alert table at the end of Chapter 1. The 15 full-length GAMSAT practice tests by Gold Standard, HEAPS-1 through HEAPS-15, contain specific cross-references to this chapter within the worked solutions. Note that the unit separating the stimulant caffeine in your online account is from HEAPS-8.

Chapter Checklist

- ☐ Access your online account to view answers, worked solutions and discussion boards.
- ☐ Reassess your 'learning objectives' for this chapter: Go back to the first page of this chapter and re-evaluate the top 3 boxes and the Introduction.
- ☐ Complete a maximum of 1 page of notes using symbols/abbreviations to represent the entire chapter based on your learning objectives. These are your Gold Notes.
- ☐ Consider your multimedia options based on your optimal way of learning:
    - ☐ Download the free Gold Standard GAMSAT app for your Android device or iPhone.
    - ☐ Create your own, tangible study cards or try the free app: Anki.
    - ☐ Record your voice reading your Gold Notes onto your smartphone (audio files, e.g., *memo* or MP3s) and listen during exercise, transportation, etc.
    - ☐ Try out the Gold Standard GAMSAT online videos at gamsat-prep.com, or you can try other options on YouTube like Khan Academy or Crash Course Organic Chemistry.
- ☐ Reassess your schedule for your full-length GAMSAT practice tests: ACER and/or HEAPS exams. Ensure that you have scheduled one full day to complete a practice test and 1-2 days for a thorough assessment of worked solutions while adding to your abbreviated Gold Notes.
- ☐ Reassess your progress in scheduling and/or evaluating stress reduction techniques such as regular exercise (sports), yoga, meditation and/or mindfulness exercises (*see* YouTube for suggestions).

Medium-level Importance

Memorise	Understand	Importance
* Nothing	* Basic theory: IR spect., NMR, mass spectrometry	**Medium level: 5% of GAMSAT Organic Chemistry** questions released by ACER are related to content in this chapter (in our estimation). * Note that approximately 60% of the questions in GAMSAT Organic Chemistry are related to just 4 chapters: 2, 6, 7 and 12.

GAMSAT-Prep.com

Introduction

Spectroscopy is the use of the absorption, emission, or scattering of electromagnetic radiation by matter to study the matter or to study physical processes. The matter can be atoms, molecules, atomic or molecular ions, or solids.

Consider the hundreds of molecules and dozens of functional groups that we have already seen in this textbook. Spectroscopy can provide evidence for which atoms compose those molecules, and how those atoms are arranged in those molecules.

Multimedia Resources at GAMSAT-Prep.com

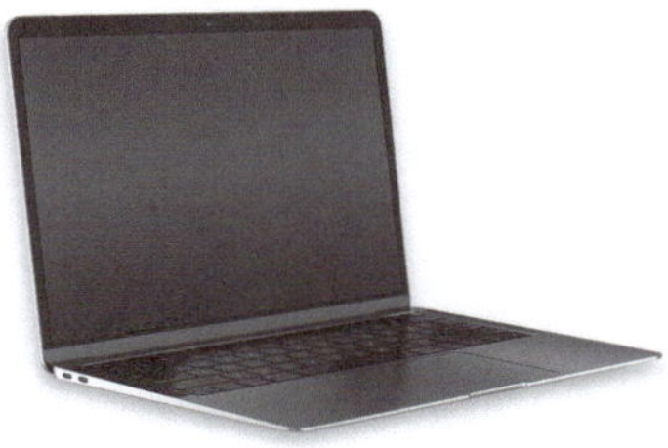

Open Discussion Boards
(*gamsat-prep.com/forum*)

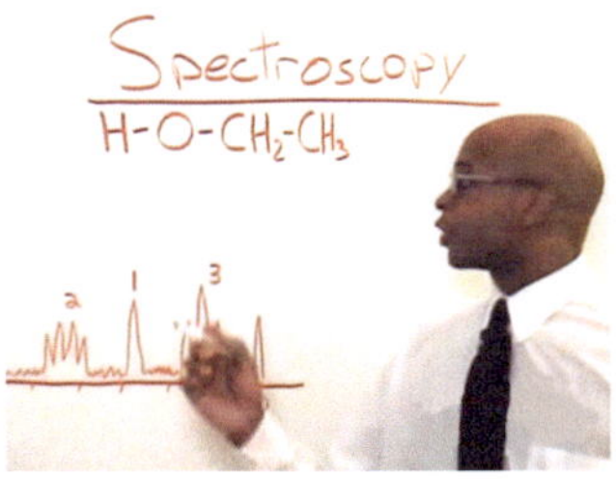

Science Preparation Videos

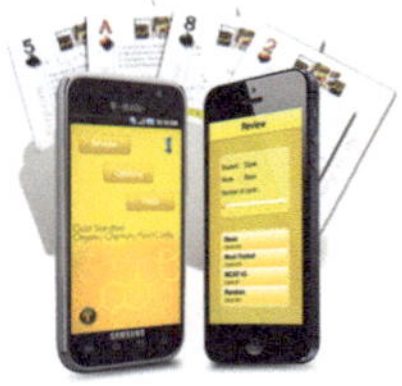

Flashcards

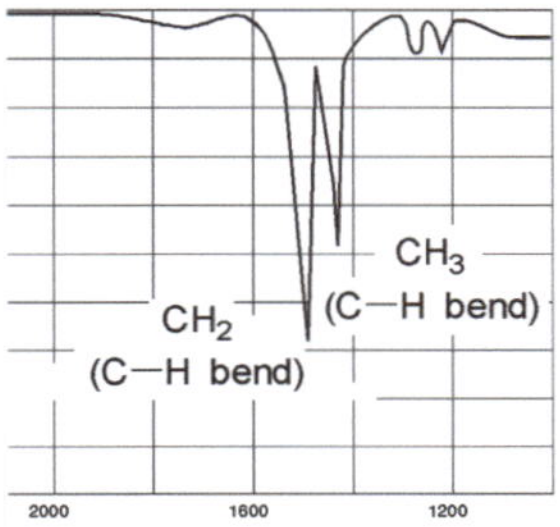

Special Guest

* The real GAMSAT may have advanced-level information presented (i.e. in a passage) but previous knowledge of said information is not required to answer the questions that would follow. Practice questions at the end of this chapter, as well as ACER and GS (HEAPS) practice GAMSATs can help you clarify this point.

14.1 IR Spectroscopy

In an infrared spectrometer, a beam of infrared (IR) radiation is passed through a sample. The spectrometer will then analyse the amount of radiation transmitted (= *% transmittance*) through the sample as the incident radiation is varied. Ultimately, a plot results as a graph showing the transmittance or absorption (*the inverse of transmittance*) versus the frequency or wavelength of the incident radiation or the wavenumber (= the reciprocal of the wavelength). IR spectroscopy is best used for the identification of functional groups.

The location of an IR absorption band (*or peak*) can be specified in *frequency units* by its wavenumber, measured in cm^{-1}. As the wave number decreases, the wavelength increases, thus the energy decreases (this can be determined using two physics equations which we have already seen, PHY 7.1.2, 9.2.4: $v = \lambda f$ and $E = hf$). A schematic representation of the IR spectrum of octane is:

Electromagnetic radiation consists of discrete units of energy called *quanta* or *photons* (PHY 7.1.3, 11.1). All organic compounds are capable of absorbing many types of electromagnetic energy. The absorption of energy leads to an increase in the amplitude of intramolecular rotations and vibrations.

Intramolecular rotations are the rotations of a molecule about its centre of gravity. The difference in rotational energy levels is inversely proportional to the moment of inertia of a molecule. Rotational energy is quantised and gives rise to absorption spectra in the microwave region of the electromagnetic spectrum.

Intramolecular vibrations are the bending and stretching motions of bonds within a molecule. The relative spacing between vibrational energy levels increases with the increasing strength of an intramolecular bond. Vibrational energy is quantised and gives rise

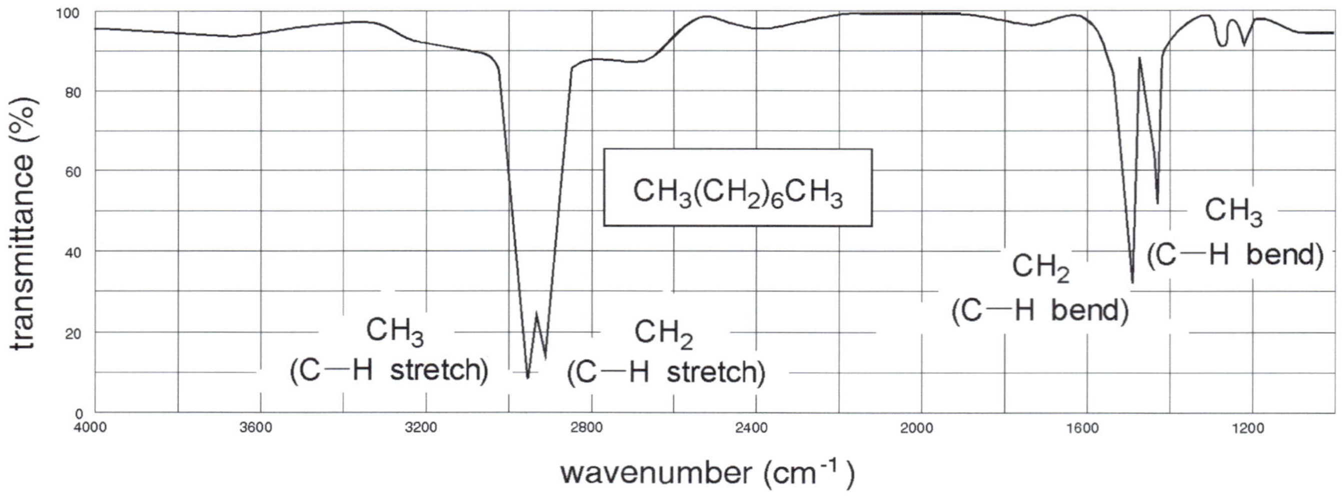

to absorption spectra in the infrared region of the electromagnetic spectrum.

Thus there are two types of bond vibration: stretching and bending. That is, after exposure to the IR radiation the bonds stretch and bend (*or contract*) to a greater degree once energy is absorbed. In general, bending vibrations will occur at lower frequencies (higher wavelengths) than stretching vibrations of the same groups. So, as seen in the sample spectra for octane, each group will have two characteristic peaks, one due to stretching, and one due to bending.

Different functional groups will have transmittances at characteristic wave numbers, which is why IR spectroscopy is useful. Some examples (*approximate values*) of characteristic absorbances are shown in the table.

By looking at the characteristic transmittances of a compound's spectrum, it is possible to identify the functional groups present in the molecule.

Symmetrical molecules or molecules composed of the same atoms do not exhibit a change in dipole moment under IR radiation and thus absorptions do not show up in IR spectra.

Group	Frequency Range (cm^{-1})
Alkyl (C–H)	2850 – 2960
Alkene (C=C)	1620 – 1680
Alkyne (C≡C)	2100 – 2260
Alcohol (O–H)	3200 – 3650
Benzene (Ar–H)	3030
Carbonyl (C=O)	1630 – 1780
▶ Aldehyde	1680 – 1750
▶ Ketone	1735 – 1750
▶ Carboxylic Acid	1710 – 1780
▶ Amide	1630 – 1690
Amine (N–H)	3300 – 3500
Nitriles (C≡N)	2220 – 2260

Most introductory level courses require students to memorise at least the absorbances for, arguably, the two most important functional groups at the introductory level: carbonyl (around 1700) and alcohol (around 3300). Knowing these 2 benchmarks may be helpful but there is no evidence that even these 2 values are required knowledge for the GAMSAT.

Medium-level Importance

14.2 Proton NMR Spectroscopy

Nuclear Magnetic Resonance (NMR) spectroscopy can be used to examine the environments of the hydrogen atoms in a molecule. In fact, using a (*proton*) NMR or

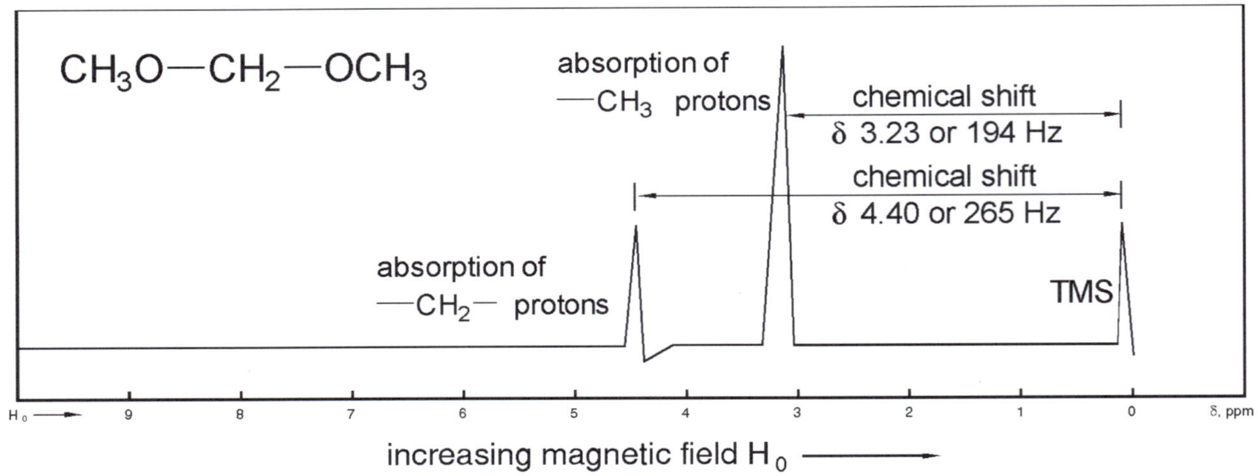

Medium-level Importance

^{1}HNMR, one can determine both the number and types of hydrogens in a molecule. The basis of this stems from the magnetic properties of the hydrogen nucleus (proton). Similar to electrons, the hydrogen proton has a nuclear spin, able to take either of two values. These values are designated as +1/2 and –1/2. As a result of this spin, the nucleus will respond to a magnetic field by being oriented in the direction of the field. NMR spectrometers measure the absorption of energy by the hydrogen nuclei in an organic compound.

A schematic representation of an NMR spectrum, that of dimethoxymethane is shown in the diagram above.

The small peak at the right is that of TMS, tetramethylsilane, shown here:

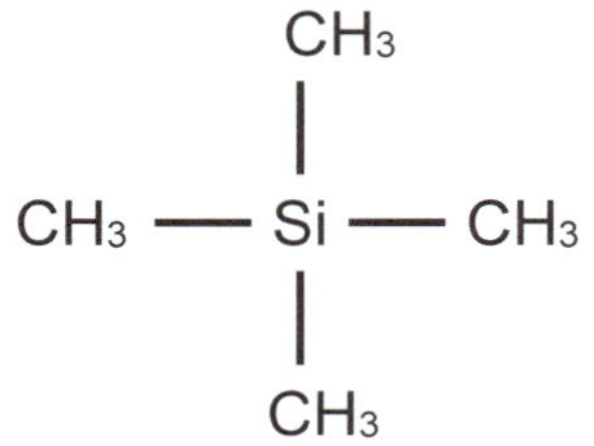

This compound is added to the sample to be used as a reference, or standard. It is volatile, inert and absorbs at a higher field than most other organic chemicals.

The position of a peak relative to the standard is referred to as its *chemical shift*. Since NMR spectroscopy differentiates between types of protons, each type will have a different chemical shift, as shown. Protons in the same environment, like the three hydrogens in $-CH_3$, are called *equivalent protons*.

Dimethoxymethane is a symmetric molecule, thus the protons on either methyl group are equivalent. So, in the example above, the absorption of $-CH_3$ protons occurs at one peak (*a singlet*) 3.23 ppm downfield from TMS. In most organic molecules, the range of absorption will be in the 0–10 ppm (= *parts per million*) range.

The area under each peak is directly related to the number of protons contributing to it, and thus may be used to determine the

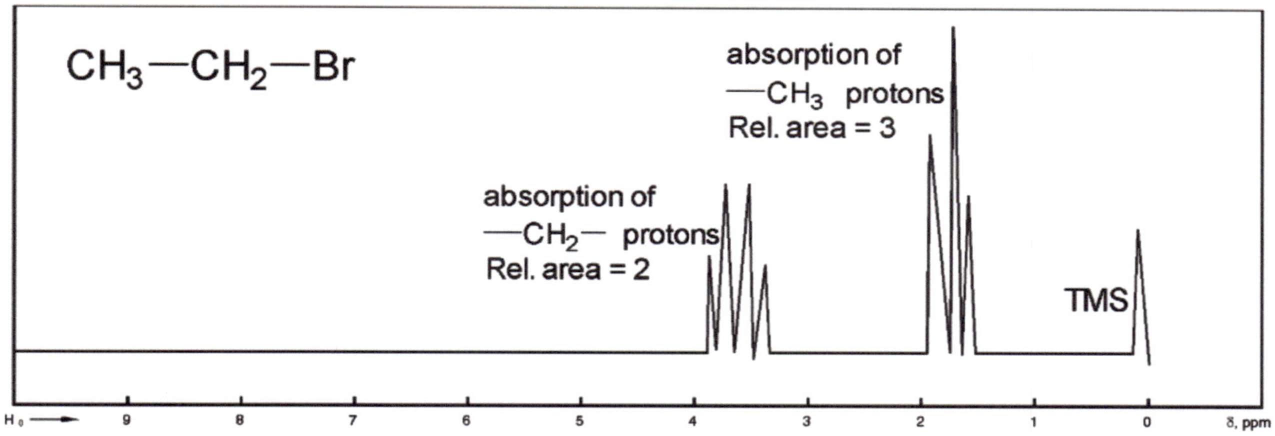

relative number of protons in the molecule. Accurate measurements of the area under the two peaks in the NMR of dimethoxymethane yield the ratio 1:3 which represents the relative number of hydrogens (i.e. 1:3 = 2:6).

Let us now examine a schematic representation of the NMR spectrum of ethyl bromide shown in the diagram above.

It is obvious that something is different. Looking at the molecule, one can see that there are two different types of protons (*either far from Br or near to Br*). However, there are more than two signals in the spectrum. As such, the NMR signal for each group is said to be split. This type of splitting is called <u>spin-spin splitting</u> (= *spin-spin coupling*) and is caused by the presence of neighboring protons (*protons on an adjacent or vicinal carbon*) that are not equivalent to the proton in question. Note that protons that are farther than two carbons apart do not exhibit a coupling effect.

The number of lines in the splitting pattern for a given set of equivalent protons depends on the number of adjacent protons according to the following rule: if there are n equivalent protons in adjacent positions, a proton NMR signal is split into $n + 1$ lines.

Therefore the NMR spectrum for ethyl bromide can be interpreted thus:

- There are two groups of lines (*two split peaks*), therefore there are two different environments for protons.
- The relative areas under each peak is 2:3, which represents the relative number of hydrogens in the molecule.
- There are 4 splits (*quartet*) in the peak which has relatively two hydrogens ($-CH_2$). Thus the number of adjacent hydrogens is $n + 1 = 4$; therefore, there are 3 hydrogens on the carbon adjacent to $-CH_2$.
- There are 3 splits (*triplet*) in the peak which has relatively three hydrogens ($-CH_3$).

Thus the number of adjacent hydrogens is $n + 1 = 3$; therefore, there are 2 hydrogens on the carbon adjacent to $-CH_3$.

The relative areas under each peak may be expressed in three ways: (i) the information may simply be provided to you (*too easy!*); (ii) the integers may be written above the signals (= *integration integers*, i.e. 2, 3 in the previous example); or (iii) a step-like *integration curve* above the signals where the relative height of each step equals the relative number of hydrogens.

14.2.1 Deuterium Exchange

Deuterium, the hydrogen isotope ^2H or D (PHY 12.2), can be used to identify substances with readily exchangeable or acidic hydrogens. Rather than H_2O, D_2O is used to identify the chemical exchange:

$$ROH + DOD \rightleftharpoons ROD + HOD$$

The previous signal due to the acidic $-O\boxed{H}$ would now disappear. However, if excess D_2O is used, a signal as a result of HOD may be observed.

Solvents may also be involved in exchange phenomena. The solvents carbon tetrachloride (CCl_4) and deuteriochloroform ($CDCl_3$) can also engage in exchange-induced decoupling of acidic hydrogens (usu. in alcohols).

Medium-level Importance

14.2.2 ^{13}C NMR

The main difference between the proton NMR and ^{13}C NMR is that most carbon 13 signals occur 0–200 δ downfield from the carbon peak of TMS. There is also very little coupling between carbon atoms as only 1.1% of carbon atoms are ^{13}C. There is coupling between carbon atoms and their adjacent protons which are directly attached to them. This coupling of one bond is similar to the three bond coupling exhibited by proton NMR.

Signals will be split into a triplet with an area of 1:2:1 when a carbon atom is attached to two protons. Another unique feature of ^{13}C NMR is a phenomenon called spin decoupling where a spectrum of singlets can be recorded - each corresponding to a singular carbon atom. This allows one to accurately determine the number of different carbons in their respective chemical environments as well as the number of adjacent hydrogens (spin-coupled only).

To remind yourself of the isotopes deuterium and carbon-13, consider revising PHY 12.2.

Mass spectrometry (the former expression "mass spectroscopy" is discouraged), unlike other forms of NMR we have seen, destroys the sample during its analysis. The analysis is carried out using a beam of electrons which ionise the sample and a detector to measure the number of particles that are deflected due to the presence of a magnetic field. The reflected particle is usually an unstable species which decomposes rapidly into a cationic fragment and a radical fragment.

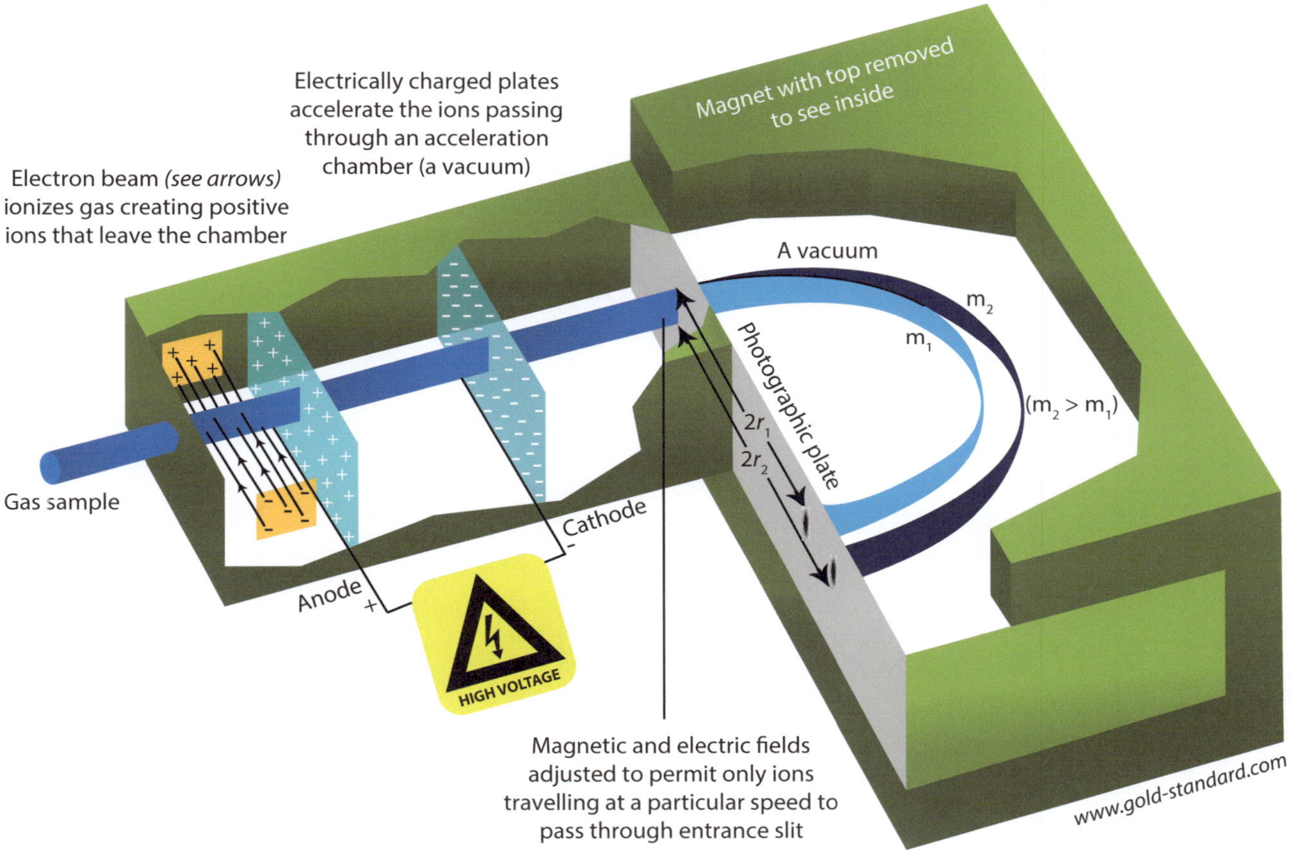

Figure IV.B.14.1: Diagrammatic representation of a mass spectrometer. Electrons stream out (beam) from a heated cathode (negatively charged orange plate) towards the anode (positively charged orange plate) thus bombarding the gas creating cations. The cations are accelerated by a high voltage electric field. Magnetic and electric fields are adjusted to permit only ions traveling at a particular speed to pass through the entrance slit (i.e. to pass through the slit between the acceleration chamber and the magnetic chamber). Notice that the heavier particles are less deviated (more inertia; PHY 4.2) and thus have a larger diameter (= 2r) from the slit to the photographic plate. Note: Questions 40-43 from ACER's GAMSAT booklet entitled *GAMSAT Practice Questions* (currently free when you register to sit the GAMSAT) form a unit based on the mass spectrometer requiring an integration of concepts including electromagnetic fields (PHY 9.1, 9.2) and, because of the path of the ions in the magnetic chamber, circular motion (PHY 3.3). Masters Series GAMSAT Physics Chapter 9 has a unit covering these issues in the GAMSAT-level practice questions at the end of the chapter. (adapted from chemeddl.org)

Since there are many ways in which the particle can decompose, a typical mass spectrum is often composed of numerous lines, with each one corresponding to a specific mass/charge ratio (m/z, sometimes symbolised as m/e or m/q). It is important to note that only cations are deflected by the magnetic field, thus only cations will appear on the spectrum which plots m/z (x-axis) vs. the abundance of the cationic fragments (y-axis). See the figure provided.

The tallest peak represents the most common ion and is also referred to as the base peak. The molecular weight can be obtained not from the base peak but rather from the peak with the highest m/z ratio, 129 in this case. This is called the parent ion peak and is designated by M+. By looking at the fragmentation pattern we can ascertain information regarding the compound's structure, something that IR spectroscopy is incapable of achieving. Note that if the charge on the ion has a magnitude of 1 (which is usually the case) then the magnitude on the x axis is simply the mass (i.e. m/z = m/1 = m = atomic mass units = amu; PHY 12.2, CHM 1.3).

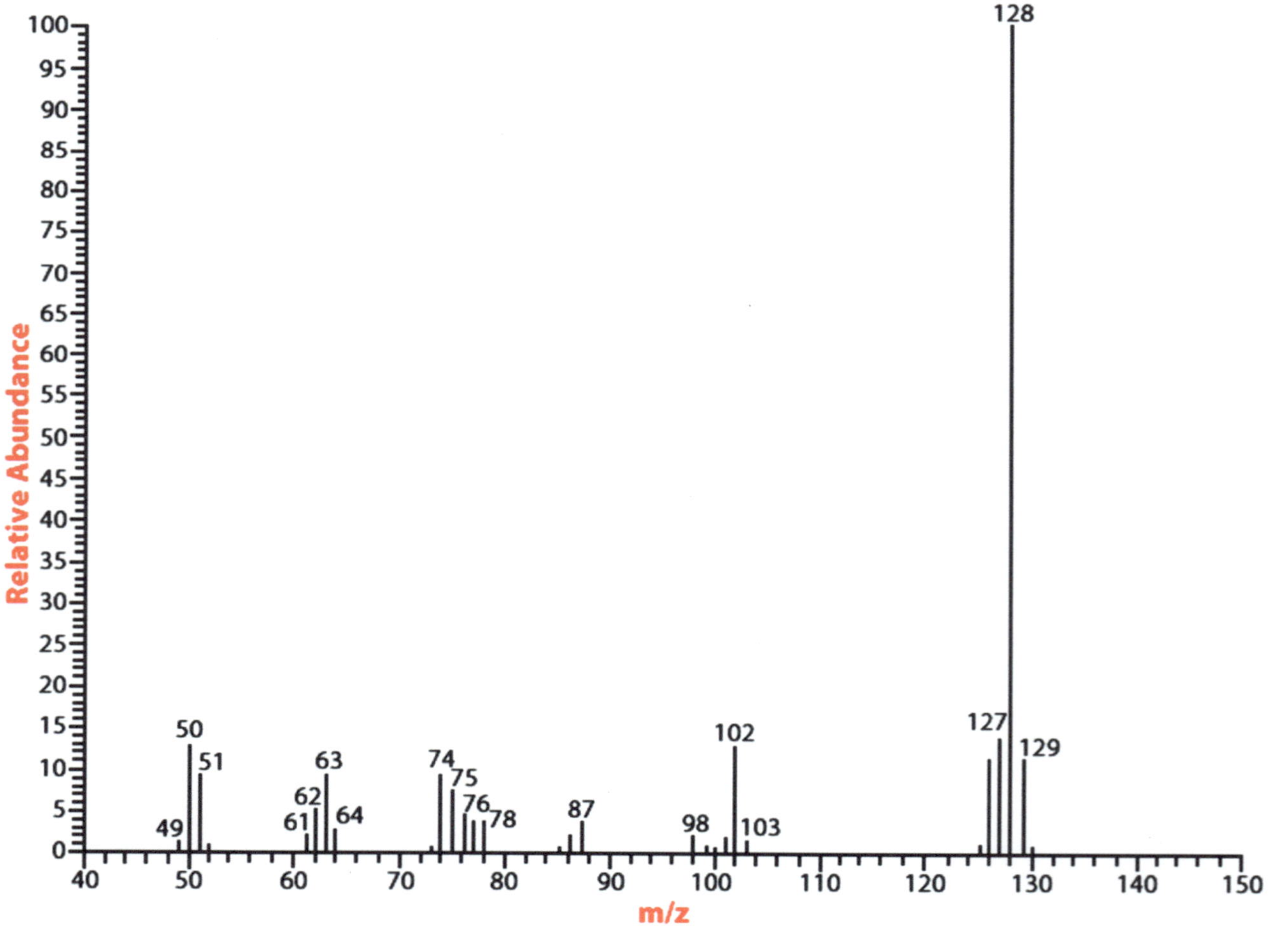

Medium-level Importance

If IR, NMR or 'mass spec.' show up on the GAMSAT, you will be reminded of the rules to apply prior to the questions (i.e. there is no need to commit the rules to memory). Ideally, moving forward, you would not focus on re-reading chapters. Rather, the bulk of your GAMSAT Organic Chemistry preparation should include affirming basic nomenclature, geometric reasoning (following substituents, bonds, etc.), applying rules (Diels-Alder, Hückel's, separations, spectroscopy), revising Gold Notes, GAMSAT videos, and of course, 'practice, practice, practice'! Speaking of which, practice questions, answers, and worked solutions for Chapter 14 are accessible through your online account.

SPOILER ALERT

Gold Standard has cross-referenced the content in this chapter to examples from ACER's official GAMSAT practice materials. It is for you to decide when you want to explore these questions since you may want to preserve some of ACER's materials for timed mock-exam practice.

Examples – This is a great, simple unit about NMR: Q26-28 of 1. The latter deserves special mention because it is one of the rare units from ACER's oldest booklet that has been reported in public forums to be reincarnated, from time to time, in similar form. The same booklet has a unit covering the physics of the machine used as a mass spectrometer: Q40-43 or 1. This unit gets special mention, but it is not counted towards the Importance of this chapter since it is dependent on your understanding of circular motion (Physics Chapter 3), electromagnetism (Physics Chapter 9), and equation manipulation. Note that "Q" is followed by the question number, and, for example, "of 1" refers to booklet number 1 which is referenced in the Spoiler Alert table at the end of Chapter 1. The 15 full-length GAMSAT practice tests by Gold Standard, HEAPS-1 through HEAPS-15, contain specific cross-references to this chapter within the worked solutions. Note that the m/z mass spectroscopy unit in your online account is from HEAPS-1, and the infrared spectroscopy unit is from HEAPS-6. Also note, as referenced in ORG 14.3, the Masters Series GAMSAT Physics Chapter 9 has a unit covering the physics of a *cyclotron* (mass spectrometer) in the GAMSAT-level practice questions at the end of the chapter.

Chapter Checklist

- ☐ Access your online account to view answers, worked solutions and discussion boards.
- ☐ Reassess your 'learning objectives' for this chapter: Go back to the first page of this chapter and re-evaluate the top 3 boxes and the Introduction.
- ☐ Complete a maximum of 1 page of notes using symbols/abbreviations to represent the entire chapter based on your learning objectives. These are your Gold Notes.
- ☐ Consider your multimedia options based on your optimal way of learning:
    - ☐ Download the free Gold Standard GAMSAT app for your Android device or iPhone.
    - ☐ Create your own, tangible study cards or try the free app: Anki.
    - ☐ Record your voice reading your Gold Notes onto your smartphone (audio files, e.g., *memo* or MP3s) and listen during exercise, transportation, etc.
    - ☐ Try out the Gold Standard GAMSAT online videos at gamsat-prep.com, or you can try other options on YouTube like Khan Academy or Crash Course Organic Chemistry.
- ☐ Reassess your schedule for your full-length GAMSAT practice tests: ACER and/or HEAPS exams. Ensure that you have scheduled one full day to complete a practice test and 1-2 days for a thorough assessment of worked solutions while adding to your abbreviated Gold Notes.
- ☐ Reassess your progress in scheduling and/or evaluating stress reduction techniques such as regular exercise (sports), yoga, meditation and/or mindfulness exercises (*see* YouTube for suggestions).